Nutrition

For Healthy Living

Fifth Edition

WENDY J. SCHIFF, MS, RDN

McGraw Hill Education

NUTRITION FOR HEALTHY LIVING, FIFTH EDITION

Published by McGraw—Hill Education, 2 Penn Plaza, New York, NY 10121. Copyright © 2019 by McGraw—Hill Education. All rights reserved. Printed in the United States of America. Previous editions © 2016, 2013, and 2011. No part of this publication may be reproduced or distributed in any form or by any means, or stored in a database or retrieval system, without the prior written consent of McGraw—Hill Education, including, but not limited to, in any network or other electronic storage or transmission, or broadcast for distance learning.

Some ancillaries, including electronic and print components, may not be available to customers outside the United States.

This book is printed on acid—free paper.

1 2 3 4 5 6 7 8 9 LMN 21 20 19 18

ISBN 978—1— 259—70997—5
MHID 1—259—70997—3

Senior Portfolio Manager: *Marija A. Magner*
Product Developer: *Darlene M. Schueller*
Marketing Manager: *Valerie Kramer*
Senior Content Project Manager: *Vicki Krug*
Lead Content Project Manager: *Jodi Banowetz*
Senior Buyer: *Laura Fuller*
Senior Designer: *Tara McDermott*
Senior Content Licensing Specialist: *Shawntel Schmitt*
Cover Image: *©Laszio Podor/Getty Images*
Compositor: *MPS Limited*

All credits appearing on page or at the end of the book are considered to be an extension of the copyright page.

Library of Congress Cataloging—in—Publication Data

Schiff, Wendy, author.
   Nutrition for healthy living/Wendy J. Schiff, MS, RDN.
   Fifth edition. | New York, NY : McGraw—Hill Education, [2019] |
   Includes index.
   LCCN 2017034402 | ISBN 9781259709975 (alk. paper)
   LCSH: Human nutrition—Textbooks.
   LCC QP141 .S3435 2019 | DDC 612.3—dc23 LC record available
   at https://lccn.loc.gov/2017034402

mheducation.com/highered

Nutrition

For Healthy Living

FIFTH EDITION

WENDY J. SCHIFF

Brief Contents

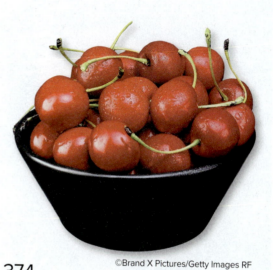

©Brand X Pictures/Getty Images RF

Meet the Author

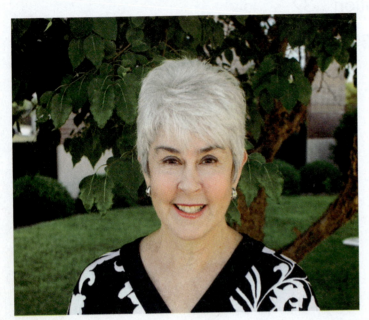

Wendy J. Schiff, MS, RDN received her BS in biological health/medical dietetics and MS in human nutrition from The Pennsylvania State University. She has taught introductory foods and nutrition courses at the University of Missouri–Columbia as well as nutrition, human biology, and personal health courses at St. Louis Community College–Meramec. She has worked as a public health nutritionist at the Allegheny County Health Department (Pittsburgh, Pennsylvania) and State Food and Nutrition Specialist for Missouri Extension at Lincoln University in Jefferson City, Missouri. In addition to authoring *Nutrition for Healthy Living* and *Nutrition Essentials: A Personal Approach,* Wendy has coauthored *Human Nutrition: Science for Healthy Living* and a college-level personal health textbook and authored many other nutrition-related educational materials. She is a registered dietitian nutritionist and a member of the Academy of Nutrition and Dietetics.

To my late father

Welcome to the Fifth Edition of *Nutrition for Healthy Living*

We think of ourselves as consumers when we purchase homes, cars, computers, and food. We are also consumers of nutrition-related information. Nearly every day, we are literally bombarded with messages in media and from acquaintances concerning nutrition, foods, and health. Much of this information is unreliable, and often it is intended to promote sales of products or services. Unfortunately, many consumers lack the knowledge and skills needed to analyze such information critically and decide whether or not to apply it to their decision-making process.

Helping students become better-informed consumers, particularly as this relates to food and nutrition, is the foundation of Nutrition for Healthy Living. This major theme flows throughout the textbook by providing students with practical information, critical thinking skills, and the scientific foundation needed to make better-informed choices about their diet and health. By reading Nutrition for Healthy Living, not only will students learn basic principles of nutrition, they will also be able to evaluate various sources of nutrition information critically and to apply sound nutrition practices to improve their lives.

Wendy J. Schiff

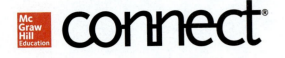 **connect®**

McGraw-Hill Connect® is a highly reliable, easy-to-use homework and learning management solution that utilizes learning science and award-winning adaptive tools to improve student results.

Homework and Adaptive Learning

- Connect's assignments help students contextualize what they've learned through application, so they can better understand the material and think critically.

- Connect will create a personalized study path customized to individual student needs through SmartBook®.

- SmartBook helps students study more efficiently by delivering an interactive reading experience through adaptive highlighting and review.

Over **7 billion questions** have been answered, making McGraw-Hill Education products more intelligent, reliable, and precise.

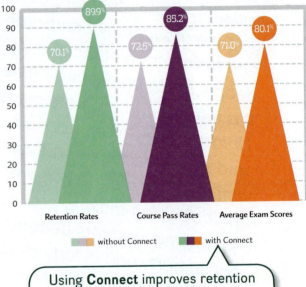

Connect's Impact on Retention Rates, Pass Rates, and Average Exam Scores

Retention Rates: 70.1% (without Connect), 89.9% (with Connect)
Course Pass Rates: 72.5% (without Connect), 85.2% (with Connect)
Average Exam Scores: 71.0% (without Connect), 80.1% (with Connect)

without Connect | with Connect

Using **Connect** improves retention rates by **19.8%**, passing rates by **12.7%**, and exam scores by **9.1%**.

73% of instructors who use **Connect** require it; instructor satisfaction **increases** by 28% when **Connect** is required.

Quality Content and Learning Resources

- Connect content is authored by the world's best subject matter experts, and is available to your class through a simple and intuitive interface.

- The Connect eBook makes it easy for students to access their reading material on smartphones and tablets. They can study on the go and don't need internet access to use the eBook as a reference, with full functionality.

- Multimedia content such as videos, simulations, and games drive student engagement and critical thinking skills.

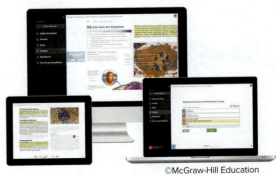

Robust Analytics and Reporting

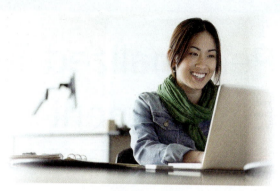

©Hero Images/Getty Images RF

- Connect Insight® generates easy-to-read reports on individual students, the class as a whole, and on specific assignments.

- The Connect Insight dashboard delivers data on performance, study behavior, and effort. Instructors can quickly identify students who struggle and focus on material that the class has yet to master.

- Connect automatically grades assignments and quizzes, providing easy-to-read reports on individual and class performance.

Impact on Final Course Grade Distribution

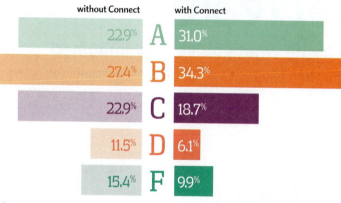

without Connect		with Connect
22.9%	A	31.0%
27.4%	B	34.3%
22.9%	C	18.7%
11.5%	D	6.1%
15.4%	F	9.9%

More students earn **As** and **Bs** when they use **Connect**.

Trusted Service and Support

- Connect integrates with your LMS to provide single sign-on and automatic syncing of grades. Integration with Blackboard®, D2L®, and Canvas also provides automatic syncing of the course calendar and assignment-level linking.

- Connect offers comprehensive service, support, and training throughout every phase of your implementation.

- If you're looking for some guidance on how to use Connect, or want to learn tips and tricks from super users, you can find tutorials as you work. Our Digital Faculty Consultants and Student Ambassadors offer insight into how to achieve the results you want with Connect.

Personalized Teaching and Learning Environment

NEW! Dietary analysis auto—graded assignments within Connect. One of the challenges many instructors face with teaching nutrition classes is having the time to grade dietary analysis projects. To help overcome that challenge, auto-graded assignments that require students to use NutritionCalc Plus and answer questions based on the generated reports have been developed. These assignments were developed and reviewed by faculty who use such assignments in their own teaching. They are designed to be relevant, current, and interesting!

"The case studies provide a neutral way for my students to explore dietary analysis. My students are engaged by the case study assignments and find them easy to use. The fact that the assignments are auto-graded gives me more time to focus on content development and instruction for my course.

I appreciate how flexible the case study assignments are. I can use the case and the diet plan, and then only assign those questions that best match my learning outcomes. I can also add my own questions to the assignments."

Hannah Thornton
Texas State University

NutritionCalc Plus is a powerful dietary analysis tool featuring more than 30,000 foods from the ESHA Research nutrient database, which is comprised of data from the latest USDA Standard Reference database, manufacturer's data, restaurant data, and data from literature sources. NutritionCalc Plus allows users to track food and activities, and then analyze their choices with a robust selection of intuitive reports. The interface was updated to accommodate ADA requirements and modern mobile experience native to today's students.

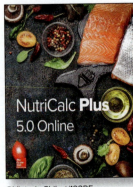
NutriCalc Plus 5.0 Online
©Victoria Shibut/123RF

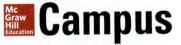
LEARNSMART®

LearnSmart® Prep is designed to get students ready for a forthcoming course by quickly and effectively addressing prerequisite knowledge gaps that may cause problems down the road.

create™

Create what you've only imagined

McGraw—Hill Create is a self—service website that allows you to create customized course materials using McGraw—Hill Education's comprehensive, cross—disciplinary content and digital products.

tegrity®

Deliver your lecture online quickly and easily. Tegrity Campus is a fully automated lecture capture solution used in traditional, hybrid, "flipped classes," and online courses to record lessons, lectures, and skills.

Campus

McGraw—Hill Campus® is a groundbreaking service that puts world—class digital learning resources just a click away. Faculty—whether or not they use a McGraw—Hill Education title—can instantly browse, search, and access the entire library of McGraw—Hill Education instructional resources and services—including eBooks, test banks, PowerPoint® slides, animations, and learning objects—from any learning management system at no additional cost to your institution. Users also have single sign—on access to McGraw—Hill Education digital platforms, including Connect, ALEKS®, Create, and Tegrity.

The ABCs of Nutrition

Who Was *Nutrition for Healthy Living* Written for?

Writing a nutrition textbook is not an easy task. Throughout the process, I relied on my experience in teaching nutrition, foods, biology, and personal health classes at both the university and the community college levels to develop a vision for a fresh approach to presenting basic information about nutrition. My teaching experiences also provided valuable insights into the diversity, as well as the needs, interests, and capabilities, of today's students. In addition, manuscript reviews by colleagues helped define the shared goals of those who teach the course, which in turn helped shape the content of this textbook.

Nutrition for Healthy Living is intended for students who are interested in learning about nutrition for personal reasons, as well as students considering majoring in nutrition, nursing, or other health– and science–related fields. Students from a wide variety of academic backgrounds often enroll in introductory nutrition courses, and in many instances, they have not taken college–level science courses prior to this nutrition course. With this in mind, I wrote the textbook with the understanding that an introductory textbook must appeal to students who represent a broad range of interests and academic backgrounds—English majors as well as nursing majors. My hope is that this introductory course, along with my textbook, can spark students' interest in adopting healthier dietary practices and possibly even inspire some students to consider nutrition as their major.

The *Nutrition for Healthy Living* Difference Is *ABC*

When I began to write this textbook, I felt strongly that I wanted to craft an alternative to established nutrition textbooks, while maintaining a focus on concepts that are fundamental to introductory nutrition courses. By building upon my experiences as coauthor of a college–level personal health textbook, I sought to develop a nutrition textbook that not only was scientifically up–to–date but also included consumer–oriented content and features. I wanted to create a textbook that would be visually appealing and fun to read, engage students' interest, be well organized, and have features that contribute to the pedagogy without being distracting. As my developmental editor gathered feedback from numerous instructors, the advantages that the new textbook would offer took shape—what my team at McGraw–Hill Education and I refer to as the **"ABCs of *Nutrition for Healthy Living*."**

A = Accessible Science

Nutrition is an "offspring" science that requires a basic understanding of certain chemical and physiological concepts and terms. Ignorance about chemistry and physiology contributes to food faddism and health quackery. By providing a solid scientific foundation, nutrition educators can more easily dispel commonly held but inaccurate beliefs, such as "When you're inactive, muscle turns into fat," and "Cellulite is a special type of body fat."

Becoming knowledgeable about nutrition involves a certain level of understanding of basic scientific principles. *Nutrition for Healthy Living* recognizes the importance of introducing such principles in a manner that every college student can understand. As my primary goal for students who use this textbook, I want students to acquire a basic understanding of nutritional science so that they can make intelligent, practical choices that can result in improved nutrition and health.

Chapter 4 (Body Basics) presents basic principles of chemistry and human physiology as they apply to the study of nutrition but at a level that students can easily understand. This chapter, for example, introduces and defines terms that relate to nutrition and foods, such as *acid*, *basic*, *enzyme*, and *solvent*. The text includes numerous illustrations to help students understand basic physiological concepts that relate to nutrition.

Because students and courses vary in the depth of scientific foundation required, this chapter features some flexibility. The chapter is divided into two main sections, chemistry and human physiology, so professors can choose to skip the chemistry section if they prefer.

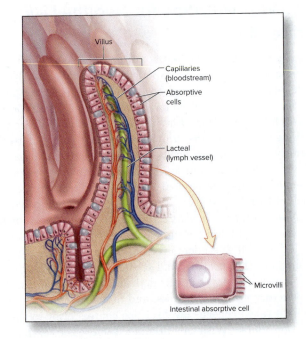

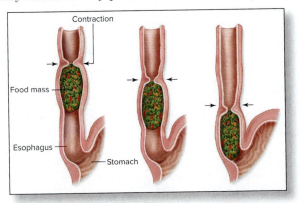

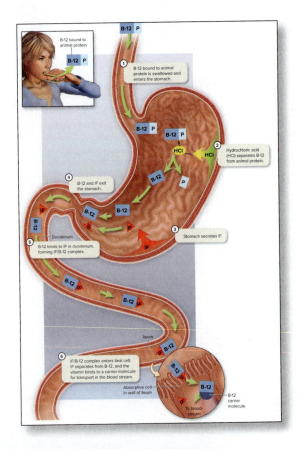

"This textbook is clearly written, in everyday language which my students can follow. It is also interesting and engaging, making use of questions incorporated throughout the reading, stories about real people, interesting facts, practical tips, and easy-to-understand visuals."

Liza Mohanty
Olive-Harvey College

B = Brief Organization

In developing the structure of this book, a new approach emerged; instructors often do not have the time to cover all the material in their textbooks. Based upon their feedback, I chose to organize the core content into 13 chapters. I believe this organization makes teaching introductory nutrition more manageable and fits the time frame of most courses better than textbooks that include 15 or more chapters. Furthermore, basic information concerning diet and heart disease, diet and cancer, and dietary supplements is incorporated where it is relevant throughout the book.

Nutrition for Healthy Living follows a more traditional approach to the study of nutrition in that the textbook's organization focuses on nutrients rather than certain functions, tissues, or diseases. Additionally, the textbook integrates health information, particularly diet—related chronic diseases, within each chapter where it is appropriate, rather than relegate it to a single chapter near the end of the textbook. For example, the chapters that discuss nutrients provide fundamental information first and then present applications, including the nutrient—related health effects of certain lifestyle practices, particularly dietary choices. Additionally, the quantity and length of boxed features in the chapters are limited, as they tend to disrupt the flow of content and students often skip reading them.

Nutrition for Healthy Living covers the core material instructors need in a format that is logical and practical for nearly all introductory nutrition courses:

- Chapter 1 introduces students to nutrition and nutrients, and presents 10 key nutrition concepts, such as "most naturally occurring foods are mixtures of nutrients" and "variety can help ensure the nutritional adequacy of a diet."
- Chapter 2 presents basic information about scientific methodology as it relates to nutrition research and provides tips for becoming a more wary consumer of nutrition— and health—related information.
- Chapter 3 discusses dietary standards and guidelines, food groups and guides, and how to use information provided on the labels of food packages.

2.4 Nutrition Matters: What Are Dietary Supplements?

Learning Outcomes

1. Explain the difference between conventional medicine and alternative health care, and identify health care practices that are either conventional or alternative.
2. Explain how the FDA regulates medicines differently than dietary supplements.
3. Discuss the risks and benefits of taking dietary supplements.

Do you take a daily vitamin or mineral pill because you are concerned about the nutritional quality of your diet? Do you use herbal pills or extracts to strengthen your immune system, boost your memory, or treat illnesses such as the common cold? If you follow any of these practices, you are not alone. According to results of a national survey, over 50% of the American population takes one or more dietary supplements regularly.[9]

According to the Dietary Supplement Health and Education Act of 1994 (DSHEA), a dietary supplement is a product (other than tobacco) that

- adds to a person's dietary intake and contains one or more dietary ingredients, including nutrients or *botani-cals* (herbs or other plant material);

Blueberries: ©PhotoAlto/Getty Images RF

- is taken by mouth; and,
- is a concentrate, metabolite, constituent, or extract.[10]

Dietary supplements include nutrient pills, protein pow-ders, and herbal extracts. Many dietary supplements are often referred to as "nutraceuticals," but there is no legal definition for this term.

In the United States, the most commonly used dietary supplements are **multivitamin/mineral (MV/M)** products.[9] There is no standard definition for the contents of a MV/M supplement, but such products may contain several vitamins and minerals. In 2012, the most popular nonvitamin, nonmineral dietary supplements among American adults were fish oil or "omega 3," glucosamine and/or chondroitin, probiotics/prebiotics, and melatonin.[11]

Some people use dietary supplements, particularly those containing nutrients, because the products are rec—ommended by their physicians or registered dietitian nutritionists. Physicians, for example, may prescribe a

©Wendy Schiff

©McGraw-Hill Education. Jill Braaten, photographer

- Chapter 4 introduces basic chemical and physiological concepts and key terms that relate to the science of nutrition. This chapter also provides basic information about human digestion and nutrient absorption.
- Chapters 5, 6, 7, 8, and 9 present basic and practical information about the nutrients, such as their major functions in the body, food sources, and roles in health.
- Chapters 10, 11, 12, and 13 focus on applying basic nutrition information for important concerns or different age groups. Chapter 10, for example, covers weight management; Chapter 11 presents information relating to physical fitness; Chapter 12 features information about food—borne illness; and Chapter 13 discusses nutrition during the life span.

Although some topics were important to cover, they did not warrant using a full chapter. Thus, topics such as global nutrition concerns, alcohol and alcohol abuse, and eating disorders are presented in the last section of chapters, called "Nutrition Matters."

C = Consumer Focus

Regardless of their backgrounds, students are consumers of nutrition information from a wide variety of sources, including popular magazines, friends, diet books, infomercials, and the Internet. Oftentimes these students arrive in class with many misconceptions about their diet and health. As nutrition educators, we seek to identify these beliefs and to impart sound, reliable nutrition and health information. We also strive to equip our students with the tools they need to make intelligent, informed food– and nutrition–related decisions beyond the classroom. Chapter 2 (Evaluating Nutrition Information) presents a practical introduction to becoming an informed consumer of nutrition and nutrition–related information. This book is unique among nutrition textbooks in its inclusion of this chapter, which provides basic information concerning scientific research and a thorough discussion of how to evaluate nutrition– and health–related sources and messages. In addition to devoting an entire chapter to evaluating nutrition–related information, the consumer emphasis is integrated throughout the book.

©Comstock/Stockbyte/Getty Images RF

Recipe for Healthy Living is a practical application of nutrition and food information that will appeal to most college students. Each chapter features an easy–to–make, kitchen–tested recipe that helps bring the chapter's content to life (e.g., "Egg Salad"). In addition to the pie graph for macronutrient content and a bar chart to illustrate % Daily Value for energy and key nutrients in a serving of the food, this feature also indicates which MyPlate food groups the major ingredients in the dish represent. By trying the recipes, students can develop basic food preparation skills and may be inspired to cook more foods from scratch.

Food & Nutrition Tips present practical suggestions that apply material discussed in a section. These tips provide information students can use every day—and for the rest of their lives.

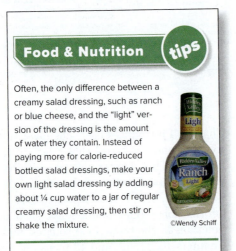

Food & Nutrition tips

Often, the only difference between a creamy salad dressing, such as ranch or blue cheese, and the "light" version of the dressing is the amount of water they contain. Instead of paying more for calorie-reduced bottled salad dressings, make your own light salad dressing by adding about ¼ cup water to a jar of regular creamy salad dressing, then stir or shake the mixture.

©Wendy Schiff

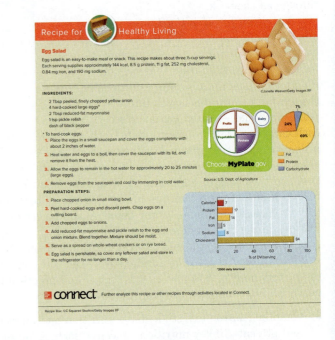

Recipe for **Healthy Living**

Egg Salad
Egg salad is an easy-to-make meal or snack. This recipe makes about three ½-cup servings. Each serving supplies approximately 144 kcal, 8.5 g protein, 11 g fat, 252 mg cholesterol, 0.84 mg iron, and 190 mg sodium.

©Jonelle Weaver/Getty Images RF

INGREDIENTS:
2 Tbsp peeled, finely chopped yellow onion
4 hard-cooked large eggs*
2 Tbsp reduced-fat mayonnaise
1 tsp pickle relish
dash of black pepper

* To hard-cook eggs:
1. Place the eggs in a small saucepan and cover the eggs completely with about 2 inches of water.
2. Heat water and eggs to a boil, then cover the saucepan with its lid, and remove it from the heat.
3. Allow the eggs to remain in the hot water for approximately 20 to 25 minutes (large eggs).
4. Remove eggs from the saucepan and cool by immersing in cold water.

PREPARATION STEPS:
1. Place chopped onion in small mixing bowl.
2. Peel hard-cooked eggs and discard peels. Chop eggs on a cutting board.
3. Add chopped eggs to onions.
4. Add reduced-fat mayonnaise and pickle relish to the egg and onion mixture. Blend together. Mixture should be moist.
5. Serve as a spread on whole-wheat crackers or on rye bread.
6. Egg salad is perishable, so cover any leftover salad and store in the refrigerator for no longer than a day.

Source: U.S. Dept. of Agriculture

*2000 daily total kcal

■ **connect** Further analyze this recipe or other recipes through activities located in Connect.

Recipe Box: ©C Squared Studios/Getty Images RF

Did You Know? This margin feature notes interesting nutrition–related tidbits that relate to information presented in that section of the chapter. Some of these features dispel commonly held beliefs about food and nutrition that are inaccurate.

Did *YOU* Know?

Many kinds of fresh fruit make quick and easy snacks that can be carried in backpacks, purses, and briefcases. Fresh fruit such as apples, oranges, tangerines, kiwifruit, and grapes can be kept for a few days at room temperature in a fruit bowl. You can store fresh fruits for longer periods by placing them in the refrigerator. Banana peels, however, turn dark brown when the fruit is refrigerated, so it is best to store bananas at room temperature, but refrigerated bananas are still good to eat.

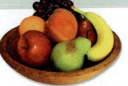

©Wendy Schiff

My Diverse Plate. This feature introduces students to foods and dietary prac–tices that are ethnically and culturally diverse.

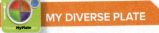

MY DIVERSE PLATE

Pico de Gallo

Pico de gallo (*pee'-ko-dee-guy'-yo*) is a Mexican salsa made with fresh ingredients, including chopped tomatoes, onions, hot peppers (such as serrano and jalapeño), fresh cilantro leaves, lime juice, and a dash of salt. The salsa is eaten as a dip for tortilla chips or served on a variety of foods, including scrambled eggs, burritos, and grilled poultry, fish, or meat. A one-half cup serving of the salsa provides 20 kcal, almost no fat, and 1 g of fiber.

©Wendy Schiff

Real People, Real Stories feature information about people who actually have recovered from or are currently living with nutrition—related conditions such as celiac disease, type 1 diabetes, and hypertension. This feature is designed to help students recognize the daily challenges people with such conditions face and the role diet and physical activity play in managing health.

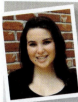

REAL PEOPLE | REAL STORIES

Stephanie Patton

Although she is only 18 years old, college freshman Stephanie Patton has a long list of accomplishments. "When I was little, I took singing, dancing, and acting lessons," she says. "I loved being on the stage, so I had my parents take me to auditions for local talent shows and theatrical performances. Since I was 7 years old, I've been in over 50 musicals and plays. I appeared in my first beauty pageant at age 10, and I recently competed for the Miss Missouri title. I placed in the top 11, won the preliminary talent award and two college scholarships for community service." Stephanie is majoring in Health Sciences at the University of Missouri-Columbia. While in college, she plans to continue competing for the title of Miss Missouri.

Stephanie manages to balance her college life with her extracurricular activities, but she also has to manage her health and diet. This impressive young lady has type 1 diabetes. Stephanie says, "Just before my fifth birthday, I lost weight and began drinking gallons of juice, water, and milk. At night, I wet the bed. My parents became

©Wendy Schiff

Key Terms and Pronunciation Guide Key terms and definitions are provided in the margins on the same two—page spread where the terms first appear in the chapter. Many unfamiliar terms have pronunciations provided within the text. A glossary of these key terms is at the end of the textbook.

suffering from chronic vitamin A deficiency, these cells accumulate keratin, and the white of the eye develops "foamy" areas (Fig. 8.10). Eventually, the epithelial cells harden and stop producing mucus. This condition is called **xerophthalmia** (*zir–op–thal'–me–a*) or "dry eye." Corneas affected by xerophthalmia can be damaged easily by dirt and bacteria. Unless a person with xerophthalmia receives vitamin A, the condition eventually leads to blindness.

xerophthalmia condition affecting the eyes that results from vitamin A deficiency

teratogen agent that causes birth defects

References *Nutrition for Healthy Living* includes in—text citations and extensive lists of references in Appendix H. References provide readers with access to sources of information for more in—depth understanding or for topics that hold particular interest.

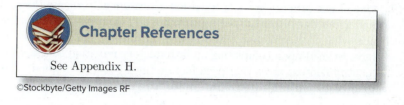

Chapter References

See Appendix H.

©Stockbyte/Getty Images RF

End—of—Chapter Summary This feature provides a brief review of the main points of each major section of the chapter.

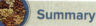

Summary

5.1 Introducing Carbohydrates

- Carbohydrates are an important source of energy for the body. Plants use energy from the sun to make carbohydrates from water and carbon dioxide. Some of the energy is stored in

©C Squared Studios/Getty Images RF

Assessment and Evaluation of Learning

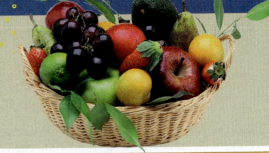

©Pixtal/age fotostock RF

One of our primary goals as nutrition educators is to ensure that our students leave the introductory nutrition course with a better understanding of the nutrition principles and concepts needed to improve their diet and health. To assess how well faculty are achieving that goal, many colleges and universities are implementing Student Learning Outcomes as a way to measure what students have learned upon completing an introductory nutrition course. Student Learning Outcomes can also be used to help instructors identify content areas that need more refined teaching methods. *Nutrition for Healthy Living* has been developed around the following coursewide outcomes.

Coursewide Student Learning Outcomes

1. Identify functions and sources of nutrients.
2. Demonstrate basic knowledge of digestion, absorption, and metabolism.
3. Apply current dietary guidelines and nutrition recommendations.
4. Analyze and evaluate nutrition information scientifically.
5. Relate roles of nutrients in good health, optimal fitness, and chronic diseases.
6. Summarize basic concepts of nutrition throughout the life span.
7. Evaluate a personal diet record using a computer database.

Additionally, each major section of a chapter opens with a list of section–specific learning outcomes that build upon the broader coursewide outcomes. The Learning Outcomes help students prepare for reading the section and clarify major concepts they are expected to learn. These measurable outcomes are further supported by assessment methods and study aids found within the chapters and in Connect.

> **Learning Outcomes**
> 1. Identify major organs of the digestive system, and describe primary functions of each organ.
> 2. Identify the accessory organs of the digestive system and the roles these organs play in digestion.
> 3. Discuss the overall processes of nutrient digestion, absorption, and transport; and waste elimination.
> 4. Discuss gut microbiota and its role in health.

Quiz Yourself

This pretest, comprised of five true–or–false questions, appears at the beginning of each chapter; answers to the quiz are provided at the end of the chapter. The purpose of Quiz Yourself is to stimulate interest in reading the chapter. By taking the quiz, students may be surprised to learn how little or how much they know about the chapter's contents.

> ## Quiz Yourself
> To test your knowledge of the material covered in Chapter 4, take the following quiz; the answers are at the end of the chapter.
> 1. The atom is the smallest living unit in the body. _____ T _____ F
> 2. The stomach produces gastric juice that contains hydrochloric acid. _____ T _____ F
> 3. Digestion begins in the stomach. _____ T _____ F

Concept Checkpoint

The Concept Checkpoint feature includes review questions, many of which involve critical thinking skills, posed at the end of major headings. Such questions enable students to test their acquisition of information presented in the section. Answers to the questions in each Concept Checkpoint are located in Appendix G.

> ## Concept CHECKPOINT
> 23. What are the signs and symptoms of iron deficiency anemia? Which members of the population are most at risk of iron deficiency?
> 24. Identify at least three signs or symptoms of hemochromatosis. How is the condition treated?
> 25. What is a goiter? What is cretinism? How can cretinism be prevented?
> 26. Prepare a table for trace minerals that includes information about each trace

Critical Thinking

The Critical Thinking feature involves higher–level cognitive skills, including applying, analyzing, synthesizing, and evaluating information. This assessment features a series of thought–provoking questions at the end of the chapter. The questions can help students develop higher–level cognitive skills using nutrition–related content. Acquiring and/or sharpening these skills can help students become better consumers of nutrition–related information.

> "I love the Critical Thinking questions! This is the real world!"
>
> Purti Gadkari
> Wharton County Junior College

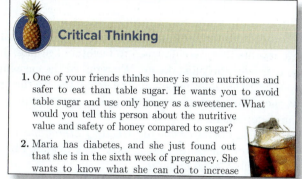

Critical Thinking

1. One of your friends thinks honey is more nutritious and safer to eat than table sugar. He wants you to avoid table sugar and use only honey as a sweetener. What would you tell this person about the nutritive value and safety of honey compared to sugar?

2. Maria has diabetes, and she just found out that she is in the sixth week of pregnancy. She wants to know what she can do to increase

©Stockbyte/Getty Images RF

Personal Dietary Analysis

Many chapters include an end–of–chapter activity for analyzing personal eating habits. Most of these activities require the use of a dietary analysis software program, such as NutritionCalc Plus. Students can gain insight into their eating behaviors by completing this activity.

> "I absolutely love these dietary analysis activities because they help the students apply the knowledge, and they help them in their own lives, too."
>
> Catherine Palmer
> Oklahoma State University–Oklahoma City

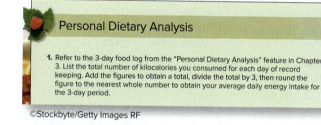

Personal Dietary Analysis

1. Refer to the 3-day food log from the "Personal Dietary Analysis" feature in Chapter 3. List the total number of kilocalories you consumed for each day of record keeping. Add the figures to obtain a total, divide the total by 3, then round the figure to the nearest whole number to obtain your average daily energy intake for the 3-day period.

©Stockbyte/Getty Images RF

Practice Test

Each chapter ends with a series of 10 or more multiple–choice questions that test students' comprehension and recall of information presented in the chapter. Answers to the test questions are in Appendix G. The multiple–choice questions prepare students for classroom exams, because they are similar in type and format to those in the test bank. In many instances, the test questions are correlated to the Coursewide Student Learning Outcomes and Learning Outcomes.

> "I love Practice Tests. I always assign these. I believe that the more questions the student is exposed to, the better they prepare."
>
> Ruby D. Johnson
> Ozarka College

Practice Test

Select the best answer.

1. Which of the following statements is false?
   a. Lean tissue contains more water than fat tissue.
   b. Water is a major solvent.
   c. Generally, young women have more body water than young men.
   d. Water does not provide energy.

2. If the extracellular fluid has an excess of sodium ions,
   a. sodium ions move into cells.
   b. intracellular fluid moves to the outside of cells.
   c. phosphate and calcium ions are eliminated in feces.
   d. blood levels of arsenic and oxalate increase.

3. Which of the following foods has the lowest percentage of water?
   a. Tomatoes
   b. Oranges
   c. Whole–grain bread
   d. Vegetable oil

4. In the United States, table salt is often fortified with
   a. iron.
   b. selenium.
   c. potassium.
   d. iodine.

5. Which of the following foods is not a good source of calcium?
   a. Butter
   b. American cheese
   c. Canned sardines
   d. Kale

6. Henry is concerned about his risk of osteoporosis. Which of the following characteristics is a modifiable risk factor for this chronic condition?
   a. Family history
   b. Racial/ethnic background
   c. Physical activity level
   d. Age

©Stockbyte/Getty Images RF

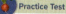

What's New in this Edition

The first edition of this textbook included beautiful, pedagogically based illustrations and creative page layouts that were designed to facilitate learning. The fifth edition maintains this energetic and visually appealing design. We retained the engaging photos that draw students' attention to the written information and relate content to the "real world." It is important to note that the use of products in photos is for example representation only and does not constitute an endorsement.

The fifth edition of *Nutrition for Healthy Living* has been updated extensively, and many of the diagrams and illustrations have been modified to increase their clarity. The following list describes some updates.

- Updated Daily Values charts in the Recipe for Healthy Living features
- Several new and/or revised practice Test and Critical Thinking questions
- New Appendix I for the Dietary Reference Intakes

Chapter 1: The Basics of Nutrition

- Updated Figure 1.2, which is a pie chart that has the 10 leading causes of death in the United States
- Figure 1.4 compares Americans' current food choices with food selections the population made in 1970.
- Redesigned Figure 1.6 (Energy and Nutrient Comparison), Figure 1.8 (Comparing Nutrient Densities), and Figure 1.9 (Energy Density) that makes the information easier for students to grasp
- My Diverse Plate feature discusses kimchi, a traditional Korean dish.

Chapter 2: Evaluation Nutrition Information

- Did You Know? feature that focuses on the sugar industry's role in influencing scientific opinions about diet and cardiovascular health in the mid−1960s
- Redesigned Figure 2.6 that makes its content easier for students to understand
- Updated Table 2.2 (Popular Non−micronutrient Dietary Supplements)

Chapter 3: Planning Nutritious Diets

- Figures that display the new Nutrition Facts panel

Chapter 4: Body Basics

- Expanded section about gut microbiota, including information about probiotics, prebiotics, and gut microbiota ("fecal") transplantation

Chapter 5: Carbohydrates

- Redesigned Figure 5.7 (Regulating Blood Glucose) that makes it easier for students to follow
- Did You Know? features about prebiotics, diabetic alert dogs, stevia, and FODMAPs

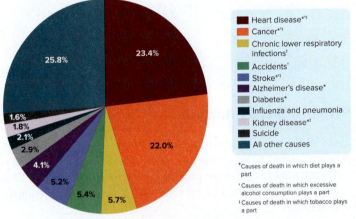

- Heart disease*†
- Cancer*†
- Chronic lower respiratory infections†
- Accidents†
- Stroke*†
- Alzheimer's disease*
- Diabetes*
- Influenza and pneumonia
- Kidney disease*†
- Suicide
- All other causes

23.4%
22.0%
25.8%
5.7%
5.4%
5.2%
4.1%
2.9%
2.1%
1.8%
1.6%

*Causes of death in which diet plays a part

†Causes of death in which excessive alcohol consumption plays a part

‡Causes of death in which tobacco plays a part

Source: National Center for *Health Statistics: Health, United States, 2016.* https://www.cdc.gov/nchs/data/hus/2016/019.pdf Accessed: June 28, 2017.

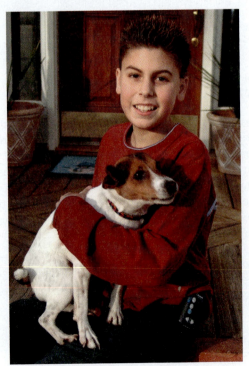

©Realistic Reflections RF

- Includes photos of food packages that highlight the added sugars line of the new Nutrition Facts panel
- Section that discusses the role of sugar–sweetened beverages in health and their association with the development of nonalcoholic fatty liver disease
- Expanded Personal Dietary Analysis feature that includes questions about added sugars intake

Chapter 6: Fats and Other Lipids

- Discussion about partially hydrogenated oils and why they have been banned from being added to foods
- Food & Nutrition Tips feature that can help students reduce their intake of sodium, solid fats, and added sugars when they prepare meals and snacks
- My Diverse Plate feature that highlights *pico de gallo*
- Self–assessment for alcohol abuse and new table for effects of blood alcohol concentration on the body

Chapter 7: Proteins

- Did You Know? features about taurine and energy drinks, peanut allergy and introducing peanuts to a baby's diet, and gluten sensitivity
- Information about gout

Chapter 8: Vitamins

- Revised Figure 8.12 (Vitamin D) makes the body's synthesis of the vitamin easier to follow
- Did You Know? features about niacin toxicity, the effects of passive exposure to cigarette smoke on a person's needs for vitamin C, raw egg white consumption and biotin deficiency, and an unusual cause of pyridoxine deficiency in infants

Chapter 9: Water and Minerals

- Did You Know? features the 2016 hurricane that battered a region of Haiti, disrupting the supply of clean water to the area: calcium–containing antacids; phytic acid and zinc bioavailability; and inorganic arsenic and rice
- My Diverse Plate feature introduces students to *kiwano*.

Chapter 10: Energy Balance and Weight Control

- Figure 10.1 (Obesity Map of the United States) has been updated to the 2015 version.
- Did You Know? features about helpful methods of reducing body weight and the association between television watching and obesity

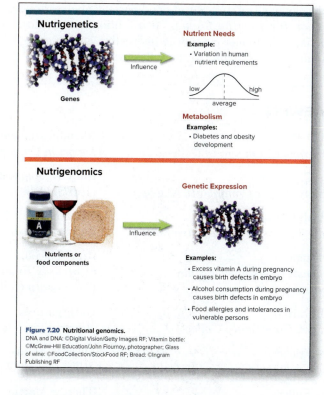

Figure 7.20 Nutritional genomics.
DNA and DNA: ©Digital Vision/Getty Images RF; Vitamin bottle: ©McGraw-Hill Education/John Flournoy, photographer; Glass of wine: ©FoodCollection/StockFood RF; Bread: ©Ingram Publishing RF

Chapter 11: Nutrition for Physically Active Lifestyles

- Did You Know? about use of hormones to increase muscle mass

Chapter 12: Food Safety Concerns

- Table 12.2 (Serious Signs and Symptoms of Food–Borne Illness: When to See a Physician)
- Did You Know? about toxic mushrooms
- New Figure 12.13 (What's Generally Safe to Eat?) shows foods and beverages that are safe and unsafe to eat when one is in a country that does not have sanitary water supplies and safe farming methods.

Chapter 13: Nutrition for a Lifetime

- Table 13.3 (Recommended Weight Gain During Pregnancy)
- Did You Know? about caffeine intake during pregnancy
- Section about introducing solid foods discusses changes in recommendations concerning preventing food allergies.
- Information about sarcopenic obesity among older adults
- Real People, Real Stories about 90–year–old Paul Appelbaum

Acknowledgments

The development of an accurate and current manuscript for *Nutrition for Healthy Living*, Fifth Edition, was facilitated by the input of numerous college instructors and emeriti. I offer my sincere thanks to the following colleagues who provided a wide range of valuable input, including reviewing chapters, class–testing chapters, and preparing supplemental materials:

Reviewers

Jennifer Bess
Hillsborough Community College

Maria C. Carles
Northern Essex Community College

Janet M. Colson
Middle Tennessee State University

Kay Daigle
Southeastern Oklahoma State University

Sarah Darrell
Ivy Tech Community College

Linda Friend
Wake Technical Community College

Jenny Fuller
Bluegrass Community and Technical College

Purti Gadkari
Wharton County Junior College

Janis E. Grimland
Hill College

Ahondju Umadjela Holmes
Langston University

Ruby D. Johnson
Ozarka College

Yanyan Li
Husson University

Anne Lincoln
Professor Emeritus, North Country Community College

Kathryn Link
Alfred State College

Mara L. Manis
Hillsborough Community College

Theresa Martin
College of San Mateo

Liza M. Mohanty
Olive–Harvey College

Catherine Palmer
Oklahoma State University–Oklahoma City

Wanda Perkins
Salisbury University

Robin Polokoff
Cal State University East Bay
Diablo Valley College
Las Positas College

Ramona S. Price
Texas State University

Linda Rankin
Idaho State University

Jan Sholes
Frederick Community College

Carole A. Sloan
Henry Ford College

Brenda Stagner
Butte College

Nicole Stob
University of Colorado Boulder

Francis Tayie
Southeast Missouri State University

We are pleased to have been able to incorporate real student data points and input, derived from our SmartBook users, to help guide our revision. SmartBook heat maps provided a quick visual snapshot of usage of portions of the text and the relative difficulty students experienced in mastering the content. With these data, we were able to hone not only our text content but also the SmartBook probes.

My very special thanks is necessary to the individuals who helped make *Nutrition for Healthy Living* more real and interesting by contributing their stories to Real People, Real Stories features.

Many McGraw–Hill Education employees invested a great deal of time and effort into the development and production of this new edition of *Nutrition for Healthy Living*. My sincerest thanks is extended to all the members of the McGraw–Hill Education editorial, design, production, and marketing team for their enthusiastic support and encouragement.

A few members of the team deserve special recognition. Marija Magner served as my Sr. Portfolio Manager. Under her very capable direction, I was able to focus my attention on the preparation of this edition. Thanks as well to Valerie Kramer,

Marketing Manager; Tara McDermott, Designer; Jodi Banowetz, Assessment Content Project Manager; Content Licensing Specialist, Shawntel Schmitt; Jerry Marshall and Elaine Kosta for their wonderful work on photo and text permissions. Vicki Krug, Content Project Manager, had the difficult task of managing my chapters as they progressed through production, and she helped convey my wishes concerning the art and layout to the compositor. Vicki's efforts were instrumental in the production of a superior textbook.

I also want to thank Thomas Timp, Managing Director, for providing support for the production of a superior textbook. Last, but not least, my Product Developer, Darlene Schueller, deserves my heartfelt gratitude for the hard work, long hours, and extraordinary dedication she invested in the production of *Nutrition for Healthy Living*.

Wendy J. Schiff

©C Squared Studios/Getty Images RF

Contents

©C Squared Studios
/Getty Images RF

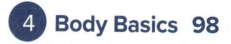
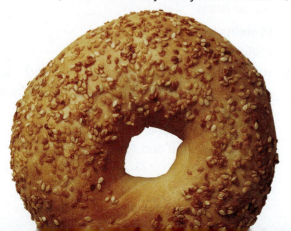

©C Squared Studios/Getty Images RF

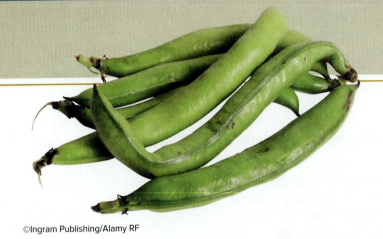
©Ingram Publishing/Alamy RF

©C Squared Studios/Getty Images RF

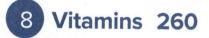

8 Vitamins   260

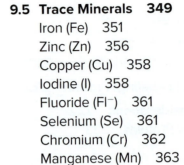

©C Squared Studios/
Getty Images RF

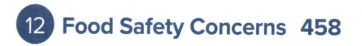

11 Nutrition for Physically Active Lifestyles   426

12 Food Safety Concerns   458

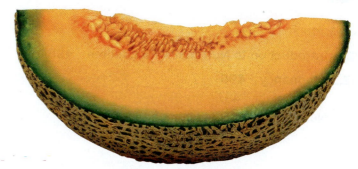

©C Squared Studios/Getty Images RF

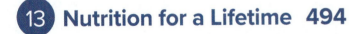

13 Nutrition for a Lifetime 494

The Basics of Nutrition

Nutrition

For Healthy Living

Fifth Edition

WENDY J. SCHIFF, MS, RDN

CHAPTER 1

The Basics of Nutrition

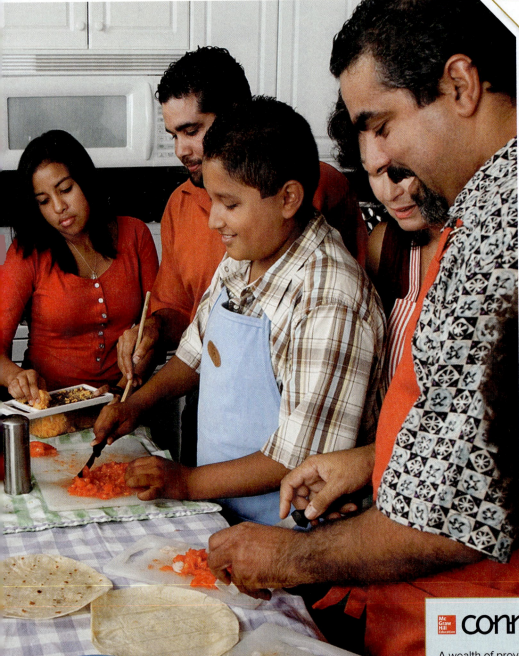

Quiz Yourself

Take the following quiz to test your basic nutrition knowledge; the answers are at the end of the chapter.

1. There are four classes of nutrients: proteins, lipids, sugars, and vitamins. _____ T _____ F

2. Proteins are the most essential class of nutrients. _____ T _____ F

3. All nutrients must be supplied by the diet because they cannot be made by the body. _____ T _____ F

4. Vitamins are a source of energy. _____ T _____ F

5. Milk, carrots, and bananas are examples of "perfect" foods that contain all nutrients. _____ T _____ F

McGraw Hill Education **connect**®

A wealth of proven resources are available on Connect® including SmartBook®, NutritionCalc Plus, and many other dynamic learning tools. Ask your instructor about Connect!

1.1 Nutrition: The Basics

Learning Outcomes

1 Explain why it is important to learn about foods and nutrition.

2 Identify factors that influence personal food choices.

3 Identify lifestyle factors that contribute to some of the leading causes of death in the United States.

4 List the six classes of nutrients, and identify a major role of each class of nutrient in the body.

5 Explain how to determine whether a substance is a phytochemical or an essential nutrient.

When you were an infant and a young child, your parents or other adult caregivers were the "gatekeepers" of your food; they chose what you ate and prepared it, and you probably ate most of it. If you balked at eating steamed broccoli or baked salmon, they may have told you, "Eat your vegetables if you expect to get dessert" or "Finish that fish. People in Africa are starving!" As you grew older, your **diet,** your usual pattern of food choices, came increasingly under your control. Today, your diet is more likely to be composed of foods that you enjoy as well as can afford and probably those you can prepare easily or obtain quickly. Your family's ethnic and cultural background may also play a role in determining what you eat regularly. For example, do you eat tamales, tripe, goat, or kimchi because you ate these foods as a child? Numerous other factors influence your food choices, including friends and food advertising, as well as your beliefs and moods (Fig. 1.1).

Food is a basic human need for survival. You become hungry and search for something to eat when your body needs **nutrients,** the life—sustaining substances in food. Nutrients are necessary for the growth, maintenance, and repair of your body's cells. However, you were not born with the ability to select the appropriate mix of nutrients your body requires for proper functioning. To eat well, you need to learn about the nutritional value of foods and the effects that your diet can have on your health.

Simply having information about nutrients and foods and their effects on health may not be enough for people to change ingrained food—related behaviors; a person must be moti—vated to make such changes. Some people become motivated to improve their diets because they want to lose or gain weight. Others are so concerned about their health, they are motivated to change their eating habits in specific ways, such as by eating fewer salty or fatty foods. Many people, however, do not care if the food they eat is beneficial or harmful to their health.

diet usual pattern of food choices

nutrients chemicals necessary for proper body functioning

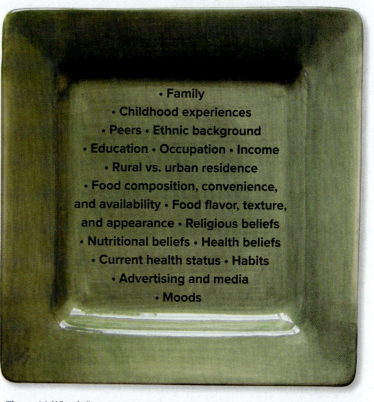

- Family
- Childhood experiences
- Peers • Ethnic background
- Education • Occupation • Income
- Rural vs. urban residence
- Food composition, convenience, and availability • Food flavor, texture, and appearance • Religious beliefs
- Nutritional beliefs • Health beliefs
- Current health status • Habits
- Advertising and media
- Moods

Figure 1.1 What influences your eating practices? Numerous factors influence food choices, including food advertising, peers, income, moods, and personal beliefs.
©Wendy Schiff

Why Learn About Nutrition

Why should you care about your diet? The foods and bever—ages you usually select for meals and snacks contribute to your health now and in the future. In the United States, poor eating habits contribute to several leading causes of death, including

MY DIVERSE PLATE

MyPlate: Source: U.S. Dept. of Agriculture

Kimchi (*kim-chee'*) is a traditional Korean food made with vegetables such as cabbage, cucumbers, or Korean radishes. A very popular kimchi uses leaves from fresh napa cabbages. The leaves are first carefully washed and then salted. The salt kills harmful bacteria and draws water out of the leaves, so they become soft and limp. Next, the leaves are rinsed to remove the salt, and then each leaf is completely smeared with a pastelike mixture that is made with hot red chili pepper flakes, garlic, ginger, brown sugar, fish or shrimp sauce, and chopped Korean radishes, green onions, and *buchu* (Asian chives). The seasoned cabbage leaves are folded and stuffed into a sealed container, and the mixture is allowed to ferment for 1 to 5 days.

Fermentation is a natural process in which bacteria or yeast break down certain nutrients, producing acids, gases, and alcohol as a result. Many foods and beverages, including pickles, sauerkraut, yogurt, wine, and beer, are produced by fermentation.

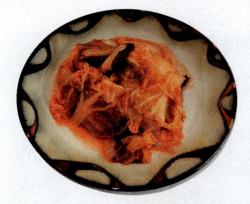

| Kimchi made with napa cabbage. ©Wendy Schiff

nutrition scientific study of nutrients and how the body uses these substances

chemistry study of the composition and characteristics of matter and changes that can occur to it

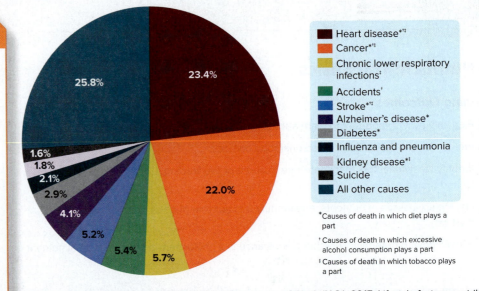

Legend:
- Heart disease*†‡
- Cancer*†‡
- Chronic lower respiratory infections‡
- Accidents†
- Stroke*†‡
- Alzheimer's disease*
- Diabetes*
- Influenza and pneumonia
- Kidney disease*‡
- Suicide
- All other causes

*Causes of death in which diet plays a part

†Causes of death in which excessive alcohol consumption plays a part

‡Causes of death in which tobacco plays a part

Figure 1.2 Approximate percentages of leading causes of death (U.S.), 2015. Lifestyle factors contribute to many of the 10 leading causes of death in the United States. Source: National Center for *Health Statistics: Health, United States, 2016.* https://www.cdc.gov/nchs/data/hus/2016/019.pdf Accessed: June 28, 2017.

heart disease, some types of cancer, stroke, and type 2 diabetes (Fig. 1.2). Results of a long−term study that followed over 215,000 adult Americans living in Hawaii and California indicated the likelihood of dying from all causes during the study was lower for subjects who followed nationally recommended dietary guidelines.[1] According to the *2015–2020 Dietary Guidelines for Americans*, people can reduce their chances of developing serious diseases that contribute to premature deaths by consuming more fruits, vegetables, unsalted nuts, fat−free or low−fat dairy products, and whole−grain cereals, as well as exercising regularly.[2]

Are you concerned about the nutritional quality of your diet? The fact that you are taking this course indicates you have a strong interest in nutrition and a desire to learn more about the topic. A major objective of this textbook is to provide you with the basic information you need to better understand how your diet can influence your health. Managing your diet is your responsibility. We will not tell you what to eat to guarantee optimal health: No one can make that promise. After reading this textbook and learning about foods and the nutrients they contain, you can use the information to make informed decisions concerning the foods you eat. Furthermore, you will be able to evaluate your diet and decide if it needs to be changed.

Each chapter of this textbook begins with "Quiz Yourself," a brief true−or−false quiz to test your knowledge of the material covered in the chapter. Each major section of a chapter ends with "Concept Checkpoints," a series of multiple−choice questions that can help you determine whether you understood the major concepts in the section. Answers to the "Concept Checkpoints" are given in Appendix G. At the end of each chapter, you will find the answers to the opener quiz, as well as a group of multiple−choice questions that test your understanding of the material in the chapter. The answers to those questions are also provided in Appendix G. References for information cited in chapters are in Appendix H.

Introduction to Nutrition

Nutrition is the scientific study of nutrients, chemicals necessary for proper body functioning, and how the body uses them. Understanding nutrition requires learning about chemistry. **Chemistry** is the study of the composition and characteristics of matter, and changes that can occur to it. Matter is anything that takes up space and has mass or weight (on Earth). The air you breathe, this textbook, and even your body con—sist of chemicals and are forms of matter. "There are chemicals in our food!" This statement may sound frightening, but it is true. Food is matter; therefore, it contains chemicals, some of which are nutrients.

There are six classes of nutrients: carbohydrates, fats and other lipids, proteins, vitamins, minerals, and water. Your body is comprised of these nutrients (Fig. 1.3). Although an average healthy young man and woman have similar amounts of vitamins, min—erals, and carbohydrates in their bodies, the young woman has less water and protein, and considerably more fat than the man.

Table 1.1 presents major roles of nutrients in your body. In general, your body uses certain nutrients for energy, growth and development, and regulation of processes, including the repair and maintenance of cells. A **cell** is the smallest living functional unit in an organism, such as a human being. There are hundreds of different types of cells in your body.

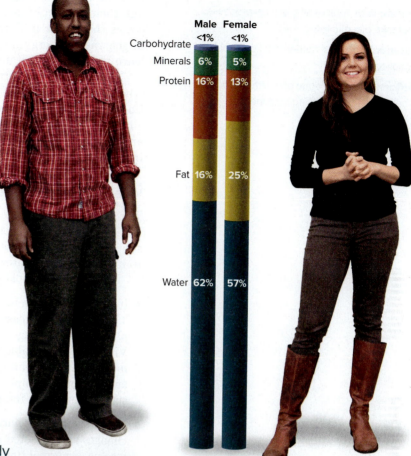

Figure 1.3 Comparing composition. These illustrations present the approximate percentages of nutrients that comprise the bodies of a healthy young man and woman. Note that the amount of vitamins in the human body is so small, it is not shown.

Man, woman: ©McGraw-Hill Education. Aaron Roeth Photography

TABLE 1.1   Major Functions of Nutrients in the Body

Nutrient	Major Functions
Carbohydrates	Energy (most forms)
Lipids	Energy (fat)
	Cellular development, physical growth and development
	Regulation of body processes (certain chemical messengers, for example)
	Absorption of certain vitamins
Proteins	Production of structural components, such as cell membranes, and functional components, such as enzymes
	Cellular development, growth, and maintenance
	Regulation of body processes (certain chemical messengers, for example)
	Immune function and fluid balance
	Energy
Vitamins	Regulation of body processes, including cell metabolism
	Maintenance of immune function, production and maintenance of tissues, and protection against agents that can damage cellular components
Minerals	Regulation of body processes, including fluid balance and metabolism; formation of certain chemical messengers; structural and functional components of various substances and tissues; physical growth, maintenance, and development
Water	Maintenance of fluid balance, regulation of body temperature, elimination of wastes, and transportation of substances
	Participant in many chemical reactions

cell smallest living functional unit in an organism

metabolism total of all chemical processes that take place in living cells

essential nutrient nutrient that must be supplied by food

deficiency disease state of health that occurs when a nutrient is missing from the diet

Cells do not need food to survive, but they need the nutrients in food to carry out their metabolic activities. **Metabolism** is the total of all chemical processes that occur in living cells, including chemical reactions (changes) involved in generating energy, making proteins, and eliminating waste products. You will learn more about metabolism in Chapter 4 (Body Basics).

Understanding nutrition also involves learning about human *physiology*, the study of how the body functions. Chapter 4 prepares you for the study of nutrition by presenting basic information about chemistry and human physiology. Chapters 5 (Carbohydrates), 6 (Fats and Other Lipids), 7 (Proteins), 8 (Vitamins), and 9 (Water and Minerals) provide information about the functions of nutrients in the body.

What Is an Essential Nutrient?

The body can synthesize (make) many nutrients, such as the lipids cholesterol and fat, but about 50 nutrients are dietary essentials. An **essential nutrient** must be supplied by food because the body does not synthesize the nutrient or make enough to meet its needs. Water is the most essential nutrient.

There are three key features that help identify an essential nutrient:

- If the nutrient is missing from the diet, a **deficiency disease** occurs as a result. The deficiency disease is a state of health characterized by certain abnormal physiological changes. (*Physiological* refers to the functioning of the body.) Visible or measurable changes are referred to as *signs* of disease. Disease signs include rashes, failure to grow properly, and elevated blood pressure. *Symptoms* are subjective complaints of ill health that are difficult to observe and measure, such as dizziness, fatigue, and headache.

- When the missing nutrient is added to the diet, the abnormal physiological changes are corrected. As a result, signs and symptoms of the deficiency disorder resolve as normal functioning is restored, and the condition is cured.

- After scientists identify the nutrient's specific roles in the body, they can explain why the abnormalities occurred when the substance was missing from the diet.

If you wanted to test your body's need for vitamin C, for example, you could avoid consuming foods or vitamin supplements that contain the vitamin. When the amount of vitamin C in your cells became too low for them to function normally, you would develop physical signs of *scurvy*, the vitamin C deficiency disease. Early in the course of the deficiency, tiny red spots that are actually signs of bleeding under the skin (tiny bruises) would appear where the elastic bands of your clothing applied pressure. When you brushed your teeth, your gums would bleed from the pressure of the toothbrush. If you cut yourself, the wound would heal slowly or not at all. If you started consuming vitamin C–containing foods again, the deficiency signs and symptoms would disappear within a few days as your body recovered. By reading about vitamin C in Chapter 8, you will learn that one of the physiological roles of vitamin C is maintaining a substance in your body that literally holds cells together. This substance is also needed to produce scar tissue for wound

©Greg Kuchik/Getty Images RF

healing. Thus, vitamin C meets all the required features of an essential nutrient.

Table 1.2 lists nutrients that are generally considered to be essential. Fortunately, the human body is designed to obtain these substances from a wide variety of foods. Chapter 3 provides information about ways to plan nutritious diets.

What Are Nonnutrients? Some foods contain nonnutrients—substances that are not nutrients, yet they may have healthful benefits. Plants make hundreds of nonnutrients called **phytochemicals** (*phyto* = plant). Caffeine, for example, is a phytochemical naturally made by coffee plants that has a stimulating effect on the body. Many phytochemicals are antioxidants that may reduce risks of heart disease and certain cancers. An **antioxidant** protects cells and their components from being damaged or destroyed by exposure to certain harmful environmental and internal factors. Some vitamins also function as antioxidants (see Chapter 8).

Not all phytochemicals have beneficial effects on the body. Some phytochemicals, such as nicotine in tobacco leaves, ricin in castor beans, and oxalic acid in rhubarb leaves, are toxic or can interfere with the absorption of nutrients. Scientific research that explores the effects of phytochemicals on the body is ongoing. Table 1.3 lists several phytochemicals that are currently under scientific investigation, identifies rich food sources of these compounds, and indicates their biological effects on the body, including possible health benefits.

TABLE 1.2 Essential Nutrients for Humans

Water	Glucose†	Fats that contain linoleic and alpha-linolenic acids
Vitamins:	**Minerals:**	
A	Calcium	
B vitamins	Chloride	
Thiamin	Chromium	
Riboflavin	Copper	**Components of proteins (amino acids):**
Niacin	Iodine	
Pantothenic acid	Iron	
Biotin	Magnesium	Histidine
Folate	Manganese	Leucine
B-6	Molybdenum	Isoleucine
B-12	Phosphorus	Lysine
Choline*	Potassium	Methionine
C	Selenium	Phenylalanine
D**	Sodium	Threonine
E	Sulfur	Tryptophan
K	Zinc	Valine

*The body makes choline but may not make enough to meet needs. Often classified as a *vitamin-like* compound.

**The body makes vitamin D after exposure to sunlight, but a dietary source of the nutrient is often necessary.

†A source of glucose is needed to supply the nervous system with energy and spare protein from being used for energy.

Dietary Supplements

Many Americans take dietary supplements such as vitamin pills and herbal extracts to improve their health. The Dietary Supplement Health and Education Act of 1994 (DSHEA) allows manufacturers to classify nutrient supplements and certain herbal products as foods.[3] The DSHEA defines a **dietary supplement** as a product (excluding tobacco) that contains a vitamin, a mineral, an herb or other plant product, an amino acid, or a dietary substance that supplements the diet by increasing total intake. According to scientific evidence, some dietary supplements, such as vitamins and certain herbs, can have beneficial effects on health. However, results of scientific testing also indicate that many popular dietary supplements are not helpful and may even be harmful. The "Nutrition Matters" feature in Chapter 2 ("What Are Dietary Supplements?") discusses dietary supplements. Information about specific dietary supplements, including those that contain phytochemicals, is also woven into chapters where it is appropriate.

phytochemicals compounds made by plants that are not nutrients

antioxidant substance that protects other compounds from being damaged or destroyed by certain factors

dietary supplements nutrient preparations, certain hormones, and herbal products that are taken to increase total dietary intake

TABLE 1.3   Phytochemicals of Scientific Interest

Classification and Examples	Rich Food Sources	Biological Effects/Possible Health Benefits
Carotenoids		Antioxidant activity; may reduce risk of macular degeneration (a major cause of blindness)
Alpha-carotene, beta-carotene, lutein, lycopene, zeaxanthin	Orange, red, yellow fruits and vegetables; egg yolks	
Phenolics		Antioxidant activity; may inhibit cancer growth, may reduce risk of heart disease
Quercetin	Apples, tea, red wine, onions, olives, raspberries, cocoa	
Catechins	Tea, chocolate, plums, apples, berries, pecans	
Anthocyanins	Red, blue, or purple fruits and vegetables	
Resveratrol	Red wine, purple grapes and grape juice, dark chocolate	
Isoflavonoids	Soybeans and other legumes	
Lignans	Flaxseed, berries, whole grains, bran, nuts	
Ellagic acid	Raspberries, strawberries, cranberries, walnuts, pomegranates	
Organosulfides		Antioxidant effects; may improve immune system functioning and reduce the risk of heart disease
Isothiocyanates, indoles, allylic sulfur compounds	Garlic, onions, cruciferous vegetables (broccoli, cauliflower, cabbage, kale, bok choy, collard and mustard greens)	
Alkaloids		Stimulant effects
Caffeine	Coffee, tea, kola nuts, cocoa	
Capsaicinoids		May provide some pain relief
Capsaicin	Chili peppers	
Fructooligosaccharides		May stimulate the growth of beneficial bacteria in the human intestinal tract
	Onions, bananas, asparagus, wheat	

Concept CHECKPOINT

1. Identify at least two of the 10 leading causes of death that are diet related.
2. Identify at least four factors that influence your eating habits.
3. List the six major classes of nutrients.
4. What are three key factors that determine whether a substance is an essential nutrient?
5. Define *phytochemical* and *dietary supplement*.

See Appendix G for responses.

1.2 Factors That Influence Americans' Health

Learning Outcomes

1 Explain why people should be concerned about their lifestyle and risk factors for chronic diseases.

2 Compare Americans' current typical eating habits to the population's typical eating habits in 1970.

3 Identify the main nutrition-related goal of *Healthy People 2020*.

As mentioned in the opener of this chapter, poor eating habits contribute to several of the leading causes of death in the United States. Note in Figure 1.2 that heart disease is the leading cause of death for all Americans, and cancer is the second leading cause of death. In 2015, these two diseases accounted for almost half of all deaths.[4]

Conditions such as heart disease and cancer are *chronic* diseases. Chronic diseases usually take many years to develop and have complex causes. A **risk factor** is a personal characteristic that increases your chances of developing a chronic disease. For example, genetic background or family history is an important risk factor for heart disease. If your father's father had a heart attack before he was 55 years old and your mother is being treated for having a high blood cholesterol level (a risk factor for heart disease), your family history indicates you have a higher-than-average risk of having a heart attack. For many people, however, having a family history of a chronic disease does not mean that they definitely will develop the condition. Other risk factors that contribute to health are age, environmental conditions, psychological factors, access to health care, and lifestyle practices.

Lifestyle is a person's usual way of living that includes dietary practices, physical activity habits, use of drugs such as tobacco and alcohol, and other typical patterns of behavior. Your lifestyle may increase or reduce your chances of developing a chronic disease or delay its occurrence for years, even decades. Poor diet, cigarette smoking, and excess alcohol consumption, for example, are risk factors that increase the likelihood of heart disease, stroke, and many forms of cancer. Cigarette smoking is the primary cause of preventable cancer deaths, but dietary habits and physical activity patterns also contribute to the development of certain cancers.[5,6] Additionally, poor diet and lack of physical activity can result in obesity, a condition characterized by the accumulation of too much body fat. Obesity is a risk factor for numerous health problems, including heart disease, certain cancers, type 2 diabetes, and *hypertension* (chronic high blood pressure).

Our Changing Eating Habits

Americans' diets have changed significantly over the past 45 years. In 2014, we ate more fruits and vegetables than Americans consumed in 1970, but we did not eat the recommended amounts.[7] We also consumed less red meat (beef, veal, pork, and lamb), eggs, and milk and yogurt, and more fish and shellfish, cheese, and chicken and turkey than in 1970 (Fig. 1.4). Our diet also supplies more food energy from flour and cereal products than in 1970, but *refined* grain foods, such as white bread and pasta, make up the majority of these products.

Did YOU Know?

Your genetic makeup influences the effects of diet on your health as well as disease susceptibility. *Nutritional genomics* is a relatively new area of nutrition research that explores complex interactions among gene functioning, diet and other lifestyle choices, and the environment. Section 7.9 provides more information about nutritional genomics.

risk factor personal characteristic that increases a person's chances of developing a disease

lifestyle usual way of living, including dietary practices and physical activity habits

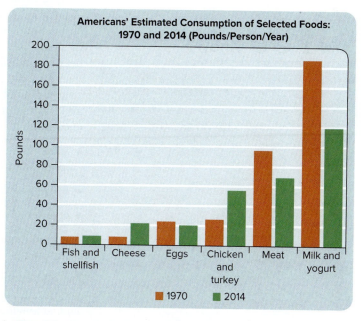

Americans' Estimated Consumption of Selected Foods: 1970 and 2014 (Pounds/Person/Year)

■ 1970   ■ 2014

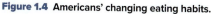

Figure 1.4 Americans' changing eating habits.

Source: U.S. Department of Agriculture, *Economic Research Service: Food availability (per capita) data system.* Last updated: November 23, 2016. Accessed: April 15, 2017, https://www.ers.usda.gov/data-products/food-availability-per-capita-data-system/food-availability-per-capita-data-system/# Loss-Adjusted Food Availability.

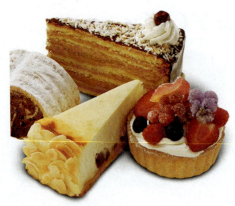

©FoodCollection/StockFood RF

TABLE 1.4   Estimated Energy Intakes (1970 and 2010)

Dietary Component (Calories per day)	1970	2010*
Total food energy	2024	2481
Added fats	346	575
Added sugars	333	373

* Data for 2010 was available in March 2017.

U.S. Department of Agriculture, Economic Research Service: Food availability (per capita) data system: *Average daily per capita calories from the U.S. food availability, adjusted for spoilage and other waste.* August 2016. https://www.ers.usda .gov/data-products/food-availability-per-capita-data-system/food-availability-per-capita-data-system/#Food Availability Accessed: April 15, 2017.

Raw foods often undergo some form of processing, such as refining, canning, freezing, or cooking, before they are eaten. Processing can make a food more nutritious, safer to eat, and less likely to spoil. However, some forms of processing remove nutrients and phytochemicals that were naturally in the food. Other forms of processing add unhealthy amounts of sodium, sugar, and certain fats to foods.

Compared to 1970, the typical American diet provided more added fats, added sugars, and total food energy in 2010, which was the last year that data were available at the time of this text's publication (Table 1.4).[7] If a person's energy intake is more than needed, especially for physical activity, his or her body fat increases. Nationwide surveys indicate that Americans are fatter than in previous decades. Dietary practices, however, should not receive all the blame for this unhealthy finding; during the same period, we have become increasingly dependent on various labor−saving gadgets and machines that make our lives easier but also reduce the amount of energy we need to expend to avoid unwanted weight gain. Chapter 10 examines weight management in detail.

Healthy People 2020

Since the late 1970s, health promotion and disease prevention have been the general focus of public health efforts in the United States. A primary component of such efforts is developing educational programs that can help people prevent chronic and infectious diseases, birth defects, and other serious health problems. In many instances, it is more practical and less expensive to prevent a serious health condition than to treat it.

In early 2011, the U.S. Department of Health and Human Services (DHHS) issued *Healthy People 2020*, a report that includes national health promotion and disease prevention objectives to be met by 2020. *Healthy People 2020* goals encourage Americans to:

- attain higher−quality, longer lives that are free of preventable disease, disability, injury, and premature death;

- achieve health equity by eliminating disparities to improve the health of all groups;

- create social and physical environments that promote good health for all; and

- promote quality of life, healthy development, and healthy behaviors across all life stages.[8]

The main nutrition−related goal of *Healthy People 2020* is to promote good health and reduce the risk of chronic disease by consuming healthful diets and achieving and maintaining healthy body weights. To help meet this goal, *Healthy People 2020* has several nutrition−related objectives, some of which are listed in Table 1.5. You can access more information about these objectives at the government's website (https://www.healthypeople.gov/2020/topics−objectives /topic/nutrition−and−weight−status/objectives).

TABLE 1.5   Some *Healthy People 2020* Objectives: Nutrition and Weight Status (NWS)

NWS Number	Objective
8	Increase the proportion of adults who have a healthy weight
9	Reduce the proportion of obese adults
10	Reduce the proportion of obese children and adolescents
14	Increase fruit intake among people who are 2 years of age and older
15	Increase the variety and intake of vegetables among people who are 2 years of age and older
16	Increase whole grain intake among people who are 2 years of age and older
17	Reduce intakes of solid fats and added sugars among people who are 2 years of age and older
18	Reduce sodium intake among people who are 2 years of age and older
19	Increase calcium intake among people who are 2 years of age and older

Source: https://www.healthypeople.gov/2020/topics-objectives/topic/nutrition-and-weight-status/objectives

Concept CHECKPOINT

6. What is a risk factor?
7. Explain how your lifestyle can affect your health.
8. Discuss how Americans' eating habits have changed since 1970.
9. Identify the main nutrition-related goal of *Healthy People 2020*.

See Appendix G for responses.

1.3 Metrics for Nutrition

Learning Outcomes

1 Identify basic units of the metric system often used in nutrition.

2 Use the caloric values of macronutrients and alcohol to estimate the amount of energy (kcal) in a food.

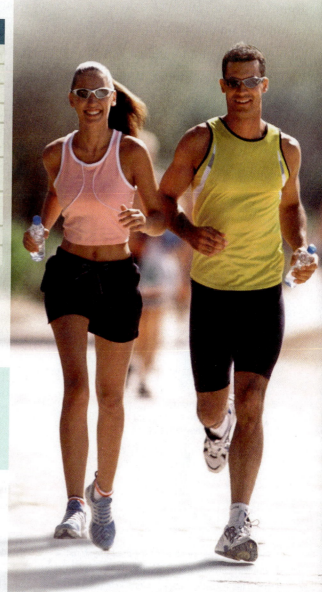

©Image Source/Getty Images RF

Scientists classify specific nutrients according to their chemical composition and major functions in the body. Nutrients can also be classified based on how much of them are in food. Americans usually refer to length in terms of inches and feet, weight in pounds, and amounts of food in familiar household measures (e.g., teaspoons, tablespoons, cups). Scientists, however, generally use metric values to report length (*meter*), weight (*gram*), and volume (*liter*). The following section provides a basic review of the metric system. Appendix A provides common English–to–metric and metric–to–household unit conversions.

Metric Basics

The metric prefixes *micro–*, *milli–*, *centi–*, *deci–*, and *kilo–* indicate whether a measurement is a fraction or a multiple of a meter (m), gram (g), or liter (l or L) (Table 1.6).

TABLE 1.6   Common Metric Prefixes in Nutrition

kilo- (k) = one thousand (1000)
deci- (d) = one-tenth (0.1)
centi- (c) = one-hundredth (0.01)
milli- (m) = one-thousandth (0.001)
micro- (mc or μ) = one-millionth (0.000001)

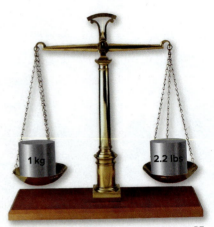

©Burke/Triolo/Brand X Pictures/Jupiter Images RF

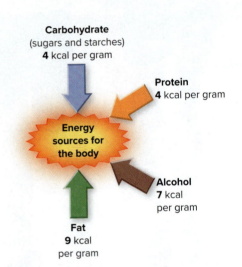

Figure 1.5 Energy sources for the body. Most forms of carbohydrate supply 4 kcal/g; protein also provides 4 kcal/g. Fat supplies 9 kcal/g, and alcohol (a nonnutrient) provides 7 kcal/g.

kilocalorie or **Calorie** heat energy needed to raise the temperature of 1 liter of water 1° Celsius; measure of food energy

macronutrients nutrients needed in gram amounts daily and that provide energy; carbohydrates, proteins, and fats

micronutrients vitamins and minerals

There are approximately 2.54 centimeters (cm) per inch. To obtain your approximate height in centimeters, multiply your height in inches by 2.54. For example, a person who is 5′5″ in height (65″) measures about 165 cm (65 × 2.54) in length. There are approximately 28 g in an ounce and 454 g in a pound. A kilogram (*kilo* = 1000) equals 1000 g or about 2.2 pounds. To determine your weight in kilograms (kg), divide your weight in pounds by 2.2. A person who weighs 130 pounds, for example, weighs about 59 kg.

Assume that a small raisin weighs 1 gram. If you cut this raisin into 1000 equal pieces, then each piece weighs 1 milligram (*milli* = 1000). Thus, 1000 milligrams (mg) equal 1 gram (g). Imagine cutting a small raisin into 1 million equal pieces. Each piece of raisin would weigh 1—millionth of a gram, or a microgram (mcg or μg). Amounts of nutrients in blood are often reported as the number of milligrams or micrograms of the substance per deciliter of blood. For example, a normal blood glucose level for a healthy fasting person is 90 milligrams/deciliter (90 mg/dl).

What's a Calorie?

Running, sitting, studying—your body uses energy even while sleeping. Every cell in your body needs energy to carry out its various activities. As long as you are alive, you are constantly using energy. You are probably familiar with the term *calorie,* the unit that describes the energy content of food. A calorie is the heat energy necessary to raise the temperature of 1 g (1 ml) of water 1° Celsius (C). A calorie is such a small unit of measurement, the amount of energy in food is reported in 1000—calorie units called kilocalories or Calories. Thus, a **kilocalorie** (kcal) or **Calorie** is the heat energy needed to raise the temperature of 1000 g (a liter) of water 1° Celsius (C). A small apple, for example, supplies 40,000 calories or 40 kcal or 40 Calories. If no number of kilocalories is specified, it is appropriate to use "calories." In this textbook, the term *calories* is interchangeable with *food energy* or simply *energy.*

A gram of carbohydrate and a gram of protein each supplies about 4 kcal; a gram of fat provides about 9 kcal (Fig. 1.5). Although alcohol is not a nutrient, it does provide energy; a gram of pure alcohol furnishes 7 kcal. If you know how many grams of carbohydrate, protein, fat, and/or alcohol are in a food, you can estimate the number of kilocalories it provides. For example, if a serving of food contains 10 g of carbohydrate, 3 g of protein, and 5 g of fat, multiply 10 g by 4 (the number of kcal each gram of carbohydrate supplies). Next, multiply 3 g by 4 (the number of kcal each gram of protein provides). Then multiply 5 g by 9 (the number of kcal each gram of fat supplies). By adding the three caloric values (40 kcal from carbohydrate, 12 kcal from protein, and 45 kcal from fat), you will determine that this food provides 97 kcal/serving.

Macronutrients and Micronutrients

Carbohydrates, fats, and proteins are referred to as **macronutrients** because the body needs relatively large amounts (grams) of these nutrients daily. Vitamins and minerals are **micronutrients,** because the body needs very small amounts (milligrams or micrograms) of them to function properly. In general, a serving of food supplies grams of carbohydrate, fat, and protein, and milligram or microgram quantities of vitamins and minerals. It is important to understand that macronutrients supply energy for cells, whereas micronutrients do not. Although the body requires large amounts of water, this nutrient provides no energy and is not usually classified as a macronutrient.

Amounts of nutrients present in different foods vary widely, and even the same food from the same source can contain different amounts of nutrients. Therefore, food composition tables and nutrient analysis software generally indicate average amounts of nutrients in foods. By using these tools, however, you can obtain approximate values for each nutrient measured and estimate your nutrient intake.

Concept CHECKPOINT

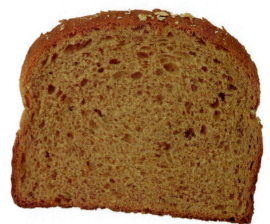

©Wendy Schiff

1.4 Key Nutrition Concepts

Learning Outcomes

1 Give examples of foods that supply a lot of empty calories and foods that are energy-dense and/or nutrient-dense.

2 Discuss key basic nutrition concepts, such as the importance of eating a variety of foods and why food is the best source of nutrients.

Before learning about the nutrients and their roles in health, it is important to grasp some key basic nutrition concepts (Table 1.7). The content in the chapters that follow will build upon these key concepts and can help you make more informed choices concerning your dietary practices.

Concept 1: Most Naturally Occurring Foods Are Mixtures of Nutrients

Which foods do you think of when you hear the words *protein* or *carbohydrate?* You probably identify meat, milk, and eggs as sources of protein; and potatoes, corn, and rice as sources of carbohydrate. Most naturally occurring foods, however, are mixtures of nutrients. In many instances, water is the major nutrient in foods. For example, 8 ounces of whole milk is about 88% water by weight, but it is an excellent source of protein and supplies carbohydrate, some fat, and several vitamins and minerals. A 6–ounce raw white potato is 79% water and only about 18% carbohydrate by weight. The potato also supplies iron and potassium (minerals) and vitamins C and niacin.

Most processed foods are also mixtures of nutrients. Sweet snacks, for example, are sources of nutrients other than sugar, a carbohydrate. Although sugar comprises about 44% of the weight of a chocolate with almonds candy bar, over one–third of the sweet snack's energy is from fat. The candy bar also contains small amounts of protein, iron, calcium, vitamin A, and the B–vitamin riboflavin. Figure 1.6 compares the energy, water, protein, carbohydrate, fat, and calcium contents of a 6–ounce baked potato, a slice of whole–wheat bread, 8 ounces of fat–free milk, and a chocolate–glazed doughnut (4–inch diameter). You can find information about the energy and nutrient contents of foods by using "What's in the Foods You Eat *Search Tool*" at the U.S. Department of Agriculture's website: www.ars.usda.gov/Services/docs.htm?docid=17032.

Concept 2: Variety Can Help Ensure the Nutritional Adequacy of a Diet

No natural food is "perfect" in that it contains all nutrients in amounts that are needed by the body. To help ensure the nutritional adequacy of your diet, choose a

TABLE 1.7 Key Basic Nutrition Concepts

- Most naturally occurring foods are mixtures of nutrients.

- Variety can help ensure the nutritional adequacy of a diet.

- There are no "good" or "bad" foods.

- Enjoy eating all foods in moderation.

- For each nutrient, there is a range of safe intake.

- Food is the best source of nutrients and phytochemicals.

- There is no "one size fits all" approach to planning a nutritionally adequate diet.

- Foods and the nutrients they contain are not cure-alls.

- Malnutrition includes *under*nutrition as well as *over*nutrition.

- Nutrition is a dynamic science.

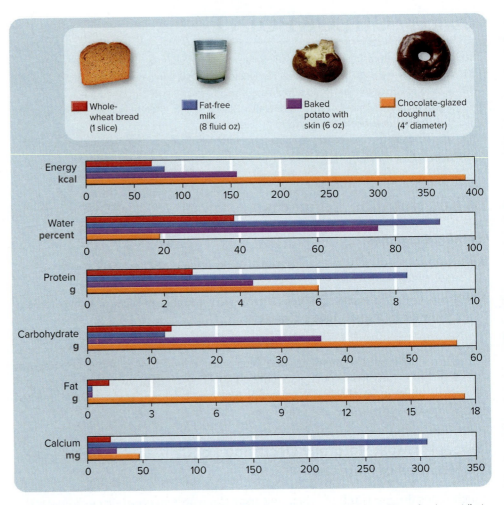

Figure 1.6 Energy and nutrient comparison. Most foods are mixtures of nutrients. These foods contribute very different amounts of energy, water, protein, carbohydrate, fat, and calcium to diets.

Bread: ©Ed Carey/Cole Group/Getty Images RF; Milk, potato: ©McGraw-Hill Education. Christopher Kerrigan, photographer; Doughnut: ©Wendy Schiff

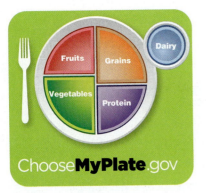

Figure 1.7 MyPlate. Source: U.S. Dept. of Agriculture

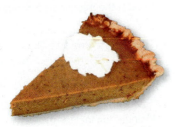

Because pumpkin pie is made with eggs and milk, this holiday favorite is a good source of protein. ©Wendy Schiff

diet that contains a variety of foods from each food group that is shown in MyPlate (Fig. 1.7), including fruits, low—fat or fat—free dairy products, and whole grains. MyPlate is a personalized approach to menu planning that can help you incorporate a variety of foods from all food groups into your daily diet. To make menu planning more interesting and dishes more appealing, try unfamiliar foods and new recipes for preparing your usual fare. Chapter 3 (Planning Nutritious Diets) provides infor—mation about the food groups and practical menu planning tools, such as MyPlate.

Concept 3: There Are No "Good" or "Bad" Foods

Are some foods "good" and others "bad" for your body? If you think there are such foods, which ones are good and which are bad? Do you sometimes feel guilty about eating "junk foods"? What is a junk food? Should pizza, chips, candy, doughnuts, ice cream, and sugar—sweetened soft drinks be classified as junk food?

All foods have nutritional value. For example, many people think pumpkin pie is a junk food. Pumpkin pie, however, is a good source of protein, the mineral iron, and the phytochemical beta—carotene that the body can convert to vitamin A. Even sugar—sweetened soft drinks provide water and the carbohydrate sugar, a source of energy. Although pies, doughnuts, and ice cream contain a lot of fat and added sugar, these foods also supply small amounts of protein, vitamins, and minerals to diets. Healthy diets, however, generally contain limited amounts of such foods.

A food *is* bad for you if it contains toxic substances or is contaminated with bacteria, viruses, or microscopic animals that cause food—borne illness. Chapter 12 (Food Safety Concerns) focuses on food safety concerns, including major types of food—borne illnesses and how to prevent them.

Empty Calories

Some foods and beverages, such as bacon, candy, pastries, snack chips, and sugar—sweetened drinks, provide much of their energy from unhealthy solid fats and added sugars. Such items are described as sources of "**empty calories.**"[9] Alcohol—containing drinks may also be considered a source of empty calories. Eating too many foods and beverages that are high in empty calories may displace more nutritious foods from the diet. Furthermore, consuming more calories than needed can result in unwanted weight gain. Therefore, people should limit their intake of foods and beverages that contain a lot of empty calories.

Nutrient Density

Certain foods are more nutritious than others. According to some nutrition experts, a **nutrient—dense** food supplies more key beneficial nutrients, such as potassium and calcium, in relation to its total calories per serving (Table 1.8). Furthermore, a nutrient—dense food has little or no solid fats, added sugars, refined starches, and sodium.[2] Broccoli, leafy greens, fat—free milk, orange juice, lean meats, and whole—grain cereals are examples of nutrient—dense foods. Figure 1.8 compares the nutritional values of 8—fluid—ounce servings of fat—free milk and a sugar—sweetened soft drink. Note that milk supplies water, protein, and certain vitamins and minerals, whereas the soft drink supplies water and carbohydrate but is a poor source of protein and micronutrients. A nutritious diet contains a variety of nutrient—dense foods.

Energy Density

Energy density describes the energy value of a food in relation to the food's weight. For example, a chocolate, cake—type frosted doughnut that weighs about 2 ounces provides 242 kcal; 5 medium strawberries also weigh about 2 ounces, but they provide only 19 kcal. You would have to eat nearly 64 of the strawberries to obtain the same amount of food energy that is in the chocolate doughnut. Therefore, the doughnut is an energy—dense food in comparison to the berries. In general, high—fat foods such as doughnuts are energy dense because they are con—centrated sources of energy. Most fruits are not energy dense, because they contain far more water than fat. Figure 1.9 compares the energy densities of a few foods.

Not all energy—dense foods are high in empty calories. Nuts, for example, are high in fat and, therefore, energy dense. However, nuts are also nutrient dense because they contribute protein, vitamins, minerals, and fiber to diets. Most forms of fiber are classified as carbohydrates.

Concept 4: Enjoy Eating All Foods in Moderation

Dietary **moderation** involves obtaining enough nutrients from food to meet one's needs and balancing calorie intake with calorie expenditure, primarily by physical activity. This can be accomplished by choosing nutrient—dense foods, limiting serving sizes of energy—dense foods, and incorporating moderate— to vigorous—intensity physical activities into your daily routine. Although moderation requires

TABLE 1.8 Nutrient Density: Key Beneficial Nutrients

Protein
Fiber
Vitamins: A, C, and E
Minerals: Calcium, iron, potassium, and magnesium

Source: Drewnowski A, Fulgoni VL (III): Nutrient density: principles and evaluation tools. *American Journal of Clinical Nutrition* 99(suppl):1223S, 2014.

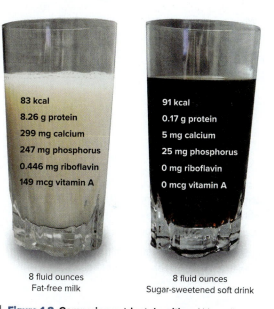

83 kcal
8.26 g protein
299 mg calcium
247 mg phosphorus
0.446 mg riboflavin
149 mcg vitamin A

91 kcal
0.17 g protein
5 mg calcium
25 mg phosphorus
0 mg riboflavin
0 mcg vitamin A

8 fluid ounces
Fat-free milk

8 fluid ounces
Sugar-sweetened soft drink

Figure 1.8 **Comparing nutrient densities.** Although the milk and soft drink have similar caloric contents, milk is a much better source of protein and micronutrients.
©Wendy Schiff

empty calories energy supplied by unhealthy solid fats, added sugars, and/or alcohol

nutrient-dense describes a food or beverage that contains more key beneficial nutrients in relation to its total calories

energy density energy value of a food in relation to the food's weight

moderation obtaining adequate amounts of nutrients while balancing calorie intake with calorie expenditure planning meals and setting aside time for physical activity daily, it can help you achieve your health and fitness goals. If, for example, you overeat during a meal or snack, you can regain dietary moderation and balance by eating less energy–dense food and exercising more intensely during the next 24 hours.

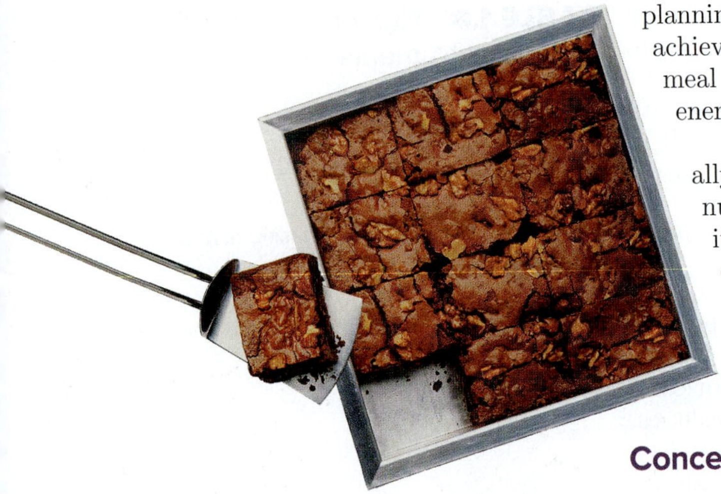

Eliminating all sources of empty calories from your diet is not generally recommended or necessary. If your core diet is comprised primarily of nutrient–dense foods and meets your nutritional needs, including some items that supply empty calories adds enjoyment to living when they are consumed in moderation. Physically active individuals, such as athletes in training programs, often find it difficult to consume enough energy from nutrient–dense foods to sustain healthy body weights, unless they include some empty calories in their diets.

When a diet meets nutritional needs, including some items that contain a lot of empty calories such as these brownies adds enjoyment when such foods are consumed in moderation. ©Michael Lamotte/Cole Group/ Getty Images RF

Concept 5: For Each Nutrient, There Is a Range of Safe Intake

By eating a variety of nutrient–dense foods, you are likely to obtain adequate and safe amounts of each nutrient. The **physiological dose** of a nutrient is the amount that is within the range of safe intake and enables the body to function optimally. Consuming less than the physiological dose can result in marginal nutritional status. In other words, the person's body has just enough of the nutrient to function adequately, but that amount is not sufficient to overcome the added stress of infection or injury. If a person's nutrient intake falls below the marginal level, the individual is at risk of developing the nutrient's deficiency disease. For example, recommended daily intakes of the B–vitamin niacin are 16 mg for men and 14 mg for women. People whose diets contain little or no niacin are at risk of developing *pellagra*, the vitamin's deficiency disease.

Most people require physiological amounts of micronutrients. A **megadose** is an amount of a vitamin or mineral that greatly exceeds the recommended amount of the nutrient. When taken in high amounts, many vitamins act like drugs and can produce unpleasant and even toxic side effects. For example, physicians sometimes use megadoses of the B–vitamin niacin to treat high blood cholesterol levels, but such amounts may cause painful facial flushing and liver damage. Minerals have very narrow ranges of safe intakes.

Many consumers take megadoses of vitamin and/or mineral supplements without consulting physicians because they think the micronutrients will prevent or treat ailments such as the common cold or heart disease. For most people, consuming amounts of nutrients that exceed what is necessary for good health is economically wasteful and could be harmful to the body. "More is not always better," when it relates to optimal nutrition.

In their natural states, most commonly eaten foods do not contain toxic levels of vitamins and minerals. You probably do not need to worry about consuming toxic levels of micronutrients, unless you are regularly eating large

physiological dose amount of a nutrient that is within the range of safe intake and enables the body to function optimally

megadose amount of a vitamin or mineral that greatly exceeds the recommended amount

Figure 1.9 Energy density. Although each of these portions of butter, broiled hamburger, cheese, and peanuts weighs about the same (2 ounces), they differ in their energy densities. For example, you would need to eat about 13 ounces of raw strawberries to consume the same amount of energy in a 2-ounce, broiled hamburger patty (10% fat).
Butter, cheese, meat patty, peanuts: ©Wendy Schiff

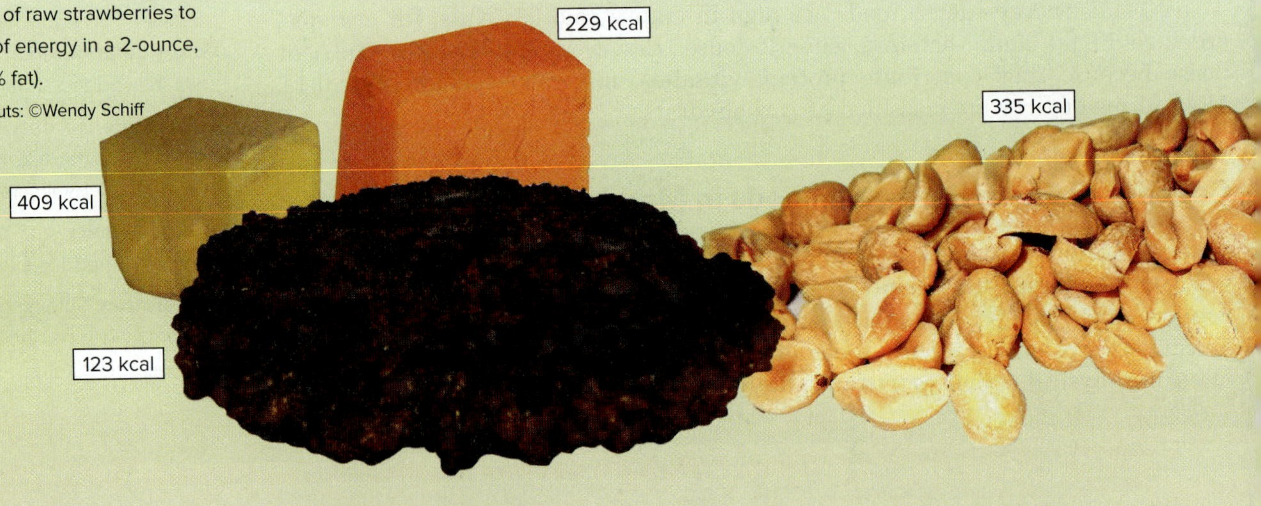

229 kcal

335 kcal

409 kcal

123 kcal

amounts of foods that are fortified with these nutrients. The diagram shown in Figure 1.10 illustrates the general concept of deficient, safe, and toxic intake ranges for nutrients such as vitamins and minerals. Chapters 8 and 9 provide more information about micronutrients, including deficiencies and toxicities.

Concept 6: Food Is the Best Source of Nutrients and Phytochemicals

The most natural, reliable, and economical way to obtain nutrients and beneficial phytochemicals is to base your diet on a variety of "whole" and minimally processed foods. Plant foods naturally contain a variety of nutrients and phytochemicals, but processing the foods often removes some of the most healthful parts. For example, a wheat kernel is stripped of its germ and outer hull (bran) during refinement into white flour (Fig. 1.11). Wheat germ is a good source of thiamin, phosphorus, magnesium, zinc, and beneficial lipids. Wheat bran contains fiber, protein, and certain phytochemicals, and it is a rich source of niacin, iron, potassium, copper, zinc, and selenium. The endosperm that remains is primarily starch (a form of carbohydrate) with some protein and very small amounts of micronutrients and fiber. By replacing refined grain products, such as white bread, with whole-grain products, you can increase the likelihood of obtaining a wide variety of nutrients and phytochemicals.

In addition to eating food, many people take nutrient supplements in the form of pills, powders, bars, wafers, or beverages. The human body, however, is designed to obtain nutrients from foods. In some instances, nutrients from food are more available, that is, more easily digested and absorbed, than those in supplements.

It is important to understand that nutrient supplements do not contain everything one needs for optimal nutrition. For example, they do not contain the wide variety of phytochemicals found in plant foods. Although dietary supplements that contain phytochemicals are available, they may not provide the same healthful benefits as consuming the plants that contain these compounds. Why? Nutrients and phytochemicals may need to be consumed together to provide the desirable effects in the body. Food naturally contains combinations of these chemicals in very small amounts and certain proportions. There is nothing "natural" about gulping down handfuls of supplements.

Some individuals have increased needs for certain nutrients, particularly micronutrients. People who have chronic illnesses, digestive disorders that interfere with nutrient absorption, and certain inherited disorders may require supplemental nutrients. Additionally, many older adults may need higher amounts of vitamins and other nutrients than those found in food. Because it is often difficult to plan and eat nutritious menus each day, taking a dietary supplement that contains a variety of vitamins may be advisable, especially for older adults. In general, there appears to be little danger in taking a supplement that provides 100% of recommended amounts of the micronutrients daily.[10]

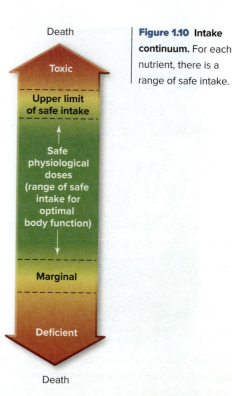

Death

Figure 1.10 **Intake continuum.** For each nutrient, there is a range of safe intake.

Toxic

Upper limit of safe intake

↑

Safe physiological doses (range of safe intake for optimal body function)

↓

Marginal

Deficient

Death

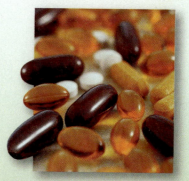

Dietary supplements should not be considered substitutes for nutrient-dense food. ©Nancy R. Cohen/ Getty Images RF

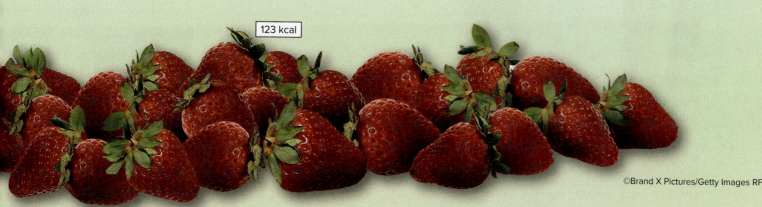

123 kcal

©Brand X Pictures/Getty Images RF

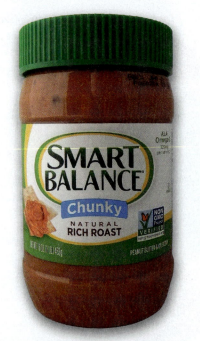

This product is a functional food because it was manufactured with oils that may reduce the risk of heart disease. ©Wendy Schiff

However, healthy adults should consider taking such supplements as a dietary "insurance policy" and not a substitute for eating a variety of nutrient–dense foods.

Concept 7: There Is No "One Size Fits All" Approach to Planning a Nutritionally Adequate Diet

By using food guides presented in Chapter 3, you can individualize your diet so that it is nutritionally adequate and suits your food likes and dislikes, budget, and lifestyle. Individualizing a diet does not mean only eating foods that "match" your blood type, hair color, personality, or shoe size. If someone promotes a diet based on such personal traits, steer clear of the diet and the promoter. Consider this: Human beings would not have survived as a species for thousands of years if their diets had to be matched to physical character–istics or personalities.

Physicians often prescribe special diets, sometimes referred to as *medical nutrition therapies*, for people with chronic health conditions such as diabetes. Even the nutritional needs of healthy people vary during different stages of their lives. Chapter 13 (Nutrition for a Lifetime) provides information about the importance of diet during pregnancy, childhood, and other stages of the lifecycle.

Concept 8: Foods and the Nutrients They Contain Are Not Cure-Alls

Although specific nutrient deficiency diseases, such as scurvy, can be cured by eating foods that contain the nutrient that is missing or in short supply, nutrients do not "cure" other ailments. Diet is only one aspect of a person that influences his or her health. By making certain dietary changes, however, a person may be able to prevent or forestall the development of certain diseases, or possibly lessen their severity if they occur.

Although there is no legal definition for "functional foods," such prod–ucts may have health benefits beyond simply helping to meet basic nutritional needs.[11] Functional foods are often manufactured to boost nutrient intakes, reduce the risk of disease, or help manage specific health problems. For example, consumers who want to increase their calcium intake can purchase orange juice that has the mineral added to it. Certain peanut butter substitutes contain oils

Figure 1.11 What is white flour? During refinement, a wheat kernel is stripped of its nutrient-rich germ and bran. The endosperm (white flour) that remains is mostly starch. Wheat: ©PhotoDisc/Getty Images RF; Flour: ©McGraw-Hill Education. Michael Scott, photographer

Bran

Endosperm

Germ

White Flour

NET WT 4LB

that may lower the risk of heart disease. Although some functional foods can help Americans improve their health, more research is needed to determine their benefits as well as possible harmful effects.

Concept 9: Malnutrition Includes *Under*nutrition as Well as *Over*nutrition

Malnutrition is a state of health that occurs when the body is improperly nourished. Everyone must consume food and water to stay alive, yet despite the abundance and variety of nutritious foods, many Americans consume nutritionally poor diets and suffer from malnutrition as a result. Some people select nutritionally inadequate diets because they lack knowledge about nutritious foods or the importance of nutrition to health. Low−income people, however, are at risk for malnutrition because they have limited financial resources for making wise food purchases. Other people who are at risk of malnutrition include those who have severe eating disorders, are addicted to drugs such as alcohol, or have certain serious medical problems. This chapter's "Nutrition Matters" feature discusses the international problem of *under*nutrition.

Although many people associate malnutrition with undernutrition and starvation, *over*nutrition, the long−term excess of energy or nutrient intake, is also a form of malnutrition. Overnutrition is often characterized by obesity (having an excessive and unhealthy amount of body fat). You may be surprised to learn that overnutrition is associated with more deaths throughout the world than undernutrition (Fig. 1.12).[12] Obesity is widespread in countries where most people have the financial means to buy plenty of food, have an ample supply of energy−dense foods, and obtain little exercise. Chapter 10 provides information about obesity.

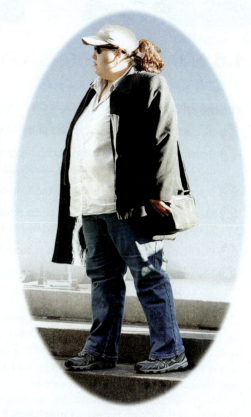

Figure 1.12 Obesity. Throughout the world, obesity is a common nutrition-related health problem.
©Lars A. Niki RF

malnutrition state of health that occurs when the body is improperly nourished

Concept 10: Nutrition Is a Dynamic Science

As researchers continue to explore the complex relationships between diets and health, nutrition information constantly evolves. As a result, dietary practices and recommendations undergo revision as new scientific evidence becomes available and is reviewed and accepted by nutrition experts. Unfortunately such changes can be confusing to the general public, who expect medical researchers to provide definite answers to their nutrition−related questions and rigid advice concerning optimal dietary practices.

Even nutrition educators find it difficult to keep up with the vast number of research articles published in scientific journals. Chapter 2 explains how nutrition research is conducted using scientific methods. Furthermore, Chapter 2 provides information to help you become a better consumer of nutrition and health information that appears in popular sources such as magazines, infomercials, and the Internet.

Concept CHECKPOINT

14. Identify at least five of the key nutrition-related concepts presented in this section.

15. What is the difference between a food that supplies a lot of empty calories and a nutrient-dense food?

16. What is the difference between a physiological dose and a megadose of a nutrient?

See Appendix G for responses.

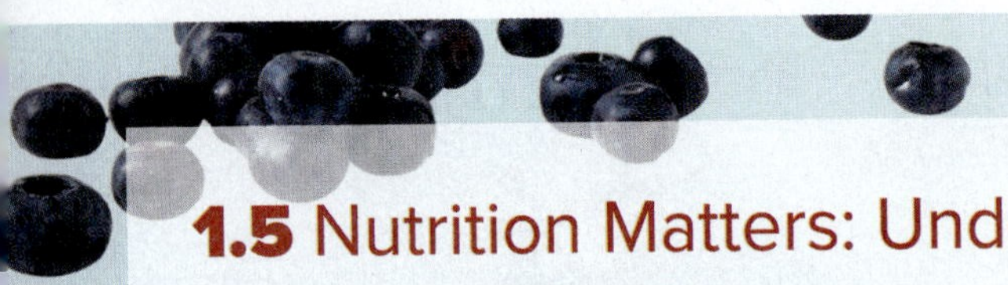

1.5 Nutrition Matters: Undernutrition—A Worldwide Concern

Learning Outcomes

1. Discuss factors that contribute to undernutrition in the world.

2. Describe how undernutrition during pregnancy and childhood can affect a child's physical and intellectual development.

3. Discuss undernutrition in the United States.

4. Identify major federal food assistance programs in the United States and the populations served by each program.

5. Define biotechnology as it relates to food production.

6. Discuss how sustainable agriculture can improve the environment.

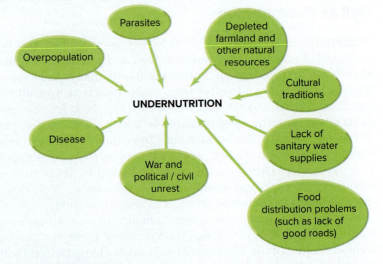

Figure 1.13 Factors that contribute to undernutrition. Many factors, including war, disease, and overpopulation, contribute to undernutrition in developing countries.

Over 6.5 billion people inhabit the Earth. In 2016, an estimated 800 million of these persons were chronically undernourished.[13] Chronic undernutrition is a condition that occurs when a person's long-term energy and nutrient intakes are insufficient to meet his or her needs.

Many factors contribute to undernutrition (Fig. 1.13). Poverty and lack of access to nutritious food are major contributors, particularly in sub-Saharan Africa and certain regions of Asia, where decades of civil unrest, wars, and the AIDS epidemic have left millions of people impoverished and living in uncertainty. Furthermore, unfavorable weather conditions and crop failures can cause regional food shortages. In 2015, over 660 million people used drinking water that may have been contaminated with feces.[14] Such water is unsafe to drink because it can contain bacteria and viruses that cause diarrhea, cholera, and polio. Every year, an estimated 502,000 people die as a result of developing diarrhea after consuming unclean water (Fig. 1.14).

Undernutrition During Periods of Growth

When undernutrition occurs during periods of rapid growth, such as pregnancy, infancy, and childhood, the long-term effects can be devastating. Each year, undernutrition contributes to 45% of deaths of children under the age of 5 years.[15] In developing countries, vitamin A deficiency causes as many as 500,000 cases of blindness among

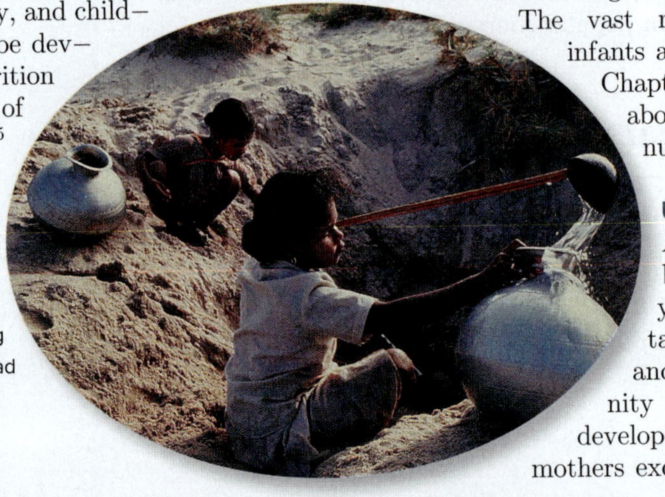

Figure 1.14 Unsafe water source. In developing countries, lack of clean cooking and drinking water contributes to the spread of potentially deadly infectious diseases.

©Digitial Vision/Getty Images RF

Blueberries: ©PhotoAlto/Getty Images RF

young children annually.[16] Half of these children die within a year of becoming blind. The vast majority of childhood deaths associated with undernutrition occur among poor populations in developing countries, particularly in sub-Saharan Africa and parts of Asia.[17]

Undernutrition During Pregnancy Women who are undernourished during pregnancy are more likely to die while giving birth than pregnant women who are adequately nourished. Furthermore, malnourished pregnant women have a high risk of giving birth to infants that are born too soon. These babies often suffer from breathing problems and have low birth weights—conditions that increase their risk of dying during their first year of life. Each year, an estimated 20 million low-birth-weight infants are born in the world.[18]

The vast majority of low-birth-weight infants are born in developing countries. Chapter 13 provides more information about the importance of adequate nutrition during pregnancy.

Undernutrition During Infancy As explained in Chapter 13, breast milk is the best food for young infants because it is sanitary, is nutritionally adequate, and provides babies with immunity to some infectious diseases. In developing countries, only 43% of new mothers exclusively breastfeed their babies for their first 6 months of life.[19] Although infant formulas are nutritious substitutes for breast milk, they do not provide immunity to diseases, and they are generally expensive. To increase the volume of infant formula that they can afford to give their children, poor parents in developing countries often add excessive amounts of water. This practice dilutes the nutritional value of the formula and increases the likelihood of contaminating it with disease–causing microbes. Infants who drink formula that has been mixed with unsanitary water can develop diarrhea that causes loss of body water (*dehydration*) and death.

Ideally, babies should be exclusively breast fed for their first 6 months and then consume breast milk in addition to solid foods well into their second year. According to the World Health Organization (WHO), 800,000 children under the age of 5 years die each year because they did not consume adequate amounts of breast milk during their first 2 years of life.[19]

Undernutrition During the Preschool Years In under–nourished children, nutrient deficiencies are responsible for stunted physical growth, delayed physical development, blindness, impaired intellectual development, and premature death (Fig. 1.15). In the United States and other developed countries, children are usually well nourished and vaccinated against common childhood diseases such as measles. In poorer nations, however, many children are malnourished and not protected against infectious agents, such as the virus that causes measles. Measles can be a life–threatening illness in undernourished children because their immune systems do not function normally.

Undernutrition in the United States

Undernutrition also occurs in wealthy, developed nations such as the United States. In some instances, undernutrition is not due to poverty in these countries. For example, many people suffering from anorexia nervosa and chronic alcoholism are undernourished despite having enough money to purchase food. Nevertheless, Americans with low incomes have a higher risk of malnutrition than members of the population who are in higher income categories. Between 2011–2015, 13.5% of the population were living at or below the U.S. Department of Health and Human Services *poverty guideline*.[20] In 2017, the poverty guideline was $24,600 for a family of four.[21] Most American households are *food secure*, which means the people in those households have access to and can purchase sufficient food to lead healthy, active lives. In 2015, **food insecurity** was reported in almost 13% of all households in the United States.[22] Food insecurity describes individuals or families who are concerned about running out of food or not having enough money to buy more food. People who are unemployed, work in low–paying jobs, or have excessive medical and housing expenses often experience food insecurity. Food insecurity may also affect elderly Americans who live on fixed incomes, especially if they are forced to choose between purchasing nutritious food and buying life–extending medications.

Charities and churches in many cities operate food pantries and "soup kitchens" to feed food–insecure people (Fig. 1.16). In addition to the help provided by the private sector, low–income individuals can obtain food aid from federal food assistance programs. Table 1.9 summarizes information about some of the major federally subsidized food programs in the United States. Although not every eligible food–insecure

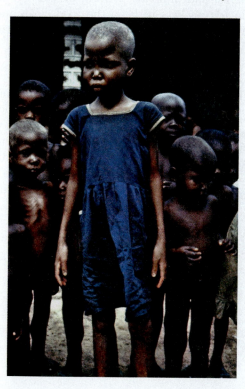

Figure 1.15 Chronic undernutrition. This photograph shows a group of undernourished children outside a Nigerian orphanage during the late 1960s. Source: Centers for Disease Control and Prevention/Dr. Lyle Conrad

food insecurity situation in which individuals or families are concerned about running out of food or not having enough money to buy more food

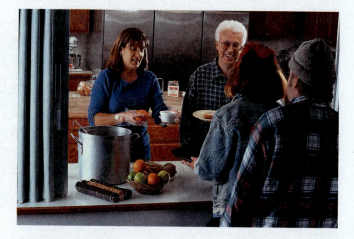

Figure 1.16 Feeding the hungry. In many cities, charities and churches operate food pantries and "soup kitchens" to feed food-insecure people.
©Getty Images RF

TABLE 1.9 Some Major Federally Subsidized Food Programs in the United States

Program	General Eligibility Requirements	Description
Supplemental Nutrition Assistance Program (SNAP)	Low-income individuals and families	Participants use an electronic benefit transfer (debit) card to purchase allowable food items.
Commodity Distribution Program	Certain low-income groups, including pregnant women, preschool-age children, and the elderly	In some states, state agencies distribute U.S. Department of Agriculture (USDA) surplus foods to eligible people.
Women, Infants, and Children (WIC)	Low-income pregnant or breastfeeding women, new mothers who are not breast-feeding, infants, and children under 5 years of age who are at nutritional risk	Participants receive checks or vouchers to purchase a variety of nutritious foods, such as milk, cheese, fruits and vegetables, certain cereals, and infant formula, at grocery stores. Nutrition education and support for breastfeeding mothers are also provided.
Child Nutrition Programs School Breakfast Program, National School Lunch Program, Summer Food Service Program, Child and Adult Care Food Program, Special Milk Program	Low-income children of school age Low-income adults (Child and Adult Care Food Program)	Certain schools and child-care facilities receive subsidies from the government to provide free or reduced-price nutritionally balanced meals and snacks.
Nutrition Program	Age 60 or older (no income guidelines)	Provides grants for sites to provide nutritious congregate and home-delivered meals
Food Distribution Program on Indian Reservations	Low-income American Indian or non-Indian households on reservations; members of federally recognized Native American tribes	Distribution of monthly food packages. This program is an alternative to SNAP and provides grants for a nutrition education component.

person has access to or takes advantage of the aid, federal food assistance programs protect most American children from hunger and undernutrition. For more information about the federal government's various food assistance programs, visit www.nutrition.gov/food−assistance−programs.

World Food Crisis: Finding Solutions

Reducing hunger through food aid programs is a major goal of the United Nations. The World Food Program and United Nations Children's Fund (UNICEF) are agencies within the United Nations that provide high−quality food for undernourished populations. UNICEF also

supports the development and distribution of ready−to−use therapeutic food (RUTF) to treat severe undernutrition among young children in developing countries. Plumpy'Nut, for example, is an energy− and nutrient−dense paste made from a mixture of peanuts, powdered milk, oil, sugar, vita−mins, and minerals. During processing, the paste is placed in foil packets to keep the food clean and make it easy to transport to remote places without refrigeration. In 2015, UNICEF acquired over 38,400 tons of RUTFs to feed starv−ing children in developing nations.[23]

The Promise of Biotechnology   **Biotechnology** involves the use of living things—plants, animals, microbes—to manu−facture new products. Biotechnology in agriculture has led to the development of crops that supply higher yields, resist pests, or are tolerant of drought conditions. By increasing food production or modifying the nutritional content of foods, biotechnology offers another way of alleviating the world food crisis.

Genetic modification methods, such as *genetic engineering*, involve scientific methods that alter an animal or plant's hereditary

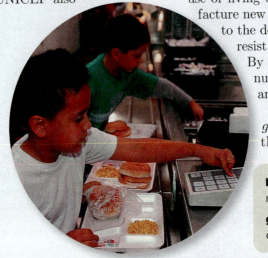

Any child who attends a school that participates in the School Lunch Program can purchase a nutritious lunch. After selecting from the menu, the child enters his or her personal identification number (PIN) into the device shown in the photo. The device records the purchase and debits the child's school lunch account. By using this system, the program protects the identity of children who receive free or reduced-price lunches. Source: USDA Photo by Ken Hammond

biotechnology using living things to manufacture new products

genetic modification techniques that alter an organism's DNA

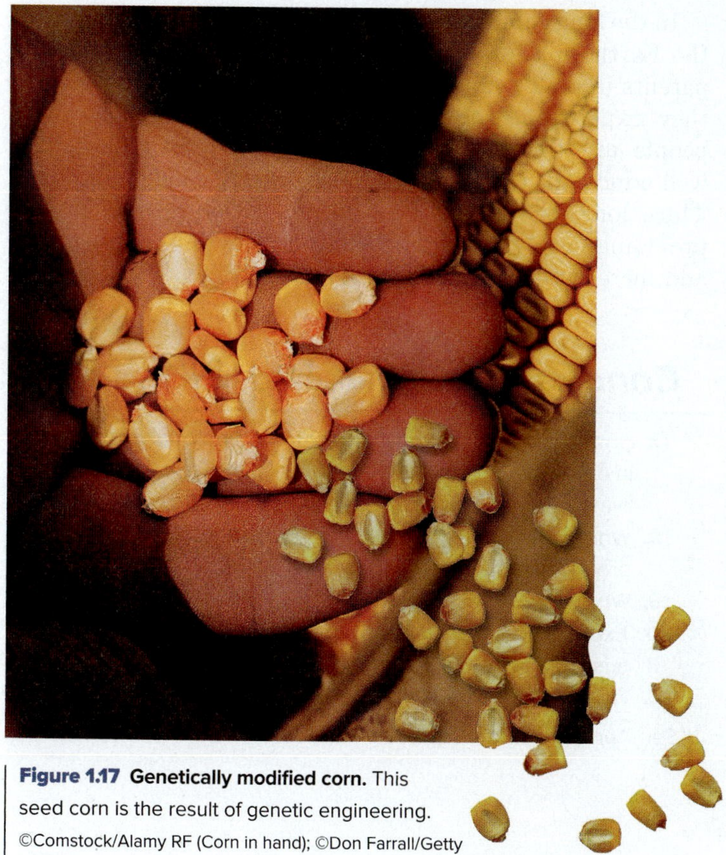

Figure 1.17 Genetically modified corn. This seed corn is the result of genetic engineering.
©Comstock/Alamy RF (Corn in hand); ©Don Farrall/Getty Images RF (Corn kernels)

material (*genes* or DNA). For example, genes that produce a desirable trait are transferred from one organism into the DNA of a second organism, altering its genes.

Cotton, corn, and soybeans are the most common genetically modified crops grown in the United States (Fig. 1.17).[24] These crops may have been genetically altered to improve their flavor, resist pests, increase yields, and improve their immunity to plant diseases. In the future, genetic engineering of food crops will provide the opportunity to enhance the plants' nutritional qualities.

Genetic engineering has also been used to improve animals. In 2015, the U.S. Food and Drug Administration (FDA) approved the application for AquAdvantage Salmon, a genetically engineered form of Atlantic salmon. These salmon will be bred in Canada and their eggs hatched in Panama; food from these salmon will be imported into the United States.[25] The FDA regulates the safety of genetically engineered foods. According to a report published by the National Academy of Sciences in 2016, there is no scientific evidence that indicates genetically engineered crops are unsafe for humans to consume or harmful to the environment.[26] Nevertheless, researchers continue to examine the long-term safety of GMOs.

Feeding the World, Protecting Natural Resources Our current system of food production relies primarily on conventional agricultural methods. In general, conventional farming requires considerable amounts of water and pesticides that can harm the environment. Irrigation systems often remove fresh water from rivers and other natural sources at a faster rate than it is restored. This activity reduces water flow to many communities. The water that runs off conventional farms can carry with it precious topsoil and pesticides that pollute waterways. Such farming methods also release greenhouse gases, especially carbon dioxide and methane, which contribute to global warming. Furthermore, the need for new farmland often requires cutting down trees so that forests can be converted to croplands. The loss of forests eliminates native animal and plant habitats. About 40% of the Earth's land (excluding Greenland and Antarctica) is used for food production; very little suitable land remains to be farmed.[27] What can be done to feed the world's population without destroying the Earth's natural resources?

What's Sustainable Agriculture? Sustainable agriculture involves farming methods that meet the demand for more food without depleting natural resources and harming the environment. The challenge is finding ways for farmers and ranchers to make the conversion from primarily conventional farming techniques to sustainable agriculture. Farming needs to be profitable for farmers and ranchers, so any switch from conventional to sustainable agricultural methods must not reduce their profit margins.

To solve the problems created by conventional agricultural methods, an international team developed the following points for establishing a universal policy:[27]

- Stop expanding agricultural activity, especially into tropical forests and grasslands.
- Find ways to improve crop yields on existing farms. Biotechnology in agriculture has led to the development of crops that supply higher yields, resist pests, or are tolerant of drought conditions. By increasing food production or modifying the nutritional content of foods, biotechnology offers a way of reducing the world food crisis.
- Find ways to use natural resources and pesticides more efficiently. Use irrigation systems that apply water directly to a plant's base instead of spraying it into the air, where much of the water evaporates.
- Rely more on nonchemical methods of pest management (see Chapter 12).
- Eat less meat. Sixty percent of the world's crops (primarily grains) are grown for human consumption. Most of the remaining crops are used to feed cattle and other farm animals. It takes about 30 pounds of grains to produce 1 pound of hamburger. By reducing

sustainable agriculture farming methods that do not deplete natural resources or harm the environment while meeting the demand for food

the consumption of meat, especially beef, more grains could be produced to feed people. Grass—fed beef also spares grains for human consumption, because grass is not eaten by people.

- Reduce food waste—about 30% of food is wasted. In many instances, the food spoils before it is eaten or it is thrown out as garbage. Smaller portion sizes and better menu planning can reduce the amount of food that people waste each day.

Taking Action Poverty and hunger have always plagued humankind; the causes of poverty and hunger are complex and, therefore, difficult to eliminate. Nevertheless, certain social, political, economic, and agricultural changes can reduce the number of people who are chronically hungry. In the short run, wealthy countries can provide food aid to keep impoverished people from starving to death. Families and small farmers in underdeveloped nations need to learn new and more efficient methods of growing, processing, preserving, and distributing nutritious regional food prod—ucts. Additionally, governments can support programs that encourage breastfeeding and fortify locally grown or com—monly consumed foods with vitamins and minerals that are often deficient in local diets.

In the long run, population control is critical for preserving the Earth's resources for future generations. Impoverished parents in poor countries often have many children because they expect only a few to survive to adulthood. When people are financially secure, adequately nourished, and well educated, they tend to have fewer, healthier children. Thus, long—term ways to slow population growth include providing well—paying jobs, improving public education, and increasing access to health care services.

Concept CHECKPOINT

17. How do unfavorable environmental and political factors in developing countries affect the health status of people living in those nations?

18. What effects can undernutrition have on the health of pregnant women and young children?

19. What is the "WIC program"?

20. Explain the difference between conventional and sustainable agricultural methods.

21. What is a genetically modified organism?

See Appendix G for responses.

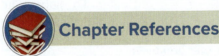

Chapter References

See Appendix H.

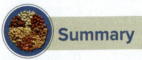

Summary

1.1 Nutrition: The Basics

- Lifestyle choices, including poor eating habits and lack of physical activity, contribute to the development of many of the leading causes of premature deaths for American adults, including heart disease, cancer, stroke, and diabetes. However, you may be able

Stacked books: ©Stockbyte/Getty Images RF; Nuts: ©C Squared Studios/Getty Images RF

©Brand X Pictures/Getty Images RF

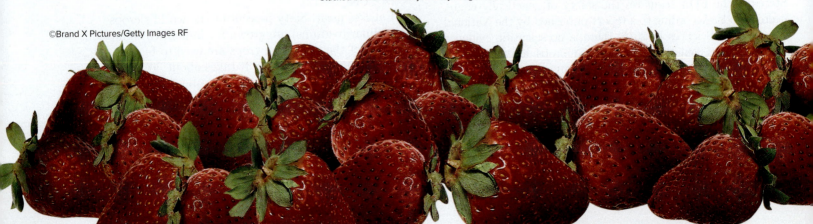

to extend your years of healthy life and improve your quality of life by applying what you learn about nutrition and the role of diet and health.

- There are six classes of nutrients: carbohydrates, lipids, proteins, vitamins, minerals, and water. The body needs certain nutrients for energy, growth and development, and regulation of processes, including the repair and maintenance of cells. The human body can synthesize many nutrients, but about 50 nutrients are dietary essentials that must be supplied by food.

- Nonnutrients, which include phytochemicals, are substances in food that may have healthful benefits. Many phytochemicals are antioxidants that protect cells from being damaged or destroyed by exposure to certain environmental factors. However, some phytochemicals are toxic. The Dietary Supplement Health and Education Act of 1994 (DSHEA) allows manufacturers to classify herbal products and nutrient supplements as dietary supplements.

1.2 Factors That Influence Americans' Health

- Heart disease is the leading cause of death for all Americans. Chronic diseases, such as heart disease, are complex conditions that have multiple risk factors. A risk factor is a personal characteristic that increases a person's chances of developing diseases. In many instances, people can live longer and healthier by modifying their diets, increasing their physical activity, and altering other aspects of their lifestyles. Objectives to improve the status of Americans' health, including nutrition-related programs, are an important focus of *Healthy People 2020*.

1.3 Metrics for Nutrition

- Scientists generally use metric values when measuring volume, weight, and length. The metric prefixes *micro-, milli-, deci-, centi-,* and *kilo-* indicate whether a measurement is a fraction or a multiple of a meter, gram, or liter. Approximately 28 grams are in an ounce and 454 grams are in a pound; a kilogram equals 1000 grams or about 2.2 pounds. Each gram equals 1000 milligrams or 1 million micrograms.

- Every cell needs energy. A Calorie is the heat energy needed to raise the temperature of 1 liter of water 1° Celsius (C). Calories or kilocalories (kcal) are used to indicate the energy value in food. If no number of kilocalories is specified, it is appropriate to use "calories." A gram of carbohydrate and a gram of protein each supply about 4 kcal; a gram of fat provides about 9 kcal. Although alcohol is not a nutrient, a gram of pure alcohol furnishes 7 kcal.

- Carbohydrates, fats, and proteins are referred to as macronutrients because the body needs relatively large amounts of these nutrients daily. Vitamins and minerals are micronutrients because the body needs very small amounts. Although the body requires large amounts of water, this nutrient provides no energy and is not usually classified as a macronutrient.

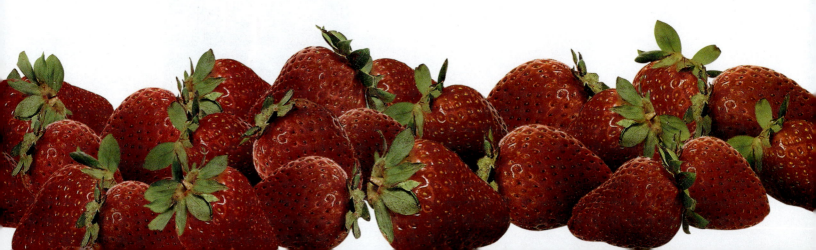

1.4 Key Nutrition Concepts

- There are several key points to understanding nutrition. Most naturally occurring foods are mixtures of nutrients, but no food contains all the nutrients needed for optimal health. Thus, nutritionally adequate diets include a variety of foods from all food groups. Instead of classifying foods as "good" or "bad," people can focus on eating all foods in moderation and limiting empty calories. For each nutrient, there is a range of safe intake. Healthy people should rely on eating a variety of foods to meet their nutrient needs instead of taking dietary supplements. Foods and the nutrients they contain are not cure-alls. There is no "one size fits all" approach to planning a nutritionally adequate diet. Malnutrition includes overnutrition as well as undernutrition. Finally, nutrition is a dynamic science; new scientific information about nutrients and their roles in health is constantly emerging. Therefore, ways the science of nutrition is applied, such as dietary recommendations, also change.

1.5 Nutrition Matters: Undernutrition—A Worldwide Concern

- Poverty and undernutrition are commonplace in many developing countries. Impoverished people must often cope with infectious diseases and polluted water supplies. In developing countries, poor sanitation practices and lack of clean cooking and drinking water contribute to diseases and deaths. In undernourished children, nutrient deficiencies are responsible for stunted physical growth, delayed physical development, blindness, impaired intellectual development, and premature death. Chronic undernutrition depresses the body's immune functioning, increasing the risk of death from infectious diseases, such as measles, especially in childhood. The vast majority of childhood deaths associated with undernutrition occur among poor populations in developing countries, particularly in sub-Saharan Africa and parts of Asia. When undernutrition occurs during the first 5 years of life, the effects can be devastating to the child's brain and result in permanent learning disabilities. Additionally, chronically undernourished children do not grow normally and tend to be shorter if they survive to adulthood.

- Reducing hunger through food aid programs is a major goal of the United Nations. Biotechnological advances in agriculture have led to the development of improved crops. Conventional farming methods can cause soil loss and add pesticides to water supplies. Sustainable agriculture refers to farming methods that do not deplete natural resources or harm the environment while meeting the demand for food.

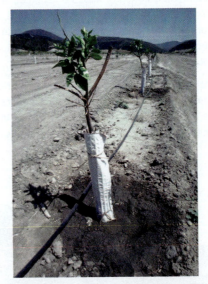

This row of young citrus trees is obtaining water via a drip irrigation system. Drip irrigation helps conserve water because it delivers small amounts of water directly to the trees over a long period and reduces the amount of irrigation water that is lost by evaporation. Source: Photo by Tim McCabe, USDA Natural Resources Conservation Service

Recipe for 🗃 Healthy Living

Food Preparation Basics (Yes, You *Can* Cook!)

By learning how to prepare dishes, experiment with recipe ingredients, and use a variety of spices and herbs as seasonings, you can make home-cooked meals that are more tasty, more appealing, and lower in fat, sugar, salt, and calories than the usual choices at fast-food restaurants. Additionally, you can save money by making your meals and snacks instead of purchasing them from restaurants and vending machines.

At the end of each chapter, you will find the "Recipe for Healthy Living," a nutritious, easy-to-prepare recipe. Each recipe includes a list of ingredients, instructions, and some information concerning the energy and selected nutrient contents in a serving of the product. The "MyPlate" icon indicates which of the USDA's food groups are primarily represented in the recipe (see Fig. 1.7). The circle graph shows approximate percentages of total calories for each macronutrient in the food. The bar graph indicates approximate percentages of Daily Values (DVs) for energy and some key nutrients. Daily Values are a set of nutrient standards used for food labeling purposes (see Chapter 3).

Even if you've had little or no cooking experience, you can learn the basics of preparing foods. Some cooks don't measure ingredients; they know from experience how to estimate amounts of foods and seasonings to add when preparing dishes. Until you feel confident with your food preparation skills, it is best to follow recipes and measure ingredients carefully.

You'll need some basic food preparation equipment to get started. You don't have to spend a lot of money, but buy well-made stainless steel (rustproof) cooking utensils and mixing bowls that will last for decades. Baking pans should also be stainless steel. A square or rectangular tempered-glass baking dish can be used for a variety of cooking needs, including heating foods in a toaster oven or microwave oven.

Understanding how to use household measurements is a good place to begin when learning how to cook. Purchase a set of metal measuring spoons that includes ⅛ teaspoon (tsp), ¼ tsp, ½ tsp, 1 tsp, and 1 tablespoon (Tbsp) measures. You'll also need a set of plastic or metal measuring cups that includes the following measures: ¼ cup, ⅓ cup, ½ cup, and 1 cup. These cups are used to measure dry ingredients such as flour or sugar. Finally, purchase a 2-cup glass or clear plastic measuring pitcher that is marked to indicate fluid ounces. This pitcher is used for measuring liquid ingredients such as water, milk, and oil.

To measure dry ingredients, fill the appropriate measuring cup or spoon to the top, and skim off the excess with the straight edge of a knife. To measure liquid ingredients, use a liquid measuring pitcher. Fill the pitcher to the desired amount, and place it on a level surface. Crouch down so you are at eye level with the fluid's level, and then carefully add more or remove some fluid as needed.

HOUSEHOLD UNITS

Common household units often used for measuring food ingredients and their commonly used abbreviations are listed below. Ounces (oz) are a measure of weight; *fluid* ounces are a measure of volume. Appendix A provides information about English-to-metric and metric-to-household unit conversions.

COMMON HOUSEHOLD UNITS FOR MEASURING FOOD INGREDIENTS

3 tsp = 1 Tbsp	1 cup = 8 fluid ounces (oz)
4 Tbsp = ¼ cup	1 cup = ½ pint
5 Tbsp + 1 tsp = ⅓ cup	2 cups = 1 pint
8 Tbsp = ½ cup	4 cups or 2 pints = 1 quart
16 Tbsp = 1 cup	4 quarts = 1 gallon

Low-Fat Applesauce Oatmeal Muffins

The following muffin recipe is simple and will give you an opportunity to practice measuring dry and liquid ingredients. This recipe makes 12 small muffins, so you'll need a muffin tin with 12 muffin cups. Each muffin supplies approximately 167 kcal, 4.6 g fat, 27.0 g digestible carbohydrates, 4.5 g protein, 1.5 g fiber, and 5.7 mg iron.

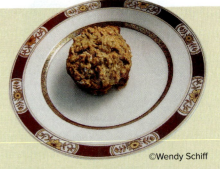
©Wendy Schiff

INGREDIENTS:

1 ½ cups quick oats, enriched, uncooked
1 ¼ cups all-purpose enriched flour
1 tsp baking powder
¾ tsp baking soda
1 tsp ground cinnamon
¼ tsp ground nutmeg
1 cup unsweetened applesauce
½ cup fat-free milk
½ cup brown sugar
3 Tbsp vegetable oil
1 medium egg
vegetable oil cooking spray

PREPARATION STEPS:

1. Preheat oven to 400° F. Spray vegetable oil spray lightly on the bottom of each cup of the muffin tin.

2. Combine oats, flour, baking powder, baking soda, and spices in a large bowl. Stir until well mixed. By using a large spoon, form a depressed area (a "well") in the center of the dry ingredients.

3. In another bowl, break the egg and use a fork to beat the egg to blend the white and yolk into a yellow mixture.

4. Add applesauce, milk, brown sugar, and oil to the beaten egg, and stir with a large spoon until ingredients are well mixed.

5. Pour the applesauce-containing mixture into the "well" of dry ingredients in the first bowl. Stir gently and just until the dry ingredients have been moistened by the applesauce mixture. Do not be concerned if small lumps of dry ingredients are in the batter. Do not beat or overmix the ingredients; otherwise, the muffins will form air tunnels and have peaked rather than rounded tops.

6. Spoon batter into muffin cups until the cup is half full of batter.

7. Bake 20 minutes or until muffins are golden brown. Use pot holders to protect your hands when taking the muffin tin out of the oven. Cool muffins for about 5 minutes before removing them from the tin. Muffins can be stored in a closed container in the refrigerator for up to a week. Before eating, warm each muffin in a microwave oven for about 15 seconds.

Tip: For easier cleanup, soak the bowl that contained the batter in cold, soapy water.

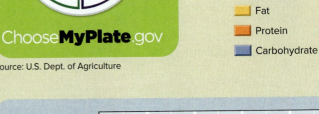
ChooseMyPlate.gov
Source: U.S. Dept. of Agriculture

64%
11%
25%

Fat
Protein
Carbohydrate

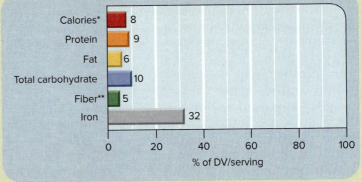

Calories* 8
Protein 9
Fat 6
Total carbohydrate 10
Fiber** 5
Iron 32

0   20   40   60   80   100
% of DV/serving

*2000 daily total kcal
**Component of Total carbohydrate

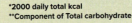 Further analyze this recipe or other recipes through activities located in Connect.

Personal Dietary Analysis

1. For 1 week, keep grocery and convenience store receipts.

   a. How much money did you spend on foods purchased at these markets?

   b. Which foods were the most expensive items purchased?

   c. How much money did you spend on foods and beverages that contain high amounts of empty calories such as salty snacks, cookies, soft drinks, and candy? _____

   d. What percentage of your food dollars were spent on foods that were rich sources of empty calories? _____ (Divide the amount of money spent on such foods by the total cost of food for the week. Move the decimal point over 2 places to the right and place a percent sign after the number.)

   e. How much money did you spend on nutrient-dense foods such as whole-grain products, fruits, and vegetables? _____

   f. What percentage of your food dollars were spent on nutrient-dense foods? _____ (Divide the amount of money spent on nutrient-dense foods by the total cost of food for the week. Move the decimal point over 2 places to the right and place a percent sign after the number.)

2. For 1 week, keep a detailed log of your usual vending machine purchases, including the item(s) purchased and amount of money spent for each purchase.

   a. What types of foods and beverages did you buy from the machines?

   b. How many soft drinks did you consume each day? _____

   c. How much money did you spend on vending machine foods and beverages? _____

   d. Based on this week's vending machine expenditures, estimate how much money you spend on such purchases in a year. _____

3. For 1 week, keep a detailed log of your usual fast-food consumption practices, including fast-food purchases at convenience stores. List the types of food and beverages you purchased and amount of money you spent.

   a. According to your weekly record, how often do you buy food from fast-food places and convenience stores? _____

   b. What types of foods did you usually buy?

   c. How much money did you spend on fast foods? _____

   d. Based on this week's expenditures, estimate how much money you spend on fast-food purchases in a year. _____

connect Complete the Personal Dietary Analysis activity located in Connect.

©Stockbyte/Getty Images RF

Raspberry: ©Stockbyte/Getty Images RF

Critical Thinking

1. Identify at least six factors that influence your food and beverage selections. Which of these factors are the three most important to you? Explain why.

2. Consider your current eating habits. Explain why you think your diet is or is not nutritionally balanced.

3. "Everything in moderation." Explain what this statement means in terms of your diet.

4. If you were at risk of developing a chronic health condition that could be prevented by changing your diet, would you make the necessary changes? Explain why or why not.

5. Have you ever used dietary supplements, such as vitamins, to treat or prevent illnesses? If you have, describe the situations and discuss which supplements were used.

6. What actions have you taken or can you take to help hungry or food–insecure people obtain adequate nutrition?

7. List five packaged foods you would donate to a local food pantry. Explain why you chose these particular foods to donate.

Practice Test

Select the best answer.

1. Diet is a

    a. practice of restricting calorie intake.
    b. technique for limiting empty calorie intake.
    c. method of reducing portion sizes.
    d. usual pattern of food choices.

2. Which of the following conditions is not one of the top 5 leading causes of death in the United States?

    a. Cancer
    b. Kidney disease
    c. Heart disease
    d. Stroke

3. The nutrients that provide energy are

    a. carbohydrates, vitamins, and lipids.
    b. lipids, proteins, and minerals.
    c. vitamins, minerals, and proteins.
    d. proteins, fats, and carbohydrates.

4. _____ refers to all chemical processes that occur in living cells.

    a. Metabolism   b. Catabolism
    c. Anatomy   d. Physiology

5. Phytochemicals

    a. are essential nutrients.
    b. may have healthful benefits.
    c. should be avoided.
    d. are in animal sources of food.

6. Which of the following foods is energy and nutrient dense?

    a. Fat–free yogurt
    b. Sugar–sweetened soft drink
    c. Peanut butter
    d. Iceberg lettuce

7. Which of the following foods is a source of phytochemicals?

    a. Hamburger
    b. Raspberries
    c. Eggs
    d. Chicken

8. An antioxidant is a(an)

    a. essential nutrient found only in animal foods.
    b. dietary supplement that is available without prescription.
    c. substance that protects cell components from being damaged or destroyed.
    d. nonnutrient produced by plants that provides health benefits.

9. In the United States, the primary cause of preventable cancer deaths is

    a. physical inactivity.
    b. tobacco use.
    c. high–fat diet.
    d. excessive alcohol intake.

10. Lena weighs 60 kg. What is her weight in pounds?

    a. 75 pounds
    b. 220 pounds
    c. 132 pounds
    d. 165 pounds

11. A serving of food contains 40 g carbohydrate, 10 g protein, and 9 g fat. Based on this information, a serving of this food supplies _____ kcal.

    a. 281
    b. 225
    c. 84
    d. 165

12. A serving of food supplies 12 g carbohydrate, 5 g protein, 7 g fat, and 50 g water. Which of the following state—ments is true about a serving of the food?

    a. Protein provides the most food energy.
    b. Carbohydrate provides the most food energy.
    c. Water provides the most food energy.
    d. Fat provides almost 50% of total calories.

13. Which of the following foods is the most nutrient dense?

    a. Potato chips
    b. Broccoli
    c. Butter
    d. Ice cream

14. Which of the following statements is false?

    a. A megadose is generally less than a physiological dose of a nutrient.
    b. Megadoses of nutrients may behave like drugs in the body.
    c. In general, physiological doses of nutrients are safe to consume daily.
    d. People should avoid taking megadose amounts of vitamin and mineral supplements.

15. The _____ Program enables eligible participants to use a special debit card to purchase food at authorized stores.

    a. Nutritious Food Purchase
    b. Supplemental Nutrition Assistance
    c. Healthy Diets for All
    d. Eat Better for Less

16. Which of the following actions has been proposed to help solve environmental problems created by conventional agricultural methods?

    a. Having populations shift to diets based primarily on meat, fish, and poultry
    b. Converting tropical jungles into much needed farmland
    c. Developing ways to use irrigation systems more effectively
    d. Resisting efforts to increase food production through biotechnology

Answers to Quiz Yourself

1. There are four classes of nutrients: proteins, lipids, sugars, and vitamins. **False** (Section 1.1)

2. Proteins are the most essential class of nutrients. **False** (Section 1.1)

3. All nutrients must be supplied by the diet because they cannot be made by the body. **False** (Section 1.1)

4. Vitamins are a source of energy. **False** (Section 1.3)

5. Milk, carrots, and bananas are examples of "perfect" foods that contain all nutrients. **False** (Section 1.4)

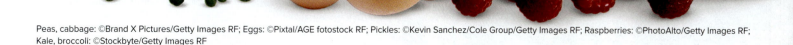

Evaluating Nutrition Information

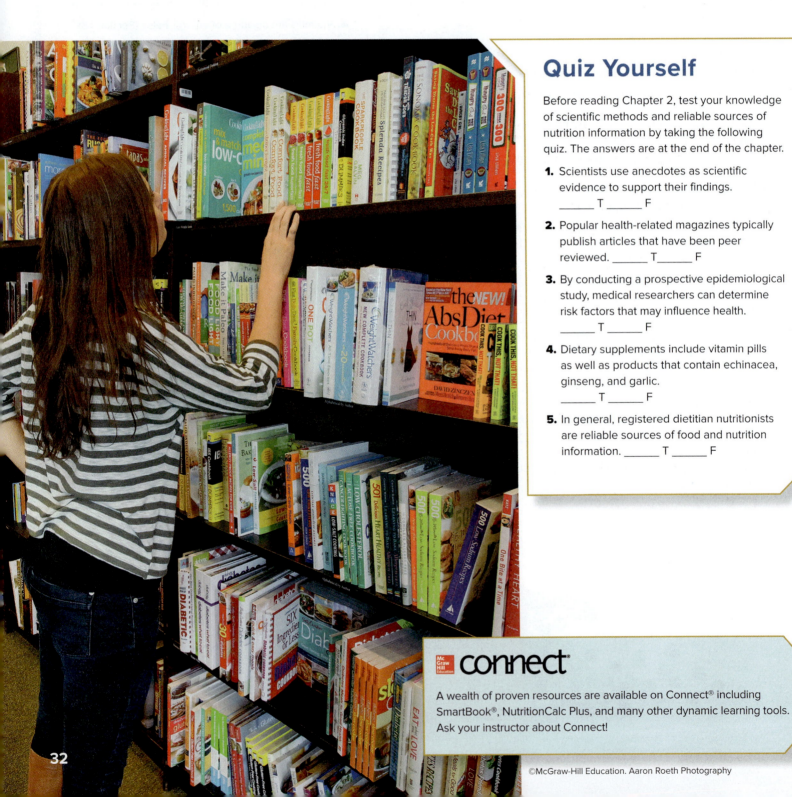

Quiz Yourself

Before reading Chapter 2, test your knowledge of scientific methods and reliable sources of nutrition information by taking the following quiz. The answers are at the end of the chapter.

1. Scientists use anecdotes as scientific evidence to support their findings.
_____ T _____ F

2. Popular health-related magazines typically publish articles that have been peer reviewed. _____ T_____ F

3. By conducting a prospective epidemiological study, medical researchers can determine risk factors that may influence health.
_____ T _____ F

4. Dietary supplements include vitamin pills as well as products that contain echinacea, ginseng, and garlic.
_____ T _____ F

5. In general, registered dietitian nutritionists are reliable sources of food and nutrition information. _____ T _____ F

Mc Graw Hill Education connect®

A wealth of proven resources are available on Connect® including SmartBook®, NutritionCalc Plus, and many other dynamic learning tools. Ask your instructor about Connect!

2.1 Nutrition: Science for Consumers

Learning Outcomes

1 Explain the basic steps of the scientific method.

2 Explain the importance of having controls when performing experiments.

3 Design a nutrition-related study that involves human subjects.

4 Explain why nutrition information derived from anecdotes is not evidence based.

5 Discuss why similar scientific studies often have different results.

We consume food, and we consume nutrition information. There seems to be no way to avoid nutrition information: If you browse shelves of books and magazines at a bookstore, surf the Internet, watch television, listen to the radio, or shop for groceries, you will encounter information about the subject. Even family mem— bers and friends contribute to the flood of nutrition information. Much of the information from such popular sources is not **evidence based,** that is, it is not supported by scientific evidence. The challenge for you and other consumers is to understand how scientists collect evidence about nutrition and health and how to analyze this information to determine whether it is factual and based on solid evidence (reliable) or misinformation that is unsupported by the facts.

How do nutrition scientists determine facts about foods, nutrients, and diets? Why do nutrition scientists seem to contradict themselves so much? How can you evaluate the reliability of nutrition information? Where can you obtain up—to—date, accurate nutrition information? This chapter will provide answers to these questions and help you become a more critical and careful consumer.

> **evidence based** information that is based on results of scientific studies
>
> **anecdotes** reports of personal experiences

Understanding the Scientific Method

In the past, nutrition facts and dietary practices were often based on intuition, common sense, "conventional wisdom" (tradition), or **anecdotes** (reports of personal experiences). Today, *registered dietitian nutritionists (RDNs)* and other nutrition experts discard conventional beliefs, explanations, and practices when the results of current scientific research no longer support them.

Scientists ask questions about the natural world, such as: "How do cells make proteins?" and "What causes stomach ulcers?" To obtain answers for their questions, researchers design studies that follow generally accepted methods. The following sections take a closer look at some common methods that scientists use to collect nutrition information and establish nutrition facts.

Laboratory Experiments

An experiment is a systematic way of testing a hypothesis (question). Because of safety and ethical concerns, nutrition scientists often conduct experiments on small mammals before performing similar research on humans. Certain kinds of mice and rats are raised for experimentation purposes (Fig. 2.1). These rodents are inexpensive to house in laboratories, and their food and other living conditions can be carefully controlled. An experiment that uses whole living organisms, such as mice, is called an *in vivo* experiment. Nutrition researchers also perform controlled laboratory experiments on cells or other components derived from living organisms. These studies are *in vitro* or "test tube" experiments.

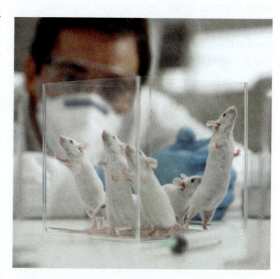

Figure 2.1 Rodents for research. Nutrition scientists often conduct *in vivo* experiments on small rodents that are raised for experimentation purposes.
©Adam Gault/Getty Images RF

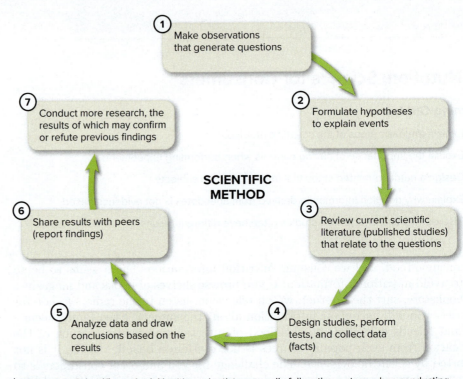

SCIENTIFIC METHOD

1. Make observations that generate questions
2. Formulate hypotheses to explain events
3. Review current scientific literature (published studies) that relate to the questions
4. Design studies, perform tests, and collect data (facts)
5. Analyze data and draw conclusions based on the results
6. Share results with peers (report findings)
7. Conduct more research, the results of which may confirm or refute previous findings

Figure 2.2 Scientific method. Nutrition scientists generally follow these steps when conducting research.

treatment group group being studied that receives a treatment

control group group being studied that does not receive a treatment

variable personal characteristic or other factor that changes and can influence an outcome

Experiments generally involve the basic steps shown in Figure 2.2. A team of nutrition scientists, for example, makes observations and generates questions that result in the development of a hypothesis. According to their hypothesis, consuming "chemical X" in charcoal–grilled meat is harmful. To test this hypothesis, the scientists divide 100 genetically similar 3–week old mice into two groups of 50 mice. One group **(treatment group)** is fed a certain amount of chemical X daily for 52 weeks; the second group **(control group)** does not receive the treatment during the period (Fig. 2.3).

Why is a control group necessary? Having a control group enables scientists to compare results between the two study groups to determine whether the treatment had any effect. A **variable** is a characteristic or other factor that can change and influence an outcome. Many variables can influence the outcome of an experimental study. Therefore, scientists who want to determine the effect or effects of a single variable, such as chemical X intake, need to control the influence of other variables. Therefore, all other conditions, including timing of feedings and amount of handling by caregivers must be the same for both groups of mice. If researchers design an experiment in which they fail to control variables that are not being tested, their findings are likely to be unclear or inaccurate.

For the duration of this study, the scientists examine the mice regularly for signs of health problems and record data (facts). If the data show that the mice in the treatment group are as healthy as the mice in the control group at the end of this experiment, the researchers may conclude that mice can safely consume the amount of chemical X used in the study on a daily basis for a year.

Researchers are cautious when drawing conclusions from results of *in vitro* experiments, because cells removed from a living thing may not function the same way they do when they are in the entire life form.

Medical researchers must also be careful when applying the results of *in vivo* animal studies to people because of the physiological differences between humans and laboratory animals. Nevertheless, scientists are often able to

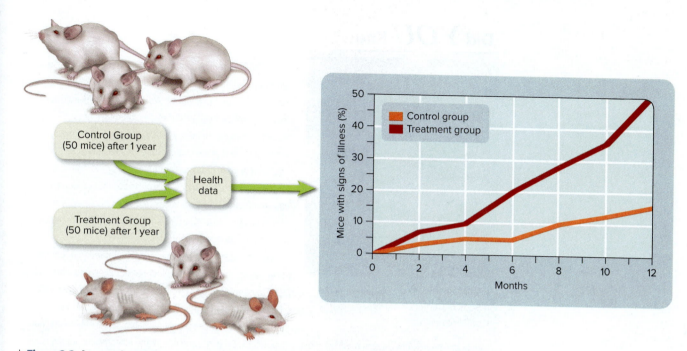

Control Group (50 mice) after 1 year	
Treatment Group (50 mice) after 1 year	Health data

Figure 2.3 **An experiment.** Based on the findings shown in the graph, is it safe for mice to consume chemical X daily for a year?

determine the safety and effectiveness of treatments by conducting research on laboratory animals before engaging in similar testing on humans. Two types of research that involve human subjects are *experimental* (intervention) studies and *observational* studies. Such investigations can provide clues about the causes, progression, and prevention of diet—related diseases.

Human Research: Experimental (Intervention) Studies

Nutrition scientists often conduct experimental studies to obtain information about health conditions (*outcomes*) that may result from specific dietary practices. When conducting an experimental study involving human subjects, researchers usually randomly divide a large group of people into treatment and control groups.

For example, every other person who enrolls in a study is placed in the treatment group. The remaining subjects become control group members. Random assignment helps ensure that the members of the treatment and control groups have similar variables, such as age and other characteristics. All subjects will be instructed to maintain their usual lifestyle during the duration of the study, except for the activities required by their participation in the research.

Then the scientists provide all study participants with the same instructions and a form of intervention, such as a dietary supplement or experimental food. However, only members of the treatment group actually receive the form of intervention. Subjects in the control group are usually given a **placebo.** Placebos are not simply "sugar pills"; they are a fake treatment, such as a sham pill, injection, or medical device. The placebo mimics the treatment. For example, a placebo dietary supplement pill looks, tastes, and smells like the supplement pill with an active ingredient that is given subjects in the treatment group. The placebo pill, however, has *inert* ingredients; that is, the pill contains substances that do not produce any measurable physical changes. Providing placebos to members of the control group enables scientists to compare the extent of the treatment's response with that of the placebo.

placebo fake treatment, such as a sham pill, injection, or medical procedure

Did *YOU* Know?

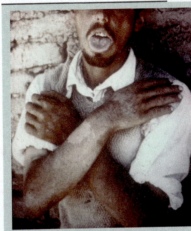

Man with pellagra
Source: Centers for Disease Control and Prevention

Today, the idea that something missing in diets can cause a nutrient deficiency disease is widely accepted. A hundred years ago, however, it was a novel idea that most medical experts dismissed because they thought only "germs" caused disease. In the early 1900s, the disease *pellagra* was widespread in the United States, especially in southern states. Each year, thousands of Americans died from this dreaded illness. Most medical experts thought pellagra was an infectious disease because it often occurred where people lived in close quarters, such as prisons, orphanages, and mental health institutions.

Joseph Goldberger, a physician who worked in a federal government laboratory, observed that not everyone who was exposed to people suffering from pellagra developed the condition. Dr. Goldberger also noted that prisoners ate a diet that was typically eaten by other people with pellagra. The diet emphasized corn bread, hominy grits (a corn product), molasses, potatoes, cabbage, and rice. At the time, this monotonous, low-protein diet was associated with poverty throughout the southern United States. He also observed that people who did not develop pellagra had higher incomes and ate more meat, milk, and fresh vegetables. Based on his observations, Goldberger rejected the medical establishment's notion that pellagra was an infectious disease. He proposed the idea that pellagra resulted from the lack of something in poor people's diet and the missing dietary factor was in meat, milk, and other foods eaten regularly by people with high incomes. To test his dietary hypothesis, Goldberger gave these foods to children in two Mississippi orphanages and patients in a Georgia mental institution who were suffering from pellagra, and they were cured of the disease. Many members of the medical establishment, however, rejected his finding that a poor diet was the cause of pellagra.

To satisfy his critics, Goldberger enrolled a group of healthy Mississippi prison inmates in an experiment that involved consuming the corn- and molasses-based diet commonly eaten in the southern states at the time. After a few months, more than half of the inmates developed pellagra. Once again, however, many of Goldberger's critics rejected his finding that poor diet was the cause of pellagra.

In 1916, Dr. Goldberger experimented on himself and some volunteers during what they called a "filth party." The group applied secretions taken from inside the nose and throat of a patient with pellagra into their noses and throats; they also swallowed pills made with flakes of skin scraped from the rashes of people with the disease. Additionally, Goldberger and one of his colleagues gave each other an injection of blood from a person who had pellagra. If pellagra were infectious, filth-party participants should have contracted the disease—but none of them did. Despite the results of Dr. Goldberger's extraordinary experiment, a few physicians still resisted the idea that pellagra was associated with diet.[1]

Dr. Goldberger died in 1929—8 years before Dr. Conrad Elvehjem and his team of scientists at the University of Wisconsin isolated a form of the vitamin niacin from liver extracts. Elvehjem and his colleagues discovered niacin cured "black tongue," a condition affecting dogs that was similar to pellagra.[2] Soon after Elvehjem's discovery, other scientists determined that niacin was effective in treating pellagra, and the medical establishment finally accepted the fact that the disease was the result of a dietary deficiency. Chapter 8 provides more information about niacin and pellagra.

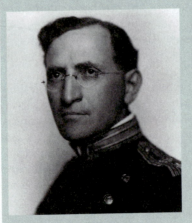

Dr. Joseph Goldberger
Source: Centers for Disease Control and Prevention

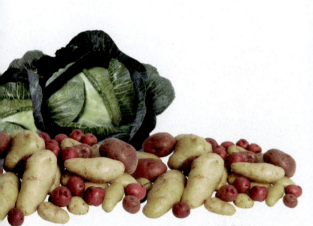

Cabbage: ©Brand X Pictures/Getty Images RF; Potatoes: ©Ingram Publishing/Alamy RF

What Is the Placebo Effect? People may report positive or negative reactions to a treatment even though they received the placebo. If a patient believes a medical treatment will improve his or her health, the patient is more likely to report positive results for the therapy. Such wishful thinking is called the **placebo effect.**

People who take certain herbal products or use other unconventional medical therapies to prevent or treat diseases are often convinced the products and treatments are effective, despite the general lack of scientific evidence to support their beliefs. Such personal findings may be examples of the placebo effect. However, placebos can produce beneficial physiological and psychological changes, particularly in conditions that involve pain.[3] Because subjects in the control group believe they are receiving a real treatment, their faith in the "treatment" can stimulate the release of chemicals in the brain that alter pain perception, reducing their discomfort. Therefore, when people report that a treatment was beneficial, they may not have been imagining the positive response, even when they were taking a placebo.

Double-Blind Studies

Human experimental studies are usually **double–blind studies;** that is, neither the investigators nor the subjects are aware of the subjects' group assignments. Codes are used to identify a subject's group membership, and this information is not revealed until the end of the study. Maintaining such secrecy is important during the course of a human study involving placebos because researchers and subjects may try to predict group assignments based on their expectations. If the investigators who interview the participants are aware of their individual group assignments during the study (a single–blind study), they may unwittingly convey clues to each subject, perhaps in the form of body language, that could influence the subject's belief about being in the experimental or control group. Subjects who suspect they are in the control group and taking a placebo may report no changes in their condition because they expect a placebo should have no effect on them. On the other hand, subjects who think they are in the treatment group could insist that they feel better or have more energy as a result of the treatment, even though the treatment may not have produced any measurable changes in their bodies. Ideally, subjects should not be able to figure out their group assignment while researchers are collecting information from them.

Human Research: Epidemiological Studies

For decades, medical researchers have noted differences in rates of chronic diseases and causes of death among various populations. The most common type of diabetes, for example, occurs more frequently among American Indian/Alaskan Native, Hispanic, and non–Hispanic African–American adults than among non–Hispanic, white American adults.[4] To understand why this difference exists, medical researchers rely on the findings of epidemiological studies.

Epidemiology (*ehp–e–dee–me–all'–uh–jee*) is the study of the occurrence, distribution, and causes of health problems in populations. For example, U.S. public health officials reported 30 new cases of lead poisoning among a state's 50,000 preschool–aged children in 2017 (*occurrence*). Epidemiologists determined that 95% of the affected children lived in a major city; the remaining children lived in smaller cities or towns (*distribution*). To determine why the city children were more likely to have lead poisoning than other children in the state, the epidemiologists compared the living conditions of the children with lead poisoning to those who were healthy. As a result of their investigation, the scientists determined that the source of the lead was the drinking water carried by the major city's old lead–lined water pipes (*cause*).

placebo effect response to a placebo

double-blind study experimental design in which neither the participants nor the researchers are aware of each participant's group assignment

epidemiology study of the occurrence, distribution, and causes of health problems in populations

Did *YOU* Know?

Prevalence refers to the number of people in a particular population who have a disease. In the United States, for example, more people have diabetes than tuberculosis, so diabetes is a prevalent disease in this country.

Epidemiologists often use physical examinations of people to obtain health data, such as height and weight. Additionally, they may collect other kinds of information by conducting surveys. Such surveys question people about their personal and family medical histories, environmental exposures, health practices, and attitudes. Since 1999, National Nutrition and Health Examination Survey (NHANES) researchers have used interviews and physical examinations to assess the health and nutritional status of a nationally representative sample of Americans. Data collected from NHANES help epidemiologists determine the prevalence of major diseases, risk factors for such diseases, and national standards for measurements that are associated with health status, including height, weight, and blood pressure.

In cases involving chronic diseases such as heart disease and cancer, it is often difficult to determine a single variable that is responsible for the development of the condition. Multiple factors, including a person's *genetic susceptibility* (inherited proneness), exposure to certain environmental conditions, and diet as well as other lifestyle practices can influence his or her likelihood of developing a disease.

By conducting studies that explore differences in dietary practices and disease occurrences among populations, nutrition epidemiologists may learn much about the influence of diet on health. If one group of people is more likely to develop a certain health disorder than another group and the two populations consume very different diets, scientists can speculate about the role diet plays in this difference.

Observational Epidemiological Studies Most epidemiological research is observational and involves either case–control study or cohort study designs. In a **case–control study**, individuals with a health condition (cases) such as heart disease or breast cancer are matched to persons with similar characteristics who do not have the condition (controls). Information such as personal and family medical histories, eating habits, and other lifestyle behaviors are collected from each participant in the study. By analyzing the results of case–control studies, researchers identify factors that may have been responsible for the illness. Scientists, for example, may be able to identify dietary practices that differ between the two groups, such as long–term fruit and vegetable intakes.

In a **cohort study** (Fig. 2.4), epidemiologists collect and analyze various kinds of information about a large group of people over time. The scientists are generally interested in making associations between exposure to a specific factor and the subsequent development of health conditions. Cohort studies can be *retrospective* or *prospective*. Retrospective means "to look back" and prospective means "to look forward" in time. (see Fig. 2.4.) In a retrospective cohort study, researchers collect information about a group's past exposures and identify current health outcomes. For example, nutritional epidemiologists might examine whether a group of people who have stomach cancer consumed more charcoal–broiled meat (the exposure) in the past than a group of people with similar characteristics who do not have stomach cancer. In a prospective cohort study, a group of healthy people are followed over a time period and any diseases that eventually develop are recorded. Scientists then try to identify links between exposures and diseases that occurred between the beginning and end of the study period.

The Framingham Heart Study that began in 1949 in Framingham, Massachusetts, is one of the most well–known prospective studies. At the beginning of the study, the over 5200 healthy participants (men and women) underwent extensive physical examinations and questioning about their family and personal medical histories as well as their lifestyle practices. Over the following years, a group of medical researchers periodically collected data concerning each participant's health and, if the person died, cause of death. The scientists analyzed this information and found relationships between a variety of personal characteristics and health outcomes. Findings from the Framingham

case-control study study in which individuals who have a health condition are compared with individuals with similar characteristics who do not have the condition

cohort study study that measures variables of a group of people over time

EPIDEMIOLOGICAL STUDIES

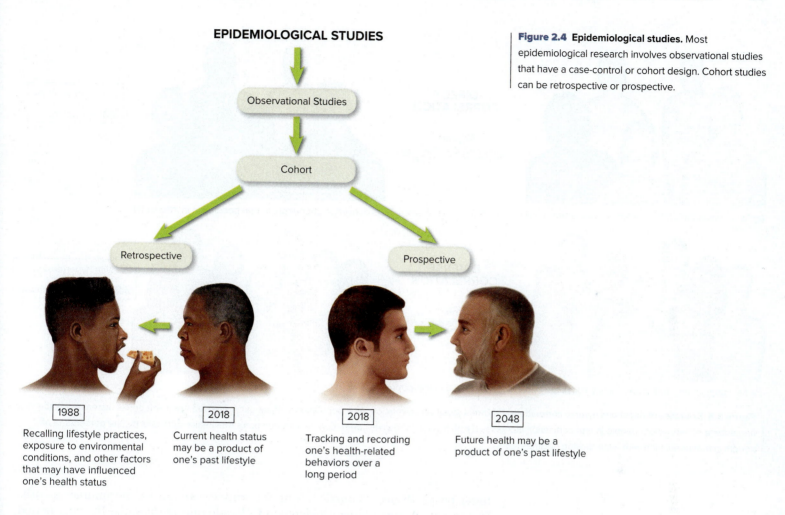

Observational Studies

Cohort

Retrospective

Prospective

| 1988 |
Recalling lifestyle practices, exposure to environmental conditions, and other factors that may have influenced one's health status

| 2018 |
Current health status may be a product of one's past lifestyle

| 2018 |
Tracking and recording one's health-related behaviors over a long period

| 2048 |
Future health may be a product of one's past lifestyle

Figure 2.4 Epidemiological studies. Most epidemiological research involves observational studies that have a case-control or cohort design. Cohort studies can be retrospective or prospective.

Heart Study identified numerous risk factors for heart disease, including elevated blood cholesterol levels, cigarette smoking, and hypertension. Today, medical researchers are still collecting information from the original Framingham Heart Study participants as well as their descendants.

Limitations of Epidemiological Studies Epidemiological studies cannot establish *causation*, that is, whether a practice is responsible for an effect. When two different natural events occur simultaneously within a population, it does not necessarily mean they are correlated. A **correlation** is a relationship between variables. A correlation occurs when two variables change over the same period; for example, when a population's intake of sugar—sweetened soft drinks increases, the percentage of overweight people in the population also increases (Fig. 2.5a). In this case, the correlation is *direct* or *positive* because the two variables—body weight and regular soft drink consumption—are changing in the same direction; they are both increasing. An *inverse* or *negative* correlation occurs when one variable increases and the other one decreases (the variables change in opposite directions). An example of an inverse correlation is the relationship between fruit intake and hypertension; as a population's fruit consumption increases, the percentage of people with hypertension in that population decreases (Fig. 2.5b).

What appears to be a correlation between a behavior and an outcome could be a coincidence, that is, a chance happening and not an indication of a *cause—and—effect* relationship between the two variables. For example, in a survey of lemonade consumption in Colorado over a 10—year period, we might observe that

correlation relationship between two variables

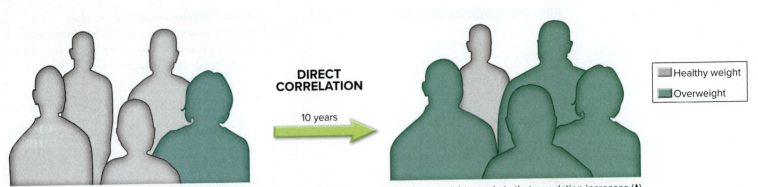

(a) As a population's intake of sugar-sweetened soft drinks increases (↑), the percentage of overweight people in that population increases (↑).

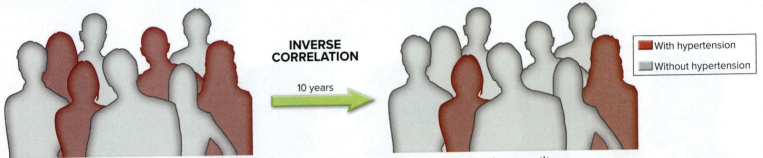

(b) As a population's fruit intake increases (↑), the percentage of people in that population with hypertension decreases (↓).

Figure 2.5 Examples of direct and inverse correlations. (a) Direct (positive) correlation: As a population's intake of sugar-sweetened soft drinks increases (↑), the percentage of overweight people in that population increases (↑). (b) Inverse (negative) correlation: As a population's fruit intake increases (↑), the percentage of people in that population with hypertension declines (↓).

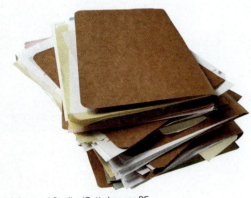

©C Squared Studios/Getty Images RF

peer review expert critical analysis of a research article before it is published

fewer people drank lemonade during the winter than during the summer months. In a survey of snow skiing accidents in Colorado during the same 10−year period, we might also find that snow skiing accidents were more likely to occur during the winter than in the summer. Thus, as lemonade consumption declined, snow skiing accidents increased. Does this mean lemonade consumption is inversely correlated to skiing accidents and people who do not drink lemonade have a greater risk of having a skiing accident at this time of year? It is more likely that the relationship between snow skiing and lemonade drinking is coincidental, because both activities are associated with seasonal weather conditions. Although this example is obviously far−fetched, it illustrates the problems scientists can have when analyzing results of epidemiological studies.

Analyzing Data, Drawing Conclusions, and Reporting Findings

Nutrition researchers use a variety of statistical methods to analyze data collected from observations and experiments. These methods may enable the researchers to find relationships between the variables and health outcomes that were studied. As a result, scientists can determine whether their hypotheses are supported by the data.

When an experiment or study is completed and the results analyzed, researchers summarize the findings and seek to publish articles with informa−tion about their investigation in scientific journals. Before articles are accepted for publication, they undergo **peer review,** a critical analysis conducted by a group of "peers." Peers are investigators who were not part of the study but are experts involved in related research. If peers agree that a study was well conducted, its results are fairly represented, and the research is of interest to the journal's readers, these scientists are likely to recommend that the journal's editors publish the article. Examples of peer–reviewed medical and nutrition journals include the *Journal of the Academy of Nutrition and Dietetics*, *The New England Journal of Medicine*, *Journal of the American Medical Association*, and *Journal of the American College of Nutrition*.

Did *YOU* Know?

By the middle of the twentieth century, the leading causes of death in the United States shifted from infectious diseases to chronic diseases, particularly heart disease. At that time, medical researchers began to suspect certain dietary components played a major role in the development of this major killer of Americans. Two scientists, John Yudkin and Ancel Keys, supported different hypotheses concerning dietary "causes" of heart disease. Yudkin thought the consumption of added sugars caused heart disease, while Keys thought the disease was caused by diets that contained too much fat, saturated fat, and cholesterol. By the 1980s, Yudkin's sugar hypothesis had been largely dismissed by medical and nutrition scientists, and many Americans heeded nationally promoted recommendations to reduce cholesterol, total fat, and saturated fat intakes.

In September 2016, a paper published in the *JAMA Internal Medicine* exposed the likelihood that in the mid-1960s, people in the sugar industry used their influence to divert attention away from sugar's role in the development of heart disease.[5] This paper revealed correspondence between individuals who worked for the Sugar Research Foundation (SRF) and a small group of well-known and respected nutrition scientists. SRF was an organization that was closely associated with the sugar industry. In 1965–1966, SRF paid the nutrition researchers to prepare a paper that reviewed scientific literature concerning the role of sugar and lipids in the development of heart disease. In 1967, *The New England Journal of Medicine* published the two-part paper, which challenged the strength and credibility of the scientific evidence that identified sugar consumption as a contributor to heart disease. The paper also blamed dietary cholesterol and saturated fat as the cause of the disease. Although the 1967 article listed the authors' affiliations and sources of support for their research, it did not mention that the authors had received money from the SRF for the paper's preparation.

Today, reliable scientific journals require authors to disclose their sources of funding, including organizations and for-profit companies established by the food and wellness industries to promote specific products. Thus, people who read articles published in reliable scientific journals can use this information to consider whether the funding sources may have influenced the authors' findings.

Research Bias   Scientists expect other researchers to avoid relying on their personal attitudes and biases ("points of view") when collecting and analyz–ing data and to evaluate and report their results objectively and honestly. This process is important because much of the scientific research that is conducted in the United States is supported financially by the federal government, nonprofit foundations, and drug companies and other private industries. Some funding sources can have certain expectations or biases about research outcomes, and as a result, they are likely to finance studies of scientists whose research efforts support their interests. The beef industry, for example, might not fund scien–tific investigations to find connections between high intakes of beef and the risk of certain cancers. On the other hand, the beef industry might be interested in supporting a team of scientists whose research indicates that a high–protein diet that contains plenty of beef is useful for people who are trying to lose weight.

Peer–reviewed journals usually require authors of articles to disclose their affiliations and sources of financial support. Such disclosures may appear on the first page or at the end of the article. By having this information, readers can decide on the reliability of the findings. Although peer review

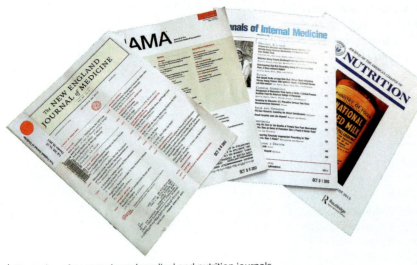

Examples of peer-reviewed medical and nutrition journals.
©Wendy Schiff

helps ensure that the scientists are as ethical and objective as possible, it is impossible to eliminate all research bias.

Spreading the News After the results of a study are published in a nutrition—related journal or reported to health professionals attending a meeting of a nutrition or medical society, the media (e.g., newspapers, magazines, Internet news sources) may receive notice of the findings. If the information is simplistic and sensational, such as a finding that drinking green tea can result in weight loss, it is more likely to be reported in the popular press. In many instances, you learn about the study's results when they are reported in a television or radio news broadcast as a 15— or 30—second "sound bite." Such sources generally provide very little information concerning the way the study was conducted or how the data were collected and analyzed.

Popular sources of nutrition information, such as magazines and the Internet, generally do not subject articles or blogs to peer review or other scientific scrutiny, and as a result, they may feature faulty, biased information. For example, a health news column in a popular magazine may report findings from a few nutrition journal articles that support the use of garlic supplements for reducing blood cholesterol levels. However, you may conclude that the column is biased if it excludes results of other studies that do not indicate such benefits. You can often distinguish a peer—reviewed scientific journal from a popular magazine simply by looking at their covers and skimming their pages. Compared to scientific journals, magazines typically have more colorful, attractive covers and photographs, and their articles are shorter and easier for the average person to read (Fig. 2.6).

It is important to keep in mind that sensational media coverage of a medical "breakthrough" is not necessarily an indication of the value or quality of research that resulted in the news story or magazine article. The results of one study are rarely enough to gain widespread acceptance for new or unusual findings or to provide a basis for nutritional recommendations. Thus, the findings obtained by one research team must be supported by those generated in other studies. If the results of several scientific investigations conducted under similar conditions confirm the original researchers' conclusions, then these findings are more likely to be accepted by other nutrition scientists.

Confusion and Conflict

One day, the news highlights dramatic health benefits from eating garlic, dark chocolate, brown rice, or cherries. A few weeks later, the news includes reports of more recent scientific investigations that do not support the earlier findings. When consumers become aware of conflicting results generated by nutrition studies, they often become confused and disappointed. As a result, some people may mistrust the scientific community and think nutrition scientists do not know what they are doing.

Consumers need to recognize that conflicting findings often result from differences in the ways various studies are designed. Even when investigating the same question, different groups of scientists often conduct their studies and analyze the results differently. For example, the numbers, ages, and physical conditions of subjects; the type and length of the study; the amount of the treatment provided;

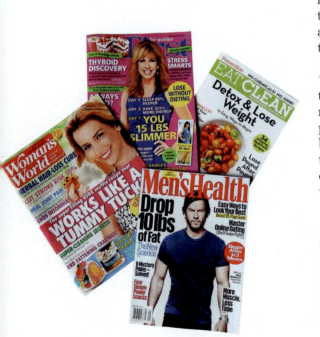

Figure 2.6 **Judging by the cover.** Consumers can be trained to look for features, such as "busy," brightly colored covers, that distinguish popular sources of nutrition information from peer-reviewed scientific journals. Also, popular sources of nutrition information, such as these magazines, are readily available at supermarkets.
©Wendy Schiff

and the statistical tests used to analyze results typically vary among studies. Additionally, individual genetic differences often contribute to a person's response to a treatment. Not only are people genetically different, they also have different lifestyles, and they typically recall dietary information and follow instructions con—cerning health care practices differently. These and other factors can influence the results of nutrition research involving human subjects.

The science of nutrition is constantly evolving; old beliefs and practices are discarded when they are not supported by more recent scientific evidence, and new principles and practices emerge from the new findings. By now you should understand that science involves asking questions, developing and testing hypotheses, gathering and analyzing data, drawing conclusions from data, and, sometimes, accepting change.

Concept CHECKPOINT

1. What is epidemiology?
2. Explain the importance of having a control group when conducting experimental research.
3. What is the major difference between a prospective study and a retrospective study?
4. What is a placebo? Why are placebos often used in studies involving human subjects?
5. What is a double-blind study?
6. What is a peer-reviewed article?
7. Explain why results of similar studies may provide different findings.

See Appendix G for responses.

2.2 Nutrition Information: Fact or Fiction

Learning Outcomes

1 Explain why there is so much nutrition misinformation.

2 Discuss how people can become more critical and careful consumers of nutrition information.

3 Identify common red flags that are signs of nutrition misinformation.

While channel surfing one afternoon, you stop and watch the host of a televised home shopping program promote FatMegaMelter, his company's brand of a dietary supplement for losing weight. According to the host, the supplement contains a chemical derived from a plant that grows naturally in South Africa. This amazing chemical reduces the appetite for fattening foods, enabling an overweight person taking FatMegaMelter to lose up to 30 pounds in 30 days, without the need to exercise more or eat less. The host interviews an attractive young actress who claims to have lost a lot of weight after she started taking FatMegaMelter pills. A few days later, a friend mentions that she has lost 3 pounds since she began taking this product a week ago. You would like to lose a few pounds without resorting to restricting your food intake or exercising. Should you take FatMegaMelter? The supplement helped the actress and your friend; will it help you?

Although the actress's health history appears to be compelling evidence that the weight—loss supplement is effective, her information is a **testimonial**, a personal endorsement of a product. People are usually paid to provide their

testimonial personal endorsement of a product

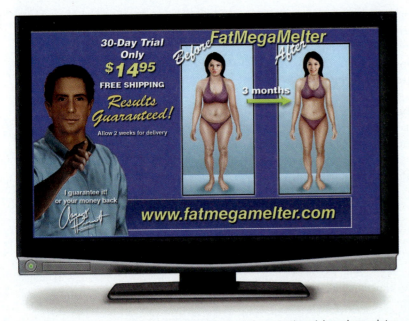

Be wary of ads for nutrition-related products that rely on testimonials and anecdotes.

testimonials for advertisements; therefore, their remarks may be biased in favor of the product. Your friend's experience with taking the same weight–loss product is intriguing, but it is an anecdote and not *proof* that Fat–MegaMelter promotes weight loss. When your source of nutrition information is a testimonial, anecdote, or adver–tisement, you cannot be sure that the information is based on scientific facts and, therefore, reliable.

Become a Critical Consumer of Nutrition Information

People may think they have learned facts about nutrition by reading popular magazine articles or best–selling books; visiting Internet websites; or watching television news, info–mercials, or home shopping programs. In many instances, however, they have been misinformed. To be a care–ful consumer, do not assume that all nutrition information presented in the popular media is reliable. The First Amendment to the U.S. Constitution guarantees freedom of the press and freedom of speech, so people can provide nutrition information that is not true. Thus, the First Amendment does not protect consumers with freedom from nutrition misinformation or false nutrition claims.

The U.S. Food and Drug Administration (FDA) can regulate nutrition–and health–related claims on product labels, but the agency cannot prevent the spread of health and nutrition misinformation published in books or pamphlets or presented in television or radio programs. As a consumer, you are responsible for questioning and researching the accuracy of nutrition information as well as the credentials of the people making nutrition–related claims.

Promoters of worthless nutrition products and services often use sophis–ticated marketing methods to lure consumers. For example, some promoters of dietary supplements claim their products are "scientifically tested," or they include citations to what appear to be scientific journal articles in their ads or articles. Consumers, however, cannot be certain the information is true. In some instances, these products have been scientifically tested, but much of the research that has been conducted using reliable methods has shown that most dietary supplements, other than vitamins and minerals, provide little or no measurable health benefits. Nevertheless, promoters of nonnutrient dietary supplements continue to sell their goods to an unsuspecting, trusting public. The "Nutrition Matters" feature at the end of this chapter focuses on dietary supplements.

Consumers also need to be alert for promoters' use of **pseudoscience,** the presentation of information masquerading as factual and obtained by scientific methods. In many instances, pseudoscientific nutrition or physiology information is presented with complex scientific–sounding terms, such as "enzymatic therapy" or "colloidal extract." Such terms are designed to convince people without science backgrounds that the nutrition–related information is true. Often, promoters of nutrition misinformation try to confuse people by weaving false information with facts into their claims, making the untrue material seem credible too.

Although people's lives have improved as a result of scientific advancements in medicine, the general public tends to mistrust scientists, medical professionals, and the pharmaceutical industry. Promoters of nutrition misinformation exploit

pseudoscience presentation of information masquerading as factual and obtained by scientific methods this mistrust to sell their products and services. For example, they may tell consumers that physicians rely on costly diagnostic methods and treatments for serious diseases because they are more interested in making money than doing what is best for their patients, such as recommending a dietary supplement. Are physicians driven by the desire to make money from their patients' illnesses, and do they hide information about natural cures from them?

Over the past 100 years, people's lives have been greatly improved by contributions of medical researchers. As a group, physicians are dedicated to improving their patients' health and saving lives. Physicians have nothing to gain from concealing a cure from the public. They strive to diagnose and treat diseases using scientifically tested and approved techniques. Moreover, a physician may face a malpractice lawsuit if he or she fails to diagnose and treat a condition effectively. Additionally, physicians have much to gain from treating their patients kindly and effectively. Consider this: If you follow a physician's advice and have positive results, are you likely to be that doctor's patient for a long time and recommend the practitioner to others?

If your car is not functioning properly, you probably would want people who have the best training, tools, and equipment to determine the problem and repair it. If you think something is wrong with your body, it is prudent to seek information and opinions from medical professionals who have the best training and experience to diagnose and treat health disorders.

Ask Questions

If you are like most people, you do not want to waste your money on things you do not need or that are useless or potentially harmful. How can you become a more careful, critical consumer of nutrition–related information or products? The following questions should help you evaluate various sources of nutrition information:

- *What motivates the authors, promoters, or sponsors to provide the information? Do you think they are more interested in your health and well–being or in selling their products?* Salespeople often have favorable biases toward the things they sell, and therefore, they may not be reliable sources of information about these products. A clerk in a dietary supplements outlet store, for example, may wear a white lab coat to look as though he or she has a science or medical educational background, but you should keep in mind that the clerk was hired to sell dietary supplements and may have little or no scientific training. Furthermore, salespeople who work in such outlets may be unwilling to inform customers about the potential health hazards of taking certain products, particularly when they earn a commission from each sale.

- *Is the source scientific, such as an article from a peer–reviewed nutrition journal?* In general, popular sources of nutrition information, such as best–selling books and articles in magazines, are not peer–reviewed by scientists. Additionally, radio or TV programs that promote nutrition information may actually be sophisticated advertisements for nutrition–related products.

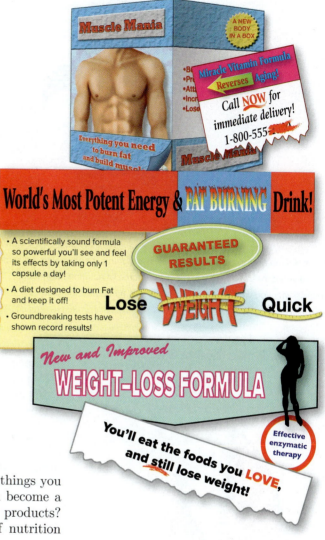

Did *YOU* Know?

In 2010, a federal district court ruled in favor of the Federal Trade Commission in a case involving companies that used unproven claims to promote "Chinese Diet Tea" and "Bio-Slim Patch." The court fined the companies nearly $2 million for claiming that the products would enable people to lose weight without diet and exercise.[6]

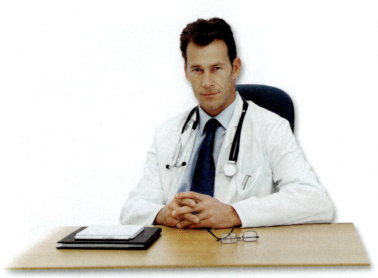

If this person appeared on a television show or in a magazine advertisement, would you consider him to be a reliable source of nutrition information? Explain why you would or would not trust his nutrition-related advice.

©Stockbyte/Getty Images RF

quackery promotion of useless medical treatments

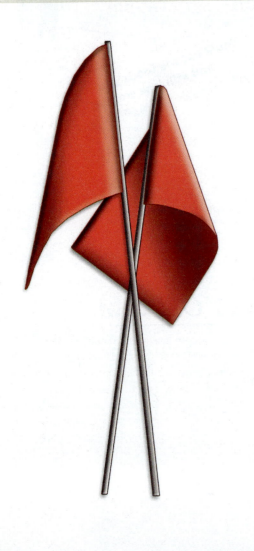

- *If a study is mentioned (cited), how was the research conducted? Did the study involve humans or animals? If people participated in the study, how many subjects were involved in the research? Who sponsored the study?* As mentioned earlier in this chapter, epidemiological studies are not useful for finding cause–and–effect relationships. Additionally, the results of studies involving large numbers of human subjects are more reliable than studies of animals. Sponsors may influence the outcomes of the studies they fund.

- *To provide scientific support for claims, does the source refer to articles in respected nutrition or medical journals or mention reliable experts?* Be careful if you see citations in popular nutrition or health books and magazines. Promoters of nutrition misinformation may refer to scientific–appearing citations from phony medical journals to convince people that their information is reliable. Furthermore, be wary of nutrition experts introduced or identified as "Doctor" because they may not be physicians or scientists. Furthermore, a so–called nutrition expert who is referred to as "Doctor" may not have a doctorate degree (Ph.D.) in human nutrition from an accredited university. Such experts may have obtained their degrees simply by purchasing them on the Internet or through a mail–order outlet, without having taken appropriate coursework or graduated from an accredited university or college.

Practicing medicine without the proper training and licensing is illegal. However, providing nutrition information and advice without the proper training and licensing is legal. **Quackery** involves promoting useless medical treatments, such as copper bracelets to treat arthritis.

To obtain information about a nutrition expert's credentials, enter the person's name at an Internet search engine and evaluate the results. For example, is the person associated with an accredited school of higher education or a government agency such as the U.S. Department of Agriculture? You can also visit www.quackwatch.org and submit an "Ask a Question" e–mail requesting information about a person's credentials from the site's sponsors.

Look for Red Flags

To become a critical consumer of nutrition information, you need to be aware of red flags, clues that indicate a source of information is unreliable. Common red flags include the following:

1. **Promises of quick and easy remedies for complex health–related problems:** "Our product helps you lose weight *without* exercising or dieting," or "Garlic cures heart disease."

2. **Claims that sound too good to be true:** "Our all–natural product blocks fat and calories from being absorbed, so you can eat everything you like and still lose weight." Such claims are rarely true. Remember, if the claim sounds too good to be true, it probably is not true.

3. **Scare tactics that include sensational, frightening, false, or misleading statements about a food, dietary practice, or health condition:** "Dairy products cause cancer," or "Eating sugar causes hyperactivity."

4. **Personal attacks on the motives and ethical standards of registered dietitian nutritionists or conventional scientists:** "Dietitians and physicians don't want you to know the facts about natural cures for cancer, diabetes, and heart disease because they'll lose money if you get well." Such statements indicate unsubstantiated biases against bona fide nutrition experts and the scientific community.

5. **Statements about the superiority of certain dietary supplements or unconventional medical practices:** "Russian scientists have discovered the countless health benefits of taking Siberian ginseng," or "Colon cleansing with herbs is the only cure for intestinal cancer."

6. **Testimonials and anecdotes as evidence of effectiveness:** "I lost 50 pounds in 30 days using this product," or "I rubbed this vitamin formula on my scar and it disappeared in days." Reliable nutrition information is based on scientific evidence, not testimonials and anecdotes.

7. **Information that promotes a product's benefits while overlooking its risks:** "Our all-natural supplement boosts your metabolism naturally so it won't harm your system." Anything you consume, even water, can be toxic in high doses. Beware of any source of information that fails to mention the possible side effects of using a dietary supplement or nutrition-related treatment.

8. **Vague, meaningless, or scientific-sounding terms to impress or confuse consumers:** "Our *all-natural, clinically tested, patented, chelated* dietary supplement works best."

9. **Sensational statements with incomplete references of sources:** "Clinical research performed at a major university and published in a distinguished medical journal indicates food manufacturers add ingredients to their products that make you hungry and fat," or "Millions of Americans suffer from various nutritional deficiencies." Which "major university" and "distinguished medical journal"? What study reported that "millions of Americans" are deficient in nutrients?

10. **Recommendations based on a single study:** "Research conducted at our private health facility proves coffee enemas can cure cancer."

11. **Information concerning nutrients or human physiology that is not supported by reliable scientific evidence:** "Now, you can combine certain foods based on your blood type," or "Most diseases are caused by undigested food that gets stuck in your guts," or "People with alkaline bodies don't develop cancer."

12. **Results disclaimers, usually in small or difficult-to-read print:** "Results may vary," or "Results not typical" (Fig. 2.7). Disclaimers are clues that the product may not live up to your expectations or the manufacturer's claims.

Using the Internet Wisely

You can find abundant sources of information about nutrition and the benefits of dietary supplements on the Internet. However, you must be careful and consider the sources. Who or what organization sponsors the site? Is the information intended to promote sales? Be wary if the site discusses benefits of dietary supplements and enables you to purchase these products online. Furthermore, a site is likely to be unreliable if it includes comprehensive disclaimers such as "The manufacturer is not responsible or obligated to verify statements." Also avoid sites that publish disclaimers such as "The nutrition and health information at this site is provided for educational purposes only and not as a substitute for the advice of a physician or registered dietitian nutritionist. The author and owner of this site are not liable for personal actions taken as a result of the site's contents."

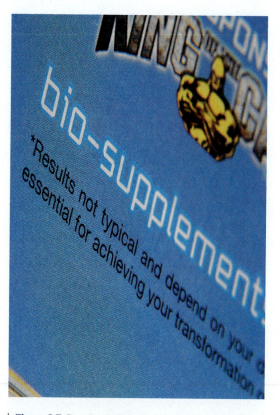

Figure 2.7 Results disclaimer. A disclaimer may be a red flag indicating a product has limited effectiveness, despite its promoter's claims.
©Wendy Schiff

TABLE 2.1   Tips for Searching Nutrition Information on the Internet

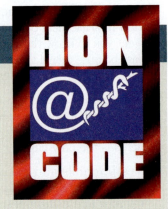

To Be a Careful Consumer of Internet Sources of Information:

1. Use multiple sites, especially government sites such as the Centers for Disease Control and Prevention (www.cdc.gov) and the Food and Drug Administration (www.fda.gov), as well as the sites of nationally recognized nutrition- or health-related associations such as the Academy of Nutrition and Dietetics (www.eatright.org), the American Diabetes Association (www.diabetes.org), and the American Heart Association (www.heart.org/HEARTORG/). Use PubMed (https://www.ncbi.nlm.nih.gov/pubmed/) as a resource when searching for science-based published articles.
2. Rely primarily on sites that are managed or reviewed by a group of qualified health professionals. Blogs might be fun and interesting to read, but they are not necessarily reliable.
3. Look for the Health on the Net symbol at the bottom of the main page of the website. The Health on the Net Foundation is a nonprofit, international organization that promotes the HONcode, a set of principles for standardizing the reliability of health information on the Internet. For more information about HONcode, you can visit the organization's website (www.hon.ch/).
4. Do not trust information at a site that does not indicate valid sources, such as well-respected peer-reviewed scientific journals or nationally recognized universities or medical centers. Contributing authors and their credentials should be identified; when they are, perform an online search of the scientific journals, as well as the authors' names and credentials, to determine their validity.
5. Be wary of sites that have surveys for you to complete, advertisements for diet-related products, and promotions in pop-up windows and that provide online diagnoses and treatments.
6. Do not trust a site that includes attacks on the trustworthiness of the medical or scientific establishment.
7. Be wary of commercial sites (*.com) with links to government sites or the sites of well-known medical, nutrition, or scientific associations. An unreliable *.com site can be linked to reliable sites without having received their endorsements.

Source: Adapted from: National Institutes of Health: *How to evaluate health information on the Internet: Questions and answers.* 2011. https://ods.od.nih.gov/Health_Information/How_To_Evaluate_Health_Information_on_the_Internet_Questions_and_Answers.aspx Accessed: July 3, 2017.

Did *YOU* Know?

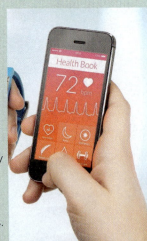

In 2014, 86% of undergraduate U.S. college students had smartphones.[7] Over 13,600 apps are available to help consumers monitor and improve their diets, energy intakes, physical activity levels, and other health-related behaviors. Choosing the most reliable apps to use can be difficult because many of these products have not been tested for effectiveness.[8] Registered dietitian nutritionists evaluated and rated some popular apps that have been developed for people who want to manage their weight, diabetes, or gluten intake. To access the reviews and ratings, visit the Academy of Nutrition and Dietetics website at http://www.eatrightpro.org/resources/media/trends-and-reviews/app-reviews.

©Alexey Boldin/Shutterstock RF

Be wary of websites that are authored or sponsored by one person, or sites that promote or sell products for profit (*.com) because such sources of information may be biased. In general, websites sponsored by nationally recognized health associations such as the Academy of Nutrition and Dietetics, (www.eatright.org) and nonprofit organizations such as the National Osteoporosis Foundation (www.nof.org) are reliable sources of nutrition information. Government agencies (*.gov) and nationally accredited colleges and universities (*.edu) are also excellent sources of credible nutrition information. Table 2.1 presents some tips for using the Internet to obtain reliable nutrition information.

The Federal Trade Commission (FTC) enforces consumer protection laws and investigates complaints about false or misleading health claims that appear on the Internet. For information to help you evaluate nutrition and health–related claims, visit the agency's website (https://www.consumer.ftc.gov/articles/0167–miracle–health–claims). To complain about a product, you can complete and submit the FTC's complaint form at the website or call the agency's toll–free line (1–877–382–4357).

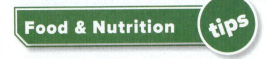

If you are looking for a recipe for guacamole, cranberry chutney, or sweet and sour cabbage, simply use the Internet—it is like having a cookbook at your fingertips. Recipes for nearly every food and from various countries and ethnic groups are available on the Internet, and you can find cooking tips from this vast resource.

When searching the Web for recipes, you need to recognize that many food manufacturers use the sites to promote their products in recipes. If the brand name of a product is mentioned in the recipe, you can usually substitute another company's product. Additionally, recipes may not provide accurate information about the nutrients and calories in a serving of food, and you cannot be certain that the recipes have been tested for quality. Therefore, it is a good idea to check more than one site for a recipe and compare the information.

Concept CHECKPOINT

2.3 Reliable Nutrition Experts

Learning Outcome

1 Explain how to identify reliable nutrition experts.

If you have questions about food or nutrition, where do you find factual answers? Although many states regulate and license people who call themselves nutritionists, you cannot always rely on someone who refers to him— or herself as a "nutrition—ist" or "nutritionalist" for reliable nutrition information because there are no stan—dard legal definitions for these descriptors. Should you ask a physician for nutrition advice? Physicians are not necessarily the best sources of nutrition information because most doctors do not have extensive college coursework in the subject.

If your university or college has a nutrition or dietetics department, you are likely to find nutrition experts, including professors, registered dietitians, and reg—istered dietitian nutritionists, who are faculty members. A **registered dietitian (RD)** or **registered dietitian nutritionist (RDN)** is a college—trained health care professional who has extensive knowledge of foods, nutrition, and *dietetics*, the application of nutrition and food information to help treat many health—related conditions. The titles "registered dietitian (RD)" and "registered dietitian nutritionist (RDN)" are legally protected. This means people cannot legally refer to themselves as RDNs unless they have been certified by the appropriate accrediting agency.

You can also locate RDNs by consulting online directories, contacting your local dietetic association or dietary department of a local hospital, or visiting the Academy of Nutrition and Dietetics website (www.eatright.org) or the Dietitians of Canada website (www.dietitians.ca).

> **registered dietitian (RD)** or **registered dietitian nutritionist (RDN)** college-trained health care professional who has extensive knowledge of foods, nutrition, and dietetics

Becoming a Registered Dietitian Nutritionist

There are three major professional divisions for RDNs: clinical dietetics, community nutrition, and food systems management. Clinical dietitians can work as members of medical teams in hospitals or clinics. Clinical dietitians can also work as community nutritionists in public health settings or as dietary counselors in private practice or with wellness programs. Food systems management dietitians direct food service systems in hospitals, schools, and settings where healthy foods are prepared and served to employees or residents of long—term care facilities. Although most RDNs work in health care settings, some are educators or researchers.

A registered dietitian nutritionist has completed a baccalaureate degree program approved by the Accreditation Council for Education in Nutrition and Dietetics (ACEND) of the Academy of Nutrition and Dietetics, the largest orga—nization of dietitians in the United States. As undergraduate students, dietetics majors are required to take a wide variety of college—level courses, including food and nutrition sciences, organic chemistry, biochemistry, anatomy, physiol—ogy, microbiology, statistics, management, and communications classes. If you are attending a major university, you can check the course or program catalog at your school to determine whether an accredited dietetics program is offered.

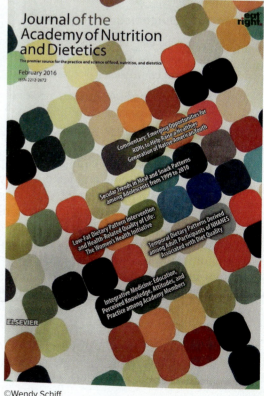

©Wendy Schiff

In addition to taking the required college coursework, the student dietitian nutritionist must obtain at least 1200 hours of supervised practice (training), which is often in a health care facility, such as a university hospital. Such train—ing (a *supervised practice program* or *SPP*) prepares the student dietitian nutritionist for an entry—level position when he or she graduates with a bac—calaureate degree in dietetics. Student dietitian nutritionists who attend colleges or universities that have accredited undergraduate dietetics programs but do not offer SSPs can apply for admittance into a *dietetic internship* (*DI*). Dietetic internships are accredited training programs that begin after the student gradu—ates. For more information about internships and their availability, visit http://www.eatrightacend.org/ACEND/.

After completing a SPP, DI, or SPPI, the student dietitian nutritionist has to pass the national registration examination to become certified as an RDN. After becoming certified, RDNs are also required to fulfill continuing educa—tion requirements to maintain their certification. The Academy of Nutrition and Dietetics provides more information about becoming an RDN and roles these professionals play in health care settings.

Concept CHECKPOINT

11. What is the difference between a nutritionist and a registered dietitian nutritionist?

12. List three ways of locating reliable nutrition experts.

See Appendix G for responses.

2.4 Nutrition Matters: What Are Dietary Supplements?

Learning Outcomes

1 Explain the difference between conventional medicine and alternative health care, and identify health care practices that are either conventional or alternative.

2 Explain how the FDA regulates medicines differently than dietary supplements.

3 Discuss the risks and benefits of taking dietary supplements.

Do you take a daily vitamin or mineral pill because you are concerned about the nutritional quality of your diet? Do you use herbal pills or extracts to strengthen your immune system, boost your memory, or treat illnesses such as the common cold? If you follow any of these practices, you are not alone. According to results of a national survey, over 50% of the American population takes one or more dietary supplements regularly.[9]

According to the Dietary Supplement Health and Education Act of 1994 (DSHEA), a dietary supplement is a product (other than tobacco) that

- adds to a person's dietary intake and contains one or more dietary ingredients, including nutrients or *botani—cals* (herbs or other plant material);

- is taken by mouth; and,
- is a concentrate, metabolite, constituent, or extract.[10]

Dietary supplements include nutrient pills, protein pow—ders, and herbal extracts. Many dietary supplements are often referred to as "nutraceuticals," but there is no legal definition for this term.

©Wendy Schiff

In the United States, the most commonly used dietary supplements are **multivitamin/mineral (MV/M)** products.[9] There is no standard definition for the contents of a MV/M supple—ment, but such products may contain several vitamins and minerals. In 2012, the most popular nonvitamin, nonmineral dietary supplements among American adults were fish oil or "omega 3," glucosamine and/or chondroitin, probiotics/prebiotics, and melatonin.[11]

Some people use dietary supplements, particularly those containing nutrients, because the products are rec—ommended by their physicians or registered dietitian nutritionists. Physicians, for example, may prescribe a

Blueberries: ©PhotoAlto/Getty Images RF

prenatal MV/M supplement for their pregnant patients. Most dietary supplements are available without the need for prescriptions, so people can take them without their doctors' knowledge and approval.

Table 2.2 provides information about some non–micronutrient dietary supplements that are popular among adult Americans. Benefits and risks of supplementing diets with micronutrients are discussed in Chapters 8 and 9.

Conventional Medicine Versus Alternative Health Care Practices

Conventional ("mainstream") medical practitioners, such as physicians and registered dietitian nutritionists, generally promote and use health care practices that have been scientifically tested and evaluated for safety and effectiveness. Examples of **conventional medical care** include surgical procedures that remove diseased tissues, FDA–approved medications that reduce high blood pressure levels, and dietary patterns that provide enough nutrients to promote good health. **Alternative health care** promotes and uses practices that may or may not have been tested scientifically for both safety and effectiveness. According to the National Institutes of Health (NIH), the use of natural products such as herbs, vitamins and minerals, and other dietary supplements is an aspect of alternative health care.[12] In 2012, approximately one–third of American adults used alternative health care, including dietary supplements, chiropractic manipulations, homeopathy, naturopathy, and massage therapy.[13]

Many forms of alternative health care are not widely accepted by physicians and other conventional health care providers because scientific studies provide little or no support for their use. However, few Americans rely only on alternative health care; most people who use alternative therapies also use conventional medical care.[12] Integrative health care refers to practices that combine certain kinds of alternative health care practices with conventional medical care. An example of integrative health care is taking a dietary supplement that contains melatonin and an anti–anxiety medication to help treat a mild sleep disorder.

Some forms of alternative health care are gaining acceptance among conventional medical practitioners, primarily because there is sufficient scientific support for the practices. For example, a type of "unfriendly" bacteria can overpopulate

the large intestine when a person takes an antibiotic for infection. The overgrowth of these bacteria can cause cramping, diarrhea, and, in severe cases, death. Physicians may recommend **probiotics** in yogurt or tablet form for patients who are taking antibiotics. Probiotics are beneficial microbes that live in the gut, but the term is also used for products that contain these microbes. Research has shown that certain probiotics can help prevent or limit diarrhea that can result from antibiotic use.[14] Chapter 4 provides more information about probiotics.

How Are Dietary Supplements Regulated?

The U.S. Food and Drug Administration (FDA) is the federal agency that is responsible for ensuring the safety and effectiveness of medications and other health–related products. The FDA strictly regulates the development, production, and marketing of new medications (drugs). A drug is a substance, natural or human–made, that alters body functions. As a result, drugs can produce beneficial as well as harmful effects on the body. Before marketing a new drug, the manufacturer must submit evidence to the FDA indicating that the product has been tested extensively and is safe and effective. If FDA experts have serious concerns about a medication's side effects or question its usefulness, the agency may reject the manufacturer's petition to sell the product.

When consumed, many dietary supplements act as drugs in the body. However, the FDA does not regulate dietary supplements as medications. Instead, the agency regulates dietary supplements as a category of foods.[15] As a result, dietary supplement manufacturers can bypass most of the strict regulations that the FDA applies to the introduction of new medications into the marketplace. Supplement manufacturers, for example, generally do not need FDA approval before manufacturing or marketing their products. Additionally, the manufacturers are not required to provide the FDA with scientific evidence indicating their products provide measurable health benefits. Manufacturers, however, must notify the FDA and provide the agency with information about the safety of any supplement that contains dietary ingredients that were not marketed in dietary supplements prior to 1994, unless the substance had been used in foods.

According to the FDA, dietary supplements are not intended to prevent, diagnose, treat, or cure diseases.[15] Thus, dietary supplement manufacturers are not allowed to make claims that are appropriate for medications, such as "reduces pain," "prevents polio," or "treats diabetes." The agency regulates the labeling of dietary supplements, including health–related claims that are permitted on labels. The "Food and Dietary Supplement Labels" section of Chapter 3 provides information about supplement labeling.

The FDA has set standards designed to help ensure the identity, purity, strength, and composition of dietary supplements. The agency, however, does not test dietary supplements to determine whether they meet such quality standards. Manufacturers of dietary supplements can have their products tested for quality by certain nongovernmental

---

multivitamin/mineral (MV/M) describes a dietary supplement that contains vitamins and minerals

conventional medical care health care practices that are widely accepted and used by mainstream medical practitioners

alternative health care health care practices that are not widely accepted and used by conventional medical practitioners

probiotics products that contain healthful microbes; beneficial gut microbes

TABLE 2.2 Some Popular Non-micronutrient Dietary Supplements

Dietary Supplement	Major Claims	Known Health Effects	
		Benefits	Risks
Alfalfa	Treats kidney problems and improves urine flow Relieves arthritis symptoms	May be effective in lowering total cholesterol and "bad" cholesterol levels, but little scientific evidence that it has other benefits	Consuming alfalfa seeds may be hazardous to health; may increase the likelihood of blood clots; and may lower blood sugar levels, which could be dangerous for people with diabetes
Bitter orange	Causes weight loss and relieves heartburn, upset stomach, and constipation	Applying the oil to skin may help certain skin infections, but there is little scientific evidence to support other health benefit claims.	May increase heart rate and blood pressure, which could result in heart attack and stroke
Chondroitin	Relieves joint damage associated with osteoarthritis	Studies show "mixed" results concerning effectiveness for treating osteoarthritis, which means results of some studies support the benefits, but results of other studies show no benefits. Often combined with glucosamine	May interfere with blood clotting; should be avoided by men who have a history of prostate cancer
Coenzyme Q-10	Increases exercise tolerance, prevents heart disease and cancer, and reverses signs of aging	May help some people with heart and blood vessel diseases	Low toxicity but may interfere with certain blood thinners
Echinacea ©Ingram Publishing/ SuperStock RF	Boosts immune system Prevents the common cold and reduces cold symptoms	Studies show "mixed" results.	Generally safe for short-term use but may provoke allergic response or intestinal upset
Evening primrose oil	Treats eczema (a common skin condition) Relieves arthritis and menopausal symptoms	Little scientific evidence to support health benefit claims	Long-term safety has not been established.
Fish oil	Prevents heart disease and stroke Cures rheumatoid arthritis Reduces depression and risk of Alzheimer's disease	Studies indicate mixed results, but consuming fatty fish may be more helpful in reducing heart disease risk than taking fish oil supplements May reduce pain and stiffness associated with rheumatoid arthritis Scientists are continuing to study the effects of fish oil on health.	May interfere with blood clotting, increasing the risk of hemorrhagic stroke
Flaxseed and flaxseed oil	Acts as a laxative (flaxseed) Reduces blood cholesterol levels	Nonanimal source of an omega-3 fatty acid Lack of scientific evidence to support flaxseed as a treatment for constipation May benefit people with heart disease, but more research is needed.	Generally safe but may cause diarrhea; seeds should be taken with plenty of water to avoid constipation.
Garlic	Lowers blood cholesterol levels	Evidence that garlic reduces blood cholesterol and blood pressure levels is weak. May slightly reduce elevated blood pressure	Raw garlic may cause allergic reaction and unpleasant body odor. May "thin" the blood (make blood clots less likely to form)
Ginger ©Stockbyte/Getty Images RF	Treats "morning sickness" and other forms of nausea Relieves stomach upsets Relieves joint and muscle pain	Can treat morning sickness and may reduce other forms of nausea More studies are needed to support other health benefit claims.	In general, few side effects when taken in small amounts; powdered ginger may cause intestinal upset. Pregnant women should consult with their physician before taking ginger.

Sources: National Institutes of Health, National Center for Complementary and Integrative Health: *Health topics A-Z.* https://nccih.nih.gov/health/atoz.htm; National Institutes of Health, National Library of Medicine, MedlinePlus: *Herbs and supplements.* https://medlineplus.gov/druginfo/herb_All.html. Accessed: July 4, 2017.

TABLE 2.2 Some Popular Non-micronutrient Dietary Supplements *(Continued)*

Dietary Supplement	Major Claims	Known Health Effects	
		Benefits	Risks
Ginkgo biloba	Improves memory Reduces the risk of Alzheimer's disease and other forms of dementia	Lack of scientific evidence to support health benefit claims	May increase the risk of bleeding and cause allergic reactions, headaches, intestinal upsets, and nausea Ginkgo seeds are toxic.
Ginseng (Asian)	Boosts overall health Treats erectile dysfunction (male impotence)	Lack of scientific evidence to support health benefit claims	May cause headaches, sleep disturbances, allergic responses, and gastrointestinal upsets Long-term use may increase risk of toxicity.
Glucosamine sulfate	Relieves joint damage associated with arthritis	Some scientific evidence supports health benefit claims, but more research is needed (frequently used with chondroitin).	Some products are not labeled accurately. Appears to be safe when taken by mouth but may cause mild gastrointestinal side effects, including nausea and heartburn
Green tea ©Wendy Schiff	Prevents or treats cancer Promotes weight loss Reduces blood cholesterol levels	Results of some laboratory studies indicate green tea protects against cancer or reduces cancer cell growth, but human studies show mixed results. Lack of reliable evidence to support other health benefit claims, including promoting weight loss	In a few cases, green tea extracts were associated with liver problems. Caffeine content may cause sleep disturbances, irritability, and digestive upset.
Kava	Reduces stress	Potential harm of using kava outweighs any benefit.	Toxic—can damage the liver May cause abnormal muscle movements, yellowed skin, and sleepiness
L-arginine	Treats heart disease Improves male sexual functioning Improves mental functioning of older adults Lowers blood pressure Increases male fertility	Amino acid (component of proteins) May improve heart function after a heart attack May reduce recovery time after surgery, reduce high blood pressure, and improve erectile function More research is needed to support other health benefits.	Probably safe when taken for short term but may cause side effects, including abdominal pain, diarrhea, gout, breathing problems, and low blood pressure Interacts with many medications May worsen recurrent herpes outbreaks Should not be taken by people who are recovering from a heart attack because the supplement may increase the risk of death after a heart attack.
Melatonin	Treats some sleep disorders Prevents jet lag Treats cancer, headaches, and irritable bowel syndrome Delays the aging process	May be effective for treating certain sleep disorders and preventing jet lag May help relieve withdrawal symptoms in smokers who quit tobacco use Lack of evidence that the supplement is useful for other conditions	Probably safe for short-term use, but long-term effects of its use are unknown. Interacts with several prescription medications and other herbs that produce sedation (calming effects) Common side effects include drowsiness, dizziness, headache, and nausea
St. John's wort Source: Jennifer Anderson/ USDA-NRCS Plants Database	Reduces depression	At this time, most studies do not support using the supplement to treat depression.	May interact with other herbal products and many medications, including prescription antidepressants and oral contraceptives

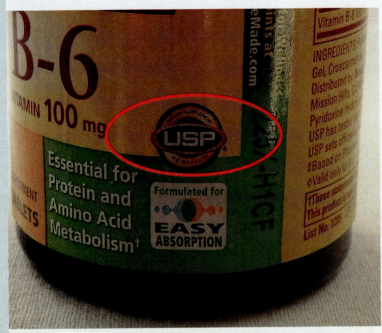

©Wendy Schiff

agencies, including U.S. Pharmacopeia and ConsumerLab .com. Products that pass this testing may include "seals of approval" on labels, but these seals are no guarantee that the dietary supplements are safe or effective.

The FDA's role in regulating dietary supplements gener— ally begins after products enter the marketplace.[16] Supple— ment manufacturers are required to keep records concerning reports they receive about serious adverse (negative) health effects that may have been caused by their products. Fur— thermore, the manufacturers must also inform the FDA about such reports. Consumers and health care professionals can also report health problems that are possibly associated with supplement use directly to the FDA.

When the FDA determines that a particular supple— ment presents a significant or unreasonable risk of harm, the agency alerts consumers about the risk and seeks to recall the product, that is, initiates efforts to have it removed from the market.[17] In most instances, the manufacturer volun— tarily recalls the product after determining there is a problem with it or being notified by the FDA about the problem. In some cases, however, the FDA requests a recall. If the FDA determines that the manufacturer's response to the recall is inadequate, the agency can take enforcement steps, such as initiating legal action against the company to seize products or stop producing the items.

Using Dietary Supplements Wisely

When used properly, many dietary supplements, particularly micronutrient products, are generally safe. Herbal supple— ments, however, are made from plants that may have toxic parts. Comfrey, pennyroyal, sassafras, kava, lobelia, and ma huang are among the plants known to be highly toxic

or cancer—causing. Products containing material from these plants should be avoided. The use of botanical products can also evoke allergic or inflammatory responses that often result in signs and symptoms of skin, sinus, or respiratory illnesses. Herbal teas may contain pollens and other parts of plants that can cause allergies, particularly in people who are sensitive to the herbs or their related species. Echinacea (purple cone flower) is related to ragweed, a plant that is often associated with seasonal respiratory allergies. When people who are allergic to ragweed pollen take supplements that contain echinacea, they may develop allergic responses that mimic symptoms of the common cold (watery eyes, runny nose, and sneezing). In some instances, inflammatory responses, such as asthma attacks, can occur after exposure to echinacea or other plants. Asthma can be a life—threatening condition. There— fore, people who have asthma or allergies should be very care— ful when using botanical supplements.

Consumers also need to be aware that medicinal herbs may contain substances that affect the usefulness or safety of prescription or over—the—counter medications as well as other herbs. Such interactions can produce unwanted and even dangerous side effects (see Table 2.2). Ginkgo biloba, for example, can interact with aspirin, increasing the risk of bleeding. Garlic, ginseng, and vitamin E supplements can also increase bleeding. Kava and valerian act as sedatives (calm— ing agents) and can amplify the effects of anesthetics and other medications used during surgery. Therefore, provide your physicians and other health care professionals with a list of the supplements you are taking.

If you use or are thinking about using one or more dietary supplements:

- Determine whether the supplement is necessary. Some people have medical reasons for taking dietary supplements that contain one or more micronutrients.
- Discuss your need for the supplement with your physician or a registered dietitian nutritionist before you purchase or use the product. This action is particularly important if you are pregnant, are breastfeeding a baby, or have a chronic medical condition such as diabetes or heart disease.
- Consult a physician before giving such products to children. Treat dietary supplements as drugs: store them away from children.
- Consult a physician as soon as you develop signs and symptoms of a serious illness. Using supplements to treat serious diseases instead of seeking conventional medical care that has proven effectiveness is a risky practice. In these instances, delaying or forgoing useful medical treatment may result in the worsening of the condition or even be life threatening.
- Be wary of claims made about a supplement's benefits and investigate the claims used to promote the product. The following government websites provide reliable information about dietary supplements:

U.S. National Library of Medicine https://medlineplus.gov/druginfo/herb_All.html

Food and Drug Adminstration www.fda.gov/food/dietarysupplements/default.htm

National Institutes of Health, National Center for Complementary and Integrative Health https://nccih.nih.gov/health/herbsataglance.htm

Office of Dietary Supplements https://ods.od.nih.gov/.

- Determine hazards associated with taking the supplement. Information about the risks and benefits of various dietary supplements can be found at the **Office of Dietary Supplements'** website: https://ods.od.nih.gov/factsheets/list−all/.
- Avoid using dietary supplements as substitutes for nutritious foods. Plant foods provide a wide array of phytochemicals, many of which may have health benefits when taken in their natural forms—foods. When these substances are isolated from plants and manufactured into supplements, they may lose their beneficial properties.

If you experience negative side effects after using a particular dietary supplement, it is a good idea to be examined by a physician immediately. Furthermore, you as well as your physician should report the problem to the FDA's MedWatch program by calling (800) FDA−1088 or visiting the agency's website: https://www.fda.gov/Safety/MedWatch/default.htm.

It is important to recognize that the manufacturing of dietary supplements is a profitable industry in the United States. According to estimates provided by the dietary supplements' industry, Americans spend several billion dollars on such products each year.[18] In many instances, however, people do not need dietary supplements, and they are wasting their money by purchasing them—money that could be better spent on natural sources of nutrients and phytochemicals, particularly fruits, vegetables, and whole−grain cereals.[19]

Concept CHECKPOINT

13. List at least three examples of alternative health care practices.

14. Explain why a prescription medication that is used to treat the common cold is not a dietary supplement.

15. List at least two examples of non-micronutrient dietary supplements.

See Appendix G for responses.

Chapter References

See Appendix H.

Summary

2.1 Nutrition: Science for Consumers

- Scientists ask questions about the natural world and follow generally accepted methods to obtain answers to these questions. Nutrition research relies on scientific methods that may involve making observations, asking questions and developing possible explanations, performing tests, collecting and analyzing data, drawing conclusions from data, and reporting on the findings. Other scientists can test the findings to confirm or reject them.

- Epidemiology is the study of the occurrence, distribution, and causes of health problems in populations. By studying differences in dietary practices and disease occurrences among populations, epidemiologists can suggest nutrition-related hypotheses for the prevalence of certain diseases. Epidemiological studies cannot indicate whether two variables are correlated because the relationship could be a coincidence.

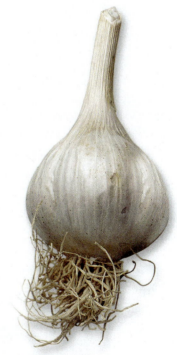

©Photodisc/Getty Images RF

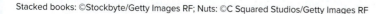

- Researchers summarize the findings and seek to publish articles with information about their investigations in scientific journals. Before articles are accepted for publication, they undergo peer review. Scientists generally do not accept a hypothesis or the results of a study until they are supported by considerable research evidence. Media coverage of a medical breakthrough is not necessarily an indication of the value or quality of research that resulted in the news story. More research is often necessary for scientists to determine whether the results are valid and can be generalized.

- Consumers may think scientists do not know what they are doing when conflicting research findings are reported in the media. Conflicting findings often result because different teams of researchers use different study designs when investigating the same hypothesis. Furthermore, each team of scientists may analyze the results differently. Other factors, such as genetic and lifestyle differences, can also influence the results of nutrition research involving human subjects. The science of nutrition is constantly evolving.

2.2 Nutrition Information: Fact or Fiction

- Although testimonials and anecdotes are often used to promote nutrition-related products and services, consumers cannot be sure that this information is reliable or based on scientific facts. Personal observations are not evidence of a cause-and-effect relationship because many factors, such as lifestyle and environment, can influence outcomes.

- Popular magazine articles, best-selling books, Internet websites, television news reports, and other forms of media are often unreliable sources of nutrition information. Consumers need to be careful and question the reliability of such sources, because the First Amendment to the U.S. Constitution guarantees freedom of the press and freedom of speech.

- Consumers need to ask questions to determine the author's reasons for promoting the information. Consumers should also look for red flags, such as scare tactics and claims that sound too good to be true.

- Much of the nutrition information that is on the Internet is unreliable and intended to promote sales. Websites sponsored by nonprofit organizations, nationally recognized health associations, government agencies, and nationally accredited colleges and universities are generally reliable sources of information.

2.3 Reliable Nutrition Experts

- Although some states regulate and license nutritionists, there is no standard legal definition for "nutritionist" in the United States. For reliable food, nutrition, and dietary information, consumers can consult persons with degrees in human nutrition from accredited institutions of higher learning, such as nutrition instructors and registered dietitian nutritionists.

2.4 Nutrition Matters: What Are Dietary Supplements?

- A dietary supplement is a product (other than tobacco) that adds to a person's dietary intake, contains one or more dietary ingredients, is taken by mouth in tablet or other forms, and may be a concentrate, metabolite, constituent, or extract.

- Dietary supplements include nutrient pills, protein powders, and herbal extracts. In many instances, people do not need dietary supplements. Healthy people should focus on obtaining nutrients and phytochemicals from foods, particularly fruits, vegetables, and whole-grain cereals. Before taking a dietary supplement, discuss the matter with your physician.

Recipe for 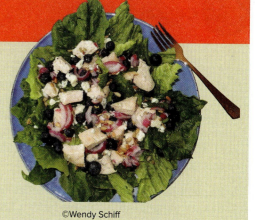 Healthy Living

Blueberry Chicken Salad

You probably have enjoyed eating fresh ripe blueberries that have been sprinkled on cereal or baked into pies. Blueberries, however, may have medicinal uses. Some people use blueberries and blueberry leaves to make remedies for a variety of common ailments, including diarrhea, sore throat, and fever. Currently, scientists are studying the effectiveness of using blueberry leaf extracts to lower high blood sugar levels in people with diabetes.[20] More research is needed to determine the safety and effectiveness of using blueberries or blueberry leaves as medicines.

The following blueberry salad recipe provides a single serving and supplies approximately 540 kcal, 50 g of protein, 9 g of fiber, 36 mg of vitamin C, and 520 RAE of vitamin A.

©Wendy Schiff

INGREDIENTS:

3 Tbsp Italian salad dressing
1/4 cup chopped red onion
3 cups romaine lettuce (small bunch), lightly packed into measuring cup
1 cup raw spinach leaves, lightly packed
1 cup, cooked, cubed, chilled chicken or turkey meat
3/4 cup fresh blueberries
1 Tbsp unsalted, roasted sunflower seeds
2 Tbsp crumbled blue cheese
Pinch of ground black pepper

PREPARATION STEPS:

1. Place chopped red onion in a small bowl and pour the Italian salad dressing over the onions. Set aside.

2. Wash greens in cold water and pat dry. Tear lettuce and spinach into small pieces, toss greens together, and arrange them on a dinner plate to form a "bed."

3. Place chopped, cooked poultry on top of the greens. Add crumbled blue cheese and blueberries.

4. Pour red onion and salad dressing mixture over the salad. Sprinkle with sunflower seeds and add dash of black pepper. Serve immediately.

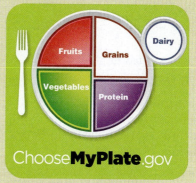

ChooseMyPlate.gov

Source: U.S. Dept. of Agriculture

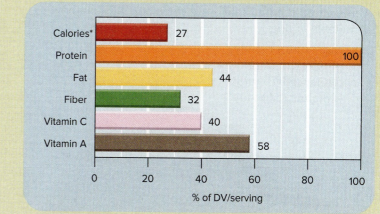

*2000 daily total kcal

Critical Thinking

1. An online health news source reports the results of a study in which people who took fish oil and vitamin E supplements daily did not reduce their risk of heart attack. Moreover, the researchers stopped the study when they determined the supplements increased the subjects' risk of stroke! Explain how you would determine whether this information is reliable.

2. Explain how you can verify the reliability of advice about dietary supplements provided at an Internet website.

3. Design a study that involves observing a nutrition-related practice of college students, such as vending machine choices or fast-food preferences, and share your idea with the class. Your study should be designed so that it is ethical and does not harm subjects physically or psychologically.

4. A group of scientists conduct a study to determine risk factors for breast cancer. According to their results, women who consume soy foods have a lower risk of breast cancer than women who do not eat soy foods. Think of two questions this finding is likely to generate that could be answered by further scientific investigation.

5. Browse through popular health-related magazines to find an article or advertisement that relates to nutrition, and make a copy of the article or advertisement. Analyze each sentence or line of the article or advertisement for signs of unreliability. Is the article or advertisement a reliable source of information? Explain why it is or why it is not.

Practice Test

Select the best answer.

1. The first step of the scientific method usually involves
   a. gathering data.
   b. developing a hypothesis.
   c. identifying relationships between variables.
   d. making observations.

2. A team of scientists conducts a survey of 1000 people who are between 60 and 75 years of age to determine whether their past consumption of seafood may have influenced their current state of health. This study is an example of a(an)
   a. case-control study.
   b. prospective study.
   c. retrospective study.
   d. experimental study.

3. An aspect of _____ involves studying causes of health problems in a population.
   a. epidemiology
   b. technobiology
   c. diseasiology
   d. censusology

4. Comparing individuals with type 2 diabetes to individuals who have very similar characteristics but are healthy would be an example of a
   a. prospective study.
   b. case-control study.
   c. retrospective study.
   d. double-blind study.

5. Generally, epidemiological studies
   a. establish causation.
   b. prove correlations.
   c. cannot determine cause-and-effect relationships.
   d. are experimental-based research efforts that examine two variables.

6. Which of the following journals does not have peer-reviewed articles?
   a. *Journal of the American Medical Association*
   b. *The New England Journal of Medicine*
   c. *Journal of the American College of Nutrition*
   d. *Men's Journal*

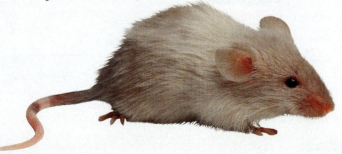

7. The government agency that enforces consumer protection laws by investigating false or misleading health-related claims is the

   a. Federal Trade Commission (FTC).
   b. Environmental Protection Agency (EPA).
   c. Agricultural Research Service (ARS).
   d. Centers for Disease Control and Prevention (CDC).

8. A testimonial is

   a. an unbiased report about a product's value.
   b. a scientifically valid claim.
   c. a personal endorsement of a product.
   d. a form of scientific evidence.

9. Which of the following websites is most likely to provide biased and unreliable nutrition information?

   a. The site of a nationally recognized health association (*.org)
   b. A site that promotes or sells dietary supplements (*.com)
   c. The site of a U.S. government agency (*.gov)
   d. An accredited college or university's site (*.edu)

10. A fake treatment is a(an)

   a. anecdote.
   b. double-blind study.
   c. pseudoscience experiment.
   d. placebo.

11. Which of the following substances would be classified as a dietary supplement according to the Dietary Supplement Health and Education Act of 1994?

   a. Tobacco   c. Chicken liver
   b. Melatonin   d. Plain yogurt

12. The _____ is the federal agency that tries to ensure the safety and effectiveness of health-related products.

   a. FDA   c. EPA
   b. FTC   d. USGS

13. Which of the following activities is an alternative health care practice?

   a. Drinking green tea to lose weight
   b. Taking ibuprofen to treat a headache
   c. Consuming more calcium-rich foods to help increase bone mass
   d. Eating fewer salty snacks to reduce sodium intake

Answers to Quiz Yourself

1. Scientists use anecdotes as scientific evidence to support their findings. **False.** (Section 2.1)

2. Popular health-related magazines typically publish articles that have been peer-reviewed. **False.** (Section 2.2)

3. By conducting a prospective epidemiological study, medical researchers can determine risk factors that may influence health. **True.** (Section 2.1)

4. Dietary supplements include vitamin pills as well as products that contain echinacea, ginseng, and garlic. **True.** (Section 2.4)

5. In general, registered dietitian nutritionists are reliable sources of food and nutrition information. **True.** (Section 2.3)

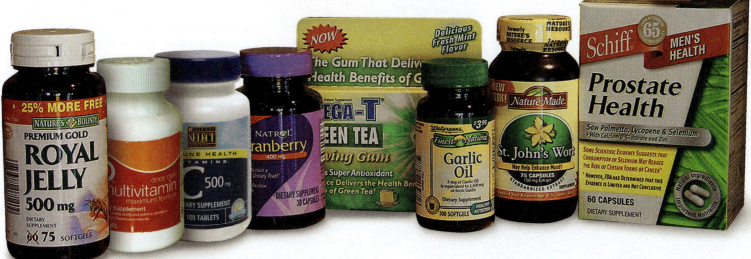

©Wendy Schiff

CHAPTER 3

Planning Nutritious Diets

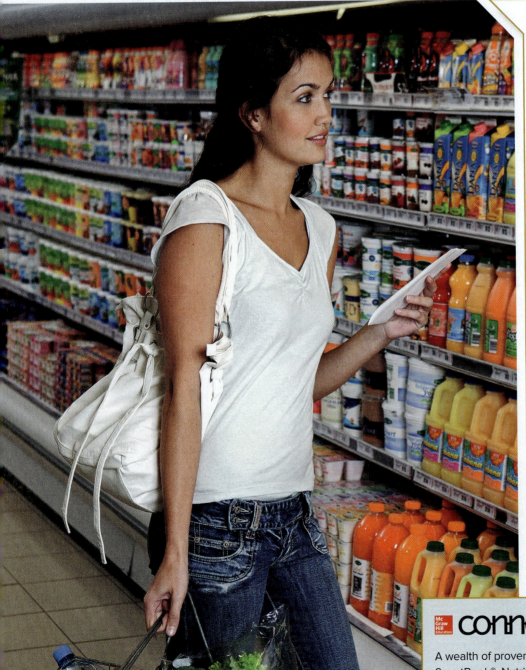

Quiz Yourself

Before reading the rest of Chapter 3, test your knowledge of dietary standards, recommendations, and guides, as well as nutrient labels, by taking the following quiz. The answers are at the end of the chapter.

1. According to the latest U.S. Department of Agriculture food guide, fruits and vegetables are combined into one food group. _____ T _____ F

2. According to the recommendations of the *2015–2020 Dietary Guidelines for Americans,* it is acceptable for certain adults to consume alcoholic beverages in moderation. _____ T _____ F

3. Last week, Colin didn't consume the recommended amount of vitamin C for a couple of days. Nevertheless, he is unlikely to develop scurvy, the vitamin C deficiency disease. _____ T _____ F

4. The Food and Drug Administration develops Dietary Guidelines for Americans. _____ T _____ F

5. The Nutrition Facts panel on a food label provides information concerning amounts of energy, fiber, and sodium that are in a serving of the food. _____ T _____ F

McGraw Hill Education **connect®**

A wealth of proven resources are available on Connect® including SmartBook®, NutritionCalc Plus, and many other dynamic learning tools. Ask your instructor about Connect!

3.1 From Requirements to Standards

Learning Outcomes

1 Explain the difference between a dietary requirement and a dietary allowance.

2 Identify the various dietary standards and explain how they can be used.

When you shop for groceries, do you sometimes feel overwhelmed by the vast array of foods that are available? If your answer is yes, your response is not surprising, considering the typical supermarket offered an average of 39,500 items in 2015.[1] Every time you enter a supermarket, you are likely to find food items that were not on the shelves during your last visit to the store. In 2016, for example, over 21,430 new food and beverage products were introduced into the marketplace.[2]

Chapter 1 introduced some key nutrition concepts, including the need for dietary adequacy, moderation, balance, and a variety of foods. Chapter 2 described how you can become a more careful consumer of nutrition information. However, you are also a consumer of food. With so many grocery items from which to choose, what are the primary factors that influence your food purchases? Do you select foods simply because they taste good, are reasonably priced, or are easy to prepare? Do you ever consider the effects certain foods may have on your health before you purchase them?

Your lifestyle reflects your health—related behaviors, including your dietary practices and physical activity habits. Americans of all ages may reduce their risk of chronic disease by adopting nutritious diets and engaging in regular physical activity. However, consumers need practical advice to help them make decisions that can promote more healthy lifestyles.

Chapter 3 discusses dietary standards, including how the standards are established and used. The information in this chapter also presents practical ways to plan a nutritionally adequate, well—balanced diet using tools such as the Dietary Guidelines and MyPlate. Furthermore, Section 3.5 explains how to interpret and use nutrition—related information that appears on food and dietary supplement labels.

What Is a Nutrient Requirement?

requirement smallest amount of a nutrient that maintains a defined level of nutritional health

By using research methods discussed in Chapter 2, scientists have been able to estimate the amount of many nutrients required by the body. A **requirement** can be defined as the smallest amount of a nutrient that maintains a defined level of nutritional health.[3] In general, this amount, when consumed daily, prevents the nutrient's deficiency disease. The requirement for a particular nutrient varies to some degree from person to person. A person's age, sex, general health status, physical activity level, and use of medications and drugs are among the factors that influence his or her nutrient requirements.

Many nutrients are stored in the body, including vitamin D and most minerals. Major storage sites include the liver, body fat, and bones. Other nutrients, such as vitamin C and most B vitamins, are not stored by the body. For optimal nutrition, you need to consume enough of those nutrients to maintain storage levels. Your body uses its nutrient stores much like you can

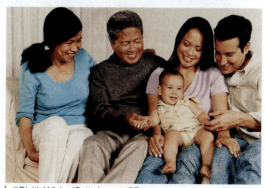

use a savings account to help manage your money. When you have some extra cash, it is wise to place the money in a savings account, so you can withdraw some of the reserves to meet future needs without going into debt. When your consumption of certain nutrients is more than enough to meet your needs, the body stores the excess. When your intake of a stored nutrient is low or needs for this nutrient become increased, such as during recovery from illness, your body withdraws some from storage. As a result of having optimal levels of stored nutrients, you may recover more quickly and avoid or delay developing deficiencies of those nutrients.

Dietary Reference Intakes

Dietary Reference Intakes (DRIs) various energy and nutrient intake standards for Americans

Food and Nutrition Board (FNB) group of nutrition scientists who develop DRIs

Estimated Average Requirement (EAR) amount of a nutrient that meets the needs of 50% of healthy people in a life stage/sex group

Estimated Energy Requirement (EER) average daily energy intake that meets the needs of a healthy person maintaining his or her weight

Dietary Reference Intakes (DRIs) encompass a variety of daily energy and nutrient intake standards that nutrition experts in the United States use as references when making dietary recommendations. DRIs are intended to help people reduce their risk of nutrient deficiencies and excesses, prevent disease, and achieve optimal health.[4] The standards (Fig. 3.1) are the Estimated Average Requirement (EAR), which includes Estimated Energy Requirement (EER); Recommended Dietary Allowance (RDA), Adequate Intake (AI), and Tolerable Upper Intake Level (UL).

A group of nutrition scientists, the **Food and Nutrition Board (FNB)** of the Institute of Medicine, develops DRIs. Periodically, members of the board adjust DRIs as new information concerning human nutritional needs and dietary adequacy becomes available. You can find tables for the latest DRIs in Appendix I of this book. The following sections provide basic information about the various DRI standards. It is important to become familiar with these terms because we refer to them in this and other chapters.

Estimated Average Requirement

An **Estimated Average Requirement (EAR)** is the daily amount of the nutrient that meets the needs of 50% of healthy people who are in a particular *life stage/sex group*. Life stage/sex groups classify people according to age, sex, and whether females are pregnant or breastfeeding. A typical 20-year-old female college student, for example, would be classified as a female, between 19 and 30 years old, and not pregnant or breastfeeding.

To establish an EAR for a nutrient, the Food and Nutrition Board identifies a physiological marker, a substance in the body that reflects proper functioning and can be measured. This marker indicates whether the level of a nutrient in the body is adequate. A marker for vitamin C, for example, is the amount of the vitamin in certain blood cells. When these cells contain nearly all the vitamin C they can hold, the body has an optimal supply of the vitamin. Thus, a physician can diagnose whether a patient is vitamin C deficient by taking a blood sample from the person and measuring the vitamin C content of certain blood cells.

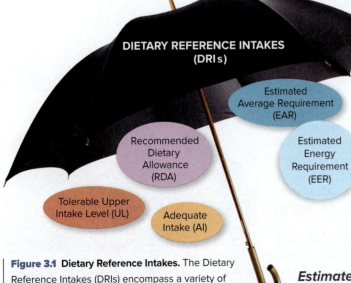

Figure 3.1 Dietary Reference Intakes. The Dietary Reference Intakes (DRIs) encompass a variety of terms that represent standards for energy and nutrient recommendations.

©Ryan McVay/Getty Images RF

Estimated Energy Requirement   The **Estimated Energy Requirement (EER)** is the average daily energy intake that meets the needs of a healthy person who is maintaining his or her weight. Registered dietitian nutritionists (RDNs) can use EERs to evaluate an individual's energy intake. The EER takes into account the person's physical activity level, height, and weight, as well as sex and life stage. Because the EER is an average figure, some people have energy needs that are higher or lower. Chapter 10 provides formulas for calculating your EER.

Recommended Dietary Allowances

The **Recommended Dietary Allowances (RDAs)** are standards for recommending daily intakes of several nutrients. RDAs meet the nutrient needs of nearly all healthy individuals (97 to 98%) in a particular life stage/sex group. To establish an RDA for a nutrient, nutrition scientists first determine its EAR. Then scientists add a "margin of safety" amount to the EAR that allows for individual variations in nutrient needs and helps maintain tissue stores (Fig. 3.2). For example, the adult EAR for vitamin C is 60 mg for women who are not pregnant or breastfeeding and 75 mg for men.[3] However, the adult RDA for vitamin C is 15 mg higher than the EAR: 75 mg for women who are not pregnant or breastfeeding and 90 mg for men. Thus, the margin of safety for vitamin C is 15 mg. Because smoking cigarettes increases the need for vitamin C, smokers should add 35 mg to their RDA for the nutrient.

Adequate Intakes

In some instances, nutrition scientists are unable to develop RDAs for nutrients because there is not enough information to determine how much is required by people. Until such information becomes available, scientists set **Adequate Intakes (AIs)** for these nutrients. To establish an AI, scientists record eating patterns of a group of healthy people and estimate the group's average daily intake of the nutrient. If the people who are being observed show no signs of the nutrient's deficiency disorder, the researchers conclude that the average level of intake must be adequate and use that value as the AI (Fig. 3.3). Vitamin K is one of the nutrients that has an AI instead of an RDA.

Tolerable Upper Intake Level

Nutrition scientists also establish a **Tolerable Upper Intake Level (Upper Level or UL)** for many vitamins and minerals. The UL is the highest average amount of a nutrient that is unlikely to harm most people when they consume that amount daily (see Fig. 3.3).[4] The risk of a toxicity disorder increases when a person regularly consumes amounts of a nutrient that is more than its UL. The UL for vitamin C, for example, is 2000 mg/day for adults.

Acceptable Macronutrient Distribution Ranges

The results of scientific research suggest that food energy sources (macronutrients) are associated with risk of developing certain diet–related chronic diseases, such as heart disease. **Acceptable Macronutrient Distribution Ranges (AMDRs)** indicate ranges of carbohydrate, fat, and protein intakes that provide adequate amounts of vitamins and minerals and may reduce the risk of diet–related chronic diseases.[4] The AMDR for carbohydrates, for example, is 45 to 65% of total energy intake. If a person's total energy intake is 2300 kcal/day, then his or her recommended carbohydrate intake is 1035 to 1495 kcal/day. To obtain the range of energy from carbohydrate, multiply total kcal/day (in this case, 2300 kcal) by 0.45 (45%) and then multiply

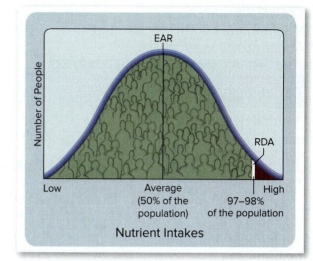

Figure 3.2 Establishing RDAs. A nutrient's RDA is high enough to meet or exceed the requirements of 97 to 98% of the population for the nutrient. In other words, about 98% of the population will have their needs for the nutrient met by just consuming the RDA amount.

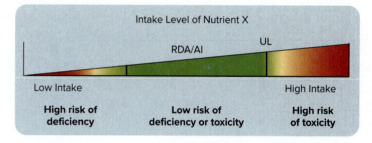

Figure 3.3 Adequate Intakes and Upper Limits. Consuming too much or not enough of a nutrient can cause health problems.

Recommended Dietary Allowances (RDAs) standards for recommending daily intakes of several nutrients

Adequate Intakes (AIs) dietary recommendations for nutrients that scientists do not have enough information about to set RDAs

Tolerable Upper Intake Level (Upper Level or UL) highest average amount of a nutrient that is unlikely to be harmful when consumed daily

Acceptable Macronutrient Distribution Ranges (AMDRs) macronutrient intake ranges that are nutritionally adequate and may reduce the risk of diet-related chronic diseases

TABLE 3.1 Acceptable Macronutrient Distribution Ranges: Adults (2000 kcal/day)

Macronutrient	AMDR (% of total energy intake)	Calories
Carbohydrate	45–65	900–1300
Protein	10–35	200–700
*Fat**	20–35	400–700

*Fat intake should include essential fatty acids (see Chapter 6).

2300 kcal by 0.65 (65%). Table 3.1 lists adult AMDRs for a person who consumes 2000 kcal/day.

Applying Nutrient Standards

Table 3.2 summarizes information about the DRIs. RDNs refer to DRIs for planning nutritious diets for groups of people and evaluating the nutritional adequacy of a population's diet. Nevertheless, RDAs and AIs are often used to evaluate an individual's dietary practices.[4] Your diet is likely to be nutritionally adequate if your average daily intake for each nutrient meets the nutrient's RDA or AI value. If your diet consistently supplies less than the EAR for a nutrient, you may be at risk of eventually developing the nutrient's deficiency disorder (see Fig. 3.3). On the other hand, if your intake of a nutrient is consistently above its UL, you are at risk of developing that nutrient's toxicity disorder. Nutrient toxicity disorders are more likely to occur when people take high doses of individual nutrient supplements, particularly vitamins and minerals. If you do not take large doses of nutrient supplements and you eat reasonable amounts of food, your risk of developing a nutrient toxicity disorder is low.

Nutritional standards have a variety of commercial applications. Pharmaceutical companies refer to DRIs when developing formulas that replace breast milk for infants and special formulas for people who cannot consume regular foods. As a result, babies can be nourished by consuming commercially prepared formulas, and adults who are unable to swallow can survive for years on formula feedings administered through tubes inserted into their bodies.

For nutrition labeling purposes, the Food and Drug Administration (FDA) uses RDAs to develop a set of standards called *Daily Values (DVs)*. Consumers may find DVs useful for comparing the nutritional contents of similar foods. The "Food and Dietary Supplement Labels" section of this chapter provides more information about nutritional labeling, including DVs.

TABLE 3.2 Summary of Dietary Reference Intakes

Standard	Definition	Example
Estimated Average Requirement (EAR)	Amount of a nutrient that meets the needs of 50% of healthy people who are in a particular life stage/sex group	**Vitamin C** 75 mg/day for males and 60 mg/day for females ages 19 through 50 years
Recommended Dietary Allowance (RDA)	Amount of a nutrient that meets the needs of nearly all healthy individuals (97.5%) in a particular life stage/sex group	**Vitamin C** 90 mg/day for males (nonsmokers) and 75 mg/day for females ages 19 through 50 years (nonsmokers)
Adequate Intake (AI)	Amount of a nutrient that is considered to be adequate based on the population's typical intakes, but there is not enough scientific information available to determine an RDA for the nutrient at this time	**Vitamin C** 40 mg/day for infants from birth through 6 months of age
Tolerable Upper Intake Level or Upper Limit (UL)	Highest average amount of a nutrient that is unlikely to harm most people when the amount is consumed daily	**Vitamin C** 2000 mg/day for adults
Acceptable Macronutrient Distribution Range (AMDR)	Range of carbohydrate, fat, and protein intakes that provide adequate amounts of micronutrients and may reduce the risk of developing certain diet-related chronic diseases	See Table 3.1

Concept CHECKPOINT

1. What is the difference between an RDA and an AI?
2. Describe how scientists establish the RDA for a nutrient.
3. Explain how an EER differs from an RDA or AI.
4. Discuss how registered dietitian nutritionists, pharmaceutical companies, and the FDA use nutrient standards.

See Appendix G for responses.

3.2 Major Food Groups

Learning Outcome

1 List major food groups, and identify foods that are typically classified in each group.

For most people, the DRIs are not practical for planning menus, so nutrition experts develop more consumer—friendly food (dietary) guides. In general, such guides classify foods into major food groups according to their natural origins and key nutrients. Major food groups are usually grains, dairy products, fruits, vegetables, and protein—rich foods. In most instances, dietary guides also provide recommendations concerning amounts of foods from each group that should be eaten daily. The following points identify major food groups and summarize key features of each group.

- *Grains* include products made from wheat, rice, and oats. Pasta, noodles, and flour tortillas are members of this group because wheat flour is their main ingredient. In general, a serving of a grain food is equivalent to 1 slice of bread, 1 cup of ready—to—eat cereal, or ½ cup of cooked rice, pasta, or cereal such as oatmeal. Although corn is a type of grain, it is often used as a vegetable in meals. Cornmeal and popcorn, however, are usually grouped with grain products.

  Carbohydrate (starch) and protein are the primary macronutrients in grains. In the United States, refined grain products can also be good sources of several vitamins and minerals when they have undergone enrichment or fortification. In general, **enrichment** replaces some of the nutrients that were lost during processing. **Fortification** is the addition of any nutrient to food to boost its nutrient content, such as adding calcium to orange juice, vitamins A and D to milk, and numerous vitamins and minerals to ready—to—eat break—fast cereals. When grains undergo processing, they can lose nutrients, particularly vitamins, minerals, and fiber. Enriched grains have specific amounts of iron and four B vitamins added to them. Although these nutrients are replaced, other nutrients that were lost during refinement are not replaced.

  Dietary guides generally recommend choosing foods made with whole grains instead of refined grains. According to the FDA, whole grains are the intact, ground, cracked, or flaked seeds of cereal grains, such as wheat, buckwheat, oats, corn, rice, wild rice, rye, and barley.[5] Compared to refined grain products, foods made from whole grains naturally contain more fiber as well as micronutrients that are not replaced during enrichment.

- *Dairy foods* include milk and products made from milk that retain (keep) their calcium content after processing, such as yogurt and hard cheeses. Dairy foods are also excellent sources of protein, phosphorus (a mineral), and riboflavin (a B vitamin). Most of the milk sold in the United States is fortified with vitamins A and D, so it is a good source of these vitamins.

  Foods and beverages made from soybeans (soy "milk" and soy "cheese") can substitute for cow's milk if they are fortified with calcium and other

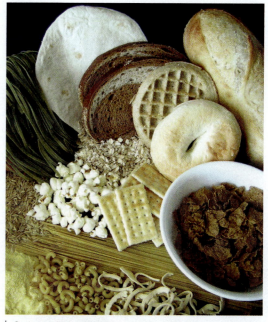

Grains include products made from wheat, rice, corn, barley, and oats. ©Wendy Schiff

enrichment replacement of some nutrients that were removed during processing

fortification addition of any nutrient to food to boost its nutritional content

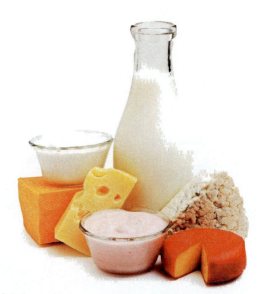

Dairy products, especially yogurt and hard cheeses, are excellent sources of calcium, protein, phosphorus, and riboflavin. Additionally, milk is often fortified with vitamins A and D. ©D. Hurst/Alamy RF

micronutrients. Milk—based desserts such as ice cream, pudding, and frozen yogurt are often grouped with dairy foods, even though they often have high added sugar and fat contents. Although cream cheese, cream, and butter are made from cow's milk, they are not included in this group because they have little or no calcium and are high in fat.

Most dietary guides, including MyPlate (U.S. Department of Agriculture [USDA]) recommend choosing dairy products that have most of the fat removed, such as fat—free or low—fat milk. (Fat—free milk may also be referred to as non—fat or skim milk.) Compared to whole milk, which is about 3.25% fat by weight, low—fat milk contains only 1% fat by weight and is often called "1% milk."

According to the USDA, 1 cup of fat—free milk generally substitutes for 1 cup of plain, low—fat yogurt or frozen yogurt; 2 cups of low—fat cottage cheese; 1½ ounces of natural cheese such as Swiss or cheddar; or 2 ounces of processed cheese, such as American cheese. To obtain about the same amount of calcium as in 1 cup of fat—free milk, you would have to eat almost 1⅔ cups of regular vanilla ice cream. This amount of ice cream provides 490 kcal and about 26 g of fat, whereas 1 cup of fat—free milk supplies about 85 kcal and less than 1 g of fat.

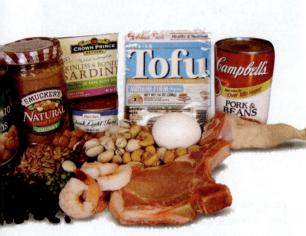

Dry beans, peas, eggs, tofu, nuts, and seeds are protein-rich foods that can substitute for meat.
©Wendy Schiff

- *Protein—rich foods* include beef, pork, lamb, fish, shellfish, liver, and poultry. Beans, eggs, nuts, and seeds are included with this group because these protein—rich foods can substitute for meats. According to the USDA, a serving of food from this group generally equals 1 ounce of meat, poultry, or fish; ¼ cup cooked dry beans or dry peas; 1 egg; 1 tablespoon of peanut butter; or ½ ounce of nuts or seeds. One—fourth cup of tofu, a food made from soybeans, can substitute for 1 ounce of meat, fish, or poultry.

  Foods in the protein group are rich sources of micronutrients, especially iron, zinc, and B vitamins. In general, the body absorbs minerals, such as iron and zinc, more easily from animal foods than from plants.

- *Fruits* include fresh, dried, frozen, sauced, and canned fruit, as well as 100% fruit juice. According to the USDA, 1 serving of food from this group generally equals 1 cup of fruit or fruit juice, or ½ cup of dried fruit, such as raisins or dried apricots.[6] Most fruits are low in fat and good sources of phytochemicals and micronutrients, especially the mineral potassium and vitamins C and folate. Additionally, whole or cut—up fruit is a good source of fiber. Although 100% juice is a source of phytochemicals and can count toward one's fruit intake, the majority of choices from this group should be whole or cut—up fruits.[7] Whole or cut—up fruits are healthier options than juices because they contain more dietary fiber.

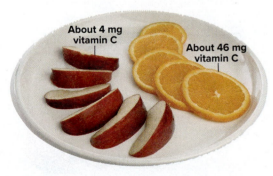

About 4 mg vitamin C

About 46 mg vitamin C

Figure 3.4 Comparing apples to oranges. The nutritional content of foods within each group often varies widely.
©McGraw-Hill Education. Christopher Kerrigan, photographer

- *Vegetables* include fresh, cooked, canned, frozen, and dried/dehydrated vegetables, and 100% vegetable juice. Vegetables may be further grouped into dark green, orange, and starchy categories. Some guides include dried beans and peas in the vegetable group as well as in the meat and meat substitutes group. According to the USDA, 1 serving of food from this group generally equals 1 cup of raw or cooked vegetables, 1 cup vegetable juice, or 2 cups of uncooked leafy greens, such as salad greens. This means if you eat 1 cup of raw carrots and drink 1 cup of tomato juice, you have consumed 2 servings from the vegetables group. Many vegetables are good sources of micronutrients, fiber, and phytochemicals. Furthermore, many vegetables are naturally low in fat and energy.

It is important to note that the nutritional content of foods within each group often varies widely. For example, 3.5 ounces of fresh sliced apples and 3.5 ounces of fresh orange slices each supply about 50 kcal. However, the apples contribute about 4 mg of vitamin C, whereas oranges supply about 46 mg of the vitamin to diets (Fig. 3.4). Therefore, dietary guides generally recommend that people choose a variety of foods from each food group when planning daily meals and snacks.

Other Foods

Food guides may include an oils group. Oils include canola, corn, and olive oils, as well as other fats that are liquid at room temperature. Certain spreadable foods made from vegetable oils, such as mayonnaise, soft or "tub" margarine, and salad dressing, are also classified as oils. Peanuts and peanut butter, walnuts, sunflower seeds, olives, avocados, and some types of fish have high fat contents, but these kinds of fat are "healthy" fats that do not contribute to heart disease (see Chapter 6). Some food guides group these foods with oils. Oils are often good sources of fat soluble vitamins.

Solid fats, such as beef fat, butter, stick margarine, and shortening, are fairly hard at room temperature. Solid fat is a source of "unhealthy" *saturated* fats that are associated with an increased risk of cardiovascular disease (CVD). Although cream and coconut oil are liquid or soft at room temperature, these foods are classified as solid fats because they are rich sources of saturated fat. Chapter 6 discusses how dietary fats can affect health.

Sugary foods ("sweets") include candy, regular soft drinks, jelly, and other foods that contain high amounts of sugar added during processing or preparation. Sugary foods and beverages typically supply energy but few or no micronutrients. The alcohol in alcohol—containing beverages is another source of empty calories.

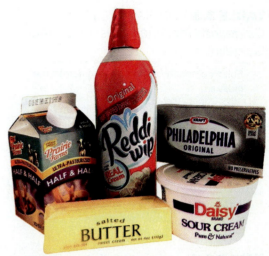
©Wendy Schiff

solid fats fats that are fairly hard at room temperature

Concept CHECKPOINT

5. List at least three foods that are generally classified as grain products.

6. What is the difference between nutrient fortification and nutrient enrichment?

7. List at least four foods that are generally classified as dairy products.

8. Why are dry beans often classified with meat?

9. According to the information in this section of Chapter 3, how many cups of dried apricots are nutritionally equivalent to 2 cups of fresh apricots?

10. Most dietary guides classify eggs and nuts with meat. Why?

11. Identify at least two foods that are classified as solid fat.

See Appendix G for responses.

3.3 Dietary Guidelines

Learning Outcome

1 List at least four overarching guidelines of the *2015–2020 Dietary Guidelines for Americans,* and provide recommendations of each one.

2 Identify features of a healthy eating pattern.

3 Apply the Dietary Guidelines to improve the nutritional quality of diets.

Heart disease, cancer, hypertension (chronically elevated blood pressure), and diabetes mellitus (commonly referred to as *diabetes*) are among the leading causes of disability and death among Americans. According to a considerable amount of scientific evidence, risk of these diseases is strongly linked with certain lifestyles, particularly poor dietary choices and lack of regular physical activity. As required by law, the U.S. Department of Health and Human Services (USDHHS) and the USDA publish the Dietary Guidelines for Americans (Dietary Guidelines), a set of general nutrition—related lifestyle recommendations that are intended for healthy people over 2 years of age.[8] The Dietary Guidelines are designed to promote good health and reduce the risk of major nutrition—related

TABLE 3.3 *2015–2020 Dietary Guidelines for Americans*: Overarching Guidelines

- Follow a healthy eating pattern across the lifespan.
- Focus on variety, nutrient density, and amount of food.
- Limit calories from added sugars and saturated fats and reduce sodium intake.
- Shift to healthier food and beverage choices.
- Support healthy eating patterns for all.

TABLE 3.4 A Healthy Eating Pattern

Includes:

- A variety of vegetables;
- Fruits, especially whole fruits;
- Grains, especially whole grains;
- Fat-free or low-fat dairy products;
- A variety of protein foods; and
- Oils.

A healthy eating pattern limits:

- Saturated fats and trans fats, added sugars, and sodium.

chronic health conditions, such as obesity and cardiovascular disease. These guidelines are updated every 5 years.

The Dietary Guidelines form the basis of the federal government's nutrition policy, which serves as a framework for national, state, and local health promotion as well as food and nutrition programs. Dietary Guidelines are also used for menu planning by individuals and health care professionals.[8] Furthermore, food and beverage manufacturers can apply the guidelines to develop healthier products that appeal to consumers.

To revise the 2010 version of the dietary guidelines, officials with the USDHHS and the USDA appointed a Dietary Guidelines Advisory Committee (DGAC) comprised of nationally recognized medical and nutrition experts. DGAC members reviewed the scientific evidence concerning the role of foods in health before preparing the *Scientific Report of the 2015 Dietary Guidelines Advisory Committee*.[9] This publication contained recommendations for the development of the *2015–2020 Dietary Guidelines for Americans*. In February 2015, the overseeing government agencies made the DGAC report available for the public to read and provide input.

According to the DGAC report, a healthy diet contains more fruits, vegetables, whole grains, low- or nonfat dairy products, seafood, legumes, and nuts than the typical diet of the general American population.[9] Additionally, a healthy diet contains fewer refined grains, red and processed meats, less sodium, and fewer sugar-sweetened foods and beverages than the typical American eating pattern. Such eating patterns should be flexible so food choices can be varied and individualized to meet a person's preferences, medical needs, and economic situation. The federal government incorporated some but not all of the DGAC's recommendations into the *2015–2020 Dietary Guidelines for Americans*.[8]

Table 3.3 indicates the overarching guidelines of the 2015–2020 Dietary Guidelines, which focus on encouraging healthy eating patterns. Table 3.4 lists key components of a healthy eating pattern, according to the Dietary Guidelines. The following information includes recommendations about each overarching guideline.[8] You can learn more about the Dietary Guidelines by visiting: http://health.gov/dietaryguidelines/2015/guidelines/.

Follow a Healthy Eating Pattern Across the Lifespan

- All food and beverage choices matter.
- People should choose a healthy eating pattern that has an appropriate number of calories to achieve and maintain a healthy body weight, is nutritionally adequate, and reduces the risk of diet-related chronic diseases.

Focus on Variety, Nutrient Density, and Amount of Food

To meet nutrient needs within calorie limits, choose a variety of nutrient-dense foods from all food groups and consume recommended amounts.

- Consume a variety of vegetables from all subgroups, including dark green, red, and orange vegetables; legumes (beans and peas); starchy; and other vegetables.
- Consume a variety of fruits, especially whole fruits.
- Consume grains, at least half of which are whole grains.
- Consume fat-free or low-fat dairy foods, including milk, yogurt, cheese, and/or fortified soy products.
- Eat a variety of protein foods, including seafood, lean meats and poultry, eggs, legumes, nuts, seeds, and soy products.
- Consume oils or cook with oils.

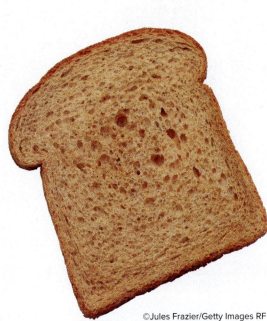
©Jules Frazier/Getty Images RF

Limit Calories from Added Sugars and Saturated Fats, and Reduce Sodium Intake

- Consume less than 10% of daily calories from added sugars. Added sugars contribute calories to foods and beverages, but they lack essential nutrients. For people consuming 2000 kcal per day, the upper limit of 10% of total calories is 200 kcal, the amount of energy in about 12 teaspoons of sugar.
- Consume less than 10% of daily calories from saturated fats.
- Consume less than 2300 mg of sodium per day. Increased sodium intake is associated with increased risk of hypertension and cardiovascular disease. Salt is the major source of sodium in diets.

Shift to Healthier Food and Beverage Choices

- Choose nutrient–dense foods and beverages from all food groups to replace less healthy products.
- Consider cultural and personal preferences when shifting foods and beverages to healthier choices.

Recommendations for Specific Population Groups

Women who can become pregnant, are pregnant, or are breastfeeding should:

- Consume 8 to 12 ounces of seafood per week from a variety of seafood types. Certain seafood contain fats that may improve an infant's health. Seafood that is rich in these particular fats includes salmon, herring, sardines, and trout.
- Not eat certain large fish, including shark, swordfish, and king mackerel, because they may contain high amounts of the toxic chemical methylmercury (see Chapter 13).
- Consume iron–rich foods or take an iron supplement, if recommended by a physician or other qualified health care provider. Iron is a "nutrient of public health concern" for pregnant females.
- Not consume alcohol.

To reduce the risk of birth defects, women who are capable of becoming pregnant should obtain 400 mcg of folic acid each day by consuming fortified foods and/or taking supplements that contain the vitamin.

Support Healthy Eating Patterns for All

- Everyone has a role in creating and supporting healthy eating patterns in multiple settings throughout the country.
- Health professionals and policymakers should use multiple strategies to promote healthy eating and physical activity behaviors across all segments of society. Such strategies can include developing educational resources that inspire individuals to take appropriate actions with regard to their food and beverage choices.

Applying the Dietary Guidelines

The Dietary Guidelines include several food and nutrition–related messages for consumers, such as "Consume more nutrient–dense vegetables" (Table 3.5). Table 3.6 suggests practical ways people can apply the Dietary Guidelines' recommendations to their usual food choices. However, making recommended dietary and other lifestyle changes does not always reduce risk factors for disease. For example, a man who has hypertension may find that his blood pressure

TABLE 3.5 Selected Messages from *2015–2020 Dietary Guidelines for Americans*

- Increase the variety of protein foods consumed, and incorporate about 8 ounces per week of various seafood into meals. Young children should eat less seafood than older children and adults.
- Consume more nutrient-dense vegetables.
- Choose more nutrient-dense fruits for snacks, desserts, or in side dishes.
- Choose enriched grain products and make at least half your grains whole grains.
- Choose lower fat versions of milk, yogurt, and cheese.
- Compare sodium in foods and choose the foods with the lowest sodium content.
- Drink water instead of sugary drinks.
- Choose foods that provide potassium, dietary fiber, calcium, and vitamin D, which are "nutrients of public health concern," because Americans tend to consume them in limited amounts.
- Achieve or maintain a healthy body weight.
- Consuming three to five 8-oz cups of coffee per day (up to 400 mg/day of caffeine) is acceptable within a healthy eating pattern.
- Consume as little cholesterol as possible while following a healthy diet.
- If one consumes alcohol, the beverage should be consumed in moderation and only by adults of legal drinking age. "Moderation" is up to one drink per day for women and up to two drinks per day for men. People should not begin to drink alcohol or drink more for any reason. Furthermore, certain individuals should not consume alcohol, especially pregnant women.

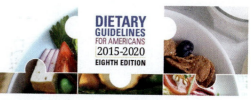

2015–2020 Dietary Guidelines for Americans. Source: U.S. Department of Agriculture, Center for Nutrition Policy and Promotion

remains dangerously elevated after several months of exercising, limiting his salt intake, and maintaining a healthy weight for his height. In this case, genetic factors may be influencing the man's health more than his lifestyle, and medication may be necessary to reduce his blood pressure.

©C Squared Studios/Getty Images RF

TABLE 3.6 Applying the Dietary Guidelines to One's Usual Food Choices

If One Usually Eats:	Consider Replacing with:
White bread and rolls	Whole-wheat bread and rolls
Sugary breakfast cereals	Low-sugar, high-fiber cereal sweetened with berries, bananas, peaches, or other fruit
Cheeseburger, French fries, and a regular (sugar-sweetened) soft drink	Roasted chicken or turkey sandwich, baked beans, fat-free or low-fat milk, or soy milk
Potato salad or cole slaw	Leafy greens or three-bean salad
Doughnuts, chips, or salty snack foods	Small bran muffin or whole-wheat bagel topped with peanut butter or soy nut butter, unsalted nuts, or dried fruit
Regular soft drinks	Water, fat-free or low-fat milk, or 100% fruit juice
Boiled vegetables	Raw or steamed vegetables (often retain more nutrients than boiled)
Breaded and fried meat, fish, or poultry	Broiled or roasted meat, fish, or poultry
Fatty meats such as barbecued ribs, sausage, and hot dogs	Chicken, turkey, or fish; lean meats such as ground round
Whole or 2% milk, cottage cheese with 4% fat, or yogurt made from whole milk	1% or fat-free milk, low-fat cottage cheese (1% fat), or low-fat yogurt
Ice cream	Frozen yogurt or "lite" ice cream
Cream cheese on a bagel	Low-fat cottage cheese (mashed) or reduced-fat cream cheese or peanut butter (if appropriate)
Creamy salad dressings or dips made with mayonnaise or sour cream	Oil and vinegar dressing, reduced-fat salad dressings, or dips made from low-fat sour cream or plain yogurt
Chocolate chip or cream-filled cookies	Fruit-filled bars, oatmeal cookies, or fresh fruit
Salt added to season foods	Herbs, spices, or lemon juice

Concept CHECKPOINT

Respond to the following points according to recommendations of the Dietary Guidelines (2015–2020 version).

12. What are two overarching guidelines of the Dietary Guidelines?

13. A healthy person who is 23 years of age should limit his sodium intake to less than _____ per day.

14. List at least three of the key recommendations of the Dietary Guidelines.

15. Replace solid fats with _____.

16. Consume less than _____% of total calories from saturated fat.

17. Consume less than _____ % of total calories from added sugars.

18. What percentage of your intake of grains foods should be whole grains?

19. An adult woman who drinks alcohol and is not pregnant should limit her alcohol intake to no more than _____ drink(s) per day.

20. Adult men who drink alcohol should limit their alcohol consumption to no more than _____ drink(s) per day.

21. Which nutrients are "of public health concern" in the American diet?

See Appendix G for responses.

©Jules Frazier/Getty Images RF

3.4 Food Guides

Learning Outcomes

1 Use MyPlate to develop nutritionally adequate daily menus.

2 Compare MyPlate with the Exchange System.

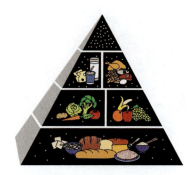

| **Figure 3.5** Food Guide Pyramid.

For over 100 years, the USDA has issued specific dietary recommendations for Americans. In 1943, the USDA published the first food guide based on RDAs for the general public to use. In the mid–1950s, the USDA simplified the original food guide to create the "Basic Four" food groups: milk, meats, fruits and vegetables, and breads and cereals. The recommendations of the Basic Four provided the foundation for an adequate diet. Although the food guide supplied only about 1200 to 1400 kcal/day, people could add extra servings of food to the basic diet plan if they had higher energy needs.

In 1992, the USDA introduced the Food Guide Pyramid (Fig. 3.5). Unlike earlier dietary guides, the Food Guide Pyramid incorporated knowledge about the health benefits and risks associated with certain foods and ranked food groups according to their emphasis in menu planning. The Food Guide Pyramid displayed the groups in a layered format with grain products at the base to establish the foundation for a healthy diet. Fruit and vegetable groups occupied the next layer of the Food Guide Pyramid, followed by a layer shared by the milk and milk products, and meat and meat substitutes groups. Fatty and sugary foods formed the small peak of the Pyramid, a visual reminder that people should limit their intake of these foods.

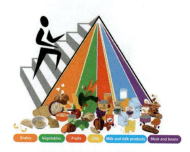

| **Figure 3.6** MyPyramid Plan.

Although the Food Guide Pyramid became a familiar feature on many packaged foods, the USDA released the *MyPyramid Plan* in 2005 (Fig. 3.6). The MyPyramid Plan was a *food guidance system*, which was based on *Dietary Guidelines for Americans, 2005*. In addition to providing foods and nutrition information, the MyPyramid.gov website emphasized the importance of physical activity and enabled consumers to monitor their activity levels. In 2011, the USDA replaced the MyPyramid Plan with *MyPlate*, another interactive dietary and menu planning guide accessible at a website.

MyPlate

MyPlate (www.choosemyplate.gov) includes a variety of food, nutrition, and physical activity resources for consumers that are based on the recommendations of the Dietary Guidelines. MyPlate differs from the Food Guide Pyramid and the MyPyramid Plan in that it no longer has six food groups shown in boxes or stripes within a pyramid (Fig. 3.7). MyPlate focuses on five different food groups: fruits, vegetables, protein foods, grains, and dairy. It is important to note that MyPlate does not have a portion of the plate for "oils" (see Figure 3.7). According to the USDA, "oils" is not a food group.[10] The government agency, however, notes the need for fat in the diet because some kinds of fat are dietary essentials.

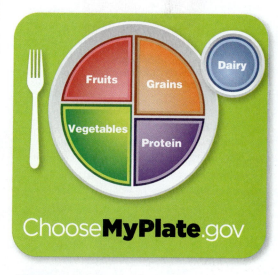

| **Figure 3.7** MyPlate. Source: U.S. Dept. of Agriculture

To learn more about MyPlate's five food groups, visit www.choosemyplate.gov and click on "MyPlate" in the menu bar to obtain a list of food groups. Click on each food group to find practical information about foods in the group, including how much food should be eaten, scientifically supported health benefits of foods, and helpful food–related tips. The site also has information and tips concerning weight management and calories, as well as physical activity.

Choosemyplate.gov has a wide variety of helpful interactive tools, including "SuperTracker," an excellent tool for developing nutritionally adequate daily food plans and recording and monitoring dietary intake and physical activity habits.

MyPlate USDA's interactive Internet dietary and menu planning guide

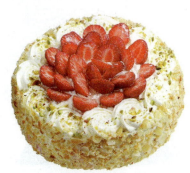

©Alamy Stock Photo RF

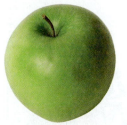

©Ingram Publishing/Alamy RF

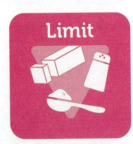

Source: USDA http://www
.www.choosemyplate.gov
/MyPlate-Daily-Checklist

The "Food Tracker" feature of SuperTracker enables people to determine the energy and nutrient contents of their favorite recipes.

Using MyPlate for Menu Planning

MyPlate has 12 different nutritionally adequate daily food patterns that supply from 1000 to 3200 kcal/day (https://www.choosemyplate.gov/MyPlate−Daily −Checklist−input). Each pattern can be individualized to meet various personal characteristics, including age, sex, physical activity level, and food likes and dislikes.

MyPlate dietary patterns include foods and beverages that contain little or no empty calories. After a person consumes recommended amounts of nutri− tious foods from each food group (and oils), a small number of calories remain. According to the Dietary Guidelines' healthy eating patterns, these extra calo− ries are "limits on calories for other uses."[8] The 2000 kcal dietary pattern, for example, has 270 kilocalories remaining, which is less than the energy in two 12−ounce sugar−sweetened soft drinks. People can use up these remaining calo− ries by choosing foods that contain a lot of solid fat and/or added sugars (empty calories) or healthy foods such as nuts, fresh fruits, and vegetables.

To use MyPlate as a personalized menu planning guide, visit http://www .choosemyplate.gov and click on "SuperTracker" and then "Create Your Profile." Fill in boxes that request information, including your age, sex, weight, height, and estimated level of physical activity. After you provide this information, MyPlate estimates your daily energy needs and indicates how much food you should eat from each of the food groups daily to meet your recommended energy level. Table 3.7 indicates MyPlate's food intake recommendations for average healthy young adults who consume 1800 to 3200 kilocalories per day.

Overall, MyPlate can be helpful for planning menus because it promotes food variety, nutritional adequacy, and moderation. You can also use MyPlate to evaluate the nutritional quality of your daily diet by recording your food and beverage choices, classifying your choices into food groups, and estimating your intake of servings from each food group.

A computer and Internet access are necessary to use the program. Many people, particularly older adults, are unfamiliar with personal computers and

Figure 3.8 Estimating portion sizes. You can use familiar items such as these to estimate portion sizes.
Dice, soap: ©McGraw-Hill Education. Christopher Kerrigan, photographer; Mouse: ©Amos Morgan/Getty Images RF; Ball: ©Wendy Schiff; Baseball: ©Ryan McVay/Getty Images RF; Yo yo: ©PhotoDisc/Getty Images RF

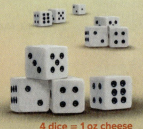

Computer mouse = 1/2 to 2/3 cup of food
(baked potato, ground or chopped food)

Tennis ball =
medium or small fruit

4 dice = 1 oz cheese

TABLE 3.7 MyPlate: Recommendations for Average, Healthy 20-Year-Old Adults

MyPlate Guidelines (Daily)	Women	Men
Kilocalories	1800–2400	2600–3200
Fruit	2 cups	2–2.5 cups
Vegetables	2.5–3 cups	3.5–4.0 cups
Grains	6–8 oz	9–10 oz
Protein foods	5.0–6.5 oz	6.5–7 oz
Dairy	3 cups	3 cups
Oils	5–7 tsp	8–11 tsp

may find the interactive www.choosemyplate.gov website challenging and frustrating to use.

How do you classify menu items that combine small amounts of foods from more than one group, such as pizza, sandwiches, and casseroles? A slice of pizza, for example, has thin crust made with wheat flour (grains), tomato sauce (vegetable), and cheese (dairy). The first step is to determine the ingredients and classify each into an appropriate food group. Estimate the number of cups or ounces of each ingredient and record the amounts contributed from a particular food group. The slice of pizza may provide ¼ cup of a vegetable, 2 ounces of grains, and ¼ cup of dairy. The Food Tracker feature of SuperTracker automatically estimates percentages of each food group that a particular food contributes to one's daily diet. Thus, Food Tracker makes it easy for consumers to monitor their intake of foods from each food group.

Another problem you may have when using MyPlate is judging portion sizes without keeping handy a battery of measuring cups and a scale for weighing foods. Figure 3.8 provides convenient ways to estimate typical portions using familiar objects, including a tennis ball and bar of soap.

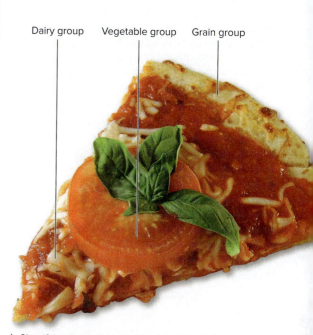

Dairy group   Vegetable group   Grain group

Classifying foods that combine ingredients that represent portions of different food groups is challenging. This slice of pizza, for example, has crust (grains), tomato sauce and tomatoes (vegetables), and cheese (dairy). ©Wendy Schiff

Baseball or human fist = 1 cup (large apple or orange, or 1 cup serving of ready-to-eat cereal)

Bar of soap or deck of cards = 3 oz meat

Small yo-yo = 1 standard bagel or English muffin

MY DIVERSE PLATE

MyPlate: Source: U.S. Dept. of Agriculture

Tomatillos

For centuries, the people of Central America have grown and eaten tomatillos ("husk-tomatoes"). After the papery husk is removed, the fruit can be roasted, chopped, and mixed with ground chili peppers to form sauces, such as salsa verde (green sauce). Three medium tomatillos provide about 33 kcal, 2 g fiber, and 12 mg vitamin C.

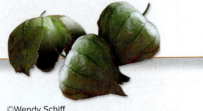

©Wendy Schiff

Exchange System method of classifying foods into lists based on macronutrient composition

MyPlate for Losing Weight

The "My Weight Manager" page at https://www.supertracker.usda.gov/MyWeight-Manager.aspx provides information about planning nutritionally adequate diets for persons who are trying to lose weight. My Weight Manager can also help a person monitor his or her weight change over time. If you would like to lose weight, start by obtaining your personalized daily food plan at https://www.supertracker.usda.gov/. Click on "Create Your Profile." In the box for "Weight," fill in your present weight; in the box for height, fill in your height. If you are too heavy for your height, the program will let you know and provide a food plan that will help you reach a healthy weight for your height (see Chapter 10). One way to reduce your calorie intake without sacrificing the nutritional adequacy of your diet is to eat smaller amounts of foods that contain a lot of empty calories or eliminate them altogether. Additionally, you can increase the amount of time that you are physically active each day.

MyPlate: Physical Activity   Although you may be busy while performing daily activities, you may not be moving your body enough to strengthen your muscles and prevent unwanted weight gain. To obtain important health benefits, you should spend at least 2.5 hours/week engaging in physical activities that are moderately intense.[11] Choosemyplate.gov includes some information about physical activity, including examples of activities that are moderate or vigorous (http://www.choosemyplate.gov/physical-activity). Chapter 11 provides more information about physical activity and the importance of a physically active lifestyle.

Other Food Guides

The USDA's original Food Guide Pyramid inspired the development of other food pyramids for people who follow cultural and ethnic food traditions that differ from the mainstream American ("Western") diet. The "Nutrition Matters" feature at the end of Chapter 3 discusses various cultural, ethnic, and religious influences on American dietary practices. The "Nutrition Matters" feature also includes illustrations of the traditional Latin American Diet (see Fig. 3.18), Mediterranean Diet (see Fig. 3.19), and the Asian Diet Pyramids (see Fig. 3.20). Health Canada, the federal agency responsible for helping Canadians achieve better health, also has a food guide, "Eating Well with Canada's Food Guide." Go to this website: http://hc-sc.gc.ca/fn-an/food-guide-aliment/index-eng.php to access this interactive guide.

Do Americans Follow Dietary Recommendations?

Analysis of government food consumption data indicates that the overall diet quality of Americans is improving, but many Americans do not follow the Dietary Guidelines.[12] In 2014, the typical diet of Americans who were 2 years of age and older did not provide recommended amounts of fruit, vegetables, and dairy foods (Fig. 3.9).[13] Furthermore, the diet generally contained too much added sugars, fats, and sodium.[12] It is apparent that the public needs to learn more about the importance of choosing a variety of foods and applying MyPlate to everyday menu planning.

The Exchange System and Carbohydrate Counting

Many serious chronic diseases require special diets to prevent or delay complications. Diabetes, for example, is easier to control when the person's diet has about the same macronutrient composition from day to day. The **Exchange System** can be used to estimate the energy, protein, carbohydrate, and fat content of foods. This menu-planning tool categorizes foods into three broad groups: carbohydrates,

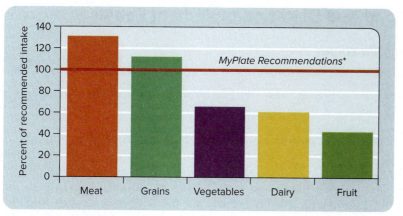

*Data based on a 2000-kcal diet.

Figure 3.9 MyPlate Recommendations. The typical American diet does not provide recommended amounts of fruit, vegetables, and dairy products. Source: U.S. Department of Agriculture, Economic Research Service: *Food availability (per capita) data system: Summary findings*. Last updated January 2017. USDA to https://www.ers.usda.gov/data-products/food-availability-per-capita-data-system/summary-findings/ Accessed: May 7, 2017.

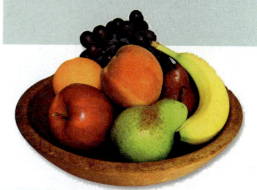

©Wendy Schiff

meat and meat substitutes, and fats.[14] The foods within each group have similar macronutrient composition, regardless of whether the food is from a plant or animal. For example, the carbohydrate group includes fruits, vegetables, and grains, as well as milk products. Nuts and seeds are grouped with fats. Meats and meat substitutes are grouped according to their fat content. Cheeses are in the meat and meat substitutes group because of their high protein and fat content. Thus, the Exchange System classifies foods differently than MyPlate does.

Within each of the three major food groups, the Exchange System provides *exchange lists* of specific types of foods. The specified amount of a food listed in an exchange list provides about the same amount of macronutrients and calories as each of the other specified amounts of foods in that list. According to the fruit list, for example, an orange is equivalent to a small apple, a kiwifruit, one–half of a fresh pear, or one–half of a large grapefruit. This equality allows people to plan a wide variety of nutritious menus by exchanging one food for another within each list.

Using the Exchange System for menu planning has lost much of its popularity. Now, many people with diabetes are using other tools, especially *carbohydrate counting* ("counting carbs"). The American Diabetes Association (http://www.diabetes.org/) offers information about counting carbohydrates (www.diabetes.org). You will learn more about diabetes in the section of Chapter 5 that discusses this serious disease in detail.

Concept CHECKPOINT

22. Americans generally do not eat enough _____ to meet MyPlate recommendations.
23. Explain how to use MyPlate to evaluate the nutritional adequacy of an individual's daily food choices.
24. Americans generally consume more _____ than MyPlate recommendations.
25. Describe how the Exchange System differs from MyPlate.

See Appendix G for responses.

3.5 Food and Dietary Supplement Labels

Learning Outcomes

1 Use the Nutrition Facts panel to make more nutritious food choices.

2 Identify nutrition-related claims the FDA allows on food and dietary supplement labels.

Consumers can use information on food labels to determine the ingredients in a packaged food or drink and to compare the number of calories (energy) and nutrient contents. In the United States, the FDA regulates and monitors information that can be placed on food labels, including claims about the health benefits of ingredients. Today, nearly all foods and beverages sold in grocery stores must have labels that provide the product's name, manufacturer's name and address, and amount of product in the package (Fig. 3.10). Producers and sellers of fresh and frozen fruits and vegetables; fresh poultry, fish, and shellfish; and a few other food items must declare the product's *country of origin* either on the packaging or where the product is located in stores. Furthermore, the ingredients list is a very important component of a label. Products that have more than one ingredient must display a list of the ingredients in descending order according to weight.

Nutrition Facts Panel

Consumers can find specific nutrition-related information about the contents of many packaged foods simply by reading the products' labels. The FDA requires food manufacturers to use a special format, the Nutrition Facts panel, to display information about the energy and nutrient contents of products (Fig. 3.11). As of June 2017, manufacturers could use either the original Nutrition Facts panel or a newer version of the panel to display the information. Unless otherwise specified, the following information refers to the newer panel format.

The Nutrition Facts panel shows the amount of a serving size, in household units, such as ounces or cups, as well as grams, and the number of servings in the entire container. The serving size is a reasonable amount of the food or beverage that a person typically consumes at one time. For example, a serving size for a 12-ounce can of soft drink is 12 ounces (the entire can).

The new Nutrition Facts panel requires most food manufacturers to provide information about the food's total fat, saturated fat, trans fat, cholesterol, sodium, total carbohydrate, fiber, total sugars, added sugars, protein, vitamin D, potassium, calcium, and iron contents in the Nutrition Facts panel. Additionally, the panel must display the total amount of energy, indicated as the number of calories, in a serving.

The panel uses grams (g) and milligrams (mg) to indicate amounts of nutrients in a serving of food. Food manufacturers can also include amounts of polyunsaturated and monounsaturated fats, as well as micronutrients that are not required to be listed on the label. If the manufacturer has fortified the food with the nutrients

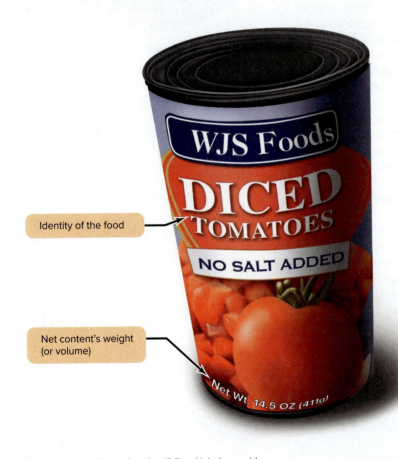

Identity of the food

Net content's weight (or volume)

Figure 3.10 What's in a food? Food labels provide specific information, including the food's identity and the container's net weight or volume.

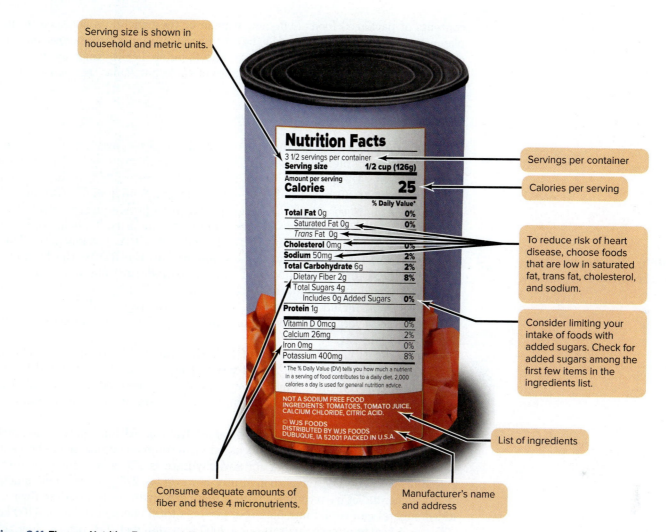

Serving size is shown in household and metric units.

Servings per container

Calories per serving

To reduce risk of heart disease, choose foods that are low in saturated fat, trans fat, cholesterol, and sodium.

Consider limiting your intake of foods with added sugars. Check for added sugars among the first few items in the ingredients list.

List of ingredients

Consume adequate amounts of fiber and these 4 micronutrients.

Manufacturer's name and address

Nutrition Facts

3 1/2 servings per container

Serving size	1/2 cup (126g)

Amount per serving
Calories 25

	% Daily Value*
Total Fat 0g	**0%**
Saturated Fat 0g	**0%**
Trans Fat 0g	
Cholesterol 0mg	**0%**
Sodium 50mg	**2%**
Total Carbohydrate 6g	**2%**
Dietary Fiber 2g	**8%**
Total Sugars 4g	
Includes 0g Added Sugars	**0%**
Protein 1g	
Vitamin D 0mcg	0%
Calcium 26mg	2%
Iron 0mg	0%
Potassium 400mg	8%

* The % Daily Value (DV) tells you how much a nutrient in a serving of food contributes to a daily diet. 2,000 calories a day is used for general nutrition advice.

NOT A SODIUM FREE FOOD
INGREDIENTS: TOMATOES, TOMATO JUICE, CALCIUM CHLORIDE, CITRIC ACID.

© WJS FOODS
DISTRIBUTED BY WJS FOODS
DUBUQUE, IA 52001 PACKED IN U.S.A.

Figure 3.11 The new Nutrition Facts panel. The new Nutrition Facts panel displays information about the serving size, servings per container, and energy and certain nutrient contents of a packaged food product.

or made claims about the product's nutrient contents, listing these particular food components is required.

Foods such as fresh fruits and vegetables, fish and shellfish, meats, and poultry are not required to have Nutrition Facts labels. However, many food suppliers and supermarket chains provide consumers with information about their products' nutritional content on posters or shelf tags displayed near the foods. In the future, fresh foods such as raw meats are likely to include Nutrition Facts panels on their labels.

The new Nutrition Facts panel displays the number of calories per serving in very bold print, so it is highly visible. Under "Total Sugars," ". . . Added Sugars," differentiates between ingredients that are added to foods or beverages to sweeten them, such as high-fructose corn syrup, from sugars that are naturally in a food or beverage, such as those in fruit and cow's milk. Such information is helpful for people who want to monitor their intake of empty calories and compare foods for their added sugar contents. The original Nutrition Facts panel provided information about the number of calories from fat. FDA officials do not require this information on the new version of the label because consumers should be more concerned about eating less unhealthy saturated and trans fats than about choosing foods that are low in total fat. Furthermore, the original Nutrition Facts panel had to include information about the vitamin A and C contents of packaged foods. The new version of the panel does not need to display amounts of vitamins C and A, but it must show amounts of potassium, calcium, iron, and vitamin D. This change reflects public health concerns that many Americans have less than adequate intakes of these particular micronutrients.

Daily Values

Nutrient standards such as the RDA and AI are sex–, age–, and life stage–specific. For example, the RDA for vitamin C is 75 mg/day and 65 mg/day for nonsmoking 18–year–old males and females, respectively. The vitamin's RDA increases to 80 mg/day for 18–year–old pregnant females. Because the RDAs and AIs are so specific, it is not practical to provide nutrient information on food labels that refers to these complex standards. To help consumers evaluate the nutritional content of food products, FDA developed the **Daily Values (DVs)** for labeling purposes. Compared to the RDAs, the DVs are a more simplified and practical set of nutrient standards. The adult DV for a nutrient is based on a standard diet that supplies 2000 kcal/day. Most nutrients have DVs, including total fat, total carbohydrate, added sugars, fiber, vitamins, and several minerals. As of April 2017, there were no DVs for total sugars and trans fat.

Appendix B lists the new set of DVs that was published in 2016. This set of DVs that applies to people over 4 years of age is used for foods and beverages that adults consume. Three other sets of DVs are used on labels of foods intended for infants, children between 1 and 4 years of age, and pregnant or breastfeeding women.

The DVs are often based on the highest RDA or AI for a particular nutrient, but in some instances, they are based on recommendations of public health experts. For example, the RDA for carbohydrate is 130 g/day for people over 1 year of age. The DV for carbohydrate, however, is 275 g/day.[15] This amount reflects general dietary recommendations that carbohydrates (other than fiber and added sugars) can contribute 55% of a person's total energy intake, or 1100 kcal (275 g × 4 kcal/g of carbohydrate) of a 2000 kcal/day diet. For people older than 1 year of age, no RDA or AI has been set for daily fat intake. However, DV for fat is 78 g/day. This amount meets the general recommendation that fat intake can be as much as 35% of a person's total energy intake for a 2000 kcal/day diet.

When evaluating or planning nutritious menus, your goal is to obtain at least 100% of the DVs for fiber, vitamins, and most minerals each day. On the other hand, you may need to limit your intake of foods that have high %DVs of total fat, saturated fat, added sugars, and sodium. High intakes of these nutrients may have negative effects on your health. Thus, your goal is to consume less than 100% of the DV for total fat, saturated fat, added sugars, and sodium each day. The general rule of thumb: A food that supplies 5%DV or less of a nutrient is a low source of the nutrient; a food that provides 20%DV or more is a high source of the nutrient.[16]

Percents of DVs are designed to help consumers compare nutrient contents of packaged foods to make more healthful choices. However, most people do not eat just packaged foods. Fresh fruits and vegetables, as well as most restaurant meals, do not have labels or menus with information about %DVs per serving. Therefore, many consumers will underestimate their nutrient intakes if they do not consider the contribution that unlabeled foods make to their diets.

It is important to note the description of a serving size and the number of servings per container when using nutritional labeling information to estimate your intakes of energy, fiber, and nutrients in the food. A common mistake people make when using a Nutrition Facts panel is assuming the information

Daily Values (DVs) set of nutrient intake standards developed for labeling purposes

applies to the entire package, which is not always true. For example, the Nutrition Facts panel on a package of food indicates there are four servings in the container. If you eat all the container's contents, you must multiply the information concerning calories, fat, and other food components by four. Why? Because you ate four servings and the nutritional information on the Nutrition Facts panel applies to only *one* serving. For some packaged foods, the FDA has developed a new Nutrition Facts label format that displays calorie and nutrient information for part as well as all of the package's contents (Fig. 3.12).

Health- and Nutrition-Related Claims

To make consumers more likely to buy their foods, manufacturers often promote products as having certain health benefits or high amounts of nutrients. A health claim describes how a food, food ingredient, or dietary supplement may reduce the risk of a nutrition–related condition. The FDA permits food manufacturers to include certain health claims on food labels (Fig. 3.13). For example, an allowable health claim may state, "Diets low in saturated fat may reduce the risk of heart disease."

The FDA only allows claims on food labels that:

- indicate the product has health benefits when it is consumed with other foods that make up a daily diet;

- are complete, easy to understand, honest, and not misleading;

- refer to a product that has 10% or more of the DVs for vitamins A and C, calcium, iron, fiber, or protein, *before* being fortified with nutrients. A food manufacturer, for example, wants to fortify its candy bar with vitamin C to boost the candy's vitamin C content from 2%DV to 30%DV. The FDA would not allow the manufacturer to place a health claim about the candy's vitamin C content on the label because the original candy had less than 10%DV for the vitamin;

- are for a product intended for people who are 2 years of age or older;

- use *may* or *might* to describe the relationship between the product and disease. For example, "Diets containing foods that are good sources of potassium and that are low in sodium may reduce the risk of high blood pressure and stroke" is an allowable claim. However, the claim "Reduces the risk of stroke" would not be permitted on a label;

- do not quantify any degree of risk reduction. For example, a claim that states, "Reduces risk of cancer by 41%" would not be allowed because it specifies the degree of risk reduction; and

- indicate that many factors influence disease.

The FDA requires specific wording for certain health claims that are allowed on labels. Table 3.8 lists some permissible health claims that can be used for labeling purposes. For more information, visit FDA's website at www.fda.gov and search for "qualified health claims."

As of April 2017, the FDA would not approve health claims for foods that contain more than 13 g of fat, 4 g of saturated fat, 60 mg of cholesterol, or 480 mg of sodium per serving.[16] For example, calcium is a mineral that strengthens bones and protects them from *osteoporosis*, a condition in which bones

Nutrition Facts

2 servings per container

Serving size			1 cup (255g)	
		Per serving	Per container	
Calories		**220**	**440**	
		% DV*		% DV*
Total Fat	5g	**6%**	10g	**13%**
Saturated Fat	2g	**10%**	4g	**20%**
Trans Fat	0g		0g	
Cholesterol	15mg	**5%**	30mg	**10%**
Sodium	240mg	**10%**	480mg	**21%**
Total Carb.	35g	**13%**	70g	**25%**
Dietary Fiber	6g	**21%**	12g	**43%**
Total Sugars	7g		14g	
Incl. Added Sugars	4g	**8%**	8g	**16%**
Protein	9g		18g	
Vitamin D	5mcg	25%	10mcg	50%
Calcium	200mg	15%	400mg	30%
Iron	1mg	6%	2mg	10%
Potassium	470mg	10%	940mg	20%

* The % Daily Value (DV) tells you how much a nutrient in a serving of food contributes to a daily diet. 2,000 Calories a day is used for general nutrition advice.

Figure 3.12 Other acceptable label formats. A Nutrition Facts label may display calorie and nutrient information for part as well as all of the package's contents. Source: http://www.fda.gov/downloads/Food /GuidanceRegulation/GuidanceDocumentsRegulatoryInformation /LabelingNutrition/UCM511964.pdf

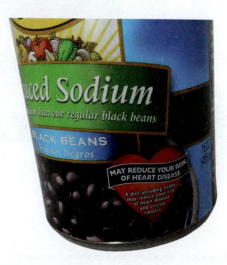

Figure 3.13 Label claims. The FDA permits food manufacturers to include certain health claims on food labels. ©Wendy Schiff

TABLE 3.8 Examples of Permissible Health Claims for Food Labels

Dietary Factor/Health Condition	Example of Permissible Health Claim
Certain lipids and heart disease	"While many factors affect heart disease, diets low in saturated fat and cholesterol may reduce the risk of this disease."
Diet and heart disease	"Diets low in saturated fat and cholesterol and rich in fruits, vegetables, and grain products that contain some types of dietary fiber, particularly soluble fiber, may reduce the risk of heart disease, a disease associated with many factors."
Calcium, exercise, and osteoporosis (a disease that weakens bones)	"Regular exercise and a healthy diet with enough calcium help teen and young adult white and Asian women maintain good bone health and may reduce their high risk of osteoporosis."
Sodium (a mineral) and high blood pressure	"Diets low in sodium may reduce the risk of high blood pressure, a disease associated with many factors."
Folate (a B vitamin) and neural tube defects (conditions in which the skull and spine do not form properly before birth)	"Healthful diets with adequate folate may reduce a woman's risk of having a child with a brain or spinal cord defect."
Fruits and vegetables and risk of cancer	"Foods that are low in fat and contain dietary fiber, vitamin A, or vitamin C may reduce the risk of some types of cancer, a disease associated with many factors. Broccoli is high in vitamins A and C, and it is a good source of dietary fiber."

Source: U.S. Food and Drug Administration: *Food labeling guide.* 2013. http://www.fda.gov/food/guidanceregulation/guidancedocumentsregulatoryinformation/labelingnutrition/ucm2006828.htm Accessed: July 7, 2017.

become brittle and break easily. Whole milk is a rich source of calcium. Never-theless, the label on a carton of whole milk cannot include a health claim about calcium and osteoporosis, because the milk contains more than 4 g of saturated fat per serving. In addition, the product must meet specific conditions that relate to the health claim. For example, a claim regarding the benefits of eating a low-fat diet is allowed only if the product contains 3 g or less of fat per serving, which is the FDA's standard definition of a low-fat food.

In 2016, FDA officials began to reevaluate the 3 g or less per serving limit for a "healthy" food. Many nuts are high in fat, but the kinds of fat they contain are considered healthy. In 2016, for example, manufacturers of peanut butter would not be allowed to place a health claim on the label of their products because peanut butter is a high-fat food (16 g of fat per serving).

Structure/Function Claims

A structure/function claim describes the role a nutrient or dietary sup-plement plays in maintaining a structure, such as bone, or promoting a normal function, such as digestion. The FDA allows structure/function claims such as "calcium builds strong bones" or "fiber maintains bowel regularity" (Fig. 3.14). Structure/function statements cannot claim that a nutrient, food, or dietary supplement can be used to prevent or treat a seri-ous health condition. For example, the FDA would not permit a claim that a product "promotes low blood pressure" because that claim implies the product has druglike effects and can treat high blood pressure.

Nutrient Content Claims

The FDA permits manufacturers to include claims on labels that describe lev-els of nutrients in packaged foods. Such nutrient content claims can use the terms *free*, *high*, or *low* to describe how much of a nutrient is in the product.

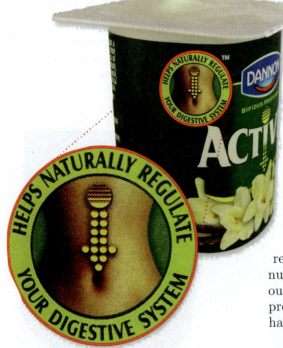

Figure 3.14 Structure/function claim. Structure/function statements cannot claim that a nutrient, food, or dietary supplement can be used to prevent or treat a serious health condition. ©Wendy Schiff

TABLE 3.9   Legal Definitions for Common Nutrient Content Claims (April 2017)

Sugar	• **Sugar free:** The product provides less than 0.5 g of sugar per serving. • **Reduced sugar:** The food contains at least 25% less sugar per serving than the reference food.
Calories	• **Calorie free:** The food provides fewer than 5 kcal per serving. • **Low calorie:** The food supplies 40 kcal or less per serving. • **Reduced or fewer calories:** The food contains at least 25% fewer kcal per serving than the reference food.
Fat	• **Fat free:** The food provides less than 0.5 g of fat per serving. • **Low fat:** The food contains 3 g or less fat per serving. Two-percent milk is not "low fat" because it has more than 3 g of fat per serving. The term *reduced fat* can be used to describe 2% milk. • **Reduced or less fat:** The food supplies at least 25% less fat per serving than the reference food.
Cholesterol	• **Cholesterol free:** The food contains less than 2 mg of cholesterol and 2 g or less of saturated fat per serving.
Fiber	• **High fiber:** The food contains 5g or more fiber per serving. Foods that include high-fiber claims on the label must also meet the definition for low fat. • **Good source of fiber:** The food supplies 2.5 to 4.9 g of fiber per serving.
Meat and poultry products regulated by USDA	• **Extra lean:** The food provides less than 5 g of fat, 2 g of saturated fat, and 95 mg of cholesterol per serving. • **Lean:** The food contains less than 10 g of fat, 4.5 g of saturated fat, and 95 mg of cholesterol per serving.

Additionally, nutrient content claims can use terms such as *more* or *reduced* to compare amounts of nutrients in a product to those in a similar product. This claim is often used for an item that substitutes for a *reference food*, which is a similar and more familiar food. For example, a "reduced–fat" salad dressing has considerably less fat than its reference food, regular salad dressing.

Table 3.9 lists some legal definitions for common nutrient content claims that are allowed on labels. Note that a product may contain a small amount of a nutrient such as fat or sugar, yet the Nutrition Facts panel can indicate the amount as "0 g." For example, the Nutrition Facts panel may indicate that a serving of food supplies "0" grams of trans fat, even though the food actually supplies less than 0.5 g of trans fat. As a result, it is possible to consume some trans fats from processed foods even though labels indicate a serving of each food does not contain this type of fat. To learn more about the FDA's regulations concerning nutrient claims, visit the agency's website (www.fda.gov) and search for "food labeling guide."

Other Descriptive Labeling Terms

According to the FDA, a *light* or *lite* food has at least one–third fewer kilocalories or half the fat of the reference food. For example, a tablespoon of lite pancake syrup has one–third fewer kcal than a tablespoon of regular pancake syrup. A tablespoon of light mayonnaise has less than half the fat of regular mayonnaise. The term *light* may also describe food characteristics such as texture and color; for example, "light brown sugar." To include the term *natural* on the label, the food must not contain food coloring agents, synthetic flavors, or other unnatural substances (as of April 2017).[17]

Dietary Supplement Labels

According to federal law, every dietary supplement container must be properly labeled (Fig. 3.15). The label must include the term "dietary supplement" or a similar term that describes the product's particular ingredient, such as "herbal

Food & Nutrition *tips*

Often, the only difference between a creamy salad dressing, such as ranch or blue cheese, and the "light" version of the dressing is the amount of water they contain. Instead of paying more for calorie-reduced bottled salad dressings, make your own light salad dressing by adding about ¼ cup water to a jar of regular creamy salad dressing, then stir or shake the mixture.

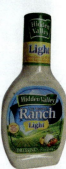

©Wendy Schiff

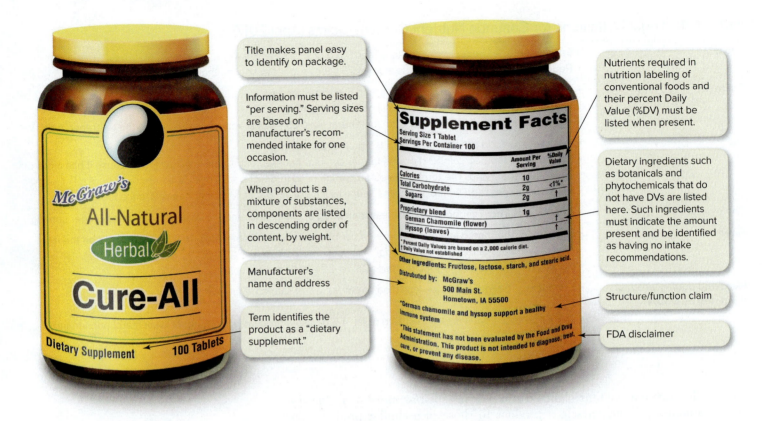

Title makes panel easy to identify on package.

Information must be listed "per serving." Serving sizes are based on manufacturer's recommended intake for one occasion.

When product is a mixture of substances, components are listed in descending order of content, by weight.

Manufacturer's name and address

Term identifies the product as a "dietary supplement."

Nutrients required in nutrition labeling of conventional foods and their percent Daily Value (%DV) must be listed when present.

Dietary ingredients such as botanicals and phytochemicals that do not have DVs are listed here. Such ingredients must indicate the amount present and be identified as having no intake recommendations.

Structure/function claim

FDA disclaimer

Figure 3.15 Supplement Facts label. A nutrient supplement label must list the product's ingredient(s), serving size, amount(s) per serving, suggested use, manufacturer and the company's address, and %DV, if one has been established. If a health claim appears on the supplement's label, the claim must be followed by the FDA disclaimer.

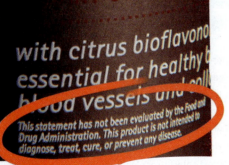

Figure 3.16 Label disclaimer. The FDA permits dietary supplement manufacturers to include certain health-related claims on their product labels. However, the label of products bearing such claims also must display this disclaimer. ©Wendy Schiff

supplement" or "vitamin C supplement." Dietary supplement labels are also required to display the list of ingredients, manufacturer's address, and suggested dosage. Furthermore, the label must include facts about the product's contents in a special format—the "Supplement Facts" panel (see Fig. 3.15). The panel provides information about the serving size; amount per serving; and percent Daily Value (%DV) for ingredients, if one has been established. Daily Values (DVs) are standard desirable or maximum intakes for many nutrients, but DVs have not been established for nonnutrient products.

According to the FDA, dietary supplements are not intended to treat, diagnose, cure, or alleviate the effects of diseases. Therefore, the agency does not permit manufacturers to market a dietary supplement product as a treatment or cure for a disease, or to relieve signs or symptoms of a disease. Although such products generally cannot prevent diseases, some can improve health or reduce the risk of certain diseases or conditions. Thus, the FDA allows supplement manufacturers to display structure/function claims on labels. Manufacturers of iron supplements, for example, may have a claim on the label that states: "Iron is necessary for healthy red blood cell formation." If the FDA has not reviewed a claim, the label must include the FDA's disclaimer indicating that the claim has not been evaluated by the agency (Fig. 3.16).

The FDA does not require dietary supplement manufacturers or sellers to provide evidence that labeling claims are accurate or truthful before they appear on product containers. However, manufacturers that include structure/ function claims on labels must notify the FDA about the claims within 30 days after introducing the products into the marketplace. If FDA officials question the safety of a dietary supplement or the truthfulness of claims that appear on supplement labels, manufacturers are responsible for providing the agency with evidence that their products are safe and the claims on labels are honest and not misleading.

The FDA requires dietary supplement manufacturers to evaluate the purity, quality, strength, and composition of their products before marketing them. The regulations are designed to result in the production of supple—ments that contain the ingredients listed on the label, are wholesome, contain standard amounts of ingredients per dose, and are properly packaged and accurately labeled.

Concept CHECKPOINT

26. Identify at least one limitation of using %DVs to determine your nutrient intakes.
27. Explain how you can use nutritional information provided on food and dietary supplement labels to become a more careful consumer.
28. What is the difference between a health claim and a structure/function claim? What is a nutrient content claim? Give an example of each type of claim.
29. Discuss the role of the FDA in protecting consumers from false nutrition and health claims on food and dietary supplement labels.

See Appendix G for responses.

3.6 Organic Food

Learning Outcomes

1 Explain differences between the production of organic foods and the production of conventional foods.

2 Discuss the USDA's three labeling categories for organic foods.

By the late twentieth century, emphasis on increasing agricultural production resulted in an inexpensive and abundant food supply in the United States. How—ever, the rise of agribusiness also resulted in social, economic, and environmental costs. Rural agricultural communities experienced a dramatic decline in the number of small farms, as the farms' owners could not compete with the production capabilities and financial resources of large, commercially run farms.

Instead of producing a variety of crops, big farms often focus on grow—ing corn, soybeans, or wheat. These crops require conventional farming methods that include heavy use of fertilizers and products to control pests (*pesticides*). In some parts of the country, large farms also need considerable amounts of water for irrigating crops. As a result, underground water supplies are being depleted in these regions.

The rise in agribusiness helped fuel interest in sustainable agriculture. Sustainable agriculture focuses on producing adequate amounts of food without reducing natural resources, such as the water supply, and harming people as well as the natural environment.[18] Such agricultural methods promote crop variety, soil and water conservation, and recycling of plant nutrients. Additionally, sustainable agriculture can support small farms, particularly organic farms.

Technically, organic substances have the element carbon bonded to hydrogen (another element) in their chemical structures. Therefore, all foods are organic

Food & Nutrition tips

According to the Environmental Protection Agency, you can reduce your exposure to pesticides in food by:

- washing and scrubbing all fresh fruits and veg-etables under running water. However, not all pesticide residues can be removed by washing;

- peeling and trimming fruits and vegetables before eating them;

- trimming fat from meat and skin of poultry and fish, because some pesticide residues accumu-late in fat; and

- eating a variety of foods; this reduces the likeli-hood of exposure to a single pesticide.[19]

TABLE 3.10 Comparing Organic and Conventional Farming Systems

Organic	Nonorganic
Synthetic fertilizers are not allowed.	Limited restrictions on fertilizers
Sewage sludge products are not allowed.	Sludge products may be used on some fields.
Restrictions on use of raw manure on fields used for food crops	Few restrictions on raw manure use for edible crop fields
Synthetic pesticides are not allowed; natural pest management practices are encouraged.	Any government-approved pesticide may be used according to label instructions. Natural pest management practices may also be used.
Genetically modified organisms (GMOs) are not allowed.	Government-approved GMOs are permitted.
Feeding livestock mammal and poultry by-products and manure is not allowed.	Certain mammal and poultry by-products are allowed in livestock feed.
Use of growth hormones and antibiotics in livestock production is not allowed.	Government-approved hormone and antibiotic treatments are permitted.
Food irradiation (a food safety method) is not allowed.	Food irradiation may be used.
Detailed record keeping and site inspections by regulators are required.	Some records are required, but no on-site checks by regulators are necessary.

organic foods foods produced without the use of antibiotics, hormones, synthetic fertilizers and pesticides, genetic improvements, or spoilage-killing radiation

because they contain substances comprised of carbon bonded with hydrogen. The term *organic*, however, also refers to certain agricultural methods that can promote sustainability. Organic farming and the production of **organic foods** do not rely on the use of antibiotics, hormones, synthetic fertilizers and pesticides, genetic improvements, or ionizing radiation.[20] Table 3.10 compares organic and conventional agricultural systems.

Over the past 40 years, the popularity of organic foods has increased in the United States as many Americans have become concerned about the environment and the safety and nutritional value of the food supply. Sales of organic foods have increased steadily since the 1990s, even though these products are usually more expensive than the same foods produced by conventional farming methods. According to the Organic Trade Association, Americans spent an estimated $43.3 billion on organic foods and beverages in 2015.[21]

People who purchase organically grown foods often think the products are better for their health and more nutritious than conventionally produced foods. Few well—designed studies have compared nutrient and phytochemical contents of organically grown foods to their conventionally grown counterparts. Nevertheless, some general trends have been determined. In general, organic food crops are not more nutritious than conventionally grown food crops.[22] Organic crops, however, may contain fewer pesticides than conventionally grown crops.[23] Nevertheless, more research is needed to determine whether there are health advantages to eating organic foods.

Labeling Organic Foods

To protect consumers, the USDA developed and implemented rules for the organic food industry. A food product cannot be labeled "organic" unless its production meets strict national standards. For labeling purposes, organic food manufacturers can use the circular "USDA Organic" symbol on the package (Fig. 3.17). This symbol indicates the products meet USDA's standards for organic food. According to the USDA, there are three organic labeling categories (Table 3.11). Note that certain foods can have the organic symbol on the pack—age, yet they may contain small amounts of ingredients that are not considered organic by the USDA. For more information about the government's organic food standards, visit the USDA's Agricultural Marketing Service's website (https://www.ams.usda.gov/grades—standards/organic—labeling—standards).

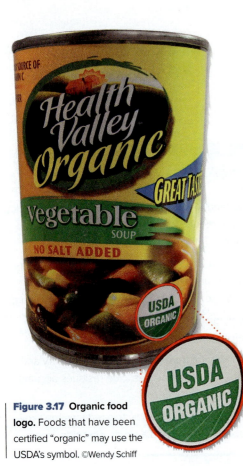

Figure 3.17 Organic food logo. Foods that have been certified "organic" may use the USDA's symbol. ©Wendy Schiff

TABLE 3.11 Organic Labeling Categories

"100% Organic" (may use USDA organic seal)	100% certified organic ingredients Must identify organic ingredients
"Organic" (may use USDA organic seal)	Contains at least 95% certifed organic ingredients Remaining 5% of ingredients are on USDA's list of allowed ingredients Must identify organic ingredients
"Made with organic _____" ***(may not use USDA organic seal)***	Contains 70 to 95% certified organic ingredients Must identify organic ingredients

Source: U.S. Department of Agriculture, Agricultural Marketing Service: *Organic labeling standards*. ND. https://www.ams.usda .gov/grades-standards/organic-labeling-standards Accessed: July 8, 2017.

Concept CHECKPOINT

30. Jeremy prefers to drink organic milk instead of milk that is not organic. What is the difference between the two types of milk?

31. Jeremy only purchases cereals that have the organic seal on the package. Explain why such cereals may not be 100% organic.

See Appendix G for responses.

3.7 Using Dietary Analysis Software

Learning Outcomes

1 Explain why different dietary analysis software programs may provide different values for energy and nutrient contents for the same food item.

2 Use the U.S. Department of Agriculture's websites to estimate the nutritional value of various foods.

How much selenium, magnesium, and niacin are in an ounce of Swiss cheese? Have you ever wanted information about nutrients in a food that are not listed on the Nutrition Facts panel? In the past, people relied on food composition tables, lists of commonly eaten foods that provide amounts of energy, fiber, macronutrients, and several micronutrients. Today, people can determine the energy and nutrient contents of their food choices by using a dietary analy— sis software program. Furthermore, people with Internet access can obtain the information from certain websites.

Dietary analysis software and websites can be quick and easy tools for determining nutrient and energy contents of a specific food. However, the values provided by these resources are not necessarily exact amounts. The same type of plant food may vary in nutrient content depending on hereditary factors, age, growing conditions, and production methods. Therefore, scientists generally analyze several samples of a particular food to determine their nutrient con— tents, and then the researchers average the results. For example, if the amount of energy in three Valencia oranges that each weighs about 4 ounces (120 g) were 55, 60, and 62 kcal, respectively, the value listed in the food composition table for a Valencia orange weighing 4 ounces would be 59 kcal, the average of the three. In many instances, values for certain nutrients are missing. This occurs when accurate data concerning the complete nutrient analysis of the food are unavailable.

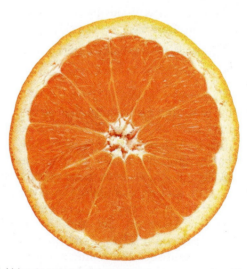

Valencia oranges and other produce may vary in nutrient content depending on numerous factors, including growing conditions. ©Savany/Getty Images RF

The following section discusses some government–sponsored websites that provide practical tools for evaluating food intakes and physical activity habits. The Personal Dietary Analysis feature at the end of this chapter provides an opportunity for you to practice using dietary analysis software.

Government-Sponsored Dietary Analysis Websites

In addition to www.choosemyplate.gov, the USDA sponsors other websites to help you assess the energy and nutrient contents of your food intake. The "What's in the Food You Eat *Search Tool*" (www.ars.usda.gov/Services/docs .htm?docid=17032) is one such site. Another USDA–sponsored site that provides extensive information regarding the energy and nutrient content of food is the National Nutrient Database for Standard Reference. You can access this nutrient database by visiting www.nal.usda.gov/fnic/foodcomp/search. To keep current, USDA–sponsored websites are updated regularly to provide information about new products and serving sizes.

Concept CHECKPOINT

32. Identify at least two reliable sources of information about the energy and nutrient contents of foods and beverages.

See Appendix G for responses.

3.8 Nutrition Matters: The Melting Pot

Learning Outcomes

1 Discuss how various ethnic and religious groups influence Americans' dietary patterns.

2 Identify religion-based dietary restrictions.

Wherever you live or travel in the United States, you're likely to find restaurants that serve a wide variety of ethnic fare, such as Italian, Thai, Vietnamese, or Middle Eastern dishes. Although your primary food selection and cooking habits probably reflect your cultural/ethnic heritage, you likely enjoy foods from other cultures and ethnic groups.

This section examines the influences that the dietary practices of certain cultures and ethnic groups have had on the American diet and the possible effects of these practices on health. Traditional ethnic diets are often based on dishes containing small amounts of animal foods and larger amounts of locally grown fruits, vegetables, and unrefined grains. However, these foods are typically the first to be abandoned as immigrants *assimilate*, that

is, blend into the general population over time. After an immigrant population has assimilated fully, the prevalence of chronic diseases such as cardiovascular disease, type 2 diabetes, and high blood pressure often increases among them, partly as a result of adopting less healthy eating practices.

Northwestern European Influences

Immigrants from northwestern European regions or countries such as the United Kingdom, Scandinavia, and Germany established the familiar "meat–and–potatoes" diet that features a large portion of beef or pork served with a smaller portion of potatoes. In the past, the potatoes were either boiled or mashed; today, they are usually fried. This mainstream American diet, often referred to as a "Western" diet, provides large amounts of animal protein and fat, and lacks fruits, whole grains, and a variety of green vegetables. Such diets are associated with high rates of serious chronic diseases, particularly CVD and type 2 diabetes, which are discussed in later chapters of this textbook.

Blueberries: ©PhotoAlto/Getty Images RF

Hispanic Influences

The Hispanic (people with Spanish ances-try) population is now the largest minority group in the United States. Many Hispanic–Americans migrated to the United States from Mexico. The traditional Mexican diet included corn, beans, chili peppers, avoca-dos, papayas, and pineapples. Many super-markets in the United States sell other plant foods that are often incorporated into Mexi-can meals, such as fresh chayote, cherimoya, jicama, plantains, and cactus leaves and fruit. Such fruits and vegetables add fiber and a variety of nutrients, phytochemicals, vivid colors, and interesting flavors to Mexican dishes (Fig. 3.18).

Authentic Mexican meals are based pri-marily on rice, tortillas, and beans, depending on the region. However, many non–Hispanic Americans do not like to eat meals limited to these inexpensive yet nutritious plant foods. To appeal to people with more Western food preferences, "Mexican" fast–food restau-rants in the United States often serve dishes that contain large portions of high–fat beef topped with sour cream and American cheese. Diets that contain high amounts of these and other solid fats are associated with excess body fat, CVD, and type 2 diabetes.

Italian and Other Mediterranean Influences

The traditional Italian diet of pasta and other grain products, olive oil, fish, nuts, fruits, and vegetables is healthier than the Western diet. Pasta, a product made from wheat flour and water, is the core of the traditional Italian diet. To many Americans, *pasta* is spaghetti topped with tomato sauce, meatballs, and grated Parmesan cheese. However, Italians eat a variety of different forms of pasta, such as penne, linguini, acini de pepe, and rotini, along with sauces that are often meatless. Pizza, a dish from southern Italy, is one of the most frequently consumed foods in the United States. Unlike traditional Italian pizza that has a thin crust and is lightly covered with tomatoes, basil (a leafy herb), and mozzarella cheese, many Americans choose thick–crust pizza topped with tomato sauce, plenty of shredded mozzarella cheese, and dotted with fatty pork sausage or pepperoni.

Dietary pyramids or plans developed by governmen-tal agencies or private organizations have plant foods as the core of a healthy diet. The Mediterranean Diet Pyramid shown in Figure 3.19 is based on traditional

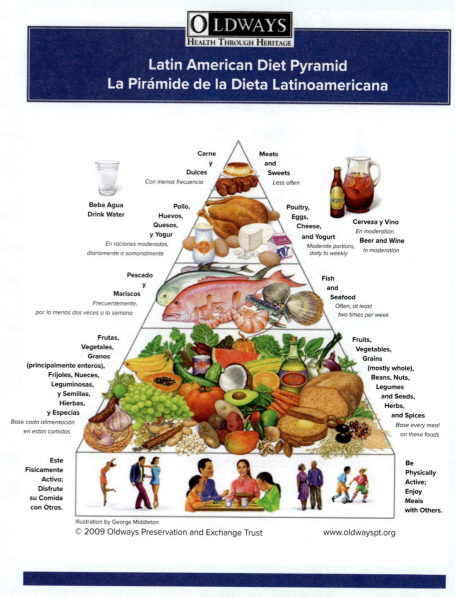

Figure 3.18 Latin American Diet Pyramid.

©2009 Oldways Preservation & Exchange Trust. Used with permission. www.oldwayspt.org

dietary practices of Mediterranean countries, such as Greece, southern Italy, and the island of Crete. Grains, fruits, and vegetables, particularly beans and potatoes, form the foundation of this diet. Red meat and sugary foods, which are at the top of the pyramid, are rarely eaten. Main dishes often include seafood and poultry, and wine may be included with meals. Although the Mediterranean Diet Pyramid allows as much as 35% of total calories as fat in the diet, much of the fat is from olive oil. Olive oil is a rich source of a type of fat that reduces rather than increases the risk of CVD. Chapter 6 provides more information about oils and fats and their roles in health.

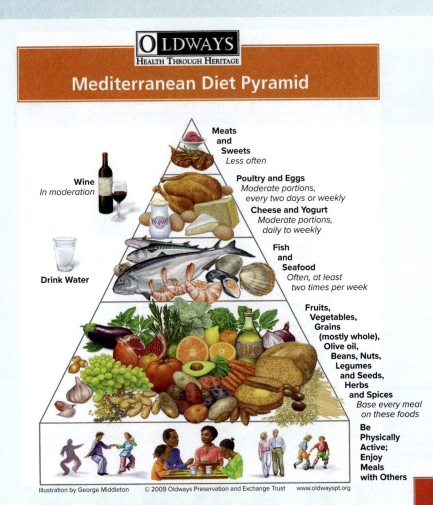

Figure 3.19 Mediterranean Diet Pyramid. The Mediterranean Diet Pyramid is based on traditional dietary practices of Greece, southern Italy, and the island of Crete. ©2009 Oldways Preservation & Exchange Trust. Used with permission. www.oldwayspt.org

African Heritage Influences

Over the past several decades, the diets of African–Americans changed significantly so they now incorporate regional food preferences. In some parts of the United States, for example, the traditional African–American diet includes sweet potato pie, fried chicken, pork, black–eyed peas, and "greens," the nutritious leafy parts of plants such as kale, collards, mustard, turnip, and dandelion. To add flavor, greens may be cooked with small pieces of smoked pork.

Although sweet potatoes, dried peas, and leafy vegetables provide fiber and a variety of vitamins and minerals, fried foods and salt–cured pork products contribute undesirable levels of fat and sodium to the diet. High–fat diets are associated with obesity, and high–sodium diets raise the risk of hypertension. You will learn more about the role of diet in the development of hypertension in Chapters 6 and 9. For more information about African heritage diets and foods, visit http://oldwayspt.org/programs/african–heritage–health#.

Asian Influences

Traditional Asian foods, such as Chinese, Japanese, Vietnamese, Thai, and Korean cuisines, are similar and generally feature large amounts of vegetables, rice, or noodles combined with small amounts of meat, fish, or shellfish. The variety of vegetables used in Asian dishes adds color, flavor, texture, phytochemicals, and nutrients to meals. Additionally, Asian dishes often include flavorful sauces and seasonings made from plants, such as soy sauce, rice wine, gingerroot, garlic, scallions, peppers, and sesame seeds. The Asian Diet Pyramid, shown in Figure 3.20, illustrates the traditional Asian dietary pattern, which generally provides inadequate amounts of calcium from milk and milk products. However, using calcium–rich or calcium–fortified foods can add the mineral to diets.

Chinese foods are popular among Americans. Many Americans, however, do not favor dishes that feature seafood and contain large portions of vegetables and grains because they believe meat should form the basis of a meal. Thus, North American Chinese restaurants that specialize in

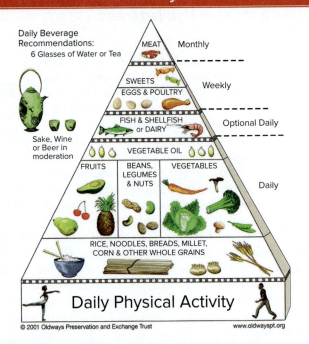

Figure 3.20 Asian Diet Pyramid. The Asian Diet Pyramid dietary pattern generally provides inadequate amounts of calcium from milk and milk products. ©2000 Oldways Preservation & Exchange Trust. Used with permission. www.oldwayspt.org

©Burke/Triolo Productions/Getty Images RF

Cantonese, Szechwan, or Mandarin cuisines typically offer menu items that contain much larger portions of animal foods such as beef and chicken than authentic dishes. Furthermore, American–Chinese foods are often prepared with far greater amounts of fat than are used in true Chinese cooking.

Traditional Chinese food preparation methods, particularly steaming and stir–frying, tend to preserve the vitamins and minerals in fresh vegetables. Stir–frying involves cooking foods in a lightly oiled, very hot pan for a short period of time. Unlike Western methods of deep–fat frying or boiling vegetables, stir–frying vegetables keeps them crisp and colorful.

Rice is the staple food in the traditional Japanese diet. Additionally, fish, poultry, pork, and foods made from soybeans provide protein in this diet. The Japanese people eat sushi, small pieces of raw fish or shellfish that are usually served rolled in or pressed into rice and served with vegetables and seaweed. American–Japanese restaurants often feature sushi, and many non–Japanese Americans like to order the dish.

Some of the longest–lived people in the world reside on Okinawa, a tiny island south of the main Japanese islands. The traditional diet of fresh vegetables, minimal amounts of salt and animal protein (mainly from pork and fish), and moderate amounts of fat may protect the island's population from premature heart disease and stroke. Younger Okinawans, however, have adopted more Western dietary practices, such as eating fast food, and as a result, their life expectancy is not as long as that of their grandparents.[24]

Traditional Asian food patterns may contain too much sodium. High sodium intakes increase the risk of hypertension. In many parts of Japan, the general population consumes too much sodium. Not surprisingly, hypertension is a serious public health problem in these areas.[25]

Native American Influences

In the past, some Native Americans were hunter–gatherers, depending on wild vegetation, fish, and game for food. Other Native Americans learned to grow vegetable crops, including tomatoes, corn, and squash. In general, the traditional Native American diet was low in sodium and fat and high in fiber. During the last half of the twentieth century, many Native Americans abandoned their traditional diets and adopted the typical Western diet. The negative health effects of this lifestyle change have been significant. Before the 1930s, for example, members of the Pima tribe in the southwestern United States primarily ate native foods that included low–fat game animals and high–fiber desert vegetation. By the end of the century, most American Pima had abandoned their native diets and had adopted a more Western diet. Today, obesity and type 2 diabetes are extremely prevalent among the Pima, whereas in the past, these conditions rarely affected tribal members.

The traditional native Alaskan diet was composed of fatty fish and sea mammals, game animals, and a few plants. Alaskan natives who still follow traditional dietary practices have CVD rates that are lower than those in the general North American population, but those who switched to a more Western diet have developed CVD at rates similar to those of the general population.

Religious Influences

Many religions require members to follow strict food handling and dietary practices that often include the prohibition of certain foods and beverages (see Table 3.12). According to Jewish dietary laws, for example, meat and poultry products must be kept separate from milk products. Milk products are not used to prepare foods that contain meat or poultry, nor are they served with them. A cheeseburger, for example, is not kosher. *Kosher* refers to a specific procedure concerning killing, butchering, and preparation activities that makes food acceptable for the religion's followers to eat. Fruits, grains, and vegetables are "neutral" foods that can be eaten with meals that contain either meat or dairy products. However, vegetables cooked with meat become a "meat" food and cannot be served with milk; peaches served with cottage cheese become a "milk" food and cannot be eaten with meat or poultry. Today many American Jews do not follow their religion's complex dietary laws as closely as their ancestors did.

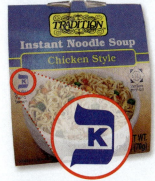

Symbol for a kosher food.
©Wendy Schiff

TABLE 3.12 Religious Influences on Dietary Practices

Religion	Dietary practices*
Buddhist	Meat is avoided; vegetarianism is encouraged.
Eastern Orthodox	Meat and fish restrictions; fasting and specific food abstinence during certain holidays
Hindu	Beef is forbidden, but dairy products are "pure" for consumption. Pork may be restricted. Alcohol is avoided. Fasting is often encouraged.
Islam	Pork; birds of prey; reptiles; insects, except locusts; most gelatins; and alcohol-containing beverages are prohibited (*ha-raam*). Ritual killing of animals that are permitted as food (*ha-lal*) Fasting from all food and drink (daytime) during month of Ramadan and certain other religious holidays
Jewish	Only kosher foods are acceptable. *Tref* (*trayf*) refers to prohibited foods. Pork and shellfish are prohibited. Eating meat with dairy is prohibited. Consuming blood is forbidden. Raw meat is soaked in cold water to remove blood, salted for 1 hour, and then rinsed. Eggs, fruits, and vegetables can be eaten with either meat or dairy foods. Eggs, however, are inspected to make sure they do not contain blood specks. Only fish with fins and scales can be eaten. Only land animals that have split hooves and chew their cud can be eaten, and only the front half of the cud-chewing animal is used. Ritual killing of certain animals is required. Fasting and specific food restrictions for certain holidays
Mormon	Alcohol, coffee, and tea are avoided. Fasting is practiced regularly.
Roman Catholic	Fasting before communion; fasting and specific food abstinence during certain holidays
Seventh Day Adventist	Animal product consumption generally limited to milk, milk products, and eggs (lacto-ovo vegetarianism) Alcohol and beverages containing stimulants are prohibited.

* Some religions have extensive rules governing food-related practices, but many people do not follow their religion's dietary guidelines fully or at all.

Bagels with smoked salmon (*lox*), pickled herring, cream cheese, dill pickles, corned beef, and pastrami are popular among the Ashkenazi, the predominant group of Jews in America. Although many non–Jews enjoy eating these traditional Ashkenazic foods, such items may be too high in sodium to be healthy.

Concept CHECKPOINT

33. Discuss how immigrants to the United States from Asia and Mexico have influenced the general population's food preferences.

34. Discuss at least two religion-related food restrictions.

See Appendix G for responses.

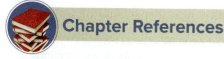

Chapter References

See Appendix H.

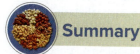

Summary

3.1 From Requirements to Standards

- A requirement is the smallest amount of a nutrient that maintains a defined level of health. Numerous factors influence nutrient requirements. Scientists use information about nutrient requirements and storage capabilities to establish specific dietary recommendations. The Dietary Reference Intakes (DRIs) are various energy and nutrient intake standards for Americans. An Estimated Average Requirement (EAR) is the amount of the nutrient that meets the needs of 50% of healthy people in a particular life stage/sex group. The Estimated Energy Requirement (EER) is used to evaluate a person's energy intake. The Recommended Dietary Allowances (RDAs) meet the needs of nearly all healthy individuals (97 to 98%) in a particular life stage/sex group. When nutrition scientists are unable to determine an RDA for a nutrient, they establish an Adequate Intake (AI) value. The Tolerable Upper Intake Level (UL) is the highest average amount of a nutrient that is unlikely to harm most people when the amount is consumed daily.

- DRIs can be used for planning nutritious diets for groups of people and evaluating the nutritional adequacy of a population's diet. RDAs and AIs are often used to evaluate an individual's dietary practices. For nutrition labeling purposes, FDA uses RDAs to develop Daily Values (DVs).

3.2 Major Food Groups

- Food guides generally classify foods into groups according to their natural origins and key nutrients. Such guides usually feature major food groups. Some food guides also include a group for oils.

3.3 Dietary Guidelines

- The Dietary Guidelines is a set of general nutrition-related lifestyle recommendations designed to promote adequate nutritional status and good health, and to reduce the risk of major chronic nutrition-related health conditions.

3.4 Food Guides

- Choosemyplate.gov is an online, interactive food intake and physical activity guide that is based on Dietary Guidelines. Most Americans do not follow the government's dietary recommendations.

- The Exchange System and carbohydrate counting are tools that people can use for planning menus.

3.5 Food and Dietary Supplement Labels

- Consumers can use information on food labels to determine ingredients and compare nutrient contents of packaged foods and beverages. The FDA regulates and monitors information that can be placed on food labels, including claims about the product's health benefits. Nearly all foods and beverages sold in supermarkets must be labeled with the product's name, manufacturer's name and address, amount of product in the package, and ingredients listed in descending order by weight. Furthermore, food labels must use a special format for listing specific information on the Nutrition Facts panel.

- The Daily Values (DVs) are a practical set of nutrient standards for labeling purposes. The nutrient content in a serving of food is listed on the label as a percentage of the DV (%DV). Most nutrients have DVs. A dietary goal is to obtain at least 100% of the DVs for fiber, vitamins, and minerals (except sodium) each day.

- The FDA permits food manufacturers to include certain health claims on food labels. However, the agency requires that health claims meet certain guidelines and, in some instances, use specific wording. A structure/function claim describes the role a nutrient plays in the body. Structure/function statements cannot claim that a nutrient or food can be used to prevent or treat a serious health condition.

- Organic foods are produced without the use of antibiotics, hormones, synthetic fertilizers and pesticides, genetic improvements, or food irradiation. In general, organic food crops are not more nutritious than similar conventionally grown foods. More research is needed to determine whether there are health advantages to eating organic foods. A food product cannot be labeled "organic" unless its production meets strict national standards.

3.6 Organic Food

- Organic farming and the production of organic foods do not rely on the use of antibiotics, hormones, synthetic fertilizers and pesticides, genetic improvements, or ionizing radiation. The USDA developed and implemented rules for the organic food industry. A food product cannot be labeled "organic" unless its production meets strict national standards.

3.7 Using Dietary Analysis Software

- Dietary analysis software and websites can be quick and easy tools for determining nutrient and energy contents of a specific food.

3.8 Nutrition Matters: The Melting Pot

- Traditional ethnic diets are often based on dishes containing small amounts of animal foods and larger amounts of locally grown fruits, vegetables, and unrefined grains. However, these foods are typically abandoned as people migrate to other countries and assimilate into the general population. After an immigrant population has assimilated fully, the prevalence of chronic diseases such as cardiovascular disease, type 2 diabetes, and high blood pressure often increases among them, partly as a result of adopting unhealthy eating practices. Many religions require members to follow strict food handling and dietary practices that often include the prohibition of certain foods and beverages.

Recipe for  Healthy Living

Mango Lassi

Lassi (*luh-see*) is a simple yogurt-based beverage that originated in India. Lassi is usually made and served before a meal, but the drink can also be a refreshing, nutritious snack. This recipe makes about four ½-cup servings. Each serving supplies approximately 97 kcal, 4 g protein, 9 g carbohydrate (excluding forms of fiber), 0.5 g fat, 1 g fiber, 122 mg calcium, and 30 mg vitamin C.

©Wendy Schiff

INGREDIENTS:

  1 ripe mango
  1 cup plain, fat-free yogurt
  1 Tbsp sugar
  6 ice cubes

PREPARATION STEPS:

1. Wash and peel mango. Remove fruit pulp from mango, and discard large seed and peel.

2. Dice mango pulp and place in blender.

3. Add yogurt, sugar, and ice cubes to blender.

4. Blend ingredients until smooth.

5. Serve immediately or refrigerate for up to 24 hours.

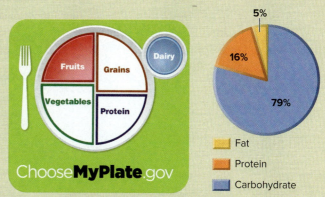

ChooseMyPlate.gov

Source: U.S. Dept. of Agriculture

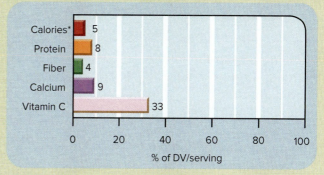

*2000 daily total kcal

Mc Graw Hill Education **connect** Further analyze this recipe or other recipes through activities located in Connect.

Personal Dietary Analysis

I. Record Keeping

A. **24-Hour Dietary Recall**

   1. Recall every food and beverage that you have eaten over the past 24 hours. Recall how much you consumed and how it was prepared.

      a. How easy or difficult was it to recall your food intake?

B. **Three-Day Diet Record**

   1. Without changing your usual diet, keep a detailed log of your food and beverage intake for 3 days; one of the days should be Friday or Saturday. Use a separate log for each day.

II. Analysis

Using nutritional analysis software, analyze your daily food intakes and answer questions in Part III of this activity. Keep the record on file for future applications.

A. **Computer-Generated Dietary Analysis**

   1. Load the software into the computer, or log on to software website.

   2. Choose the DRIs or related nutrient standard from Appendix I of this book, based on your life stage, sex, height, and weight.

   3. Enter the information from the 3-day food intake record. Be sure to enter each food and drink and the specific amounts.

   4. The software program will give you the following results:

      a. The appropriate RDA (or related standard) for each nutrient

      b. The total amount of each nutrient and the kilocalories consumed for each day

      c. The percentage intake compared with the standard amount for each nutrient that you consumed each day

   5. Keep this assessment for activities in other chapters.

III. Evaluation of Nutrient Intakes

Remember it is not necessary to consume the maximum of your nutrient recommendations every day. A general standard is meeting at least 70% of the standards averaged over several days. It is best not to exceed the Upper Level (if set) over the long term to avoid potential toxic effects of some nutrients.

A. For which nutrients did your average intake fall below the recommended amounts, that is, to less than 70% of the RDA/AI?

B. For which nutrients did your average intake exceed the Upper Level (if a UL has been set)?

IV. MyPlate

This activity determines how your diet stacks up when compared to the amounts of foods from each food group that are recommended by MyPlate.

A. Refer to your 3-day diet record. Classify each food item in the appropriate food group of MyPlate. For each food group, indicate whether you ate the recommended amount daily for your sex, age, height, weight, and physical activity level. Note that some of your food choices—pizza, for example—may contribute to more than one food group. Enter a minus sign (–) if your total falls below the MyPlate recommendation or a plus sign (+) if it equals or exceeds the daily recommendation for each food group.

connect Complete the Personal Dietary Analysis activity located in Connect.

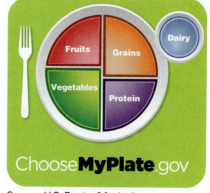

Source: U.S. Dept. of Agriculture

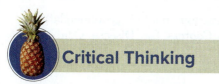

Critical Thinking

1. Your friend takes several dietary supplements daily, and as a result, his vitamin B–6 intake is 50 times higher than the RDA for the vitamin. You would like to convince him to stop taking the supplements. To support your advice, which nutrient standards would you show him? Explain why.

2. Why should consumers use MyPlate to plan menus instead of the DRIs?

3. How do your added sugars, sodium, and saturated fat intakes compare to the recommendations of the latest Dietary Guidelines?

4. Examine Table 3.6. Which foods in the left–hand column do you eat regularly? Why are those foods listed in that column?

5. The ingredient list on a package of crackers includes vegetable oil. What can you do to learn which type of vegetable oil is in the product?

6. Visit the USDA's website (www.ars.usda.gov/Services/docs.htm?docid=17032) to access "What's in the Foods You Eat *Search Tool*," a database for searching the nutritional content of foods. To practice using this search tool, find the number of kilocalories and the amounts of fiber, vitamin C, iron, and caffeine in 1 cup of raw jicama, 1 cup of 2% milk with added vitamin A, and ¼ cup of dry roasted, salt–added sunflower seed kernels (no hulls).

7. According to an article in a food science journal, an 8–oz serving of fat–free milk contains 15 mcg of folate (a B vitamin). An article in a different food science journal reports that an 8–oz serving of fat–free milk contains 12 mcg of folate. Explain why both sources of information can be correct.

8. Consider the ingredients that are used to make a typical cheese pizza. What changes can you make to the pizza recipe to make the food more healthy?

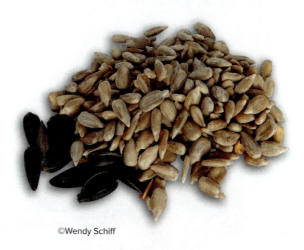

©Wendy Schiff

Pineapple: ©Stockbyte/Getty Images RF

Select the best answer.

1. The amount of a nutrient that should meet the needs of almost all healthy people in a particular group is the
   a. Estimated Average Requirement (EAR).
   b. Recommended Dietary Allowance (RDA).
   c. Nutrient Requirement (NR).
   d. Tolerable Upper Intake Level (UL).

2. Which of the following statements is true?
   a. AMDRs have been developed for all nutrients.
   b. ULs meet the nutrient needs of nearly all healthy people.
   c. RDAs contain a margin of safety.
   d. AIs are requirements for certain nutrients.

3. The Estimated Energy Requirement (EER)
   a. has a margin of safety.
   b. does not account for a person's height, weight, or physical activity level.
   c. is based on the average daily energy needs of a healthy person.
   d. reflects a person's actual daily energy needs.

4. A diet is likely to be safe and nutritionally adequate if
   a. average daily intakes for nutrients meet RDA or AI values.
   b. intakes of various nutrients are consistently less than EAR amounts.
   c. nutrient intakes are consistently above ULs.
   d. vitamin supplements are included.

5. Nutritional standards, such as the RDAs, are not
   a. used to develop formula food products.
   b. the basis for establishing DVs.
   c. used to evaluate the nutritional adequacy of diets.
   d. the basis for developing AIs.

6. According to the MyPlate plan, which of the following foods is grouped with dairy products?
   a. Cheese   c. Butter
   b. Egg   d. Cream

7. Which of the following foods is a good source of protein and contains a lot of saturated fat?
   a. Avocado   c. Cheese
   b. Dry peas   d. Peanuts

8. Fruit is generally a good source of all of the following substances, except
   a. fiber.   c. phytochemicals.
   b. vitamin C.   d. protein.

9. The Dietary Guidelines for Americans is
   a. revised every year.
   b. a set of general nutrition–related recommendations.
   c. published by the Centers for Disease Control and Prevention.
   d. used to develop DVs.

10. Which of the following foods would be classified as a source of empty calories by MyPlate?
    a. Whole milk   c. Whole–grain bread
    b. Grape jelly   d. Corn oil

11. Which of the following statements is true?
    a. According to MyPlate, vegetable oils are grouped into the "Fats and Oils" food group.
    b. The MyPlate menu planning guide cannot be individualized to meet a person's food preferences.
    c. A person can use MyPlate to evaluate his or her diet's nutritional adequacy.
    d. MyPlate was the first food guide developed for Americans.

12. The Exchange System
    a. classifies foods in the same groups as MyPlate.
    b. has exchange lists based on macronutrient contents.
    c. is useful only for people who have diabetes.
    d. incorporates high–protein foods with high–carbohydrate foods.

13. Which of the following information is not provided by the Nutrition Facts panel?
    a. Percentage of calories from alcohol
    b. Amount of total carbohydrate per serving
    c. Serving size
    d. Amount of trans fat per serving

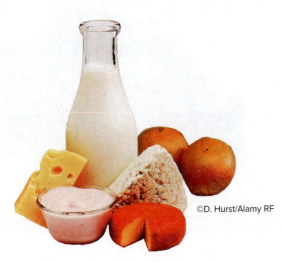
©D. Hurst/Alamy RF

14. Daily Values are
    a. for people who consume 1200 to 1500 kilocalorie diets.
    b. based on the lowest UL for each nutrient.
    c. dietary standards developed for food—labeling purposes.
    d. used to evaluate the nutritional adequacy of a popu—lation's diet.

15. People who follow Jewish dietary rules will not consume

    a. tea.   c. beef.
    b. rice.   d. shellfish.

16. Badih is a devout follower of Islam. Therefore, he will not consume

    a. red meat.
    b. beer.
    c. enriched grains.
    d. coffee.

Answers to Quiz Yourself

1. According to the latest U.S. Department of Agriculture food guide, fruits and vegetables are combined into one food group. **False.** (Section 3.4)

2. According to the recommendations of the *2015–2020 Dietary Guidelines for Americans,* it is acceptable for certain adults to consume alcoholic beverages in moderation. **True.** (Section 3.3)

3. Last week, Colin didn't consume the recommended amount of vitamin C for a couple of days. Nevertheless, he is unlikely to develop scurvy, the vitamin C deficiency disease. **True.** (Section 3.1)

4. The Food and Drug Administration develops Dietary Guidelines for Americans. **False.** (Section 3.3)

5. The Nutrition Facts panel on a food label provides information concerning amounts of energy, fiber, and sodium that are in a serving of the food. **True.** (Section 3.5)

CHAPTER 4

Body Basics

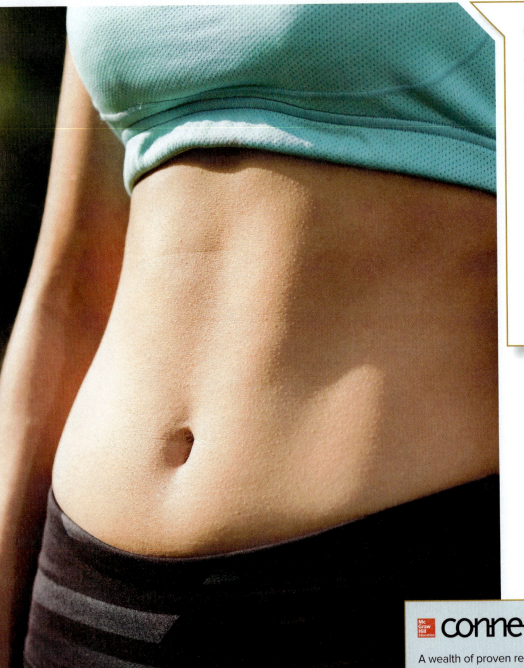

Quiz Yourself

To test your knowledge of the material covered in Chapter 4, take the following quiz; the answers are at the end of the chapter.

1. The atom is the smallest living unit in the body. _____ T _____ F

2. The stomach produces gastric juice that contains hydrochloric acid. _____ T _____ F

3. Digestion begins in the stomach. _____ T _____ F

4. A vast number of bacteria normally live in the large intestine. _____ T _____ F

5. Undigested food rots in your stomach, causing toxic materials to build up in your tissues. _____ T _____ F

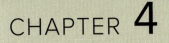 **connect®**

A wealth of proven resources are available on Connect® including SmartBook®, NutritionCalc Plus, and many other dynamic learning tools. Ask your instructor about Connect!

4.1 Nutrition: Chemistry Foundations

Learning Outcomes

1 Define key basic chemistry terms, including *element, ion, chemical bond,* and *enzyme.*

2 Explain the difference between an acid and a base.

3 Explain the role of enzymes in many chemical reactions.

In Chapter 1, we defined chemistry as the study of the composition and charac-teristics of matter, and the changes that it can undergo. We also defined human physiology as the study of how the human body functions. Principles of chemistry and human physiology form the foundation for the scientific study of nutrition. The foods you eat and the air you breathe provide nutrients and oxygen, the raw materials (matter) that your cells need to survive and function. By reading sec-tion 4.1, you will learn some basic chemistry concepts to help you understand how the matter in food becomes the raw materials for building, fueling, and sustaining healthy bodies. In section 4.2, you will learn about body structures and functions so you can understand the roles of nutrients in the body and why these particular chemicals are so important. Section 4.3 focuses on the digestive system and how it functions. Finally, section 4.4 covers some common health problems that affect the digestive system, including heartburn and irritable bowel syndrome.

Parts of this chapter may seem to be filled with unfamiliar terms and their definitions. However, learning the meaning of these terms can help you under-stand nutrition information that is in the following chapters.

Basic Chemistry Concepts

Do you or does someone you know avoid eating foods that are not labeled organic because they contain chemicals such as additives or pesticides? It is true that chem-icals are in your food, but they are not necessarily harmful. Chemicals make up food as well as every other aspect of your environment; air, water, rocks, and other forms of matter contain chemicals. In fact, you are a complex collection of chemicals, much of which is organized into cells. The following sections provide basic information about some chemistry concepts that apply to the study of nutrition.

From Atoms to Compounds

Matter is comprised of atoms that contain certain particles, including protons and electrons (Fig. 4.1). **Protons** are positively charged particles in the *nucleus,* the central region of an atom. **Electrons** are small negatively charged particles that form a cloud surrounding the nucleus. The number of electrons surrounding the nucleus equals the number of protons within the nucleus. Thus, the negative and positive charges cancel out each other, making an atom neutral, which means it has no electrical charge.

More than 100 different types of atoms exist, and each type is an **element,** a substance that cannot be separated into simpler substances by ordinary chemical or physical means. Elements are the "building blocks" of matter. Table 4.1 lists several elements, most of which are essential for human nutrition. An element is essential if the body cannot function normally without it and the element must be supplied by the diet. Note that chemists use letters as symbols to represent elements. For exam-ple, the symbols for carbon, nitrogen, and sodium are C, N, and Na, respectively.

protons positively charged particles in the nucleus of an atom

electrons small, negatively charged particles that surround the nucleus of an atom

element each type of atom; substance that cannot be separated into simpler substances by ordinary chemical or physical means

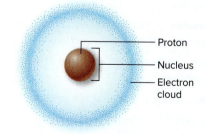

Figure 4.1 An atom. Matter is comprised of atoms that contain particles, including protons and electrons. The nucleus of this hydrogen atom contains one positively charged proton.

TABLE 4.1 Nutrition-related Elements in the Body

Element	Symbol
Hydrogen	H
Oxygen	O
Carbon	C
Nitrogen	N
Calcium	Ca
Phosphorus	P
Potassium	K
Sulfur	S
Sodium	Na
Chloride	Cl$^-$
Magnesium	Mg
Iron	Fe
Iodine	I
Copper	Cu
Zinc	Zn
Manganese	Mn
Cobalt	Co
Chromium	Cr
Selenium	Se
Molybdenum	Mo
Fluoride*	F$^-$

*Although fluoride is not essential, the mineral helps strengthen teeth and bones.

minerals elements that are found in the Earth's crust

chemical bond attraction that holds atoms together

molecule matter that forms when two or more atoms interact and are held together by a chemical bond

compounds molecules that contain two or more different elements in specific proportions

solution evenly distributed mixture of two or more compounds

solvent primary component of a solution

solute lesser component of a solution that dissolves in solvent

solubility describes a substance's ability to dissolve and form a solution

Minerals are elements, such as calcium, iron, and potassium, that are found in the Earth's crust. Many minerals are essential nutrients. However, not every mineral is in living things or is necessary for life. Your external environment has natural and human—made forms of matter that may contain elements such as mercury (Hg), aluminum (Al), and cadmium (Cd). The human body does not need these minerals to function properly, and they can be quite toxic. Chapter 9 discusses the importance of various minerals to health.

Molecules When atoms interact, they may share electrons and rearrange them—selves, forming a chemical bond. A **chemical bond** is an attraction that holds atoms together and forms a **molecule.** When illustrating the structure of molecules, chemists often use straight lines to show the bonds (Fig. 4.2a).

Molecules can contain the same element or different elements. For example, an oxygen molecule forms when two oxygen atoms bind together, whereas a water molecule forms when two hydrogen atoms bond to an oxygen atom. To identify a particular molecule without using lines to draw its chemical structure, chemists use a chemical formula. The chemical formula for an oxygen molecule is O_2; the subscript "2" indicates the presence of 2 oxygen atoms. The chemical formula for a water molecule is H_2O. The chemical formula for the simple sugar *glucose* is $C_6H_{12}O_6$. Judging from its formula, how many carbon, hydrogen, and oxygen atoms are in a glucose molecule?

Some atoms form single bonds, but a few atoms can form multiple bonds. Each carbon atom (C) has four bonding sites, and as a result, carbon atoms can bond to each other by single, double (Fig. 4.2b), and even triple bonds (Fig. 4.2c). Carbon's ability to bond to other carbon atoms as well as form multiple bonds with a neighboring carbon atom contributes to the formation of a vast array of organic (carbon—containing) compounds. **Compounds** are molecules that contain two or more different elements in specific proportions.

Solutions A **solution** is an evenly distributed mixture of two or more compounds. In living things, water is often the **solvent,** the primary component of solutions. Your body, for example, is about 60% water. A substance that dissolves in the solvent is a **solute.** Many beverages and foods are solutions that have water as the solvent (Fig. 4.3a). A sports drink, for example, is a solution that is mostly water, the solvent. The drink has relatively small amounts of sugar, minerals, colorings, and flavorings (solutes) dissolved in the water.

The **solubility** of a substance describes its ability to dissolve, that is, form a solution, in a solvent. Many naturally occurring substances, including simple carbohydrates such as sugar and all mineral elements, dissolve in water. Other substances, such as fat, are insoluble and will not dissolve in water (Fig. 4.3b). Your blood has high water content, a characteristic that makes it easier for the body to transport and eliminate water—soluble substances than water—insoluble materials.

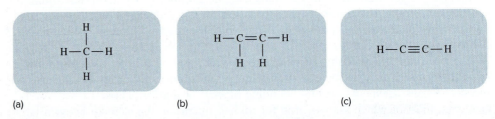

(a)   (b)   (c)

Figure 4.2 Chemical bonds. Some atoms form single bonds (*a*), but a few atoms can form multiple bonds. Carbon atoms can bond to each other by single, double (*b*), and even triple bonds (*c*).

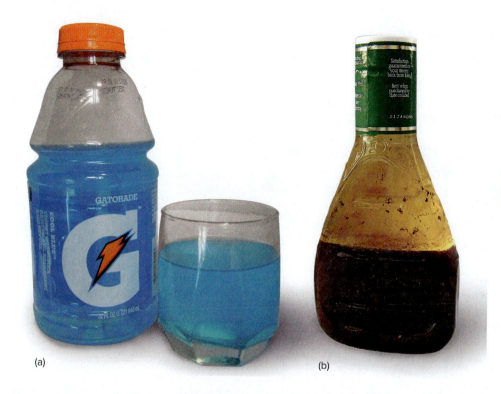

(a)   (b)

Figure 4.3 **Solubility.** The solubility of a compound describes how easily it forms a solution. Many substances, including table sugar, dissolve in water. (*a*) Sports drinks are beverages in which sugar remains dissolved in water. Other substances, such as fat, are insoluble in water and will not dissolve in it. (*b*) Vinaigrette is an example of a food in which oil and water (balsamic vinegar) do not form a solution. In this particular product, note how the oil separates from the vinegar and forms a layer on top of the darker balsamic vinegar layer.

Gatorade and Salad dressing: ©Wendy Schiff

Ions When an atom (or group of atoms) gains or loses one or more electrons, it has an electrical charge and is called an **ion** (Fig. 4.4). If an atom gains one electron, it becomes an ion with a negative charge, because electrons are negatively charged. If an atom loses an electron, it becomes an ion with a positive charge, because it has an extra proton and protons are positively charged. A negative charge is indicated with a minus sign ($^-$), and a positive charge is indicated with a plus sign ($^+$) after the chemical symbol or formula. For example, a molecule of ammonia is neutral, that is, has no electrical charge, because it has the same number of protons and electrons. If the molecule loses an electron, it becomes the positively charged ion, ammonium. The formula for the positively charged *hydrogen ion* is simply H^+.

When most mineral elements, including sodium and potassium, dissolve in water, they form solutions containing ions that can conduct electricity. Thus, sodium and potassium are called **electrolytes.** Electrolytes have many important functions in the body, including helping to maintain proper fluid balance.

What Are Acids and Bases? **Acids** are substances that lose H^+ when dissolved in water; **bases** are substances that remove and accept H^+ when dissolved in water. Many of the chemicals you encounter daily are either acidic or basic (alkaline). As you can tell by their names, phosphoric acid in soft drinks and ascorbic acid

ion atom or group of atoms that has a positive or negative charge

H^+ chemical symbol for hydrogen ion

electrolytes ions of minerals that conduct electricity when they are dissolved in water

acids substances that donate hydrogen ions

bases substances that accept hydrogen ions

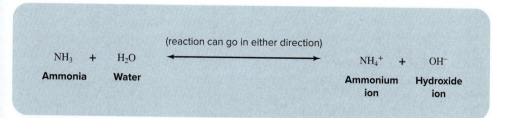

(reaction can go in either direction)

NH_3 + H_2O ⟷ NH_4^+ + OH^-

Ammonia **Water** **Ammonium ion** **Hydroxide ion**

Figure 4.4 **What is an ion?** An ion is an atom or group of atoms that loses or gains one or more electrons and, as a result, has an electrical charge. In this reaction, ammonia and water react to form the positively charged ammonium ion and the negatively charged hydroxide ion.

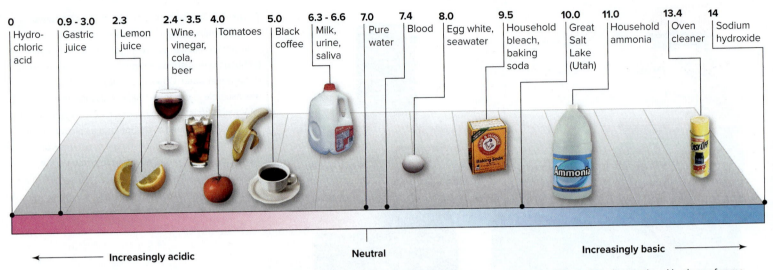

0	0.9 - 3.0	2.3	2.4 - 3.5	4.0	5.0	6.3 - 6.6	7.0	7.4	8.0	9.5	10.0	11.0	13.4	14
Hydro-chloric acid	Gastric juice	Lemon juice	Wine, vinegar, cola, beer	Tomatoes	Black coffee	Milk, urine, saliva	Pure water	Blood	Egg white, seawater	Household bleach, baking soda	Great Salt Lake (Utah)	Household ammonia	Oven cleaner	Sodium hydroxide

← Increasingly acidic   Neutral   Increasingly basic →

Figure 4.5 pH scale. Chemists measure the concentration of hydrogen ions in a watery solution by using the pH scale. This scale indicates the pH values of some substances, including foods. Substances with low pH values are more acidic than substances with high pH values (bases).

Lemon and Wine: ©Brand X Pictures/Getty Images RF; Cola: ©FoodCollection/StockFood RF; Tomato and Banana: ©Stockbyte/Getty Images RF; Coffee: ©Fuse/Getty Images RF; Milk: ©McGraw-Hill Education. Bob Coyle, photographer; Egg: ©Siede Preis/Getty Images RF; Household products: ©McGraw-Hill Education. Stephen Frisch, photographer; Ammonia: ©McGraw-Hill Education. Jacques Cornell, photographer; Oven cleaner: ©McGraw-Hill Education. Ken Karp, photographer

pH measure of the acidity or alkalinity of a solution

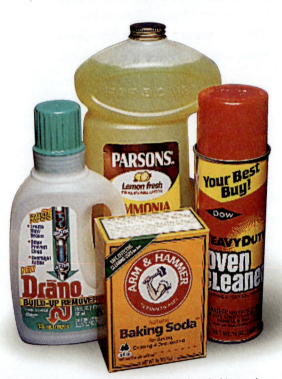

Common household products such as baking soda, household ammonia, and certain oven cleaners are bases. ©McGraw-Hill Education. Stephen Frisch, photographer

(better known as vitamin C) are acids. Baking soda and sodium hydroxide, an ingredient of many hair removal products, are bases.

Chemists measure the concentration of hydrogen ions (**pH**) in a watery solution by using the pH scale. The scale ranges from 0 to 14. With each whole number increase within the scale, the H^+ concentration decreases 10 times. Examine the pH scale shown in Figure 4.5. Note that black coffee has a pH of about 5.0 and tomatoes have a pH of about 4.0. Thus, tomatoes are 10 times more acidic than black coffee. Although it may seem confusing, a solution with a pH of 2.0 has a *higher* H^+ concentration and is *more* acidic than a solution with a pH of 12.0.

Pure water has equal concentrations of H^+ and OH^-, so it is neither acidic nor basic. Thus, pure water has a pH of 7 and is neutral. By combining an acid with a base, the pH of a solution can become 7.

Your body must maintain its *acid–base balance* to function properly. Under normal conditions, the pH of your blood ranges from 7.35 to 7.45, which is slightly alkaline. To control its pH within normal limits, blood contains buffers—ions or molecules that accept excess OH^- or H^+ when necessary. Acids form naturally as by–products of cellular activity, but if the pH of blood begins to fall, the excess H^+ must be eliminated to prevent *acidosis*, a condition that can be deadly. The lungs remove excess H^+ from blood by means of chemical reactions that result in the release of carbon dioxide (CO_2) and H_2O in exhaled air. Kidneys also partici-pate in the buffering system by removing excess H^+ from the blood when forming urine. As a result, urine is an acidic fluid.

Did *YOU* Know?

Blueberries, raspberries, red cabbage, and strawberries contain the pigment *anthocyanin*. This pigment is used as a natural dye for coloring yarns and can also be used as a crude pH meter. Anthocyanin is red when it is in solutions that have a pH of less than 4; this pigment loses its red color at higher pH values and appears blue-green or green. Aside from being an interesting pigment, anthocyanin has antioxidant activity and may provide health benefits as a result (see Table 1.3).

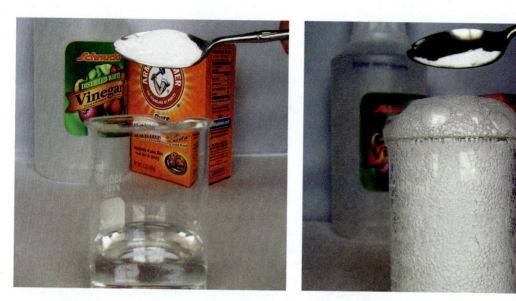

Figure 4.6 Chemical reaction. A chemical reaction occurs when vinegar (an acid) combines with baking soda (a base). This reaction forms sodium acetate (a salt), water, and carbon dioxide. Beaker and Foaming fluid: ©Wendy Schiff

What Is a Chemical Reaction?

Most molecules can undergo **chemical reactions,** processes that change the arrangement of atoms in the molecules. The elements that comprise the molecules that react are never destroyed, but they combine with other elements to form new molecules or compounds. When elements or compounds combine to form new substances, a synthetic reaction has occurred. The new substances often have physical and chemical characteristics (properties) that are quite different from those of the reactants. Decomposition reactions involve the breaking down of molecules. **Digestion,** the process by which large molecules in food are broken down into smaller ones, requires decomposition reactions.

You can observe a simple chemical reaction by combining the reactants vinegar (an acid) and baking soda (a base). As soon as the vinegar makes contact with the soda, the powdery baking soda disappears and a fizzy liquid forms (Fig. 4.6). This particular reaction produces carbon dioxide gas that forms bubbles in the fizzy liquid and sodium acetate. Thus, carbon dioxide and sodium acetate are two of the products that result when vinegar and baking soda react. Sodium acetate is a **salt,** a substance that forms when an acid reacts with a base. Table salt (sodium chloride) is actually one type of salt. Sodium chloride forms when an acid, such as hydrochloric acid (HCl), reacts with a base, such as sodium hydroxide (NaOH) (Fig. 4.7).

In recipes for baked goods that require baking soda, you will find an acid ingredient such as lemon juice, buttermilk, or cream of tartar (tartaric acid) included to react with the soda. The carbon dioxide gas that forms "raises" the mixture, giving it a light, airy structure after baking.

Metabolism Metabolism refers to the sum of all chemical reactions that occur in living cells. *Catabolic reactions* involve breaking down molecules. Catabolism, for example, occurs during digestion. *Anabolic reactions* involve synthesizing new compounds. Repairing damaged muscle tissue after injury is an example of anabolism.

Enzymes Living things contain thousands of chemicals, and life depends upon chemical reactions. However, many of these reactions occur slowly or do not occur spontaneously. An **enzyme** is a molecule (usually a protein) that *catalyzes* (speeds up) a particular chemical reaction. Enzymes are recyclable; they do not become part of the products of a reaction, and as a result, one enzyme molecule can catalyze many reactions. Figure 4.8 illustrates an enzyme's action.

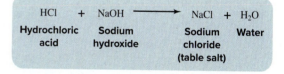

$$HCl + NaOH \longrightarrow NaCl + H_2O$$

Hydrochloric acid | **Sodium hydroxide** | **Sodium chloride (table salt)** | **Water**

Figure 4.7 What is a salt? A salt forms when an acid reacts with a base. For example, sodium chloride (NaCl) and H_2O form when hydrochloric acid (HCl) reacts with sodium hydroxide (NaOH).

chemical reactions processes that change the atomic arrangements of molecules

digestion process by which large food molecules are mechanically and chemically broken down

salt substance that forms when an acid combines with a base

enzyme molecule (usually a protein) that speeds up a particular chemical reaction

Figure 4.8 Enzyme action. In this reaction, the
enzyme sucrase is necessary to break down
sucrose into glucose and fructose.
©Wendy Schiff

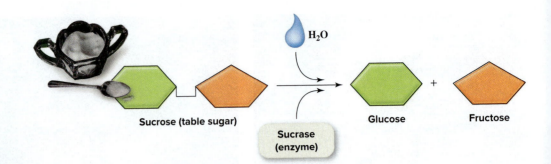

Figure 4.8 Enzyme action. In this reaction, the enzyme sucrase is necessary to break down sucrose into glucose and fructose.
©Wendy Schiff

Sucrose (table sugar) · Sucrase (enzyme) · Glucose + Fructose · H_2O

Food & Nutrition tips

Gelatin is an animal protein that dissolves in boiled water. As it cools, gelatin holds the water and thickens, forming a gel, a solution that takes the shape of its container. Pineapple, papaya, kiwifruit, and guava naturally contain enzymes that break down gelatin. Therefore, when using gelatin in recipes, don't add fresh or frozen forms of these fruits because the enzymes will break down gelatin and the mixture will not gel. Heating destroys these enzymes; thus, you can make a molded gelatin salad or dessert that contains canned pineapple. (Foods undergo heating during the canning process.)

In general, the names of most enzymes end with −*ase*. Sucrase, for example, is the enzyme that catalyzes the reaction that breaks down the carbohydrate sucrose (table sugar) to its component simple sugars, glucose and fructose (see Fig. 4.8). Additionally, each enzyme usually has a specific action. For example, sucrase breaks down sucrose, but the enzyme does not affect lactose, the type of sugar in milk.

Enzymes are sensitive to environmental conditions, including pH, temperature, and the presence of certain vitamins and minerals. If the pH or temperature is too high or too low, the enzyme will not function. Raw food contains enzymes, but cook−ing food usually destroys them.

Concept CHECKPOINT

1. Define the following terms: *electron, proton, element, chemical bond, molecule, compound, solution, solvent,* and *solute.*
2. What is an ion?
3. Explain the difference between an acid and a base.
4. What is pH?
5. What is a chemical reaction?
6. What is an enzyme?
7. What factors can alter an enzyme's activity?

See Appendix G for responses.

4.2 Basic Physiology Concepts

Learning Outcomes

1 Define *cell, tissue, organ,* and *organ systems.*

2 List the organ systems, identify major organs or tissues in each system, and describe primary functions of each system.

The human body is often compared to a complex machine, such as a car. Like a car, the body has numerous interrelated working parts and requires a source of fuel to operate. Additionally, the body has to be able to cool itself, eliminate waste products, and rely on lubrication to keep operating smoothly. Unlike most machines, however, the human body can make many of its spare parts, enabling the body to repair and maintain itself for long periods. When the body functions properly, this wondrous machine may be taken for granted and expected to perform optimally. Nevertheless, the quality of the fuel that powers the human body can affect performance, much like the quality of gasoline that runs a car.

Anatomy is the scientific study of cells and other body structures; **physiology** is the scientific study of how cells and body structures function.

anatomy scientific study of cells and other body structures

physiology scientific study of the functioning of cells and other body structures

This section provides some basic information about human anatomy and physi-ology, including the organization of the body into systems. By learning about human anatomy and physiology, you may appreciate the complexity of your body and be amazed at the variety of metabolic activities that occur within you to keep you alive, physically active, mentally alert, and healthy.

The Cell

A cell is the smallest living functional unit in an organism. Your body has about 100 trillion cells that can be classified into numerous cell types. Each type of cell has a specific function. For example, muscle cells are necessary for movement, red blood cells transport oxygen, and certain white blood cells protect the body from disease—causing bacteria and viruses.

Most human cells contain several different types of **organelles,** structures that have specific functions (Fig. 4.9). The nucleus, for example, is an organelle that contains **DNA,** the molecule that provides coded instructions for making proteins. DNA enables the nucleus to control various cellular activities, including cell division and enzyme production. Mitochondria are organelles that play a major role in the generation of energy. Ribosomes are structures involved in the assembly of proteins. The nucleus, mitochondria, and other organelles are surrounded by a watery fluid called cytoplasm. Many chemical reactions take place in the cytoplasm, including some reactions necessary to make proteins. Each human cell has a plasma mem-brane that defines the boundaries of the cell and holds the cytoplasm in place. The plasma membrane also controls the passage of materials into and out of the cell.

organelles structures in cells that have specific functions

DNA molecule that contains coded instructions for making proteins

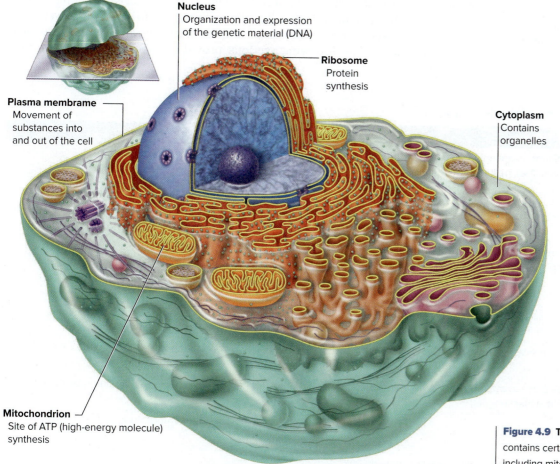

Nucleus
Organization and expression of the genetic material (DNA)

Ribosome
Protein synthesis

Plasma membrame
Movement of substances into and out of the cell

Cytoplasm
Contains organelles

Mitochondrion
Site of ATP (high-energy molecule) synthesis

Figure 4.9 Typical human cell. A typical human cell contains certain structures and various organelles, including mitochondria, ribosomes, and a nucleus.

From Cells to Systems

Cells that have similar characteristics and functions are usually joined together into larger masses called **tissues.** There are four basic types of tissues: epithelial (*ep'–ih–the'–le–al*), connective, muscle, and nervous. The cells that line every body surface, including skin and the inside of blood vessels, are epithelial tissues. Fat, bone, and blood are types of connective tissue.

An **organ** is composed of various tissues that function in a related fashion. The brain, for example, is an organ because it contains different forms of nervous tissue that work together to interpret information from the environment, find meaning from this information, and signal responses, such as muscle movements. An **organ system** is a group of organs that work together for a similar purpose. The urinary system, for example, includes two organs, the kidneys and the bladder. The major functions of the urinary system are filtering blood and excreting wastes in urine. A living person is a complete individual life form comprised of organ systems that function together (Table 4.2). Figure 4.10 illustrates how cells in the body are organized into tissues, organs, and systems.

All systems in your body must work together in a coordinated manner to maintain good health. When one system fails to function correctly, the functioning of the other systems is soon affected. The body's ability to maintain **homeostasis,** an internal chemical and physical environment that supports life and good health, is critical. Internal conditions such as body temperature and blood pressure normally fluctuate throughout the day, but the body strives to maintain such factors within fairly specific limits. Changes in the cell's internal and external environment can disrupt homeostasis, and sickness and even death can result if the abnormality persists. A healthy body, however, uses various mechanisms to regain its normal internal status. As you read about the nutrients, you will recognize how many play crucial roles in homeostasis, including maintaining proper body temperature, acid–base balance, and tissue fluid levels.

Table 4.2 lists each system's major organs or tissues and summarizes their primary functions. The following sections provide a brief description of each organ system.

tissues masses of cells that have similar characteristics and functions

organ collection of tissues that function in a related fashion

organ system group of organs that work together for a similar purpose

homeostasis maintenance of an internal chemical and physical environment that is critical for good health and survival

TABLE 4.2 The Organ Systems of the Human Body

System	Major Organs or Tissues	Primary Functions
Digestive	Mouth, salivary glands, esophagus, stomach, intestines, pancreas, liver, gallbladder	Digestion and absorption of nutrients; elimination of wastes
Cardiovascular	Heart, blood vessels, blood	Circulation of blood throughout the body
Respiratory	Nose, pharynx, larynx, trachea, bronchi, lungs	Exchange of oxygen and carbon dioxide
Lymphatic and Immune system	Lymphatic fluid, white blood cells, lymph vessels and nodes, spleen, thymus, fat cells	Defense and immunity against infectious agents, fluid balance, white blood cell production, absorption of fat-soluble nutrients from intestinal tract
Urinary	Kidneys, bladder	Elimination of salts, water, and wastes; maintenance of fluid balance
Muscular	Muscles	Movement and stability of the body
Skeletal	Bones, tendons, ligaments	Support, movement, protection, and production of blood cells
Nervous	Brain, spinal cord, nerves, sensory receptors	Thought processes, regulation and coordination of various body activities, detection of changes in external and internal environments
Endocrine	Glands or tissues that secrete hormones (chemical messengers)	Regulation and coordination of many body activities, including growth, nutrient balance, and reproduction
Integumentary	Skin, hair, nails	Protection and immunity, regulation of body temperature, vitamin D synthesis
Reproductive	Gonads and genitals	Procreation (having children)

Source: Adapted from Widmaier, EP et al., *Vander's Human Physiology*, 4th ed. Boston: McGraw-Hill, 2016.

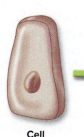

Cell

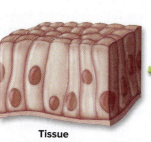

Tissue
Collection of
similar cells

Organ
Collection of various types of
tissues with related functions

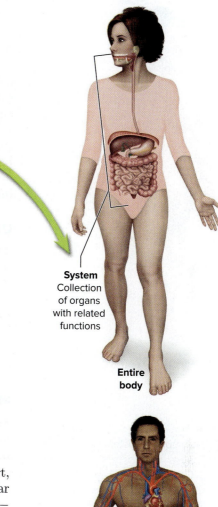

System
Collection
of organs
with related
functions

**Entire
body**

Figure 4.10 Organization of the human body. Cells in
the body are organized into tissues, organs, and organ
systems. A living organism is a complete individual
comprised of organ systems that function together.

Cardiovascular System

The major components of the cardiovascular ("circulatory") system are the heart, blood, and blood vessels (Fig. 4.11). The main function of the cardiovascular system is circulating blood throughout the body. The human heart is a four–chambered muscular pump that keeps blood moving through blood vessels. Blood contains red and white blood cells, nutrients, other substances, and *plasma*, the watery portion of the blood. Blood vessels form a network of tubes that help circulate blood throughout the body. **Arteries** carry blood away from the heart. Arteries branch into smaller and smaller vessels until they form **capillaries,** a network of tiny blood vessels with walls that are only one cell thick. The thin capillary walls enable nutrients and oxygen to move out of the blood and into cells, and carbon dioxide and other waste products to pass from cells and into the blood. After this exchange occurs, the deoxygenated (oxygen–poor) blood enters **veins** for the return trip to the heart.

After entering the right side of the heart, deoxygenated blood is pumped to the lungs, via the pulmonary arteries. In the lungs, red blood cells release carbon dioxide, a cellular waste product, and pick up oxygen from inhaled air. Cells need oxygen to obtain energy. Hemoglobin, an iron–containing protein in red blood cells, carries most of the oxygen in blood. The oxygenated (oxygen–rich) blood then returns to the heart via the pulmonary veins, so it can be pumped to the rest of the body's cells.

Respiratory System

Lungs, the primary structures of the respiratory system, enable the body to exchange gases, particularly oxygen and carbon dioxide (Fig. 4.12). As mentioned in the previous paragraph blood circulates through the lungs, picks up oxygen from inhaled air, and releases carbon dioxide, a waste product that forms when cells obtain energy. By exhaling, you eliminate carbon dioxide from your body.

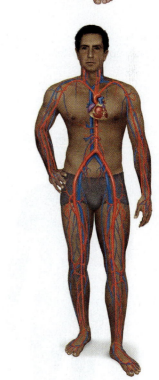

Figure 4.11 **Cardiovascular system.**

arteries vessels that carry blood away from the heart

capillaries smallest blood vessels

veins vessels that return blood to the heart

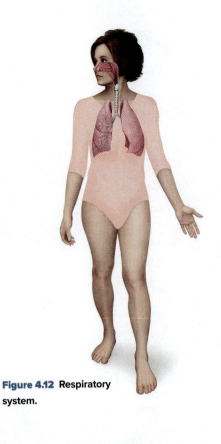

Figure 4.12 Respiratory system.

lymph fluid in the lymphatic system

Lymphatic and Immune System

This system includes a network of lymphatic vessels and lymph nodes (Fig. 4.13). As blood circulates in the body, some fluid (plasma) leaks out of capillaries and into spaces between cells. Under normal conditions, the extra fluid, called **lymph,** collects in tiny lymphatic capillaries and is transported by lymphatic vessels that eventually drain into major veins near the heart, where it enters the general circulation.

The lymphatic and immune system helps defend the body against diseases (immune function). As lymph moves through lymph vessels, lymph nodes remove bacteria and other harmful microbes from the fluid and destroys them. Fat cells are also components of this system, because they produce substances that have immune function.

Urinary System

The urinary system includes the kidneys and bladder (Fig. 4.14). The major role of the kidneys is filtering unneeded substances from blood and maintaining proper fluid balance. As blood circulates, it passes through the kidneys, two bean—shaped organs that remove waste products as well as excess water and water—soluble nutrients from the bloodstream. This filtration process forms urine that moves from each kidney by a tube for storage in the bladder. Urine is mostly water, but it also contains dissolved substances such as urea, a byproduct of protein metabolism, and excess minerals and water—soluble vitamins.

Muscular System

Muscles are the main organs of the muscular system (Fig. 4.15). Muscles enable movement to occur, and they also provide stability for the body. Furthermore, muscles generate heat that helps maintain normal body temperature.

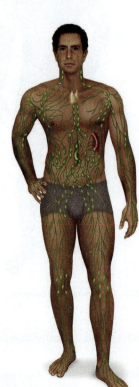

Figure 4.13
Lymphatic and Immune system.

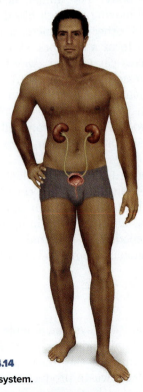

Figure 4.14
Urinary system.

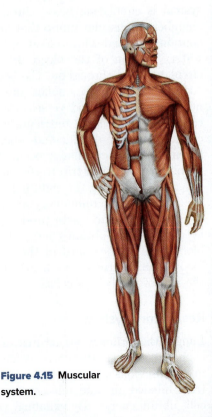

Figure 4.15 Muscular system.

Skeletal System

Bones, tendons, and ligaments are the principal organs of the skeletal system (Fig. 4.16). These structures provide support, movement, and protection for the body. Additionally, bones store excesses of several minerals and produce blood cells.

Nervous System

The brain, spinal cord, and nerves throughout the rest of the body make up the nervous system (Fig. 4.17). The brain produces a variety of intellectual functions and emotional responses, including thoughts, memories, and emotions. The brain also controls and regulates many body functions, including hunger, muscle con−tractions, and physical responses to danger. Nervous system cells (*neurons*) transmit information and responses by electrical and chemical signals.

Endocrine System

The endocrine system is comprised of organs (glands) and tissues, such as fat cells, that produce a variety of chemical messengers called hormones. When released into the bloodstream, a hormone signals cells that can respond (target cells). For example, the thyroid gland contains cells that respond to a hormone, which is released from the pituitary gland, a small organ located near the brain. When stimulated by the pituitary's hormone, the thyroid releases (secretes) a hormone that it makes, which increases the body's metabolic rate. Hormones regulate a variety of physiological activities, including metabolism, digestion, maintenance of fluid balance, and the maturation of reproductive organs that occurs during puberty. The glands of the endocrine system are shown in Figure 4.18.

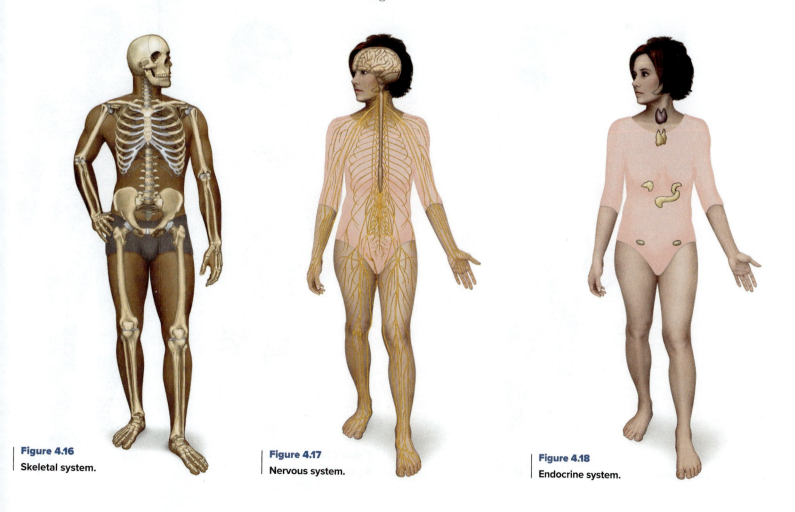

Figure 4.16
Skeletal system.

Figure 4.17
Nervous system.

Figure 4.18
Endocrine system.

Integumentary System

Hair, nails, and skin, the largest organ of your body, are structures of the integumentary system (Fig. 4.19). Skin protects against minor injuries and invading disease—causing agents, such as bacteria. Skin also helps maintain body temperature, primarily by perspiration.

Healthy skin needs many nutrients for its maintenance, including vitamin A, several types of B vitamins, and the mineral zinc. Each day, the dead cells that form the outermost layer of skin are shed, and new skin cells form that will eventually replace them. Because new skin cells are constantly being produced, skin tissue has a high need for nutrients. Therefore, the early signs of many nutritional deficiency disorders often appear as skin abnormalities such as roughened, dry skin.

Reproductive System

The main function of the reproductive system is to produce children (Fig. 4.20). Adequate nutrition is essential for fertility, healthy pregnancies, and healthy newborns. Compared to women whose diets are nutritionally adequate before and during pregnancy, poorly nourished pregnant women have higher risks of miscarriage and stillbirths (infants who are born dead), as well as of giving birth to babies with birth defects and low birth weights. During their first year of life, severely underweight infants are more likely to die than infants whose weights are normal.

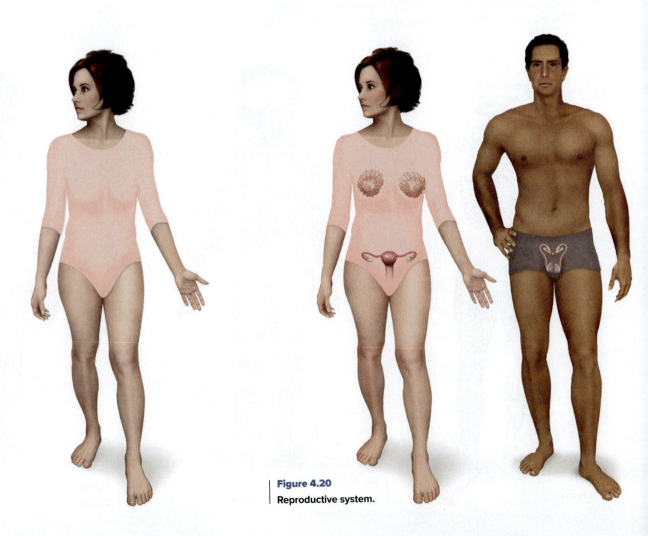

Figure 4.19
Integumentary system.

Figure 4.20
Reproductive system.

Digestive System

Your cells do not need food to carry out their metabolic activities; they need nutrients that are in food. The primary roles of the digestive system are the breakdown of large food molecules into smaller components (nutrients) and the **absorption** of nutrients into the bloodstream or lymphatic system (Fig. 4.21). Section 4.3 focuses on the process of digestion and absorption.

Concept CHECKPOINT

8. Define *cell, organelle, DNA,* and *tissue.*

9. Define *homeostasis.*

10. List at least six of the organ systems that comprise the human body and indicate at least one major function of each organ system listed.

See Appendix G for responses.

4.3 The Digestive System

Learning Outcomes

1 Identify major organs of the digestive system, and describe primary functions of each organ.

2 Identify the accessory organs of the digestive system and the roles these organs play in digestion.

3 Discuss the overall processes of nutrient digestion, absorption, and transport; and waste elimination.

4 Discuss gut microbiota and its role in health.

The mouth, esophagus, stomach, and small and large intestines are the major structures of the digestive system, which is often referred to as the **gastrointestinal (GI) tract.** In a living person, the GI tract is a hollow, muscular tube that extends approximately 16 feet from the mouth to the anus (see Fig. 4.21).[1] The length is longer in a *cadaver* (dead body), because there is no muscle tone.

The process of digestion converts large food molecules, such as protein, starch, and fat, into smaller substances that can be absorbed. Nutrients that are already in their simplest form, which include water, cholesterol, minerals, and most vitamins, are not digested but are absorbed intact.

It is important to recognize that many foods need to undergo some processing before they are eaten. Although some nutrients can be lost during food preparation, practices such as removing inedible parts or cooking raw foods often make them more digestible and safe to eat. Additionally, cooking food can enhance the absorption of its nutrients. **Bioavailability** refers to the extent to which the digestive tract absorbs a nutrient and how well the body uses it.

The teeth, tongue, salivary glands, liver, gallbladder, and pancreas are *accessory organs* of the digestive system that assist the GI tract in food digestion, nutrient absorption and distribution, and waste elimination. This section of Chapter 4 describes the digestive system, including accessory organs and their basic functions. More detailed information about digestion and absorption can be found in chapters that discuss specific classes of nutrients, such as Chapters 5, 6, and 7.

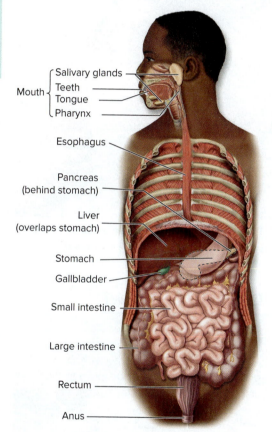

Salivary glands
Mouth { Teeth
Tongue
Pharynx

Esophagus

Pancreas (behind stomach)

Liver (overlaps stomach)

Stomach

Gallbladder

Small intestine

Large intestine

Rectum

Anus

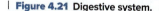

Figure 4.21 Digestive system.

absorption process by which substances are taken up from the GI tract and enter the bloodstream or the lymph

gastrointestinal (GI) tract muscular tube that extends from the mouth to the anus

bioavailability extent to which the digestive tract absorbs a nutrient and how well the body uses it

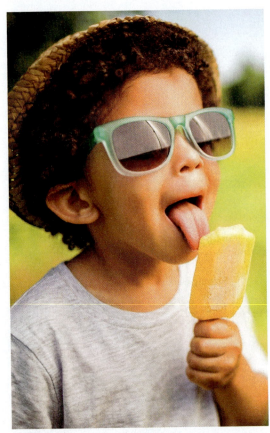

The tongue has regions that are more sensitive to a particular taste. ©wundervisuals/Getty Images RF

Did *YOU* Know?

Children have more taste buds than adults, which may explain why they often reject strong-flavored foods such as liver, cooked broccoli, and raw onion. As people age, their ability to detect certain tastes, particularly bitter and salty tastes, declines.[3] Medications, diseases, and rare inherited conditions may also interfere with the ability to taste foods.

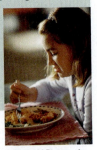

©Brand X Pictures/ PunchStock RF

esophagus structure of the GI tract that connects the pharynx with the stomach

epiglottis flap of tissue that folds down over the windpipe to keep food from entering the respiratory system during swallowing

Mouth

Digestion actually starts in the mouth. The mouth controls the intake of food; teeth begin the mechanical digestion of food by biting, tearing, and grinding food into smaller chunks that are easier to swallow. The tongue helps direct food to the back of the mouth where it can be swallowed.

Chemical digestion refers to the chemical breakdown of foods by substances secreted into the GI tract. As you chew, watery saliva from salivary glands mixes with food and lubricates it. Saliva contains the enzymes *salivary amylase* and *lingual lipase*. (See Section 4.1 for general information about enzymes.) Salivary amylase enables a minor amount of starch digestion to occur in the mouth. Lingual lipase does not begin to digest fat until the food reaches the stomach. In addition to playing an important role in digestion, the mouth senses the taste and texture of foods.

When food comes in contact with saliva or other watery fluids, certain molecules in the food dissolve. When these chemicals are in solution, they stimulate sensory structures called *taste buds* that are located primarily on the tongue. Taste buds have specialized cells that help you distinguish sweet, sour, salty, bitter, and umami (*ew–mom'–e*) tastes. Taste buds relay information about the chemicals dissolved in saliva to a part of the brain that identifies the particular taste based on past experiences. The entire tongue can detect all five tastes, but certain areas are more sensitive to specific tastes than other tastes.[1] The tip of the tongue is most likely to detect sweet–tasting foods and beverages; the sides of the tongue are more sensitive to salty and sour items; and the rear portion of the tongue is more likely to detect bitter things than other regions of the organ.

What benefits do you gain from being able to detect various tastes? The sense of taste is important for stimulating appetite and detecting nutrients or toxic substances in substances that enter the mouth. Foods that taste sweet usually contain carbohydrates, major energy sources for your cells. Chemicals that elicit a bitter taste are often poisonous, so you are more likely to eat sweet–tasting foods and reject bitter–tasting ones. The sour taste can indicate the presence of ascorbic acid, more commonly known as vitamin C. You may like foods that taste tart or sour, especially when they are teamed up with sweet ingredients. Sodium ions stimulate your taste buds to detect a salty taste; a food that tastes salty may contain other mineral nutrients as well. The umami or savory taste is often associated with meat and is detected when certain amino acids stimulate taste buds.[1] Foods that produce the umami taste may be protein–rich; protein is another important component of a healthy diet. There may be a sixth sense of taste. Scientists are studying the possibility that human taste buds can also detect certain fats in foods.[2]

The sense of smell also contributes to your ability to sense the taste of food. As you chew food, it releases chemicals that become airborne and stimulate your nasal passages. Your brain combines such information with taste sensations from your mouth to identify foods' flavors. Thus, favorite foods may seem tasteless and unappealing when you have an upper respiratory tract infection and the inside of your nose is congested.

Esophagus

The **esophagus** (*eh–sof'–ah–gus*) is a muscular tube that extends about 10 inches from the back of the mouth, the pharynx, to the top of the stomach. The primary function of the esophagus is to transfer a mass of swallowed food into the stomach. The entrance to the esophagus is near the voicebox (larynx) and the opening of the windpipe (trachea). The **epiglottis** (*ep–eh–glot'–tis*)

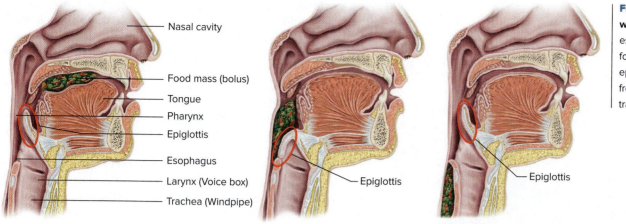

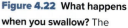

Figure 4.22 What happens when you swallow? The esophagus transfers food into the stomach. The epiglottis prevents the food from entering the larynx and trachea.

is a flap of tough tissue that prevents the food from entering the larynx and trachea (Fig. 4.22). When you swallow, breathing automatically stops and the food normally lands on the epiglottis, making it cover the opening of the larynx. These responses keep swallowed food from entering your trachea and choking you. Now you know why it is not a good idea to talk while you are eating!

Swallowing signals the GI tract that food is being eaten and stimulates **peristalsis** (*per'−uh−stall'−sis*), waves of muscular activity that help propel material through the digestive tract. In the esophagus, each muscular contraction is followed by a brief period of muscle relaxation. Peristalsis moves small amounts of food and beverage from the esophagus into the stomach (Fig. 4.23). Peristalsis is an involuntary response, which means the move−ments happen without the need to think about them.

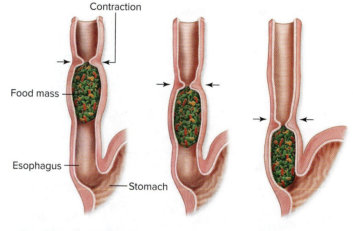

| **Figure 4.23** Peristalsis.

Stomach

The stomach is a muscular sac that can expand and hold about 4 to 6 cups of food after a typical meal.[1] The **gastroesophageal sphincter** (*gas'−tro−eh−sof−ah−jee'−al sfink'−ter*) is the section of esophagus that is next to the stomach (Fig. 4.24). After food enters the stomach, this sphincter constricts, closing the opening between the esophagus and the stomach.

As food enters the stomach, certain cells within the organ secrete *gastric juice*, a watery solution that contains hydrochloric acid (HCl) and some enzymes. HCl helps convert a chemically inactive digestive enzyme (pepsinogen) to its active form (pepsin) and makes proteins easier to digest. The acid also kills many dangerous disease−causing microorganisms that may be in food. Note, as shown in Figure 4.5, that gastric juice is very acidic.

Stimulated by the presence of food, the stomach's muscular walls respond with waves of muscular contractions ("mixing waves") and peristalsis. The churn−ing movements mix food with gastric juice, and as a result of this mechanical and chemical activity, some of the protein and fat in food breaks down. At this point, the stomach contents are a semisolid liquid called **chyme** (*kime*). Although the stomach absorbs very few nutrients from chyme, a few drugs, including some alcohol, can pass through the organ's walls and enter the bloodstream.

Stomach walls consist of muscle proteins. So how does the stomach avoid digesting itself? Special cells that line the inside of the stomach produce a thick layer of **mucus.** Mucus is a slippery alkaline substance that protects the stomach

peristalsis type of muscular contraction of the gastrointestinal tract

gastroesophageal sphincter section of esophagus next to the stomach that controls the opening to the stomach

chyme mixture of gastric juice and partially digested food

mucus fluid that lubricates and protects certain cells

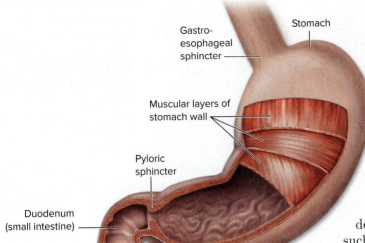

Gastro-esophageal sphincter

Stomach

Muscular layers of stomach wall

Pyloric sphincter

Duodenum (small intestine)

| **Figure 4.24** **The stomach and duodenum.**

from its acid and digestive enzymes. If the layer of mucus breaks down, HCl and gastric enzymes can reach the stomach wall, destroying the tissue. Such destruction can cause one or more sores (ulcers) to form. If the gastroesophageal sphincter does not function properly and relaxes while food is still in the stomach, reflux, the backflow of irritating stomach contents into the esophagus, can occur and cause heartburn. For more information about factors that increase the risk of gastro—intestinal tract ulcers and heartburn, read the "Nutrition Matters" feature at the end of this chapter.

The *pyloric* (*pie—lor'—ic*) sphincter, a ring of muscular tissue at the base of the stomach, controls the rate at which chyme is released into the small intestine (see Fig. 4.24). Following a meal, the stomach empties in about 4 hours, depending on the contents and size of the meal.[1] Watery meals such as soups spend less time in the stomach; fatty meals spend more time there.

Did *YOU* Know?

When you eat foods or drink beverages, you swallow some air. Burping expels most of this air before it enters the stomach. If some air manages to enter your stomach and small intestine, it mixes with chyme and bubbles through it, often producing rather loud, gurgling sounds that can be embarrassing.

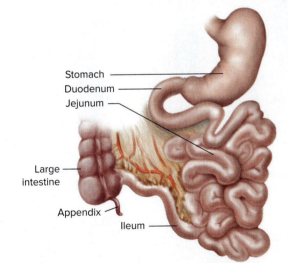

Stomach
Duodenum
Jejunum

Large intestine

Appendix

Ileum

Figure 4.25 **Small intestine.** The small intestine is tightly coiled within the abdominal cavity. Although the appendix may have immune function, you can live without it.

Small Intestine

The small intestine is a coiled hollow tube that extends from the stomach to the large intestine. The organ measures about 16 feet long because of the effects of muscle tone in living persons.[1] The small intestine is "small" because the tube's diameter is only about 1 inch, about half the width of the large intestine.

The small intestine has three sections (Fig. 4.25). The first, the **duodenum** (*do—wah—dee'—num*), is only about 10 inches long. Within the duodenum, the acidic stomach contents mix with alkaline fluids secreted by the pancreas and gallbladder. This process neutralizes the acidity of chyme and enables enzymes that function in more alkaline conditions to work. The middle segment of the small intestine is the **jejunum** (*jeh—ju'—num*). Most digestion and nutrient absorption occurs in the upper part of the small intestine, primarily in the jejunum.[1] The last portion of the small intestine is the **ileum** (*il'—lee—um*).

A **lumen** is a hollow space in an organ or structure that is surrounded by walls, such as the lumen of the small and large intestines. Each day, the small intestine secretes approximately 1½ quarts (1500 ml) of watery fluids into the lumen. This fluid lubricates the intestinal walls, facilitating the passage of chyme. The cells lining the small intestine also produce mucus that protects the tissue from being damaged by chyme as it moves through the tract.

Many of the major chemical reactions that occur during digestion are *hydrolytic* (*hydro* = water; *lytic* = breakdown) because water molecules are necessary for the reactions to occur. Water in intestinal fluid contributes H^+ and OH^- ions. These ions react with certain nutrients and become part of the products. Sucrose, for example, undergoes hydrolysis in the small intestine (see Fig. 4.8).

duodenum first segment of the small intestine

jejunum middle segment of the small intestine

ileum last segment of the small intestine

lumen open space within a structure such as the small intestine

The small intestine relies on peristalsis and *segmentation* to help digestion. Segmentation involves regular contractions of ringlike intestinal muscles followed by muscular relaxations to mix chyme within a short portion of the small intestine (Fig. 4.26). The alternating pressure forces chyme to move back and forth within the segment.

As chyme passes through the lumen of the small intestine, enzymes break down the large compounds in chyme and the intestinal cells into smaller fragments and individual nutrients that can be absorbed. The cells also contain enzymes that are added to chyme and contribute to the digestive process. By the time chyme reaches the middle part of the ileum, most of its nutrient contents have been digested and absorbed. It takes about 3 to 5 hours for chyme to move from the duodenum to the end of the ileum.[4]

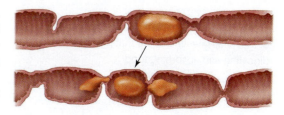

Figure 4.26 Segmentation. Segmentation helps mix chyme in the small intestine.

The Liver, Gallbladder, and Pancreas

The liver, gallbladder, and pancreas are accessory organs of the GI tract that play major roles in digestion, even though chyme does not move through them (Fig. 4.27). The liver processes and stores many nutrients. This organ also makes cholesterol and uses this lipid to make **bile,** a substance that prepares fat and fat-soluble vitamins for digestion and absorption. Bile flows from the liver into the gallbladder, where it is stored until needed. When food and, particularly, fat are in the duodenum, the small intestine sends a hormonal signal to the gallbladder, and as a result, the gallbladder contracts, releasing bile into the duodenum. Chapter 6 provides more information concerning bile's role in digestion.

In the United States, many adults develop gallstones within their gallbladders. Gallstones usually consist of cholesterol; they can be small and grainy, like particles of sand, or as large as a coin (Fig. 4.28). When a gallbladder that contains stones contracts or a gallstone lodges in one of the ducts that carry bile from the gallbladder to the small intestine, it causes considerable pain in the right upper part of the abdomen. If the stone moves out of the duct, the discomfort ends, but in some cases, the duct remains blocked and bile backs up into the liver or pancreas. When this occurs, surgery to remove the diseased gallbladder is necessary to prevent damage to the liver or pancreas. After surgery, bile drips from the liver directly into the small intestine. Having excess body fat increases the risk of gallstones, so keeping your weight at a healthy level can reduce your chances of developing the condition.

The pancreas produces and secretes most of the enzymes that break down carbohydrates, protein, and fat in the GI tract. Additionally, the pancreas secretes *bicarbonate ions* (HCO_3^-) that neutralize HCl in chyme when it enters the duodenum. This is a critical step in the digestion process because the enzymes that function in the small intestine do not work in acidic conditions.

When chyme is in the duodenum, its fat and protein content triggers the release of a hormone *cholecystokinin (co'–lee–sis'–toe–ky'–nin)* from small intestinal cells. Cholecystokinin enters the bloodstream and circulates to the pancreas, where it stimulates the organ to secrete digestive enzymes into the duodenum.

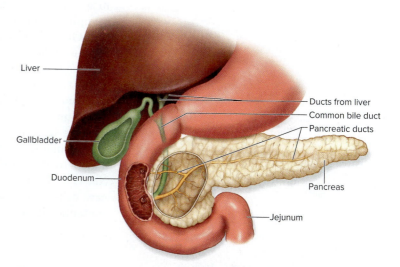

Liver — Ducts from liver — Common bile duct — Pancreatic ducts — Gallbladder — Duodenum — Pancreas — Jejunum

Figure 4.27 Liver, gallbladder, and pancreas. The liver, gallbladder, and pancreas play important roles in digestion. *Ducts* are small tubes that convey fluids, such as bile or pancreatic juice, from one structure to another.

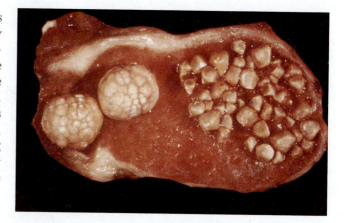

Figure 4.28 Gallstones. This diseased gallbladder has been cut open to show gallstones, which can vary in size. The stones usually consist of cholesterol. ©Biophoto Associates/Science Source

bile substance that is produced by the liver to prepare fat and fat-soluble vitamins for digestion and absorption

villi (singular, villus) tiny, fingerlike projections of the small intestinal lining that participate in digesting and absorbing food

Absorbing and Transporting Nutrients

The lining of the small intestine is not smooth. It has circular folds that look like rings, and the surface is covered by tiny, fingerlike projections called **villi** (singular, villus). Each villus has an outer layer of epithelial cells called *absorptive cells* (Fig. 4.29). Each absorptive cell has tiny, hairlike *microvilli* at the end that faces the lumen of the small intestine (see Fig. 4.29). The intestinal folds, villi, and microvilli increase the surface area of the lumen, which helps increase nutrient absorption.

Absorptive cells complete digestion and remove nutrients from chyme and transfer them into capillaries or lymph vessels (see Fig. 4.29). This process occurs in a variety of ways. Some nutrients require the help of transport proteins or pumping mechanisms within the absorptive cell's plasma membrane to enter the cell. Other kinds of nutrients can simply *diffuse* into these cells. Such diffusion happens when the concentration of a particular nutrient is higher in the lumen of the small intestine than in the absorptive cells. In a few instances, a segment of an absorptive cell's plasma membrane surrounds and "swallows" relatively large substances, such as entire protein molecules. This process, for example, enables an infant's intestinal tract to absorb whole proteins in human milk that provide immune benefits.

While digestion is occurring, absorptive cells are shed into the lumen and added to the contents of chyme. The old cells are digested along with chyme. Newly formed absorptive cells constantly replace those that have been shed. The new cells can absorb nutrients from the older cells and recycle some of their contents. However, the small intestine's high cell turnover rate leads to relatively

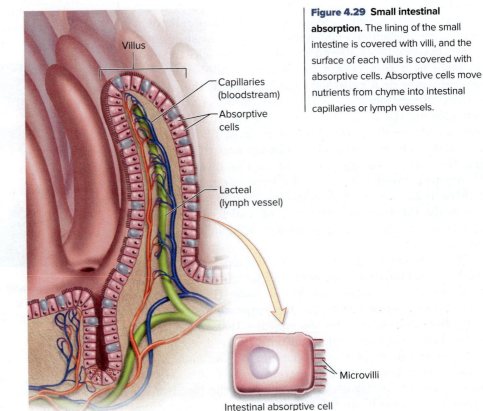

Villus

Capillaries (bloodstream)

Absorptive cells

Lacteal (lymph vessel)

Microvilli

Intestinal absorptive cell

Figure 4.29 Small intestinal absorption. The lining of the small intestine is covered with villi, and the surface of each villus is covered with absorptive cells. Absorptive cells move nutrients from chyme into intestinal capillaries or lymph vessels.

high nutrient needs for these tissues. If the nutrients needed for cell division are lacking, fewer absorptive cells can be replaced, and nutrient *malabsorption* (*mal*=poor) can occur as a result.

After being absorbed, water–soluble nutrients enter the villus's capillary and, eventually, the hepatic portal vein. This vein delivers nutrients directly to the liver, where many undergo processing before they enter the general circulation (Fig. 4.30). Most of the absorbed lipids are coated with a layer that contains protein, forming a **chylomicron** (*ky'–lo–my'–cron*). Chylomicrons move into a **lacteal,** a type of lymphatic system structure in each villus (see Fig. 4.29). Chylomicrons are transported by lymph and eventually enter the bloodstream via a vein near the heart.

About 7.6 to 8.5 quarts (8 to 9 liters) of water from ingested foods and beverages and the secretions of intestinal cells enter into the GI tract daily. Most of the water is absorbed along with other nutrients in the small intestine. Any remaining water and the undigested material that reaches the end of the small intestine must pass through another sphincter before entering the large intestine. This sphincter prevents the contents of the large intestine from reentering the small intestine.

Cystic Fibrosis Cystic fibrosis (CF) is an inherited incurable disease that is usually diagnosed in early childhood. In CF, certain cells produce thick, sticky

chylomicron particle formed by small intestinal cells that transports lipids in the bloodstream

lacteal lymph vessel in villus that absorbs most lipids

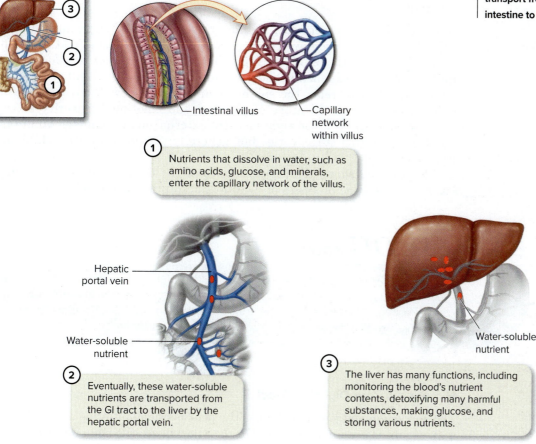

Figure 4.30 Nutrient transport from the small intestine to the liver.

Intestinal villus

Capillary network within villus

1 Nutrients that dissolve in water, such as amino acids, glucose, and minerals, enter the capillary network of the villus.

Hepatic portal vein

Water-soluble nutrient

Water-soluble nutrient

2 Eventually, these water-soluble nutrients are transported from the GI tract to the liver by the hepatic portal vein.

3 The liver has many functions, including monitoring the blood's nutrient contents, detoxifying many harmful substances, making glucose, and storing various nutrients.

mucus that blocks passageways, particularly in the respiratory and diges—tive systems. People with CF often suffer from serious breathing problems and respiratory infections. The pancreatic ducts of an affected person may also become blocked by thick mucus, which interferes with the organ's ability to deliver digestive enzymes to the small intestine. As a result, the diges—tion of nutrients, especially fat, is impaired. To overcome the malabsorption problem, patients with cystic fibrosis can take capsules that contain pancre—atic enzymes with their meals. The capsules protect the enzymes from being destroyed by stomach acid.

Large Intestine

The large intestine is shorter than the small intestine (about 5 feet long in a cadaver)[1], but as you can see in Figure 4.25, its diameter is wider. The large intestine's major sections are the *colon* and the *rectum* (Fig. 4.31). Under nor—mal circumstances, very little carbohydrate, protein, and fat escape digestion and absorption in the small intestine and enter the large intestine. However, the large intestine has no villi, so little additional absorption other than some water and minerals takes place in this structure.

As chyme passes through the large intestine, the residue becomes semisolid and is called stools or *feces*. About 30% of feces (its dry weight) consists of bac—teria that normally live in the large intestine.[4] Feces also contain undigested fiber from plant foods; a small amount of water, protein, and fat; and some mucus and cells shed from the walls of the intestinal tract.

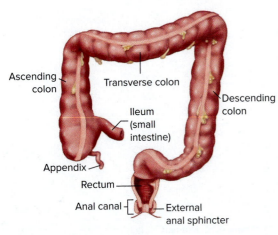

Ascending colon

Transverse colon

Descending colon

Ileum (small intestine)

Appendix

Rectum

Anal canal

External anal sphincter

| **Figure 4.31** Large intestine.

rectum lower section of the large intestine

Elimination

Feces remain in the **rectum,** the lower section of the large intestine, until muscular contractions move the material into the anal canal and then out of the body through the anus (see Fig. 4.31). The *external anal sphincter* that allows feces to be expelled is under voluntary control, so a healthy person can determine when to relax the sphincter and have a bowel movement. Young children must reach the stage of physical and emotional maturity in which they are able to relax or tighten their external anal sphincter voluntarily. The timing of this stage varies but generally occurs in healthy children by 4 years of age.

Figure 4.32 shows the key structures of the digestion system. This figure also summarizes the processes of digestion, absorption, and elimination.

Did *YOU* Know?

Using "high colonics" and other types of enemas (coffee enemas, for example) to "cleanse" your colon is not necessary because the large intestine does not need to be cleansed. Fur—thermore, frequent enemas may deplete the body of vital minerals, including sodium and potassium. Check with your physician before trying enema treatments.

Microbes in Your Digestive Tract

The duodenum and jejunum of a healthy person's small intestine usually have few microorganisms residing in them. On the other hand, the large intestine is home to vast numbers of various *species* (types) of bacteria, which are collectively

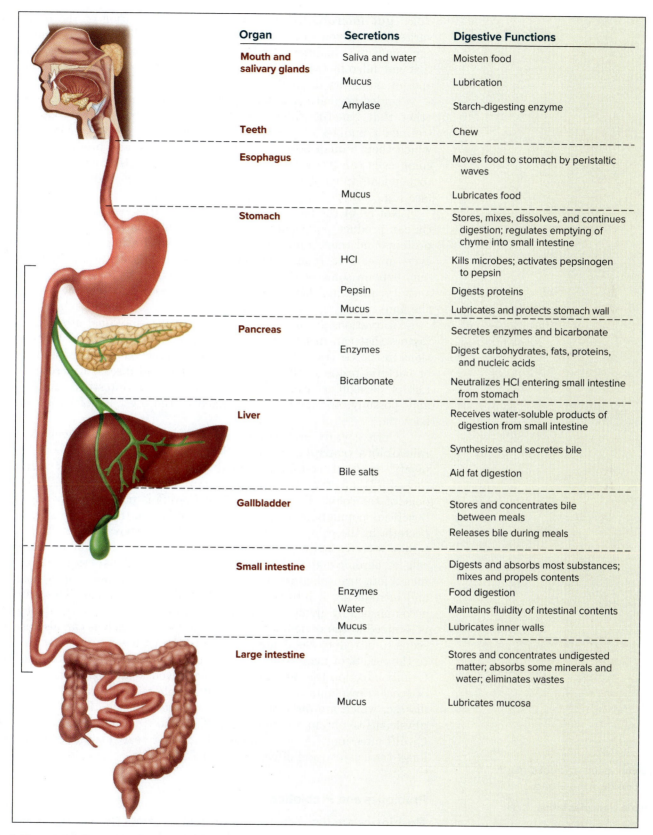

Organ	Secretions	Digestive Functions
Mouth and salivary glands	Saliva and water	Moisten food
	Mucus	Lubrication
	Amylase	Starch-digesting enzyme
Teeth		Chew
Esophagus		Moves food to stomach by peristaltic waves
	Mucus	Lubricates food
Stomach		Stores, mixes, dissolves, and continues digestion; regulates emptying of chyme into small intestine
	HCl	Kills microbes; activates pepsinogen to pepsin
	Pepsin	Digests proteins
	Mucus	Lubricates and protects stomach wall
Pancreas		Secretes enzymes and bicarbonate
	Enzymes	Digest carbohydrates, fats, proteins, and nucleic acids
	Bicarbonate	Neutralizes HCl entering small intestine from stomach
Liver		Receives water-soluble products of digestion from small intestine
		Synthesizes and secretes bile
	Bile salts	Aid fat digestion
Gallbladder		Stores and concentrates bile between meals
		Releases bile during meals
Small intestine		Digests and absorbs most substances; mixes and propels contents
	Enzymes	Food digestion
	Water	Maintains fluidity of intestinal contents
	Mucus	Lubricates inner walls
Large intestine		Stores and concentrates undigested matter; absorbs some minerals and water; eliminates wastes
	Mucus	Lubricates mucosa

Figure 4.32 Summary of digestive system organs and their functions.

called **gut microbiota.** Interestingly, the composition of the bacterial species varies from person to person, due to individual differences, including diet, age, environmental conditions, and medication use.[5] Scientists are studying the roles that gut microbiota play in the prevention and treatment of certain infectious and inflammatory diseases.

Under normal conditions, gut microbiota maintain a balance with each other that benefits their human host. Intestinal bacteria can break down (ferment) undigested food; make vitamins K, B−12, thiamin, and biotin, which their human host may be able to absorb; and produce substances that colon cells can use for energy. Gut microbiota also metabolize certain phytochemicals (phenols) into forms that can be absorbed and used by the body (see Fig. 1.3).[6]

Not all of the bacteria's metabolic activities benefit the host. The bacteria can produce potentially harmful products, particularly when they ferment proteins and their components (amino acids). Eating a high−fiber diet, however, appears to reduce the level of protein fermentation in the gut, which may explain some of fiber's healthful benefits. As a result of their metabolic activity, intestinal bacteria also produce gases that may be expelled through the anus.

Starvation, antibiotic use, and excessive emotional stress are among the factors that can upset the normal balance and diversity of bacterial populations in the GI tract. When the normal balance is disrupted and fewer species of bacteria reside in the gut, inflammation and disease can result. A person's risk of developing heart disease, certain chronic intestinal and liver diseases, and, possibly, obesity has been linked to the diversity of his or her intestinal bacteria.[5,6]

Currently, researchers are testing the safety and effectiveness of using **gut microbiota transplantation (GMT),** commonly referred to as "fecal transplant," to treat certain intestinal disorders, such as *Clostridium difficile* ("C−diff") infection. C−diff bacteria are a usual but potentially harmful resident of the colon. The population of C−diff is normally kept in check by the beneficial populations of gut bacteria. When antibiotic use kills most of the bacteria in the colon, C−diff is often able to survive and multiply. This bacterium secretes toxins that inflame and destroy tissues of the large intestine, causing chronic diarrhea that resists many conventional forms of treatment. Gut microbiota transplantation involves taking some feces from a healthy person and introducing it into the large intestine of the patient. The transfer can be accomplished by giving the patient an enema that contains the donor's feces and is retained in the patient's colon for a period.[6] Physicians can also use a colonoscope to introduce the donor's feces into the patient's large intestine. According to the results of many studies, GMT is a highly effective treatment for cases of C−diff infection that are not cured by conventional medical therapies.[5] The use of fecal transplants may also benefit people with ulcerative colitis or Crohn's disease, which are discussed later in this section. The FDA, however, requires physicians to obtain a permit to use GMT to treat diseases other than resistant C−diff infections.[5] As is often the case, more research is needed to determine the long−term safety and effectiveness of GMT.

Probiotics and Prebiotics

Probiotics are live, beneficial intestinal microbes (primarily bacteria or yeast) that have been grown (*cultured*) under laboratory conditions. Products that contain these microbes are also referred to as probiotics. Many brands of yogurt, for example, are probiotics because they contain "live and active"

gut microbiota various microbes, mostly bacteria, that reside in the GI tract

gut microbiota transplantation fecal transplants

probiotics products that contain healthful microbes; beneficial gut microbes

cultures of the beneficial bacteria (see the Recipe for Healthy Living at the end of this chapter). Probiotics are also available in pills (dietary supplements). *Lactobacillus* and *Bifidobacterium* are the groups of bacteria that are most often used in probiotics.[7] When consumed, adequate amounts of the bacteria must survive the acidic conditions of the stomach and digestive enzymes in the upper small intestine before reaching the large intestine, where they can grow and multiply.

According to studies, probiotics may help prevent the diarrhea that often occurs when antibiotics are taken, and probiotics may be useful in treating people with irritable bowel syndrome (see Section 4.4).[7] However, scientific information about the long−term safety and effectiveness of using probiotics is lacking. Thus, the FDA has not approved any health claims for probiotics.

A person's diet influences the kinds of bacteria that make up his or her gut microbiota. **Prebiotics** are forms of dietary fiber that are poorly digested by humans but support and promote the growth of probiotics in the colon. Prebiotics are in a wide variety of foods, particularly fruits, vegetables, and whole grains. Soybeans, berries, garlic, barley, kale, and legumes are rich sources of prebiotics. Chapter 5 discusses fiber, including prebiotics.

Some species of the gut microbiota can be harmful if they enter other parts of the body or contaminate food. People should wash their hands after having bowel movements to reduce the likelihood of spreading dangerous microbes from their intestinal tract to others. Chapter 12 discusses microor−ganisms that cause common food−borne infections and ways to limit exposure to them.

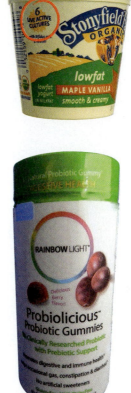

These products are probiotics. ©Wendy Schiff

Inflammatory Bowel Disease Inflammatory bowel disease (IBD) is the gen−eral name for a group of diseases that cause inflammation and swelling of the intestines. The inflammation disrupts digestion and nutrient absorption, and damages the intestines. The cause of IBD is unknown, but a faulty immune response that damages the walls of the intestines appears to contribute to the disease.[8] Ulcerative colitis and Crohn's disease are the two most common forms of IBD. Taking probiotics that contain specific bacteria can help people with ulcerative colitis, but probiotics do not relieve the symptoms of Crohn's disease.[8] The "Real People, Real Stories" feature highlights Matthew Lang, a young man who has ulcerative colitis.

Did *YOU* Know?

Sometimes popular diet "experts" claim that the human GI tract is not designed to digest animal foods. Others claim that eating certain combinations of foods is unhealthy or undi-gested food "rots" in the intestinal tract, causing blockages. Such information is simply not true.

A human being is an **omnivore,** an organism that can digest and absorb nutrients from plants, animals, fungi, and even bacteria. Additionally, the healthy human GI tract responds to dietary changes, such as alterations in the nutritional composition or amounts of food consumed, by increasing the production of various digestive enzymes. Consider this: How would people be able to survive in extreme environments, including deserts and perma-nently frozen regions, if they were unable to digest foods from a wide variety of sources? And finally, a healthy digestive tract does not become blocked by rotted or undigested food.

prebiotics forms of dietary fiber that are poorly digested by humans but support the growth of beneficial gut microbes

omnivore organism that can digest and absorb nutrients from plants, animals, fungi, and bacteria

REAL PEOPLE | REAL STORIES

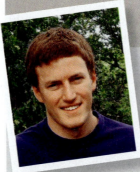

©Wendy Schiff

Matthew Lang

Matthew Lang is a college student who used to take the health of his intestinal tract for granted. When he was 20 and living on campus, he noticed a large amount of blood in his stools after having a bowel movement. Over the next few days, Matthew continued to pass blood in his stools, and he had severe "stomach" cramps. He felt unusually tired, and his friends told him that he "looked pale." After visiting the student health center on campus, Matthew was told that he had *anemia,* a condition characterized by an insufficient number of red blood cells, the cells that transport oxygen in blood to other cells in the body. When the body's cells do not have enough oxygen, they cannot function properly. Matthew's lack of energy and pale skin color are among the signs and symptoms of anemia. His form of anemia was unusual in young men and a sign of chronic blood loss.

Within a few days after visiting the student health center, Matthew had a *colonoscopy,* a procedure in which a *colonoscope,* a long, narrow, flexible tube with a video camera on the end, is inserted into the anal opening and carefully guided through the rectum and colon. The camera enables a physician to see the condition of walls of the rectum and colon. Additionally, the physician can insert small surgical instruments into the colonoscope to perform *biopsies,* the removal of small pieces of abnormal-appearing or damaged intestinal tract tissues. These tissues are sent to a laboratory and studied microscopically for evidence of inflammation or disease.

According to the results of Matthew's biopsy, his colon was inflamed and slightly ulcerated. The young man was told that he had a type of inflammatory bowel disease (IBD) called *ulcerative colitis.* At present, there is no cure for ulcerative colitis, but the condition can be controlled with anti-inflammatory drugs, such as mesalamine (Asacol®). Matthew takes four mesalamine pills a day, and as a result of the treatment, he is able to function normally and feel good.

Medical experts do not know what causes ulcerative colitis, but emotional stress and genetic factors are thought to play major roles in its development. Matthew recalls being very "stressed out" during his sophomore year in college, and the ulcerative colitis was severe enough to send him to the student health center around midterm exams. He notices that his symptoms seem to improve when he is able to relax. Additionally, he has been able to link eating certain foods with "flares," bouts of painful cramping associated with ulcerative colitis. For example, he has determined that consuming red meat, carbonated beverages, and large amounts of cheese and milk seem to trigger his intestinal discomfort.

Matthew recognizes that he will need to monitor his intestinal health, maintain a healthy diet, and probably take medication for the rest of his life. "It's annoying to take all these pills every day, but I'm getting used to it," he said. "I know it's necessary, along with following a good diet for the rest of my life. Having ulcerative colitis has made me realize the benefits of a good diet. Even people who don't have IBD should improve their eating habits. They might feel better, too."

Concept CHECKPOINT

11. Describe what happens to a cheese sandwich after it is eaten and as it moves through the digestive tract.
12. Provide an example of mechanical digestion and chemical digestion.
13. Identify four different tastes.
14. Eliot choked on a piece of hot dog. Explain why choking can occur while eating.
15. What functional aspect of a healthy digestive system prevents food from becoming "stuck" in the tract?
16. What keeps stomach contents from reentering the esophagus?
17. List the sections of the small intestine. Where does most digestion and absorption occur?
18. How would removal of the pancreas affect digestion?
19. Describe at least two different ways that nutrients can enter villi.

See Appendix G for responses.

4.4 Nutrition Matters: Gut Reaction

Learning Outcome

1. Identify some common gastrointestinal health problems, and discuss preventive measures and treatments for these conditions.

Even though you may be healthy, you have probably experienced occasional bouts of constipation, vomiting, diarrhea, or heartburn. After being miserable and uncomfortable for a while, you recovered and returned to your usual routine. This section provides general information about common intestinal problems, including peptic ulcers.

Constipation

Many Americans, especially older adults, think they are constipated if they do not have a bowel movement at least once a day. According to the American Gastroenterological Association, it is not necessary to have a daily bowel movement. Although the normal frequency of bowel movements varies individually, a healthy person should have a bowel movement at least every three days.[9] When bowel movements occur less frequently and/or are difficult to eliminate, the condition is called constipation.

Many factors influence the frequency of bowel movements. Lack of dietary fiber; low water intake; anxiety, depression, and other psychological disturbances; and changes in your typical routine, such as taking a long trip or having major surgery, can alter your usual pattern of bowel movements. Furthermore, constipation can result when people regularly ignore their normal bowel urges

and avoid making a trip to the bathroom when it's not convenient.

Although occasional constipation is a common health problem, chronic constipation can cause discomfort and may contribute to the development of inflamed hemorrhoids and diverticula. Chapter 5 provides more information on these common conditions.

If you feel uncomfortable because your bowel habits have changed or you have hard, dry stools that are difficult to eliminate, discuss the matter with your physician. In many instances, adding more fiber–rich foods to your diet is the first step to becoming more "regular." Chapter 5 provides information about dietary fiber, including rich food sources.

Diarrhea

Diarrhea is a condition characterized by frequent bowel movements with loose stools. Diarrhea occurs when more water than normal is secreted into the GI tract, and the extra water softens and dilutes the stools. In most cases, diarrhea results from bacterial or viral infections of the intestinal tract. The infectious bacteria or viruses produce irritating or toxic substances that increase the movements (motility) of the GI tract. As a result, the GI tract propels chyme more rapidly through it, absorbing less water than normal in the process. Increased GI motility also enables the large intestine to eliminate the watery feces and the toxic material it contains rapidly.

Cases of severe diarrhea require medical attention because frequent watery stools can deplete the body's fluid volume, causing dehydration and excessive losses of electrolytes, such as sodium and potassium. Therefore, treatment of severe diarrhea generally includes drinking replacement fluids that contain sodium, potassium, and simple sugars such as glucose. It's also prudent to avoid eating solid foods until the condition resolves. Prompt treatment of severe diarrhea—within 24 to 48 hours—is especially crucial for infants and older adults because they can become dehydrated quickly by the loss of body water. In adults, diarrhea that is accompanied by bloody stools or lasts more than 7 days may be a sign of a serious intestinal disease, and a physician should be consulted.

Vomiting

Not long after eating something toxic or drinking too much alcohol, you begin to feel queasy or "sick to your stomach." You soon become well aware that your body has an effective way of removing the harmful food or beverage—vomiting. Although vomiting is an unpleasant experience, it often prevents toxic substances from entering your small intestine, where they can do more harm or be absorbed. Vomiting can also be a response to intense pain, food allergies, rotating movements of the head (motion sickness), hormonal changes in pregnancy (morning sickness), and migraine headaches.[10]

Vomiting occurs when the vomiting center in the brain interprets information from various nervous system receptors concerning the physical and chemical conditions of the stomach, small intestine, and bloodstream. When a toxic chemical is detected, the center initiates vomiting by contracting the abdominal muscles, expelling the contents of the stomach and duodenum forcefully out of the body via the mouth.

Vomiting generally does not last more than 24 hours. Repeated vomiting, however, can result in dehydration and the loss of electrolytes, especially if it's accompanied by diarrhea. Treatment includes avoiding solid food until the condition resolves. Additionally, sipping small amounts of water or clear liquids, including noncarbonated soft drinks such as sports drinks, can help prevent dehydration. If the affected person is able to retain small amounts of fluid, then he or she can try to drink increasing amounts of fluid until the vomiting subsides completely.

Adults should contact a physician if their vomiting lasts for more than a day and they have signs of dehydration, such as increased thirst, decreased urination, sunken eyes, and dry mouth.[10] Contact a physician immediately if the vomit is bloody (looks like coffee grounds) or vomiting is accompanied by other signs and symptoms, such as confusion, fever, or severe abdominal pain (see Table 4.3). Children who suffer from vomiting and/or diarrhea are likely to develop dehydration more rapidly than adults who are suffering from these conditions. Signs of dehydration in young

TABLE 4.3 Vomiting Danger Signs

Contact a physician when vomiting:
1. lasts longer than a few hours (children under 6 years of age);
2. lasts longer than a day (people over 6 years of age);
3. is accompanied by:
   - blood in vomit (looks like coffee grounds)
   - signs of dehydration
   - diarrhea
   - fever
   - weakness
   - headache or stiff neck
   - severe abdominal pain
   - confusion or decreased alertness

children include sunken eyes, dry mouth, and decreased urination. Contact a physician if a child has vomiting and diarrhea that persists for more than a few hours and shows signs of dehydration.

Gastroesophageal Reflux Disease (GERD)

Many American adults complain of having occasional heartburn ("acid indigestion"), a gnawing pain or burning sensation generally felt in the upper chest, under the breastbone. This discomfort is not the result of a heart problem but is caused by the passage of acidic contents from the stomach into the esophagus ("acid reflux"). Because the esophageal lining does not produce as much protective mucus as the stomach, the acid quickly destroys the tissue, causing pain and, sometimes, bleeding (Fig. 4.33). Many factors can contribute to heartburn or worsen the condition, including being pregnant; smoking cigarettes; having excess body fat; drinking alcohol; and consuming certain foods.

Although many people think heartburn is a trivial health problem, frequent chronic heartburn can be a symptom of

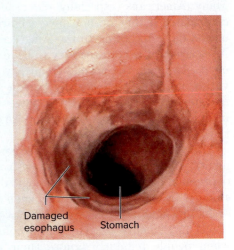

Figure 4.33 Acid reflux damage. An endoscopic view of the esophagus near the opening to the stomach. The reddened areas are signs of damage caused by acid reflux.
©David M. Martin, M.D. /Science Source

Damaged esophagus   Stomach

TABLE 4.4 Recommendations to Reduce the Risk of Heartburn

1. If you have too much body fat, lose the excess weight.
2. Do not lie down within 3 hours after eating a meal.
3. Do not overeat at mealtimes.
4. Avoid smoking cigarettes.
5. Elevate the head of your bed 6 to 8 inches higher than the foot of the bed.
6. Do not wear tight belts or clothes with tight waistbands.
7. Learn to recognize foods that cause heartburn.

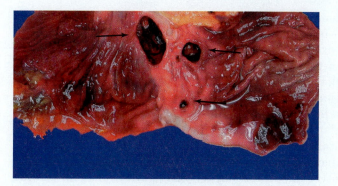

Figure 4.34 Gastric ulcers. This photo shows a portion of the inside of a stomach that has at least three peptic ulcers. Source: Courtesy of Dr. Jill Urban, Dallas County Medical Examiner's Office, Dallas, TX

gastroesophageal reflux disease (GERD). Symptoms of GERD include frequent heartburn and may include nausea, gagging, coughing, or hoarseness. If not treated properly, acid reflux damages the lining of the lower esophagus and contributes to the development of esophageal ulcers (sores). Such ulcers can damage blood vessels in the wall of the esophagus, causing bleeding. Signs of bleeding from the esophagus and stomach include black, tarry stools and iron-deficiency anemia. In severe cases, the loss of blood from a bleeding ulcer can be deadly.

People who suffer from GERD have a higher risk of esophageal cancer than people who do not have a history of this condition. If you or someone you know has GERD, typical dietary advice for treating the condition includes consuming smaller, more frequent meals that are low in fat; not overeating at mealtimes; and limiting intake of foods that relax the gastroesophageal sphincter, such as spicy or greasy foods, tomatoes and tomato products, peppermint, caffeine, alcohol, and chocolate.[11] Additionally, you should wait about 3 hours after meals before lying down because remaining upright reduces the likelihood that stomach contents will push against the gastroesophageal sphincter and move into your esophagus. Table 4.4 lists these and other recommendations for reducing the risk of heartburn and managing GERD. Taking over-the-counter antacids can neutralize excess stomach acid and relieve the discomfort of heartburn within minutes, but these products do not prevent heartburn. People who have GERD can take other medications that inhibit stomach acid production, preventing heartburn.

Peptic Ulcer

A peptic ulcer is a sore that occurs primarily in the lining of the stomach or the upper small intestine (Fig. 4.34). The typical symptoms of a peptic ulcer are dull or burning pain

gastroesophageal reflux disease (GERD) condition that can result when acid reflux damages the wall of the lower esophagus and causes ulcers

in the upper abdominal area that occurs when the stomach is empty, such as between meals or during the night. The pain is relieved briefly by taking antacids or eating. The pain results when HCl acid in the stomach comes in contact with and digests the lining of the organ, forming one or more sores. It is not unusual for the sores to damage the wall of a blood vessel, causing bleeding; thus, untreated peptic ulcers may result in iron-deficiency anemia. Furthermore, an ulcer may erode through the stomach or intestinal wall and allow GI contents to leak into the abdominal cavity, resulting in a potentially life-threatening infection. Therefore, it is important to recognize ulcer symptoms and obtain treatment early.

Physicians detect peptic ulcers by performing a clinical examination called upper endoscopy. The first step of this procedure involves administering a medication that relaxes the patient. Then the physician inserts a special flexible scope into the mouth, down the esophagus, and into the stomach and upper small intestine. The scope is equipped with a video camera that transmits images of the lining of the esophagus, stomach, and upper small intestine to a screen that the physician views for the presence of ulcers, eroded areas, or cancerous tumors. The scope also enables the physician to use tools to treat areas of bleeding or remove pieces of tissue (biopsy) for microscopic examination.

At one time, medical experts thought excessive emotional stress caused peptic ulcers. By the 1990s, however, researchers determined that in many cases, *Helicobacter pylori* (*H. pylori*), a type of bacteria that can live in parts of the stomach, was responsible for the development of stomach ulcers. *H. pylori* damages the protective mucous coating that covers the lining of the stomach. When this occurs, stomach acid comes in contact with the stomach lining and destroys it. In addition to infection with *H. pylori*, other factors are associated with the development of peptic ulcers, particularly smoking cigarettes, heavy consumption of alcohol, and use of NSAIDs (nonsteroidal anti−inflammatory drugs) such as aspirin, ibuprofen, and naproxen.[12] Note that stress is no longer considered a risk factor for ulcer formation.

Dietary approaches do not seem to help in the prevention or treatment of peptic ulcers.[12] Instead, people may be able to prevent peptic ulcers by avoiding the regular use of NSAIDs. People infected with *H. pylori* can take antibiotics, as well as medications that reduce stomach acid production. This treatment is highly effective for combating *H. pylori* infections and healing peptic ulcers.

Irritable Bowel Syndrome (IBS)

About 1 in 6 Americans suffers from irritable bowel syndrome (IBS), a condition characterized by intestinal cramps and abnormal bowel function, particularly diarrhea, constipation, or alternating episodes of both.[13] After bowel movements, the affected person may feel as though elimination of stools was incomplete.

The cause of IBS is unknown, but gastrointestinal infections, certain foods, and emotional stress may trigger the disorder. The colons of people with IBS may be more sensitive to nervous stimulation that the colons of people who do not have this condition.[13] Researchers are investigating the role of the nervous system in stimulating these abnormal intestinal tract movements.

Therapy is individualized and may include elimination diets that focus on determining which foods are most likely to contribute to IBS symptoms. A low−FODMAP diet may help some people with IBS.[14] FODMAPs are poorly digested forms of carbohydrate, including fructose in fruit, table sugar, and high−fructose corn syrup. Chapter 5 provides more information about FODMAPs. Treatment may also include learning stress management strategies, obtaining psychological counseling, and taking antidepressants and other medications.

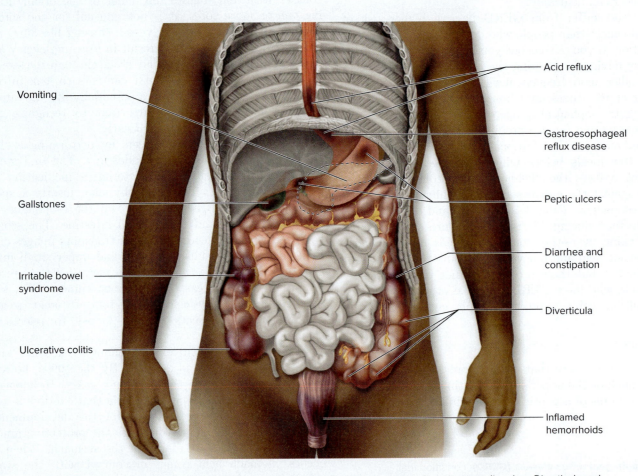

Vomiting

Gallstones

Irritable bowel syndrome

Ulcerative colitis

Acid reflux

Gastroesophageal reflux disease

Peptic ulcers

Diarrhea and constipation

Diverticula

Inflamed hemorrhoids

This illustration shows areas of the digestive system that are affected by common digestive tract disorders. Diverticula and inflamed hemorrhoids are discussed in Chapter 5.

Although irritable bowel syndrome can be uncomfortable and upsetting, the condition does not appear to inflame the tissue of the large intestine or increase the risk of colorectal cancer.[13] For more information about this condition, visit the website www.ibsgroup.org.

Concept CHECKPOINT

20. Explain why excessive diarrhea and vomiting can be dangerous.

21. Describe at least three steps people can take to reduce their risk of heartburn and GERD.

22. Discuss at least three steps people can take to reduce their risk of peptic ulcers.

23. Describe common signs and symptoms of irritable bowel syndrome.

See Appendix G for responses.

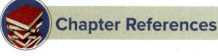

Chapter References

See Appendix H.

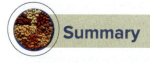

Summary

4.1 Nutrition: Chemistry Foundations

• Matter is composed of chemicals. Over 100 different types of atoms exist, and each type is an element. Atoms of elements may react with each other to form chemical bonds that hold the atoms together in a new arrangement called a molecule. Molecules that contain two or more different elements are called compounds. A solution is an evenly distributed mixture of two compounds. In living things, water is the solvent, the primary compound of a solution.

• Ions, acids, and bases play important physiological roles in the body. An ion is an atom or group of atoms that has a positive or negative electrical charge. Electrolytes are ions with minerals that can conduct electricity. An acid is a molecule that donates hydrogen ions (H^+); a base is a molecule that accepts H^+. Chemists use the pH scale to describe the H^+ concentration of a watery solution.

• Most molecules undergo chemical reactions that change their arrangement of atoms, forming new molecules or compounds. When elements or compounds combine to form new substances, a synthetic reaction has occurred. The new substances often have physical and chemical properties that are quite different from those of the reactants. Decomposition reactions, such as those occurring during digestion, involve the breaking down of molecules. Enzymes are molecules (usually proteins) that speed up rates of chemical reactions. Enzymes do not become part of the products of a reaction and, as a result, can catalyze many reactions.

4.2 Basic Physiology Concepts

• Anatomy is the scientific study of cells and other body structures; physiology is the scientific study of how cells and body structures function. A cell is the smallest functioning unit in a living organism. Cells that have similar characteristics and functions are usually joined together into larger masses called tissues. An organ is composed of various tissues that function in a related fashion. An organ system is a group of organs that work together for a similar purpose.

- The cardiovascular system involves the pumping action of the heart to circulate blood in blood vessels throughout the body. Arteries carry blood away from the heart; veins convey blood back to the heart. The thin walls of capillaries allow nutrients and oxygen to move out of the blood and into cells, and carbon dioxide and other waste products to pass from cells and into the blood.

- The respiratory system enables the body to obtain oxygen and eliminate carbon dioxide. The lymphatic system helps maintain fluid balance, absorb certain nutrients, and defend the body against infectious disease. The urinary system filters and excretes unneeded substances from blood and maintains proper fluid balance.

- The muscular and skeletal systems enable the body to move within its environment and provide support and protection for the body. The nervous system produces intellectual and emotional responses, and controls and regulates many body functions. The endocrine system produces hormones that convey information to target cells; hormones regulate a variety of physiological activities. Hair, nails, and skin are structures of the integumentary system. Skin protects against minor injuries and infectious disease-causing agents, and helps maintain body temperature. The main function of the reproductive organs is to produce children.

- To be healthy, all organ systems must work together in a coordinated manner to maintain homeostasis. When homeostasis is disrupted, the body uses various mechanisms to regain its normal internal status, but sickness and even death can result if the abnormality persists.

- Your cells do not need food to carry out their metabolic activities; they need nutrients that are in food. The primary roles of the digestive system are the breakdown of large food molecules into smaller components (nutrients) and the absorption of nutrients into the bloodstream.

4.3 The Digestive System

- Digestion is a mechanical and chemical process that breaks down large food components into nutrients that can be absorbed. The mechanical aspects of digestion include the chewing action of teeth as well as involuntary muscular activity, including peristalsis. Chemical digestion includes the actions of enzymes and substances such as hydrochloric acid and bile.

- Digestion begins in the mouth with the mechanical action of teeth and some minor chemical action of salivary amylase. The esophagus conveys food from the mouth to the stomach, where it mixes with gastric juice and is referred to as chyme. The chyme moves from the stomach to the duodenum of the small intestine. In the small intestine, enzymes complete the process of digestion. In the small intestine, cells of villi absorb the end products of digestion and transfer them to blood or lymph. Any remaining undigested material, some water, and intestinal bacteria are eliminated from the body as feces.

- The human intestinal tract contains vast numbers of microbes, particularly bacteria that reside in the large intestine. Gut microbiota play important roles in health, and imbalances in the diversity and numbers of the bacteria can cause infection and, possibly, certain chronic diseases.

4.4 Nutrition Matters: Gut Reaction

- Common gastrointestinal disorders include constipation, vomiting, diarrhea, heartburn, peptic ulcer, and irritable bowel syndrome. Chronic constipation can cause discomfort and may contribute to the development of diverticula. Frequent chronic heartburn can be a symptom of GERD. People with GERD are at risk of esophageal cancer. Peptic ulcers can cause life-threatening bleeding. In addition to infection with *H. pylori,* smoking cigarettes, heavy consumption of alcohol, and use of nonsteroidal anti-inflammatory drugs increase the risk of peptic ulcer. Although irritable bowel syndrome is common, the condition does not result in inflammation of the large intestine.

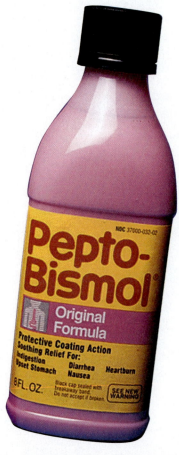

The active ingredient in this product is bismuth subsalicylate (*biz'-muth, sub'-sa-lis'-eh-late*), which is taken by mouth to treat gastroesophageal reflux for people who are 12 years of age and older. ©McGraw-Hill Education. Pat Watson, photographer

Recipe for Healthy Living

Easy Orange-Strawberry Smoothie

When made with low-fat yogurt that contains "live and active" cultures, smoothies are a tasty, low-fat, calcium- and potassium-rich snack. They are also easy to prepare: This recipe takes less than 10 minutes to make. For variety, substitute a banana, a mango, or raspberries for the strawberries, or use lime sherbet instead of orange sherbet. Experimenting with different fruits and flavored sherbets makes it easy to individualize smoothies, depending on your preferences and the fruit that's available. You'll need a sturdy blender to combine the ingredients.

The following recipe makes about three 8-fluid-ounce servings. Each serving supplies approximately 214 kcal, 9 g protein, 2 g fat, 290 mg calcium, 607 mg potassium, 125 mg sodium, 1.6 mg zinc, and 6 mcg selenium.

INGREDIENTS:

¼ cup frozen orange juice concentrate, calcium fortified
1 cup orange sherbet
1 ½ cups low-fat, plain yogurt that has live and active cultures
1 cup fresh strawberries, washed with leafy "caps" removed
   (can substitute frozen strawberries)
2 ice cubes

PREPARATION STEPS:

1. Place all ingredients, except ice cubes, in blender.

2. Blend until smooth. Add ice cubes and blend again, until ice is crushed.

3. Serve.

4. Refrigerate or freeze unused portion in a covered container. Partially thaw frozen smoothie before blending again.

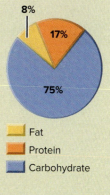

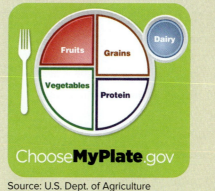

ChooseMyPlate.gov

Source: U.S. Dept. of Agriculture

8%
17%
75%

- Fat
- Protein
- Carbohydrate

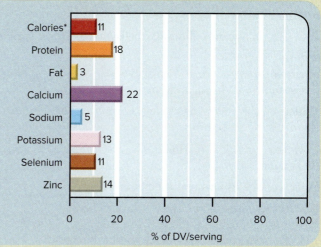

Calories* — 11
Protein — 18
Fat — 3
Calcium — 22
Sodium — 5
Potassium — 13
Selenium — 11
Zinc — 14

% of DV/serving

*2000 daily total kcal

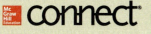

Further analyze this recipe or other recipes through activities located in Connect.

Critical Thinking

1. When your grandmother forgot to buy her heartburn medication, she added a teaspoon of baking soda to a cup of water and drank the solution to relieve her "acid indi—gestion." Explain why this remedy works, even though physicians do not recommend it (baking soda contains unhealthy amounts of sodium).

2. Why would a person's stomach feel uncomfortably full several hours after eating a bacon—topped double cheese—burger, a large serving of French fries, and a milkshake?

3. Explain why the label for a multivitamin supplement recommends taking the pill with meals, particularly meals that contain some fat.

4. Miguel had a serious condition that required removal of the upper third of his small intestine. Based on this information, is Miguel at risk for developing multiple nutrient deficiencies? Explain why or why not.

5. Your mother complains of having persistent heartburn, but she does not think her discomfort is serious enough to be investigated by her physician. Do you agree or disagree with her attitude about heartburn? Explain your position.

©Wendy Schiff

Practice Test

Select the best answer.

1. Which of the following substances is insoluble in water?

   a. Iron
   b. Sugar
   c. Fat
   d. Sodium

2. Which of the following substances has the lowest pH?

   a. Gastric juice
   b. Household ammonia
   c. Tomatoes
   d. Milk

3. A _____ is a group of similar cells that perform similar functions.

   a. ribosome
   b. tissue
   c. cytoplasm
   d. system

4. Which of the following organs is an accessory organ of the digestive system?

   a. Heart
   b. Tongue
   c. Bladder
   d. Spleen

5. Which of the following statements is true?

   a. Arteries carry blood away from the heart.
   b. Hemoglobin carries most of the enzymes in the blood.
   c. Cells need carbon monoxide to obtain energy.
   d. The liver is the primary organ of the cardiovascular system.

6. Chemical digestion begins in the

   a. liver.
   b. stomach.
   c. mouth.
   d. pancreas.

7. Two or more atoms that are held together by a chemical bond form a

   a. pH.
   b. molecule.
   c. proton.
   d. nucleus.

8. A salt forms when an _____ combines with a _____.

   a. electrolyte; proton
   b. acid; base
   c. element; pH
   d. enzyme; mineral

9. Chemical messengers in the body are

   a. enzymes.
   b. cells.
   c. capillaries.
   d. hormones.

10. Tiny, fingerlike projections of the small intestine that absorb nutrients are called

   a. salivary glands.
   b. lymph nodes.
   c. villi.
   d. organelles.

11. A lacteal is a

    a. lymph vessel within each villus.
    b. form of carbohydrate in milk.
    c. muscular structure that regulates digestion in the large intestine.
    d. specialized cell.

12. A _____ transports lipids in the bloodstream.

    a. hormone
    b. cholecystokinin
    c. chylomicron
    d. sphincter

13. The stomach secretes

    a. salivary amylase.
    b. hydrochloric acid.
    c. bile.
    d. cholecystokinin.

14. Peristalsis

    a. is a common intestinal infection.
    b. interferes with lipid absorption in the small intestine.
    c. stimulates red blood cell formation in bone marrow.
    d. helps move food/chyme through the digestive tract.

15. Which of the following conditions primarily affects the large intestine?

    a. Ulcerative colitis.
    b. GERD.
    c. Gallstones.
    d. Peptic ulcers.

16. Which of the following practices increases the risk of peptic ulcer?

    a. Chewing gum
    b. Smoking cigarettes
    c. Drinking orange juice
    d. Eating a low—fiber diet

Answers to Quiz Yourself

1. The atom is the smallest living unit in the body. **False.** (Section 4.2)

2. The stomach produces gastric juice that contains hydrochloric acid. **True.** (Section 4.3)

3. Digestion begins in the stomach. **False.** (Section 4.3)

4. A vast number of bacteria normally live in the large intestine. **True.** (Section 4.3)

5. Undigested food rots in your stomach, causing toxic materials to build up in your tissues. **False.** (Section 4.3)

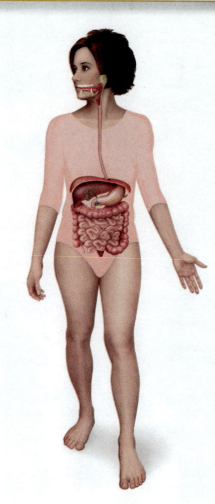

CHAPTER 5

Carbohydrates

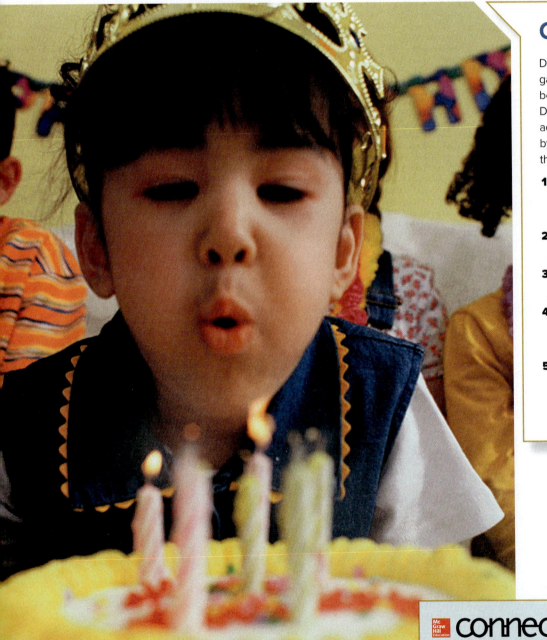

Quiz Yourself

Do "carbs" cause diabetes or unwanted weight gain? Would sweetening your cereal with honey be a healthier choice than using table sugar? Does eating sugary foods make children hyperactive? Check your knowledge of carbohydrates by taking the following quiz. The answers are at the end of the chapter.

1. Compared to table sugar, honey is a natural and far more nutritious sweetener.
_____ T _____ F

2. Ounce per ounce, sugar provides more energy than starch. _____ T _____ F

3. Eating a high-fiber diet may reduce your blood cholesterol level. _____ T _____ F

4. The average American consumes 80% of his or her energy intake as refined sugars.
_____ T _____ F

5. The results of clinical studies indicate that eating too much sugar makes children hyperactive. _____ T _____ F

McGraw Hill Education **connect®**

A wealth of proven resources are available on Connect® including SmartBook®, NutritionCalc Plus, and many other dynamic learning tools. Ask your instructor about Connect!

5.1 Introducing Carbohydrates

Learning Outcomes

1. Identify the two major kinds of carbohydrates in human diets.
2. Explain how plants make carbohydrates.
3. Identify roles of carbohydrates in the body.

When you are bored, excited, or in a good or bad mood, do you reach for something sweet to eat? Can you imagine celebrating birthdays, weddings, or holidays without cakes, candies, or cookies? If you are like many Americans, you enjoy eating sweets and may even describe yourself as having a "sweet tooth."

Why do humans, even newborn infants, prefer foods that taste sweet? The pleasant and sometimes irresistible taste of sugar is a clue that the food contains **carbohydrates.** Carbohydrates are a class of nutrients that includes substances cells can use for energy. Without a steady supply of energy, cells cannot function and they die.

Carbohydrates are generally grouped into simple or complex forms. **Simple carbohydrates** ("sugars" or "simple sugars") include *glucose*. Glucose is a very important simple carbohydrate because it is a primary energy source for human cells. Starches and most kinds of fiber (dietary fiber) are *complex carbohydrates* because they contain many simple carbohydrate molecules. Plants make sugars, starches, and fiber by using the sun's energy to combine the carbon, oxygen, and hydrogen atoms from carbon dioxide (*carbo–*) and water (*–hydrate*) (Fig. 5.1).

carbohydrates class of nutrients that includes glucose, a major source of energy for the body

simple carbohydrates group of carbohydrates that includes sugars

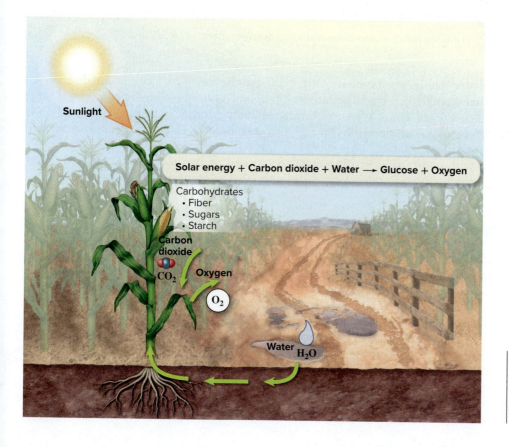

Sunlight

Solar energy + Carbon dioxide + Water ⟶ Glucose + Oxygen

Carbohydrates
• Fiber
• Sugars
• Starch

Carbon dioxide

CO_2 Oxygen

O_2

Water H_2O

Figure 5.1 Carbohydrates. Plants use the sun's energy to combine carbon, oxygen, and hydrogen atoms from carbon dioxide and water to make glucose. As a result of this process, oxygen gas is released. Plants can use glucose to make fiber, starch, and other sugars.

133

high-fructose corn syrup (HFCS) caloric sweetener that is often added to food

monosaccharide simple sugar that is the basic chemical unit of carbohydrates

disaccharide simple sugar comprised of two monosaccharides

glucose monosaccharide that is a primary fuel for muscles and other cells; "dextrose" or "blood sugar"

Some of the energy from the sun is stored in the bonds that hold the carbon and hydrogen atoms together. Human cells can break down some of those bonds, releasing energy that powers various forms of cellular work, including contracting muscles, making vital compounds, and building bone tissue.

On average, each American consumed about 115 pounds of *added* caloric sweeteners, in 2015.[1] Such sweeteners include **high—fructose corn syrup (HFCS)**, as well as honey and table sugar. Added caloric sweeteners are sources of empty calories that offer little nutritional value other than simple carbohydrates to diets. Although people need some glucose for energy, consuming too much carbohydrate, as well as the other macronutrients, can lead to extra body fat.

This chapter provides information about the major roles of carbohydrates in the body and rich food sources of carbohydrates, including simple sugars and complex carbohydrates.

Concept CHECKPOINT

1. What substances do plants need to make carbohydrates?
2. Explain why a plant will die if it is not exposed to light.
3. Why does a human cell need glucose?

See Appendix G for responses.

5.2 Simple Carbohydrates: Sugars

Learning Outcomes

1 List the three most important dietary monosaccharides for humans.

2 Identify the basic monosaccharide components of sucrose, maltose, and lactose.

3 Explain the difference between a nutritive sweetener and a nonnutritive sweetener.

4 List three nutritive and three nonnutritive sweeteners.

You probably are familiar with sugar as the sweet, white, granulated crystals often sprinkled on cereal or into iced tea, but table sugar is only one type of sugar. There are different types of sugars, including forms in milk, blood, and DNA, the genetic material in cells. The simplest type of sugar, the **monosaccharide** (*mono* = one; *saccharide* = sugar), is the basic chemical unit of carbohydrates. A **disaccharide** (*di* = two) is a sugar comprised of two monosaccharides. By combining monosaccharides, plants and animals can form complex carbohydrates.

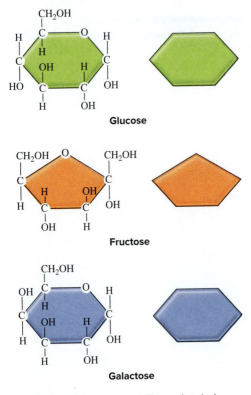

Monosaccharides

The three most important dietary monosaccharides are glucose, fructose, and galactose. Figure 5.2 shows the chemical structures of glucose, fructose, and galactose, as well as the geometric symbols used to represent them in this text—book. The chemical names of carbohydrates, particularly sugars, often end in *ose*. Gluc*ose*, fruct*ose*, and sucr*ose* are sugars commonly found in foods.

Fruits and vegetables, especially berries, grapes, corn, and carrots, are good food sources of **glucose.** Glucose is the most important monosaccharide in the human body because it is a primary fuel for muscle and other cells. In fact, red blood and nervous system cells, including brain cells, must use glucose for energy under normal conditions. Thus, a healthy body maintains its *blood glucose* levels carefully. Glucose is also called dextrose and may be referred to as blood sugar.

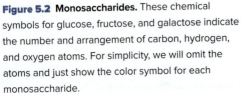

Figure 5.2 Monosaccharides. These chemical symbols for glucose, fructose, and galactose indicate the number and arrangement of carbon, hydrogen, and oxygen atoms. For simplicity, we will omit the atoms and just show the color symbol for each monosaccharide.

Fructose (fruit sugar or levulose) is naturally found in fruit, honey, and a few vegetables, particularly cabbage, green beans, and asparagus. Since fructose tastes much sweeter than glucose and is easily made from corn, food manufacturers use large amounts of high–fructose corn syrup (HFCS) as a food additive to satisfy Americans' demand for "regular" soft drinks, candies, and baked goods. The body has little need for fructose, but it can convert the monosaccharide to fat or glucose.

Unlike glucose and fructose, **galactose** is not commonly found in foods. Galactose is a component of lactose, the form of carbohydrate in milk. After a woman gives birth, special glands in her breasts convert glucose into galactose, which is necessary for production of lactose, the form of carbohydrate in breast milk.

fructose monosaccharide in fruits, honey, and certain vegetables; "levulose" or "fruit sugar"

galactose monosaccharide that is a component of lactose

maltose disaccharide comprised of two glucose molecules; "malt sugar"

sucrose disaccharide comprised of a glucose and a fructose molecule; "table sugar"

lactose disaccharide comprised of a glucose and a galactose molecule; "milk sugar"

Disaccharides

Disaccharides include maltose, sucrose, and lactose. **Maltose** (malt sugar) has two glucose molecules bonded together (Fig. 5.3a). Few foods naturally contain maltose. **Sucrose** (table sugar) consists of a molecule of glucose and one of fructose (Fig. 5.3b). **Lactose** (milk sugar) forms when a galactose molecule bonds to a glucose molecule (Fig. 5.3c). Although most animal foods are not sources of carbohydrate, milk and some products made from milk, such as yogurt and ice cream, contain lactose.

Sucrose

Although sucrose occurs naturally in honey, maple syrup, carrots, and pineapples, much of the sucrose in the American diet is refined from sugar cane and sugar beets. The refining process strips away the small amounts of vitamins and minerals in sugar cane and sugar beets. "Raw sugar," turbinado sugar, and some forms of brown sugar are not as fully processed from sugar cane as white sugar. These sweeteners contain a small amount of molasses, which contributes to their flavor, color, and nutritional value. Since refined sucrose has the reputation of being a "junk food," some manufacturers have used creative names, such as "evaporated cane juice," to disguise the presence of table sugar in their product's ingredients list. In 2016, the FDA advised food manufacturers to identify the sweetener as "cane sugar" or "sugar" instead of "evaporated cane sugar."[2]

Some people claim that refined white sugar is poisonous and honey is nutritionally superior to table sugar. However, these claims are not true. Table sugar does not contain toxic substances; in fact, it is almost 100% carbohydrate. Table 5.1 compares the nutritional value of honey with certain forms of sucrose. Note that none of the sweeteners is a good source of protein, vitamins, or minerals. The simple sugars in honey are not superior to those that comprise sucrose, and your body does not distinguish whether glucose or fructose came from honey or table sugar.

A tablespoon of white table sugar is almost 100% sucrose; a tablespoon of honey has glucose, fructose, water, and a small amount of sucrose. A tablespoon of honey contains more protein and micronutrients than a tablespoon of white sugar, but the amounts are insignificant. For example, you would have to eat a cup of honey to obtain 1.0 g of protein, 1.7 mg of vitamin C, and 1.4 mg of iron. That amount of honey supplies over 1000 kcal! Although honey contains phytochemicals, substances in plant foods that may provide health benefits, the amounts are too small to make this sticky sweetener a valuable source of these compounds. Table sugar and honey are sources of empty calories.

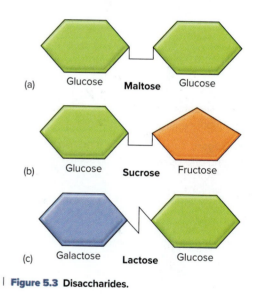

(a) Glucose **Maltose** Glucose

(b) Glucose **Sucrose** Fructose

(c) Galactose **Lactose** Glucose

Figure 5.3 Disaccharides.

Did *YOU* Know?

Bees make honey by consuming the sucrose-rich nectar from flowers and digesting most of it into glucose and fructose. The bees regurgitate (vomit) this material within the beehive, and eventually, it is collected by beekeepers for human processing and packaging.

©Allan & Sandy Carey/Getty Images RF

TABLE 5.1 Nutritional Comparison of Selected Sweeteners

Sugar/Syrup 1 Tablespoon	Water %	Kcal	Protein g	Carb g	Vit. C mg	Calcium mg	Niacin mg	Potassium mg	Iron mg	Zinc mg
Honey	17	64	0.06	17.3	0.1	1	0.025	11	0.09	0.05
White granulated sugar	0	49	0	12.6	0	0	0	0	0.01	0
Maple syrup (100% maple)	32	52	0.01	13.4	0	20	0.016	42	0.02	0.29
High fructose corn syrup (HFCS)	24	53	0	14.4	0	0	0	0	0.01	0
Brown sugar	1	52	0.02	13.5	0	11	0.015	18	0.10	0
Molasses	22	58	0	15.0	0	41	0.186	293	0.94	0.06

Source: Data from USDA National nutrient database for standard reference, release 28

Nutritive and Nonnutritive Sweeteners

Sugars are **nutritive sweeteners** because they are carbohydrates that contribute energy to foods. Each gram of a mono— or disaccharide supplies 4 kcal. **Added sugars** ("added sweeteners"), such as sucrose and HFCS, which is chemically similar to sucrose, are often added to foods during processing or preparation. In baked cereal products, added sugars contribute to the browning and tenderness of the food. Sugar also serves as a preservative by inhibiting the growth of molds and bacteria that would otherwise cause food spoilage. If one of the nutritive sweeteners listed in Table 5.2 is the first or second ingredient listed on a product's label, the food probably contains a high amount of added sugar. Table 5.3 indicates the amounts of added sugars that are in typical servings of commonly consumed foods and beverages. The following section provides information about other kinds of sweeteners.

nutritive sweeteners substances that sweeten and contribute energy to foods

added sugars sugars added to foods during processing or preparation

TABLE 5.2 Sugars and Other Nutritive Sweeteners

Brown sugar	Glucose	Polydextrose
Confectioner's or powdered sugar		Raw sugar
Corn sweeteners, corn syrup, high-fructose corn syrup (HFCS), cultured corn syrup	Honey	Sorbitol*
	Invert sugar	Mannitol*
Date sugar	Lactose	Xylitol*
Dextrose	Maltose, high-maltose corn syrup	Table sugar (sucrose)
Fructose (levulose)	Maltodextrin	Turbinado sugar
Fruit juice concentrate or concentrated fruit juice sweetener	Maple syrup	
	Molasses	

©Wendy Schiff

*Alcohol forms of sugars

TABLE 5.3 How Much Added Sugar Is in That Food?

Food	Serving Size	Kcal	Approximate Teaspoons Added Sugars
Doughnut, cake, plain	3 ¼″ diameter	226	2
Chocolate chip cookies, commercial brand	2 medium (50 g)	239	4
Sugar-frosted cornflakes	¾ cup	114	3
Chocolate-flavored 2% milk	1 cup	158	3
Ice cream, vanilla, light, soft-serve	½ cup	111	2
Chocolate candy bar with almonds	1.76 oz	235	5
Apple pie, double crust	⅛ of an 8″ diameter pie	277	4
Snack sponge cake with cream filling	1 cake (43g)	157	4
Yogurt, vanilla low-fat	8 oz	193	4
Cola, sugar-sweetened, canned	12 fl oz	136	8
Fruit punch drink	12 fl oz	175	10
Chocolate milkshake, fast food	16 fl oz	580	10

Source of data: Krebs-Smith, SM, "Choose beverages and foods to moderate your intake of sugars: Measurement requires quantification," *Journal of Nutrition* 131:527S, 2006.

Alternative nutritive sweeteners include sugar alcohols: *sorbitol, xylitol* (*zigh′–lih–tol*), and *mannitol*. Unlike sugars, sugar alcohols do not promote dental decay. Thus, these compounds are used to replace sucrose in products such as sugar–free chewing gums, breath mints, and "diabetic" candies. Sugar alcohols are not fully absorbed by the intestinal tract, and as a result, they supply an average of 2 kcal/g. However, sugar alcohols may cause diarrhea when consumed.

Nonnutritive Sweeteners

Some people try to control their caloric intake by reducing their consumption of foods and beverages sweetened with nutritive sweeteners such as sugar. **Nonnutritive sweeteners** (also referred to as sugar replacers, sugar substitutes, or "artificial" sweeteners) are substances added to food that sweeten the item while providing few or no kilocalories. **High–intensity sweeteners** are a group of nonnutritive sweeteners that have an extremely sweet taste when compared to the same amount of table sugar. Thus, a very small amount of a high–intensity sweetener is needed to sweeten a food, and such sweeteners supply little or no energy per serving.

Nonnutritive sweeteners may help people control their energy intake and manage their body weight.[4] Consumers, however, need to recognize that most "sugar–free" or "diabetic" foods are not calorie free. Furthermore, results of some studies suggest that artificially sweetened foods and beverages can pro–mote excess calorie consumption. Why? More research is needed, but the taste of products that contain artificial sweeteners may interfere with a person's ability to regulate his or her intake of sugary foods and beverages.[5]

Honey can contain spores, the inactive life stage, of the deadly bacterium *Clostridium botulinum* that resist being destroyed by food preservation methods. These spores can become active bacteria within an infant's intestinal tract and produce a poison that is extremely toxic to nerves. According to experts at the Centers for Disease Control and Prevention (CDC), honey should not be fed to children younger than 12 months of age or used to sweeten infant foods because it may cause botulism poisoning.[3] Older children and adults can eat honey without being concerned about botulism because the mature stomach produces enough acid to destroy the bacterial spores.

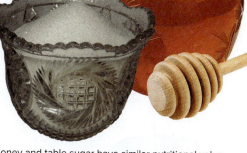

Honey and table sugar have similar nutritional value.

Sugar bowl: ©Wendy Schiff; Honey: ©Brand X Pictures/Getty Images RF

nonnutritive sweeteners substances that sweeten foods while providing few or no kilocalories

high-intensity sweeteners group of nonnutritive sweeteners that are extremely sweet tasting compared to the same amount of sugar

TABLE 5.4 Comparing Nonnutritive Sweeteners

Sweetener	Comparison to Sugar/ Serving*	Brand Name	Kilocalories/ serving
Aspartame	200 times sweeter	NutraSweet®, Equal®	Nearly 0
Saccharin	200-700 times sweeter	Sweet'N Low®, Sugar Twin®, Necta Sweet®	0
Acesulfame-K	200 times sweeter	Sunett®, Sweet One®	0
Neotame	7000–13,000 times sweeter	Neotame	0
Sucralose	600 times sweeter	Splenda®	0
Highly purified stevia leaf extracts such as rebaudioside A	200–400 times sweeter	Truvia®, SweetLeaf®, Rebiana	0
Advantame	20,000 times sweeter	Advantame	0

©Wendy Schiff

*Source: U.S. Food and Drug Administration: *Additional information about high-intensity sweeteners permitted for use in food in the United States.* 2015. https://www.fda.gov/Food/IngredientsPackagingLabeling/FoodAdditivesIngredients/ucm397725.htm#Advantame Accessed: July 6, 2017.

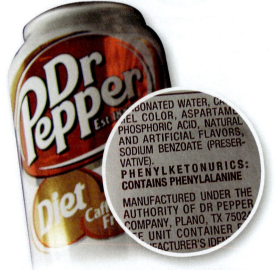

Figure 5.4 Warning label for people with PKU. People with PKU need to be concerned about their phenylalanine intake. Artificially sweetened foods that contain aspartame carry this warning on the label because aspartame contains phenylalanine.
©Wendy Schiff

The Food and Drug Administration (FDA) has approved the use of six high-intensity sweeteners: saccharin, aspartame, acesulfame–K, sucralose, neotame, and Advantame.[6] The agency has also approved the use of commercially purified extracts (steviol glycosides) from leaves of the stevia plant. Table 5.4 provides information about FDA–approved high–intensity sweeteners. As of June 2016, FDA approval for the use of extracts from *Siraitia grosvenorii* Swingle fruit (luohan guo or monk fruit) was pending.

In the United States, the safety of nonnutritive sweeteners has been under public and scientific scrutiny for decades. In 1970, the FDA banned the nonnutritive sweetener *cyclamate* after research indicated that the substance caused bladder cancer in mice. In the 1980s, panels of experts at the FDA and the National Academy of Sciences reviewed the scientific evidence and determined that cyclamate did not increase the risk of cancer in humans. Nevertheless, the ban on this food additive continues in the United States. Although *saccharin* has been in use for over 100 years, its safety has also been questioned. Despite the concern, most of the scientific evidence indicates that saccharin is safe when consumed in typical amounts.

Aspartame, better known by its trade names "NutraSweet®" or "Equal®," consists of phenylalanine and aspartic acid, two amino acids, the molecules that comprise proteins. Some people must avoid aspartame and certain protein–rich foods because they have phenylketonuria (PKU) (*fen'–nul–keet'–en–yur'–e–ah*), a rare inherited disorder. People with PKU cannot metabolize phenylalanine properly. If an infant with PKU is not treated with a special diet, phenylalanine and its metabolic by–products accumulate in the child's bloodstream and cause severe brain damage. To alert people with PKU about the presence of aspartame in foods, the FDA requires manufacturers of products containing the nonnutritive sweetener to include a warning on the label (Fig. 5.4). The "Real People, Real Stories" feature in Chapter 7 is about a college student who has PKU.

Aspartame has been blamed for causing a variety of health problems, including cancer, certain immune system diseases, and chronic headaches. However, no scientifically reliable studies have linked aspartame to any health disorder.[4]

TABLE 5.5 Acceptable Daily Intakes for Nonnutritive Sweeteners

Nonnutritive Sweetener	Amount*
Aspartame	75 packets
Saccharin	45 packets
Advantame	4,920 packets
Acesulfame-K	23 packets
Sucralose	23 packets

*Number of table top packets for a person who weighs 132 pounds

Source: U.S. Food and Drug Administration: *Additional information about high-intensity sweeteners permitted for use in food in the United States.* 2015. http://www.fda.gov/Food/IngredientsPackagingLabeling/FoodAdditivesIngredients/ucm 397725.htm#Advantame Accessed: July 20, 2017.

Sucralose, sold under the brand name "Splenda®," is made from a molecule of sucrose that has been chemically modified to escape digestion and absorption. As a result, sucralose sweetens foods and beverages without increasing their caloric value. Since the sweetener is not digested or absorbed by the intestinal tract, it is excreted in feces unchanged. During normal cooking conditions, sucralose is not destroyed by heat, a feature that makes it better for sweetening baked products than aspartame.

Do nonnutritive sweeteners pose a danger to health? A group of international health and safety organizations, including the FDA, has established *Acceptable Daily Intakes (ADI)* for certain nonnutritive sweeteners (Table 5.5). According to the Academy of Nutrition and Dietetics, nonnutritive sweeteners are safe when consumed "within acceptable daily intakes, even during pregnancy."[4] Nevertheless, researchers continue to investigate the safety and usefulness of artificial sweeteners.

Did *YOU* Know?

For hundreds of years, people have used extracts made from the leaves of the South American shrub *Stevia rebaudiana* Bertoni ("stevia") to sweeten foods. As of June 2016, however, the FDA did not permit food manufacturers to add stevia leaves or *crude* stevia extracts to their products to sweeten them. The agency, however, does permit the use of highly purified extracts from stevia leaves (*steviol glycosides*, such as Rebaudioside A and Stevioside) as sweeteners.[6]

Concept CHECKPOINT

4. Identify the three most important dietary monosaccharides.
5. What are the chemical names for blood sugar, table sugar, milk sugar, and malt sugar? Which monosaccharides comprise each molecule of maltose, lactose, and sucrose?
6. What is the difference between a nutritive sweetener and a nonnutritive sweetener?
7. Parents of a child with PKU can give their child either a beverage sweetened with sucralose or one containing aspartame. Which drink should they choose? Explain your answer.

See Appendix G for responses.

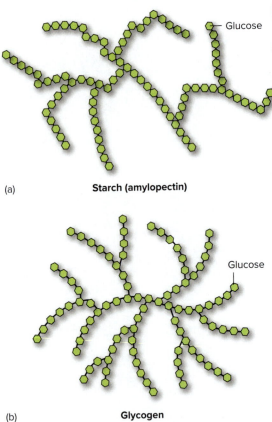

Glucose

(a) **Starch (amylopectin)**

Glucose

(b) **Glycogen**

Figure 5.5 **Starch and glycogen.** (a) Amylopectin is the major form of starch made by plants. (b) The chains of glycogen are more highly branched than those of amylopectin.

5.3 Complex Carbohydrates

Learning Outcomes

1. Explain the difference between a simple sugar and a polysaccharide.

2. Explain the difference between starch and glycogen.

3. Identify rich food sources of starch, soluble fiber, and insoluble fiber.

Complex carbohydrates (polysaccharides) are comprised of 10 or more monosaccharides bonded together. Plants and animals use complex carbohy—drates to store energy or make certain structural components such as stems and leaves. The most common dietary polysaccharides consist of hundreds of glucose molecules and include digestible and nondigestible forms.

Starch and Glycogen

Starch and **glycogen** are polysaccharides that contain hundreds of glucose molecules bound together into large chainlike structures (Fig. 5.5). Plants store glucose as starch, primarily in the form of amylopectin, in their seeds, roots, and fleshy underground stems called tubers (Fig. 5.5a). Rich food sources of starch include bread and cereal products made from wheat, rice, barley, and oats; veg—etables such as corn, squash, beans, and peas; and tubers such as potatoes, yams, taro, cassava, and jicama. Sports drinks and sports or energy bars often include *modified starches* such as maltodextrin and dextrin. Regardless of its source, each gram of starch supplies 4 kcal.

The human body stores limited amounts of glucose as glycogen (see Fig. 5.5b). Muscles and the liver are the major sites for glycogen formation and storage. Although muscles contain glycogen, most animal foods (for example, meat or the flesh of fish and poultry) are not sources of this complex carbohydrate because muscle glycogen breaks down soon after an animal dies.

Fiber

In addition to storing energy as starch, plants use complex carbohydrates to make supportive structures and protective seed coats that contribute to the fiber content of your diet. Most forms of **dietary fiber (fiber)** are complex carbo—hydrates comprised of monosaccharides. The monosaccharides are connected to each other by bonds that humans cannot digest. Cellulose, hemicellulose, pectin, gums, and mucilages are carbohydrate forms of fiber; lignin is the only type of fiber that is not carbohydrate. Although fiber is not digested, it may be metabo—lized (fermented) by gut microbiota (see Chapter 4). Any fiber that is not used by the microbes contributes to stools (fecal residue) that are eventually elimi—nated during bowel movements.

There are two types of dietary fiber, **soluble fiber** and **insoluble fiber.** Soluble types of fiber, such as pectins and gums, dissolve or swell in water. Insoluble forms of fiber, such as cellulose and lignin, generally do not dissolve in water. Oat bran and oatmeal, beans, apples, carrots, oranges and other citrus fruits, and psyllium (*sill'—e—um*) seeds are rich sources of soluble fiber; whole—grain products, including brown rice, contain high amounts of insoluble fiber. Table 5.6 provides information about the solubility of various types of fiber, effects of fiber in the body, and major food sources of soluble and insoluble fiber. Although the foods listed in Table 5.6 are rich sources of either soluble or insoluble fiber, plant foods usually contain both forms.

complex carbohydrates (polysaccharides) compounds comprised of 10 or more monosaccharides bonded together

starch storage polysaccharide in plants

glycogen storage polysaccharide in animals

dietary fiber (fiber) nondigestible plant material; most types are polysaccharides

soluble fiber forms of dietary fiber that dissolve or swell in water

insoluble fiber forms of dietary fiber that generally do not dissolve in water

TABLE 5.6 Classifying Fiber

Type	Component(s)	Physiological Effects	Food Sources
Insoluble	Cellulose, hemicelluloses	Increases fecal bulk and speeds fecal passage through GI tract	All plants Wheat, rye, brown rice, vegetables
	Lignin	Increases fecal bulk, may ease bowel movements	Whole grains, wheat bran
Soluble	Pectins, gums, mucilages, some hemicelluloses	Delays stomach emptying; slows glucose absorption; can lower blood cholesterol	Apples, bananas, citrus fruits, carrots, oats, barley, psyllium seeds, beans, and thickeners added to foods

Did *YOU* Know?

The fiber content of different forms of a food can vary widely. For example, an unpeeled raw apple that weighs 6 ounces (about 3 inches in diameter) has 4.4 g of fiber. However, 6 ounces of applesauce contains 2.0 g of fiber, and a 6-ounce serving of apple juice provides only 0.4 g of fiber.

©Kovaleva_Ka/iStockphoto/Getty Images RF

According to food labeling guidelines issued by the FDA, whole grains are the intact, ground, cracked, or flaked seeds of cereal grains. Such grains may include wheat, buckwheat, oats, corn, rice, wild rice, rye, barley, bulgur, millet, and sorghum. If a "whole-grain" product is made from ground, cracked, or flaked cereal grains, the forms must contain the starchy endosperm, oily germ, and fiber-rich bran seed components in the same relative proportions as they exist in the intact grain.[7] (Figure 1.11 is an illustration of a whole-grain kernel that shows the endosperm, germ, and bran components.)

Although fiber is not digested by humans, soluble and insoluble fiber provide important health benefits. Soluble fiber can help reduce blood cholesterol levels, and insoluble fiber may ease bowel movements. The "Carbohydrates and Health" section of this chapter provides information about the benefits of adding more fiber to your diet and practical ways to increase your fiber intake.

Table 5.7 lists common foods that are sources of dietary fiber. Note that only plant foods provide fiber; animal flesh contains muscle fibers, which are digestible proteins.

Most plant foods contain both soluble and insoluble fiber.
©Cole Group/Getty Images RF

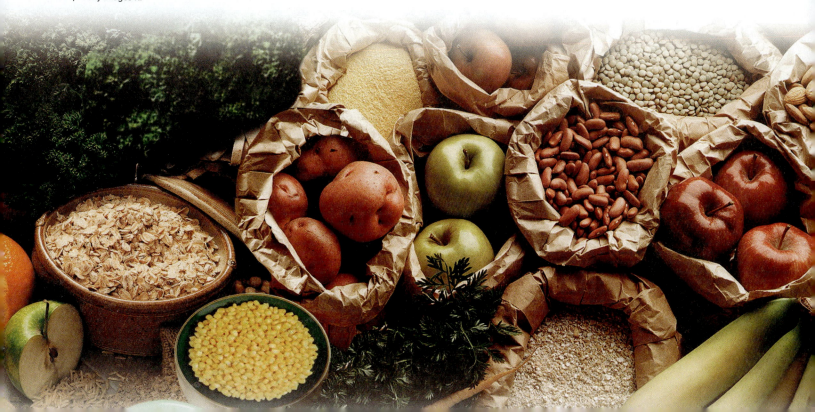

TABLE 5.7 Dietary Fiber Content of Common Foods

Food	Fiber (g)	Food	Fiber (g)
Split peas, cooked (1 cup)	16.3	Beans, green snap, cooked (1 cup)	4.0
Black beans, cooked (1 cup)	15.0	Banana, sliced (1 cup)	3.9
Oat bran, raw (1 cup)	14.5	Prunes, dried uncooked (5 prunes)	3.5
Kidney beans, canned (1 cup)	11.0	Orange, raw (1 orange)	3.4
Chickpeas, canned (1 cup)	10.6	Strawberries, raw, sliced (1 cup)	3.3
Baked beans, canned (1 cup)	10.4	Carrots, raw, grated (½ cup)	3.1
Kellogg's All-Bran cereal (½ cup)	9.1	Barley, cooked (½ cup)	3.0
Raspberries, raw (1 cup)	8.0	Almonds (1 ounce)	2.8
Blackberries (1 cup)	7.6	Broccoli, chopped, cooked (½ cup)	2.6
Green peas, frozen, cooked (½ cup)	7.2	Whole-grain bread, toasted (1 slice)	1.9
Kellogg's Raisin Bran (1 cup)	6.7	Romaine lettuce, shredded (1 cup)	1.0
Apple, raw with skin 3″ diameter	4.4	Iceberg lettuce, shredded (1 cup)	0.9
Baked potato, with skin (approx. 6 ½ oz)	4.0	White bread (1 slice)	0.8

Source: Data from U.S. Department of Agriculture, Agricultural Research Service, USDA Nutrient Data Laboratory: *USDA Nutrient database for standard reference, release* 28. 2015.

Carrots: ©C Squared Studios/Getty Images RF; Lettuce, Raspberries and Strawberries: ©Brand X Pictures/Getty Images RF; Potato: ©McGraw-Hill Education. Christopher Kerrigan, photographer; Banana: ©Stockbyte/Getty Images RF; Soybeans: ©Siede Preis/Getty Images RF

Concept CHECKPOINT

8. What is starch? What is glycogen?
9. What is dietary fiber? Identify at least two rich food sources of soluble fiber and two rich food sources of insoluble fiber.

See Appendix G for responses.

5.4 What Happens to Carbohydrates in the Body?

Learning Outcomes

1 Describe the major steps involved in digesting and absorbing starches and sugars.

2 Explain how the body regulates blood glucose.

3 Explain what happens when cells do not have glucose to use for energy.

If you eat cooked oatmeal made with milk and sweetened with a little brown sugar for breakfast, what happens to the carbohydrates in these foods? The carbohydrates in oats are primarily starch and fiber; mixing milk and brown sugar with the cereal adds lactose and sucrose. Figure 5.6 summarizes what happens to carbohydrates in the digestive tract.

The small intestine is the main site for carbohydrate digestion and absorption, but a minor amount of starch digestion begins in the mouth, as **salivary amylase** converts some of the oat starch molecules into maltose. Salivary amylase does not function when it is in an acid environment. Thus, starch digestion stops soon after the food enters the stomach.

Starch digestion resumes in the small intestine. In the small intestine, an amylase secreted by the pancreas **(pancreatic amylase)** breaks down the remaining polysaccharides in oat starch into maltose molecules. The enzyme **maltase** digests maltose into glucose molecules. The final products of starch digestion, glucose molecules, are absorbed into the intestinal bloodstream and transported to the liver via the hepatic portal vein. Under normal conditions, the process is very efficient and nearly all the starch is digested. The complex carbo-hydrates that remain are primarily forms of fiber.

The molecules of sucrose in brown sugar and lactose in milk are too large to enter the bloodstream directly from the intestinal tract. The small intesti-nal enzyme **sucrase** splits each sucrose molecule, forming one glucose and one fructose molecule in the process (see Fig. 5.6). Additionally, the enzyme **lactase** breaks down the lactose from milk into glucose and galactose molecules. Intesti-nal cells absorb the monosaccharides, and the hepatic portal vein transports them to the liver. The liver can use the simple sugars to make glycogen or fat, but if the body needs energy, the organ releases glucose into the bloodstream.

salivary amylase enzyme secreted by salivary glands that begins starch digestion

pancreatic amylase enzyme secreted by pancreas that breaks down starch into maltose molecules

maltase enzyme that splits maltose molecule

sucrase enzyme that splits sucrose molecule

lactase enzyme that splits lactose molecule

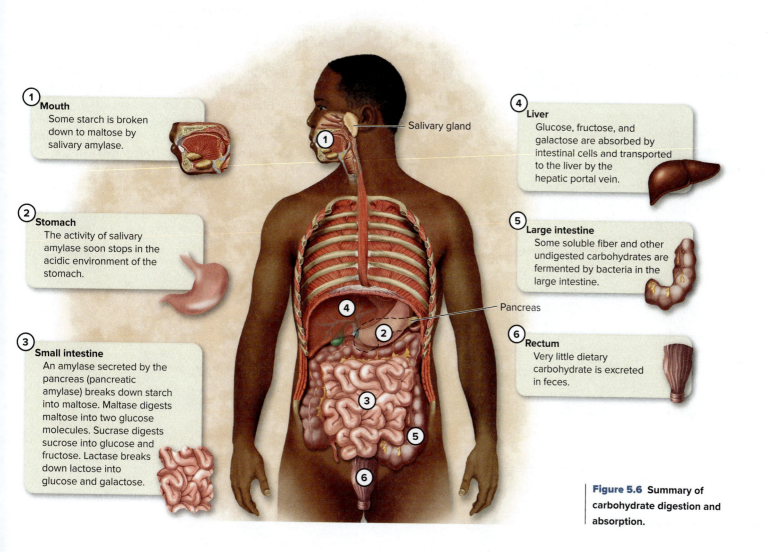

1 Mouth
Some starch is broken down to maltose by salivary amylase.

Salivary gland

2 Stomach
The activity of salivary amylase soon stops in the acidic environment of the stomach.

3 Small intestine
An amylase secreted by the pancreas (pancreatic amylase) breaks down starch into maltose. Maltase digests maltose into two glucose molecules. Sucrase digests sucrose into glucose and fructose. Lactase breaks down lactose into glucose and galactose.

4 Liver
Glucose, fructose, and galactose are absorbed by intestinal cells and transported to the liver by the hepatic portal vein.

5 Large intestine
Some soluble fiber and other undigested carbohydrates are fermented by bacteria in the large intestine.

Pancreas

6 Rectum
Very little dietary carbohydrate is excreted in feces.

Figure 5.6 Summary of carbohydrate digestion and absorption.

Did *YOU* Know?

insulin hormone that helps regulate blood glucose levels

glucagon hormone that helps regulate blood glucose levels

The fiber in oats is not digested by your small intestine, and it eventually enters the large intestine. The "friendly" intestinal bacteria that reside in the large intestine can break down (ferment) the soluble fiber and metabolize the fermentation products for energy. Soluble fiber is sometimes referred to as *viscous fiber*, because it usually forms a gooey, semisolid mass in the intestinal tract that is rapidly fermented by bacterial action. On the other hand, insoluble or fermentation—resistant fiber does not break down completely and, as a result, contributes to softer and easier—to—eliminate bowel movements.

At one time, scientists thought fiber was a nonnutrient because it had no nutritional value. Recent scientific evidence indicates that the body, particularly the cells that line the large intestine, can use by—products produced by the bacterial metabolism of fiber for energy. According to estimates, a gram of fiber adds less than 3 kcal to human diets.[8] The average American who is 2 years of age and older consumes only 17.1 g of fiber daily; therefore, fiber contributes relatively little to a typical person's energy intake.[9]

Maintaining Blood Glucose Levels

Glucose is such an important cellular fuel, its blood level is carefully maintained by hormones. Hormones are chemicals that convey messages concerning specific responses to target cells. The pancreas, a digestive system organ shown in Figure 4.27, contains beta cells, clusters of special cells that produce **insulin,** and groups of alpha cells that produce **glucagon.** These two hormones play key roles in regulating blood glucose levels. Figure 5.7 illustrates the effects of insulin and glucagon on blood glucose levels in a healthy person, after a meal that is followed by fasting.

If you do not have diabetes, your body maintains your blood glucose level at between 110 and 140 milligrams per deciliter of blood (mg/dl) during the day. If you have not eaten for a while, your blood glucose level begins to fall, you start to feel hungry, and your stomach growls. You may grab an apple or a cheese sandwich to eat, and as the carbohydrates in these foods are digested, the glucose from these foods is absorbed into your bloodstream and transported to the liver.

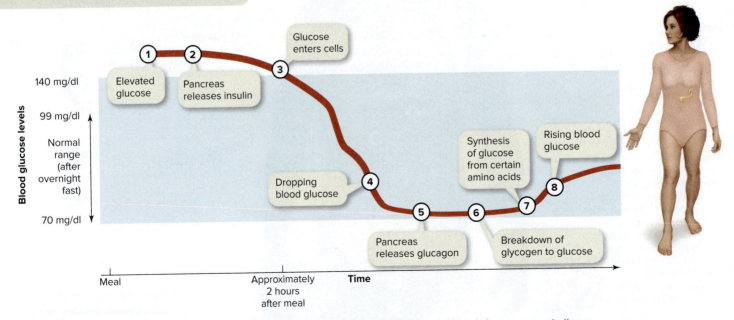

| **Figure 5.7 Regulating blood glucose.** Insulin and glucagon are key hormones in maintaining normal blood glucose concentration.

As your blood glucose level begins to rise, your pancreas responds by secreting insulin into the bloodstream (see Fig. 5.7). Insulin helps regulate blood glucose levels because the hormone enables glucose to enter most cells.

Insulin also influences fat and protein metabolism. The hormone enhances energy storage by promoting fat, glycogen, and protein production. Another effect of insulin's action: you feel satisfied with your snack or meal and are no longer hungry.

If you ignore the hunger signals and do not eat, the alpha cells in your pancreas secrete glucagon. Glucagon opposes insulin's effects by promoting the breakdown of glycogen. This process, called **glycogenolysis** (*lysis* = break down), releases glucose into the bloodstream, which helps maintain your blood glucose level in the normal range (see Fig. 5.7). Glucagon also stimulates liver and kidney cells to produce glucose from certain *amino acids*, the basic molecules that make up proteins. Furthermore, glucagon stimulates **lipolysis** (*lipo* = fat), the breakdown of triglyceride (fat) into *glycerol* and *fatty acids*. As a result, glycerol and fatty acids rapidly enter into the bloodstream. The liver uses glycerol to produce glucose, and most cells, including muscle cells, can metabolize fatty acids for energy. Although the body can convert certain amino acids into glucose, it cannot use fatty acids to make glucose.

What happens to glucose? Its fate depends on the state of your body. If your muscles and other cells that use glucose need energy, glucose enters the cells and is metabolized for energy. When you are well fed and resting, your body stores the extra glucose as glycogen. When glycogen storage reaches maximum capacity, your liver can convert some excess glucose into fat and releases it into the bloodstream. Adipose (*ad'−eh−pose*) (fat) cells remove and store the fat.

Glucose for Energy

Cells metabolize glucose to release the energy stored in the molecule's chemical bonds. As a result of this process, cells form carbon dioxide and water (Fig. 5.8). Glucose is a primary fuel for the body's cells. Furthermore, red blood cells as well as brain and other nervous system cells burn mostly glucose for energy.

Cells need a small amount of glucose to metabolize fat for energy properly. When a person is fasting or starving, or follows a very low−carbohydrate/high−protein diet (the Atkins diet, for example), his or her cells must use greater−than−normal amounts of fat for energy. Under these conditions, there is not enough glucose available for cells to metabolize the fat efficiently, and cells form more *ketone bodies* than usual. **Ketone bodies** are chemicals that result from the incomplete breakdown of fat. Muscle and brain cells can use ketone bodies for energy, but a condition commonly called *ketosis* occurs when these compounds accumulate in the blood. In cases of poorly controlled type 1 diabetes, the production of ketone bodies can be so excessive that the blood becomes acidic, and **ketoacidosis** results. If not treated, ketoacidosis can cause loss of consciousness and even death. The "Type 1 Diabetes" section of this chapter provides more information about ketoacidosis.

The Recommended Dietary Allowance (RDA) for carbohydrate is 130 g/day.[8] This amount of carbohydrate is enough to prevent ketosis. (The RDAs and other DRIs were discussed in Chapter 3.) To estimate your daily carbohydrate intake, complete the Personal Dietary Analysis at the end of this chapter.

Under normal conditions, human cells obtain a small proportion of their energy needs by converting certain amino acids, the components of proteins, into glucose. Starvation, however, dramatically alters the body's energy metabolism. Starvation diets lack sources of energy such as glucose and amino acids. The body, however, needs glucose to fuel vital activities such as breathing, trans−mitting nerve impulses, and pumping blood. To meet the body's energy needs,

glycogenolysis glycogen breakdown

lipolysis fat breakdown

ketone bodies chemicals that result from incomplete fat breakdown

ketoacidosis condition that occurs when the body forms excessive ketone bodies

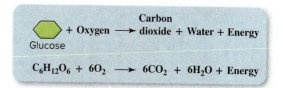

$$\text{Glucose} + \text{Oxygen} \longrightarrow \text{Carbon dioxide} + \text{Water} + \text{Energy}$$

$$C_6H_{12}O_6 + 6O_2 \longrightarrow 6CO_2 + 6H_2O + \text{Energy}$$

Figure 5.8 Releasing energy from glucose. Cells use oxygen to release the energy stored in glucose. As a result of this process, cells produce carbon dioxide and water.

the starving person's skeletal muscles sacrifice amino acids from their proteins for glucose production. Using muscle proteins as a source of energy extends the starving person's survival time but results in muscle wasting, weakness, and, eventually, death. Chapter 7 provides information about proteins.

Concept CHECKPOINT

10. Sherita ate some whole-wheat crackers with grape jelly for a snack. As this snack passed through her digestive tract, discuss what happened to the starch, sucrose, and fiber in the food.
11. What effects do insulin and glucagon have on blood glucose levels?
12. What is a ketone body? Under what conditions does the body form excessive ketone bodies?

See Appendix G for responses.

5.5 Carbohydrate Consumption Patterns

Learning Outcomes

1. Identify the major sources of added sugars in American diets.
2. List three practical ways to reduce a person's added sugar consumption.

In developing nations, millions of people rely on diets that supply the majority of their energy from relatively unprocessed carbohydrates, especially complex carbohydrates from whole grains, beans, potatoes, corn, and other starchy vegetables. In industrialized nations, people tend to eat more highly refined starches and added sugars. Nutritionally adequate diets should provide 45 to 65% of total energy from carbohydrates.[8] The typical diet of adult Americans supplies about 48% of calories from carbohydrates, much of which is sugars (nutritive sweeteners) added to foods during processing (Fig. 5.9).

As mentioned in Chapter 1, added sugars are sources of empty calories. In 2015, the average American consumed about 22 teaspoons of added sugars per day, which is almost 18% of the energy in a diet that supplies 2000 kcal/day.[1] According to the Dietary Guidelines, people who follow a 2000 kcal/day diet should limit their intake of added sugars to no more than 12 teaspoons per day (about 200 kcal).[11]

A 12-ounce can of a cola-flavored, sugar-sweetened soft drink contains about 37 g of added sugar.[12] Each gram of sugar supplies 4 kcal, so this soft drink contributes about 150 kcal of added sugars to the diet. By drinking only one can of the cola, a person who needs 2000 kcal daily will meet three-quarters of his or her daily limit for the intake of added sugars.

A 12-ounce serving of 100% orange juice supplies about the same amount of carbohydrate as 12 ounces of a sugar-sweetened cola. Because they both contain simple sugars, should you drink regular soft drinks instead of fruit juices? Unlike colas and other soft drinks, 100% fruit juices, such as orange, grapefruit, and cranberry juice, contribute water-soluble vitamins and antioxidant phytochemicals to your diet. Thus, the sugars that are naturally in fruit are not considered added sugars (empty calories).

The main sources of added sugars in Americans' diets are sugar-sweetened beverages, snacks, and "sweets."[10] Sugar-sweetened beverages include carbonated "regular" soft drinks, fruit "ades," flavored vitamin-water products, and

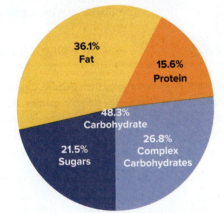

Average Percentage of Calories per Person (Adult Americans, One Day)

- 36.1% Fat
- 15.6% Protein
- 48.3% Carbohydrate
- 21.5% Sugars
- 26.8% Complex Carbohydrates

Figure 5.9 Average macronutrient intakes. This graph shows the adult American's average intake of macronutrients as approximate percentages of total kilocalories from macronutrients (2064) on one day in 2013–2014. (Percentage of total energy from alcohol is not included.) Source: U.S. Department of Agriculture, Agricultural Research Service, "Nutrient Intakes from food and beverages: Mean amounts consumed by individuals: By gender and age," *What We Eat in America,* NHANES 2013-2014, 2016. https://www.ars.usda.gov/ARSUserFiles/80400530/pdf/1314/Table_1_NIN_GEN_13.pdf

sports and energy drinks. Although energy drink consumption has increased, carbonated soft drink consumption has declined since 1999–2000. How many fluid ounces of energy, sports, and/or sugar–sweetened soft drinks do you consume each day?

Reducing Your Intake of Refined Carbohydrates

Sugar–sweetened beverages, cookies, chips, and many other types of processed snack foods contain large amounts of refined carbohydrates, including added sugars. Such foods may satisfy your hunger and thirst, but they may be crowding out more nutritious items from your diet. If you frequently purchase foods and beverages from vending machines, convenience stores, or fast–food restaurants, you are probably eating unhealthy amounts of refined carbohydrates. Some fast–food restaurants and college cafeterias sell yogurt, fresh fruit, and fat–free or low–fat milk as well as unsweetened fruit juices. With a little advance planning, you can prepare your own portable, tasty, and nutritious snacks. For example, place whole fresh fruit or small plastic containers filled with chunks of fresh fruit and pieces of vegetables into your purse or backpack to eat during the day. At home, keep a bowl of fresh grapes, apples, bananas, or other easy–to–eat fruit available for handy snacks, and eat fresh fruit for dessert. Most fruits contain a variety of antioxidants, and they have less fat and more fiber, vitamins, and minerals than pastries or chips.

Concept CHECKPOINT

13. What are the main sources of added sugars in American diets?

14. Instead of drinking orange juice, should you choose a beverage called "Orange-Ade"? Explain why or why not.

See Appendix G for responses.

5.6 Understanding Nutrient Labeling: Carbohydrates and Fiber

Learning Outcome

1 Compare carbohydrate contents of packaged foods by using the Nutrition Facts panel.

Consumers can learn how much total carbohydrate, sugars, and dietary fiber are in packaged foods and beverages by reading the Nutrition Facts panel of a food label. As indicated in Figure 5.10, grams of total carbohydrate in a serving (5 cookies) are listed, and under it, grams of fiber, total sugar, and added sugars.

According to the label shown in Figure 5.10, 24 g of total carbohydrate are in one serving; of this amount, there are 11 g of total sugars and 10 grams of added sugars. Each serving supplies no grams of fiber. How can you estimate the grams of starch in the serving of the food? In this example, add the number of grams of total sugars (11 g) with that of fiber (0 g) and subtract this amount from grams of total carbohydrate (24 g), and you will find that starch comprises 13 g of the carbohydrate in a serving of the food.

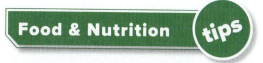

- Replace soft drinks with plain water.
- Make plain water more interesting to drink by adding to it a slice of lemon or lime, or a few fresh or frozen berries.
- Add 1 part club soda to 1 part orange or other 100% fruit juice to make a refreshing carbonated drink.
- Read the label for information about juice content when selecting a fruit juice product. Fruit "drinks," "punches," "blends," "cocktails," or "ades" often contain added sugars and only 10% fruit juice.

Nutrition Facts
About 5 servings per container
Serving Size 5 Cookies (32g)

Amount per serving
Calories 150

	% Daily Value*
Total Fat 5g	**6%**
Saturated Fat 2g	**10%**
Trans Fat 0g	
Polyunsaturated Fat 1.5g	
Monounsaturated Fat 1g	
Cholesterol 0mg	**0%**
Sodium 130mg	**6%**
Total Carbohydrate 24g	**9%**
Dietary Fiber 0g	**0%**
Total Sugars 11g	
Includes 10g Added Sugars	**20%**
Protein 2g	

Vit. D 0mcg 0%	•	Calcium 10mg 0%
Iron 0.8mg 4%	•	Potas. 30mg 0%

* The % Daily Value (DV) tells you how much a nutrient in a serving of food contributes to a daily diet. 2000 calories a day is used for general nutrition advice.

Ingredients: Enriched flour (wheat flour, niacin, reduced iron, vitamin B1 [thiamin mononitrate], vitamin B2 [riboflavin], folic acid), sugar, vegetable oil (soybean, palm and palm kernel), dextrose, invert sugar, contains 2% or less of cornstarch, whey, corn syrup solids, salt, leavening (baking soda, monocalcium phosphate), natural and artificial flavors, milk, lemon juice solids, nonfat milk, citric acid, lemon oil, soy lecithin, annatto extract color.

CONTAINS WHEAT, MILK AND SOY INGREDIENTS. MAY CONTAIN TREE NUTS.

Figure 5.10 Nutrition Facts panel (new version).
©Wendy Schiff

INGREDIENTS: Whole-wheat flour, Water, Brown sugar, Wheat gluten, Cracked wheat, Wheat bran, Yeast, Salt, Molasses, Soybean oil, Calcium propionate (preservative), Mono–and diglycerides, Lecithin, Reduced-fat milk

Figure 5.11 **Ingredients list.** Note the different sources of carbohydrate that are in these crackers.

If you are interested in the kinds of added sugars used to make a product, read the ingredients list at the bottom of the panel. Consider the ingredients used to make crackers (Fig. 5.11). Can you identify the added sugars in the product?

Concept CHECKPOINT

15. According to the Nutrition Facts panel, a serving of ready-to-eat cereal contains 44 g of total carbohydrate, 5 g of dietary fiber, 15 g of total sugars, and 3 g of added sugars. Estimate the grams of starch in the serving of the cereal.

See Appendix G for responses.

5.7 Carbohydrates and Health

Learning Outcomes

1 Discuss the effects of excess carbohydrate consumption on health.

2 Discuss differences between type 1 and type 2 diabetes, including treatments.

3 List at least three signs or symptoms of diabetes.

4 List at least four risk factors for developing type 2 diabetes and ways to reduce the likelihood of developing the disease.

5 List at least four serious health problems associated with poorly controlled diabetes, including poorly controlled diabetes during pregnancy.

6 Compare hyperglycemia with hypoglycemia.

7 Identify the primary signs of metabolic syndrome, the impact the condition has on health, and how one can reduce the risk of developing the syndrome.

8 Explain the difference between lactose intolerance and milk allergy.

9 Discuss the health benefits of including fiber-rich foods in one's diet.

Carbohydrates seem to get a lot of "bad press." Promoters of low–carbohydrate/high–protein diets often blame sugars and starches for causing unwanted weight gain and diabetes. Many Americans think consuming sugary foods causes depression and hyperactive behavior. On the other hand, "carbs" are welcomed by athletes as an inexpensive and efficient source of energy. What have scientists learned about the roles of carbohydrates in health?

Are Carbohydrates Fattening?

Americans are fatter now than they were 30 years ago. To lose the excess weight, many people follow low–carbohydrate diets, such as the Atkins diet or the Paleo diet. Are carbohydrates responsible for the epidemic of excess body fat in the United States? Are low–carbohydrate diets useful for weight loss?

"Calories do count," because people gain body fat when their intake of food energy from macronutrients and the nonnutrient alcohol exceeds their output of energy for various physiological needs. Regardless of whether people eat a low–carbohydrate, high–fat, or high–protein diet, they will maintain their weight as long as their energy intake matches their energy output.

Foods that contain large amounts of refined carbohydrates, however, do not satisfy hunger as well as those that contain more protein or fat. As a result, a person may become hungrier sooner after eating a meal or snack that contains a lot of added sugars and refined starches than if he or she ate a high–protein, high–fat meal or

Did *YOU* Know?

Tooth decay is clearly associated with consuming certain carbohydrates, particularly simple sugars that stick to teeth. If a person does not follow good dental hygiene practices, the debris becomes food for bacteria that live on teeth. As the bacteria metabolize carbohydrate for their energy needs, the acid they produce damages tooth enamel and results in decay.

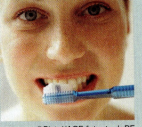
©Pixtal/AGE fotostock RF

snack. Thus, people following a high–protein, high–fat diet can lose weight in the short term because the diet keeps their appetite under control by reducing hunger.

Metabolism plays a major role in the development of obesity, a chronic health condition characterized by unhealthy amounts of body fat. When a person consumes excess carbohydrate, his or her body converts some of the glucose into fat, but much of the excess is "burned" as a biological fuel. As a result, dietary fat is spared from being used as a fuel and stored in fat cells.[13] Thus, eating too much carbohydrate indirectly contributes to excess body fat.

Combining Carbohydrate with Fat

Foods that contain a lot of added sugars and solid fats tend to be energy dense. Thus, people can reduce their energy intake by eating fewer energy–dense foods. Fats supply 9 kcal/g compared to only 4 kcal/g of carbohydrates, so adding even small amounts of fat to food can dramatically increase its energy content. People, however, tend to blame carbohydrates for their unwanted weight gain because starches and sugars are often combined with hidden fats such as butter or shortening in processed foods. Fats make foods taste rich, creamy, and difficult to resist. Moreover, the sweet taste of sugar masks the bland taste of fat. Although you would not consider eating spoonfuls of plain sugar, flour, shortening, or butter, your mouth waters at the sight of candy bars, fruit pies, doughnuts, and other baked or fried foods. If you are like many people, you probably find it is difficult to resist eating these foods.

Although consumption of added sugars has increased over the past several years, other dietary changes have occurred as well. Americans consume an excess of calories from all foods, and the higher intake contributes to the increased prevalence of obesity in the United States. In 2013–2014, adult males consumed an average of 2477 kcal/day, and adult females consumed an average of 1825 kcal/day.[9] These amounts were 323 and 328 kcal higher, respectively, than the average daily calorie intakes of adult males and females about 25 years earlier.[14] Therefore, overall dietary habits may be partly to blame for rising rates of overweight and obesity among the U.S. population.

Sugar-Sweetened Beverages

Over the past 35 years, the percentage of obese Americans rose dramatically. Some nutrition scientists think Americans' intake of added sugars is largely responsible for the population's rising rates of obesity as well as type 2 diabetes. Sugar–sweetened soft drinks are one of the major sources of added sugars in the diets of Americans who are 6 years of age and older.[15]

According to results of large epidemiological studies, risks of obesity, type 2 diabetes, heart disease, and stroke are associated with the highest intakes of sugar–sweetened beverages.[16] People who drink sugar–sweetened beverages do not reduce their consumption of solid foods enough to avoid gaining weight.[17] Excess body fat is a risk factor for type 2 diabetes, heart disease, and stroke. Furthermore, consuming high amounts of fructose may harm the liver. According to results of one study, people who drank 32 ounces of a sugar–sweetened cola daily for 6 months gained body fat, including fat in their liver, compared to people who drank the same amount of diet cola, water, or milk each day for 6 months.[17] When experimental diets supply excess energy and high amounts of fructose (100 grams or more/day), weight gain, abnormal blood lipid levels, and a condition commonly called "fatty liver" may occur.[16] Such health problems, however, could be the result of excessive caloric intake rather than excessive fructose consumption. Consuming fructose in amounts that support the recommendations of the

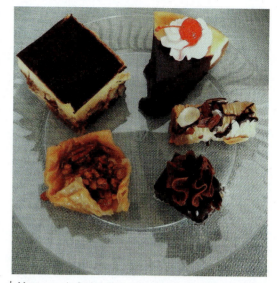
Many people find it difficult to resist foods that contain a lot of sugar and fat, such as these pastries. ©Wendy Schiff

Did YOU Know?

Many people think sucrose is addictive. Addiction is characterized by an uncontrolled need (compulsion) to take a substance and the development of withdrawal signs and symptoms when the substance is not taken.

There is no scientific evidence that people can become addicted to foods, particularly those containing sucrose, as cigarette smokers become addicted to nicotine. Certain nervous system cells make a chemical messenger called *dopamine* that is associated with pleasurable sensations. Eating a tasty food causes the release of dopamine in the reward areas of the brain, similar to the response that occurs in the brain of a person using an addictive drug, such as nicotine. The release of dopamine, however, is not enough of a response to cause addiction.[18]

Factors that regulate eating behavior are very complex and include a person's hormones, environment, past experiences, senses, and mood.[18] What appears to be an "addiction" to a particular food or type of food may be a learned response to situations that the person thinks are difficult and stressful, such as worrying about a test. Nevertheless, researchers are continuing to study the possible effects of eating certain foods, particularly chocolate and "sweets," on mental health.

Dietary Guidelines (less than 10% of total calories) is not likely to contribute to the risk of chronic diseases, particularly obesity or fatty liver.

Nonalcoholic Fatty Liver Disease

Under normal conditions, the liver does not store fat, but the organ can accumulate the lipid in response to alcohol consumption and develop fatty liver. Fatty liver also occurs in people who drink little or no alcohol but are obese or have diabetes (**nonalcoholic fatty liver disease [NAFLD]**). Although there is no specific treatment for NAFLD, losing excess body fat, avoiding alcohol, and eating a healthy diet may allow the liver to heal and avoid inflammation. According to experts at the National Institutes of Health, an estimated 30 to 40 percent of adult Americans have NAFLD.[19]

If people with NAFLD continue to have fat accumulate in their liver, the fat damages liver cells, causing inflammation of the organ (*nonalcoholic steatohepatitis* [*stee'–a–toe–hep'–ah–tie'–tis*]). The inflammation can result in cirrhosis (*sear–hoe'–sis*) of the liver, a condition in which liver cells die and are replaced with scar tissue that has no metabolic function. Eventually, the scar tissue hardens, and the affected person experiences liver failure. People with liver failure require a liver transplant to survive. An estimated 3 to 12 percent of Americans have nonalcoholic steatohepatitis.[19]

What Is Diabetes?

Diabetes mellitus (diabetes) is a group of serious chronic diseases characterized by abnormal glucose, fat, and protein metabolism. There are two major types of diabetes mellitus: type 1 and type 2 diabetes. About 5% of people with diabetes have type 1; in the past, this form of diabetes was called "juvenile diabetes" because it was diagnosed more often in children and young adults. Although type 1 diabetes is more likely to occur in children and young adults, the disease can strike at any age.[20] The majority of people with diabetes have type 2, which used to be called "adult–onset diabetes."

The primary sign of diabetes is **hyperglycemia** (*hyper =* excess; *glycemia =* blood glucose), abnormally elevated blood glucose levels. A person's blood glucose levels are usually measured after he or she has not eaten (has fasted) for about 12 hours. Normal fasting blood glucose levels are 70 to 99 mg/dl (Table 5.8). People with **pre-diabetes** ("impaired glucose tolerance")

nonalcoholic fatty liver disease (NAFLD) abnormal fat accumulation in the liver that is not related to alcohol intake

diabetes mellitus (diabetes) group of serious chronic diseases characterized by abnormal glucose, fat, and protein metabolism

hyperglycemia abnormally high blood glucose level

pre-diabetes condition characterized by fasting blood glucose levels that are 100 to 125 mg/dl

TABLE 5.8 Classifying Diabetes Mellitus

Blood Glucose Level (Fasting)	Classification
70 to 99 mg/dl	Normal
100 to 125 mg/dl	Pre-diabetes
126 mg/dl or more	Diabetes

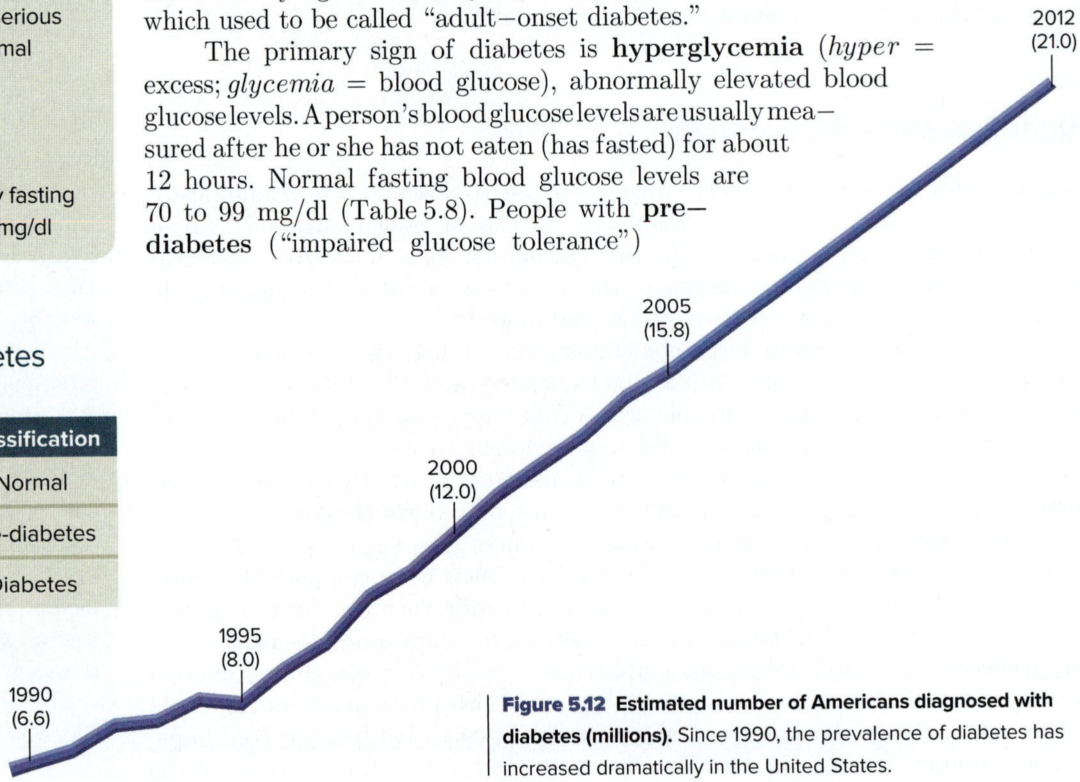

Figure 5.12 Estimated number of Americans diagnosed with diabetes (millions). Since 1990, the prevalence of diabetes has increased dramatically in the United States.

1990 (6.6) · 1995 (8.0) · 2000 (12.0) · 2005 (15.8) · 2012 (21.0)

have fasting blood glucose levels that are between 100 and 125 mg/dl. Although a person with pre–diabetes does not have diabetes, he or she has a high risk of cardiovascular disease and eventually developing type 2 diabetes. Individuals who have fasting blood glucose levels of 126 mg/dl or more have diabetes.

Some people with diabetes experience hyperglycemia because their beta cells do not produce any insulin or do not produce enough to meet their needs. In other cases, the affected person produces some insulin, but his or her body does not respond properly to the hormone (*insulin resistance*), and hyperglycemia results. Major signs and symptoms of hyperglycemia include excessive thirst, frequent urination, blurred vision, and poor wound healing (Table 5.9). Over time, hyperglycemia damages nerves, organs, and blood vessels. In fact, poorly controlled diabetes is a major cause of heart disease, kidney failure, blindness, and lower limb amputations. In 2014, diabetes was the seventh leading cause of death in the United States.[21]

In the United States, the prevalence of diabetes is increasing at an alarm–ing rate (Fig. 5.12). In 2012, an estimated 29.1 million Americans had diabetes; 21 million of these persons were diagnosed with diabetes, and the remainder did not know they had the disease.[20] In 2012, an estimated 86 million adult Americans had pre–diabetes. The prevalence of diabetes increases with advancing age; an estimated 25% of Americans who are 65 years of age or older have diabetes.[20] Public health officials are very concerned about the increasing number of children and adolescents who have diabetes, particularly type 2 diabetes.

Type 1 Diabetes

Type 1 diabetes is an *autoimmune* disease that occurs when certain immune system cells malfunction and do not recognize the body's own beta cells. As a result, the immune system cells attack and destroy many of the beta cells, and the affected person must obtain insulin, usually by injecting the hormone into his or her body, regularly (Fig. 5.13). It is not clear why the immune cells of some individuals malfunction, but genetic susceptibility and environmental factors, particularly exposure to certain viral intestinal infections, are associated with the development of type 1 diabetes. Furthermore, infants who drink cow's milk or cow's milk–based formulas have a greater risk of developing type 1 diabetes than breastfed babies.[22] The role of dietary factors in the development of type 1 diabetes continues to undergo scientific study.

People with undiagnosed or poorly managed type 1 diabetes usually develop ketoacidosis. Signs and symptoms of ketoacidosis include excessive thirst, fre–quent urination, and a blood glucose level of more than 250 mg/dl. Individuals with the condition may also have nausea, vomiting, fatigue, and confusion. The breath of a person with ketoacidosis typically has a "fruity" or acetone odor; acetone is a chemical that is often in fingernail polish remover. Ketoacidosis is a potentially life–threatening condition that requires immediate medical care. If untreated, ketoacidosis can lead to coma (loss of consciousness) and death. Proper management of diabetes, including regular testing of blood glucose levels, is crucial for preventing ketoacidosis.

At present, there is no cure for type 1 diabetes, but the disease can be managed. Stephanie Patton has type 1 diabetes. You can learn about her and how she manages her health by reading the "Real People, Real Stories" feature in this chapter.

TABLE 5.9 Signs and Symptoms of Diabetes Mellitus

Elevated blood glucose levels
Excessive thirst
Frequent urination
Blurry vision
Vaginal yeast infections (adult women)
Foot pain, abdominal pain
Numbness, especially in the feet
Impotence (male)
Sores that do not heal
Increased appetite with weight loss*
Breath that smells like fruit*
Fatigues easily*
Confusion*

* Typical symptoms of poorly controlled type 1 rather than type 2 diabetes.

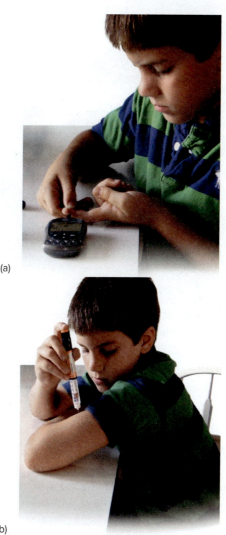

(a)

(b)

Figure 5.13 Managing diabetes. Nine-year-old Carson Smith was diagnosed with type 1 diabetes when he was 5 years of age. (*a*) Carson checks his blood glucose at least four times a day. (*b*) After obtaining information about Carson's blood glucose level, his parents determine the amount and type of insulin he needs, and Carson uses a special device to inject the insulin into his body.
©Wendy Schiff

Type 2 Diabetes

The most common form of diabetes is type 2 diabetes. Beta cells of people with type 2 diabetes usually produce insulin, but the hormone's target cells are insulin—resistant, which means they do not respond properly to the hormone and do not allow glucose to enter them. As a result, the level of glucose in the bloodstream becomes abnormally elevated and the typical signs and symptoms of diabetes occur (see Table 5.9).

Over the past 30 years, the number of adults and children with type 2 diabetes has reached epidemic proportions in the United States. Certain people have greater risk of type 2 diabetes than others. Individuals who are physically inactive (sedentary), have excess body fat, and are genetically related to a close family member with type 2 diabetes are more likely to develop the disease than persons who do not have these characteristics. Additionally, Americans who have Hispanic, Native American, Asian, African, or Pacific Islander ancestry are more likely to develop type 2 diabetes than Americans who are not members of these racial/ethnic groups.[20] The American Diabetes Association has an online questionnaire that you can take to assess your risk of type 2 diabetes http://www.diabetes.org/are—you—at—risk/diabetes—risk—test/.

Diabetes During Pregnancy During pregnancy, a woman with poorly controlled diabetes and her developing offspring (*embryo* or *fetus*) can develop serious health problems. The first 8 weeks of pregnancy are a critical period in a human embryo's development because its organs are forming. If a woman with diabetes lacks good control of her blood glucose level, her embryo can develop birth defects as a result. By managing her blood glucose properly, however, the pregnant diabetic woman can reduce her chances of giving birth to a baby with birth defects. Additionally, she will be less likely to experience serious health problems, such as high blood pressure, during pregnancy.

About 9% of pregnant American women develop a form of diabetes (**gestational diabetes**), usually after the fifth month of pregnancy.[23] Pregnant women who have a family history of type 2 diabetes, are overweight, or have high blood pressure are more likely to experience gestational diabetes than pregnant women who do not have these characteristics. The fetus of a woman with gestational diabetes receives too much glucose from its hyperglycemic mother. As a result of obtaining the excess glucose, the fetus gains weight rapidly and can be abnormally heavy at birth, weighing about 9 pounds or more. Giving birth to such a large infant is risky for the mother as well as the infant, because it may prolong the birth process and cause the baby to be injured during delivery.

After giving birth, most women who had gestational diabetes recover and have normal blood glucose levels. Although the new mothers are healthy, they have an increased risk of developing type 2 diabetes later.[24]

A healthy pregnancy typically lasts about 40 weeks. Pregnant women with poorly controlled diabetes or gestational diabetes are more likely to have miscarriages (death of an embryo/fetus before the 20th week of pregnancy), stillbirths (delivery of a dead baby), and premature (born before the 37th week of pregnancy) deliveries than women with diabetes who manage their blood glucose properly. Furthermore, women with poorly controlled diabetes or gestational diabetes are more likely to give birth to babies who are too large and have difficulty controlling their own blood glucose levels than mothers who do not have diabetes or develop the condition during pregnancy. Thus, pregnant women who have diabetes are encouraged to monitor blood glucose levels carefully to minimize risks to both themselves and their fetuses.

Women who have adequate *prenatal* (before birth) medical care during pregnancy usually undergo screening to detect gestational diabetes. Treatment for women who are diagnosed with gestational diabetes generally includes a

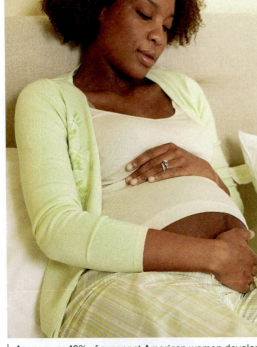

As many as 10% of pregnant American women develop gestational diabetes. ©Brand X Pictures/JupiterImages RF

gestational diabetes form of diabetes that pregnant women can develop

special diet to help manage blood glucose levels and regular physical activity. Some mothers—to—be will also need to monitor their blood glucose levels and give insulin injections to themselves regularly.

Controlling Diabetes

To avoid or delay serious health complications, people who have diabetes need to achieve and maintain normal or near—normal blood glucose levels. Many people with diabetes rely on daily blood testing to monitor their blood glucose levels (see Fig. 5.13a). Physicians can measure *glycated hemoglobin*, also called glycosylated hemoglobin or *hemoglobin A1c* ("HbA1c"), to determine their patients' average blood glucose levels over longer periods. Results of this blood test can provide information about a patient's long—term management of the condition.

Hemoglobin is the compound in red blood cells that carries oxygen. HbA1c is a component of hemoglobin that attracts some glucose that is in blood. About 4.5 to 5.7% of a healthy person's hemoglobin is HbA1c. A person with poorly controlled diabetes often has blood glucose levels that are much higher than normal (Table 5.10). As a result, this individual's hemoglobin will have a higher percentage of HbA1c. Most people with diabetes should strive to maintain their HbA1c level below 7%.[25]

Proper blood glucose management involves monitoring blood glucose levels regularly and carefully following a special diet that usually includes counting grams of carbohydrates. Including physical activity in one's daily routine is also recommended. People with pre—diabetes and type 2 diabetes who are overweight can often reduce their insulin resistance by losing small amounts of excess body fat. Additionally, exercise increases glucose uptake by muscles, reducing blood glucose levels and improving the body's insulin response. In some instances, however, people with type 2 diabetes need oral medication to stimulate their bodies' insulin production, or they must receive insulin injections.

Promoters of certain weight reduction diets claim that people can lose weight or control diabetes by following *low glycemic index* diets. However, some medical experts question the value of the glycemic index for predicting the body's blood glucose level after eating. To learn more about the glycemic index and glycemic load, read the "Nutrition Matters" section of this chapter.

Can Diabetes Be Prevented?

There is no way to prevent type 1 diabetes. By losing some excess body fat and increasing physical activity levels, people with pre—diabetes can prevent or delay the onset of type 2 diabetes and lower their risk of heart disease and stroke.[26] Medical experts refer to these actions as *therapeutic lifestyle changes (TLC)*.

Certain eating habits may help prevent type 2 diabetes. The typical American diet ("Western diet") contains high amounts of saturated fat, and refined sugars and starches. Such diets may increase the risk for type 2 diabetes and other serious chronic diseases. On the other hand, diets that contain fewer sugar—sweetened drinks and less saturated fat, and more fiber—rich whole grains, fruits, and vegetables are healthier than the Western diet.[27] The "Mediterranean diet" is a healthy eating pattern that may help prevent type 2 diabetes or delay its onset.[28] The Mediterranean diet pyramid is illustrated in Figure 3.19.

TABLE 5.10 Classifying Diabetes According to A1c Values

Diagnosis*	A1c Level
Normal	4.5 to 5.7%
Pre-diabetes	5.7 to 6.4%
Diabetes	6.5% or above

*Any test for diagnosing diabetes requires a second test to confirm the diagnosis, unless the patient has signs and symptoms of diabetes.

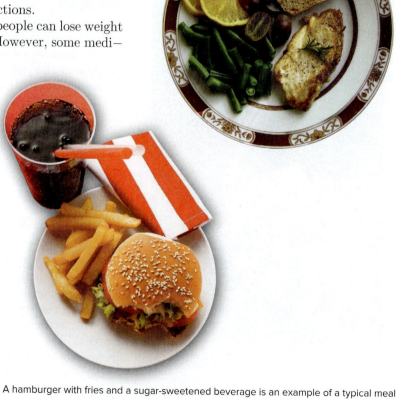

A hamburger with fries and a sugar-sweetened beverage is an example of a typical meal for a "Western" diet. Baked chicken served with a whole-grain roll and a variety of fruits and vegetables is an example of a healthier meal.

Lean meal: ©Wendy Schiff; Hamburger meal: ©FoodCollection/StockFood RF

Did *YOU* Know?

A diabetic alert dog (DAD) is a service dog that can save the life of an individual with type 1 diabetes by alerting other people when the diabetic person's blood sugar level is abnormal.[29] People with type 1 diabetes can develop hypoglycemia ("low blood sugar") quickly, and the effects of hypoglycemia can be dangerous, even deadly. To learn how to detect hypoglycemia, dogs being trained to become DADs are exposed to samples of perspiration and exhaled breath that are provided by people with diabetes who are experiencing hypoglycemia.[30] In small study of eight women with type 1 diabetes who were hypoglycemic, scientists found high levels of a particular chemical (*isoprene*) in samples of the women's exhaled air.[31] Additional research is needed to determine whether isoprene can be used to train DADs effectively.

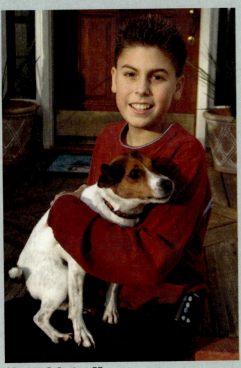

©Realistic Reflections RF

hypoglycemia condition that occurs when the blood glucose level is abnormally low

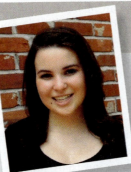

©Wendy Schiff

REAL PEOPLE | REAL STORIES

Stephanie Patton

Stephanie Patton has a long list of accomplishments. "When I was little, I took singing, dancing, and acting lessons," she says. "I loved being on the stage, so I had my parents take me to auditions for local talent shows and theatrical performances. Since I was 7 years old, I've been in over 50 musicals and plays. I appeared in my first beauty pageant at age 10, and I recently competed for the Miss Missouri title. I placed in the top 11, won the preliminary talent award and two college scholarships for community service."

This impressive young lady has type 1 diabetes. Stephanie says, "Just before my fifth birthday, I lost weight and began drinking gallons of juice, water, and milk. At night, I wet the bed. My parents became alarmed, because I have some cousins with type 1 diabetes, and they were worried that I had the disease, too." On her fifth birthday, Stephanie's parents took her to the doctor for a checkup, and her physician told her parents to have her admitted immediately to the local children's hospital. While Stephanie was in the hospital, her parents learned about diabetes and how to take care of their daughter's condition. "At first, my parents gave the insulin shots to me," says Stephanie, "but in a few months, I learned to inject myself and 'count carbs.' An apple was 15 carbs, and my body needed 1 unit of insulin to handle every 15 carbs. I also learned that I had to eat on a set schedule because of the way insulin worked in my body.

"In first grade, the kids avoided me. They didn't understand that you don't 'catch' diabetes like the flu. I was miserable, so my parents placed me in a new school. Since then, I learned that I'm different, and that's OK. I also became determined to educate my friends and the public about diabetes. I was always a very outgoing kid, so after I was diagnosed, my parents started volunteering for the Juvenile Diabetes Research Foundation, and I became one of the organization's child ambassadors. I'd give speeches about the importance of finding a cure for diabetes, and I raised thousands of dollars for this cause. Diabetes doesn't get in my way; I don't let diabetes define who I am."

What Is Hypoglycemia?

Hypoglycemia (*hypo* = low) is a condition that occurs when the blood glucose level is too low to provide enough energy for cells. Hypoglycemia may be diagnosed when the blood glucose level is less than 70 mg/dl.[32]

In response to rapidly declining blood glucose levels, the adrenal glands secrete epinephrine (see Fig. 4.18 [endocrine system]). You may be more familiar with epinephrine's common name, *adrenaline*. Like glucagon, epinephrine increases the supply of glucose and fatty acids in the bloodstream, but the hormone can also make a person with hypoglycemia feel irritable, restless, shaky, hungry, and sweaty. If the blood glucose level drops too low, the affected person can develop seizures, and he or she may lose consciousness and die.

Hypoglycemia is a major concern for people who give themselves insulin injections or take medication to raise the amount of insulin made by their bodies. Having too much insulin in the bloodstream contributes to hypoglycemia.

Treating hypoglycemia generally includes taking pills or a gel that contains glucose or consuming a serving of food or beverage that supplies 15 g of sugar.[32] Eating a tablespoon of sugar or honey, for example, can help raise the blood glucose level to normal. To prevent hypoglycemia, people with diabetes should eat regular meals and snacks that contain appropriate amounts of carbohydrate and monitor their blood glucose levels as often as recommended by their healthcare professionals.[32]

Metabolic Syndrome

Do you or does someone you know have a "spare tire," "beer belly," "muffin tops," or an "apple shape"? People who are too fat often have excess abdominal fat, which can be dangerous, especially when it is accompanied by insulin resistance, hypertension, and elevated blood lipid (triglyceride and cholesterol) levels.

An estimated one in three Americans has **metabolic syndrome,** a condition characterized by three or more of the signs listed in Table 5.11.[33] A **syndrome** is a group of signs and symptoms that occur together and indicate a specific health problem. Compared to people who do not have metabolic syndrome, individuals with this condition have five times the risk of type 2 diabetes and almost twice the risk of heart and blood vessel (cardiovascular) disease.[34]

Although genetic factors play a major role in the development of metabolic syndrome, excess abdominal fat, lack of physical activity, and insulin resistance are the primary risk factors for the condition.[35] People may lower their likelihood of developing metabolic syndrome by avoiding obesity, being physically active, and increasing their intake of fruits, vegetables, and other fiber-rich foods, such as whole-grain cereals.

TABLE 5.11 Signs of Metabolic Syndrome

Sign	Defining Value
Large waist circumference	≥ 40 inches (men) ≥ 35 inches (women)
Chronically elevated blood pressure (hypertension)	≥ 130 mm Hg systolic (upper value) or ≥ 85 mm Hg diastolic (lower value) or Drug treatment for hypertension
Chronically elevated fasting blood fats (triglycerides)	≥ 150 mg/dl or Drug treatment for elevated triglycerides
Low fasting high-density lipoprotein cholesterol (HDL cholesterol)	< 40 mg/dl (men) < 50 mg/dl (women) or Drug treatment for reduced HDL
High fasting blood glucose	≥ 100 mg/dl or Drug treatment for elevated glucose

Source: Data from Grundy, SM and others: "Diagnosis and management of the metabolic syndrome, An American Heart Association/National Heart, Lung, and Blood Institute scientific statement: Executive summary," *Circulation* 112:e285, 2005.

Did YOU Know?

For over 50 years, medical researchers have been testing the effectiveness of transplanting a pancreas or pancreatic islet (*i'-let*) cells, which contain insulin-producing beta cells, into the bodies of people with type 1 diabetes. The expectation was to help patients achieve good control over their blood glucose levels while reducing their need to have daily insulin injections. A major limitation of such procedures has been the need to place the donor's islet cells into the patient's liver, which does not have the same blood supply as the pancreas.

In 2017, scientists at the University of Miami's medical school published a report in *The New England Journal of Medicine* that described a 43-year-old woman who had been using insulin for over 2 decades to treat type 1 diabetes.[34] The woman had bouts of severe hypoglycemia, and she was often not aware that her blood glucose level was too low. In an experimental treatment, islet cells were taken from a person who had died and transplanted into the *omentum* of the woman with diabetes. The omentum is a fatty structure that drapes over the stomach and small intestine (see Figure 10.3). Unlike the liver, the omentum has the same blood supply as the pancreas.

After the procedure, the patient was given medication to suppress rejection of the transplanted cells. She is likely to need anti-rejection medications for the rest of her life. Within 3 weeks after the surgery, the patient was able to stop giving herself insulin injections. After one year, she still had good control over her blood glucose levels and had not experienced hypoglycemic episodes. The scientists involved in this experiment will continue to follow their patient's progress to determine whether this method of transplanting islet cells is both safe and effective as a long-term treatment for type 1 diabetes.

metabolic syndrome condition that increases risk of type 2 diabetes and CVD

syndrome group of signs and symptoms that occur together and indicate a specific health problem

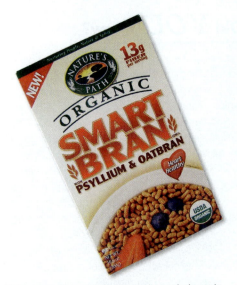

Eating more fiber-rich foods, such as whole-grain cereals, may reduce the risk of metabolic syndrome.
©Wendy Schiff

lactose intolerance inability to digest lactose properly

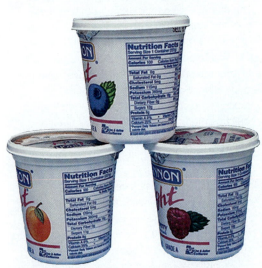

Lactose-intolerant people may be able to eat yogurt without experiencing digestive tract discomfort.
©McGraw-Hill Education. Bob Coyle, photographer

Did YOU Know?

People who have severe lactose intolerance should read food labels carefully because lactose-containing substances may be listed as ingredients. Products contain lactose if they include whey, curds, milk by-products, dry milk solids, and nonfat dry milk powder.

Individuals who already have metabolic syndrome may reduce their risk of cardiovascular disease (CVD) by lowering their elevated blood pressure, glucose, insulin, and triglyceride levels. Lifestyle changes that can help manage these levels include losing excess weight, exercising regularly, and reducing intakes of salt, saturated fat, and simple sugars. If such changes do not alleviate the condition, medication may be necessary to manage blood pressure and blood lipid levels. Chapter 6 provides more information about cardiovascular disease and "heart healthy" eating patterns.

Lactose Intolerance

Millions of Americans suffer from **lactose intolerance** (also referred to as lactose maldigestion or malabsorption), the inability to digest lactose completely. Lactose—intolerant people do not produce enough lactase, the enzyme that breaks lactose into glucose and galactose. When a lactose—intolerant person consumes lactose, the disaccharide is not completely digested and absorbed by the time it enters the large intestine. Bacteria that reside in the large intestine break down lactose and produce irritating gases and acids as metabolic by—products. As a result, a lactose—intolerant person usually experiences intestinal cramps, bloating, gas, and diarrhea within 30 minutes to 2 hours after consuming milk or other lactose—containing products.

Normally, infants produce lactase, but by the time children are 2 years old, their small intestine begins to produce less of the enzyme. Many older children and adults, particularly those with African, Asian, and Eastern European ancestry, are lactose intolerant and experience some degree of abdominal discomfort after drinking milk.

Lactose intolerance is not the same as milk allergy, which is an immune system response to cow's milk proteins. Milk allergy is most likely to occur during infancy; lactose intolerance is more likely to occur during adolescence (the teen years) or in adulthood.[36]

Milk and milk products are often excellent sources of protein, many vitamins, and the minerals calcium and phosphorus. What can people with lactose intolerance do to achieve a nutritionally adequate diet without drinking milk? Lactose—intolerant people are often able to eat hard cheeses and yogurt without experiencing any digestive tract discomfort. Milk loses most of its lactose content when it is processed to make aged cheeses, such as cheddar and Swiss. The bacteria used to make yogurt convert much of the lactose in milk to lactic acid, and the microbes assist with the digestion of the remaining lactose even after the yogurt is eaten.[37]

Many people with lactose intolerance can consume small amounts of milk without experiencing intestinal discomfort. People who cannot tolerate even limited amounts of fresh fluid milk can probably drink milk that has been pre—treated with lactase to reduce its lactose content. Most large supermarkets sell fresh lactase—treated milk in the dairy food section (Fig. 5.14). Also, lactase—containing solutions and pills are available without prescription. A lactose—intolerant person simply adds a small amount of the solution to milk 24 hours before drinking the beverage or takes one of the pills with lactose—containing food. People who cannot tolerate lactose can substitute soy milk for cows' milk because soy milk does not contain lactose.

Does Sugar Cause Hyperactivity?

If you have ever been in charge of a 7—year—old child's birthday party or observed third graders preparing for their Halloween celebration, you can understand why people often blame sugary foods for causing unruly and "hyperactive" behavior. Attention deficit hyperactivity disorder (ADHD) is characterized by impulsivity, hyperactivity, and difficulty paying attention.[38] According to estimates provided by the Centers for Disease Control and Prevention, about 11% of American children have ADHD.[39] Many children do not outgrow the condition by the time they reach adulthood.

Although scientists do not know what causes ADHD, it probably involves genetic and environmental factors. The results of scientific studies do not indicate that eating sugary foods or drinks increases children's physical activity levels, causes ADHD, or has any other negative effects on their behavior.[38] Birthday and school parties are exciting and happy occasions that typically involve a radical change from a child's usual routine. In these situations, a youngster's excitement and more active behavior is more likely to be the result of the occasion rather than a particular food.

Fiber and Health

Technically, fiber is not an essential nutrient, because the human body can live without it. You can live *better*, however, by adding fiber–rich foods to your diet. Eating high–fiber foods may reduce your risk of obesity, diabetes, certain intestinal tract disorders, and cardiovascular disease, which includes heart disease and stroke.

A person's diet, particularly its fiber content, affects his or her bowel habits. Some kinds of fiber in food attract water and swell in the digestive tract, forming a large, soft mass that applies pressure to the inner muscular walls of the large intestine, stimulating the muscles to push the residue quickly through the tract. People who often eat foods that contain adequate amounts of fiber have softer stools and more regular bowel movements, and they are less likely to strain while having bowel movements than people whose diets lack fiber. Thus, people generally do not need to rely on over–the–counter laxatives to treat constipation. Eating more fiber–rich foods is the natural way to become "regular."

Diverticula and Swollen Hemorrhoids

Diverticula are marble–size sacs that form in the lining of the colon (Fig. 5.15). In most people, diverticula do not produce symptoms, but they can bleed or become painfully inflamed when bacteria or feces are trapped within them. When this condition (*diverticulitis*) occurs, the affected person may need surgery to remove the damaged section of large intestine. The causes of diverticula are unknown, but age is a factor because the sacs are more likely to form in older adults.[40] At one time, health care providers advised people with diverticular disease to not eat certain high–fiber foods, including popcorn, nuts, and sunflower seeds. Now, no special diet is recommended, but individuals with the disease should learn to avoid foods that seem to aggravate the condition.

Hemorrhoids are clusters of small rectal veins that can become swollen and inflamed, making them likely to bleed and cause discomfort and itching (Fig. 5.16). This condition commonly affects adults and may be more likely to occur when a person sits for long periods or strains during bowel movements. Although swollen hemorrhoids are generally not a sign of a serious health problem, you should consult a physician if you experience any bleeding during bowel movements because it may also be a sign of colorectal cancer, a major cancer site for Americans.

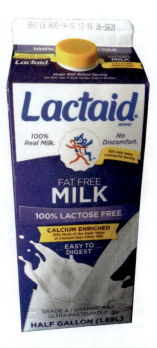

Figure 5.14 Lactase-treated milk. Fresh lactase-treated milk is often available in the dairy section of supermarkets.
©Wendy Schiff

diverticula abnormal, small sacs that form in wall of colon

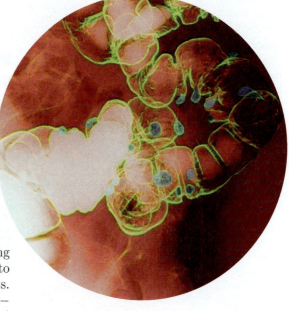

Figure 5.15 Diverticula. In this color-enhanced x-ray, the blue areas are diverticula.
©Du Cane Medical Imaging Ltd/Science Source

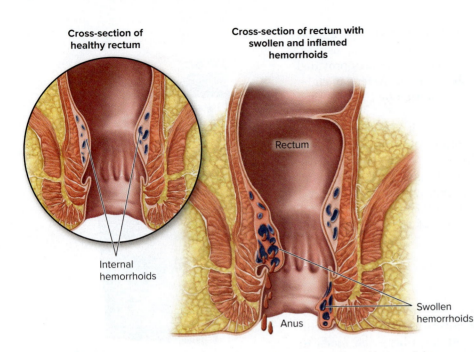

Cross-section of healthy rectum

Cross-section of rectum with swollen and inflamed hemorrhoids

Rectum

Internal hemorrhoids

Anus

Swollen hemorrhoids

| **Figure 5.16** **Hemorrhoids.** Swollen hemorrhoids can bleed, cause pain, and become itchy.

Did *YOU* Know?

Dried plums (*Prunus domestica* L.) are commonly called prunes. The fruit contains fiber, the sugar alcohol sorbitol, and other substances that are mild natural laxatives. Prune juice provides the laxative effect of prunes but lacks the whole fruit's fiber content.

Source: Scott Bauer/ARS/USDA

Fiber and Colorectal Cancer

In the United States and throughout the world, colon or *colorectal* cancer (cancer of the two lower portions of the large intestine) is one of the most common cancers.[41] In the early 1970s, a group of scientists noted that rural African populations who typically ate high−fiber diets rarely developed colorectal cancer. When these populations moved to urban areas and adopted relatively low−fiber Western diets, their risk of colorectal cancer increased. As a result of these observations, the scientists suggested that high−fiber diets were protective against colorectal cancer. Today, scientists think a healthy diet that supplies high−fiber foods, such as whole grains, fruits, and vegetables, may reduce the risk of colorectal cancer.[42]

Fiber and Heart Health

Diets rich in fiber, particularly soluble types of fiber, can reduce the risk of cardiovascular disease by reducing blood cholesterol levels. High blood levels of certain forms of blood cholesterol are associated with increased risks of cardiovascular disease. The liver uses cholesterol to make bile, a substance that helps digest fats. The gallbladder stores bile and releases the substance into the small intestine during meals. Instead of eliminating bile along with fecal matter in bowel movements, the intestinal tract breaks it down and absorbs its components, which eventually enter the liver. The liver recycles the "used" bile components to make new bile. When you eat oat cereal, the soluble fiber in oats interferes with this recycling process because it binds to the used bile components in the intestinal tract and prevents them from being absorbed. (See Fig. 6.12.) Thus, the used bile components are eliminated during bowel movements. As a result, blood cholesterol levels drop as the liver removes cholesterol from the blood to make new bile. The "Recipe for Healthy Living" feature of this chapter has a hot oatmeal recipe.

Fiber and Weight Control

If you are trying to lose excess body fat, you may find it helpful to add more fiber−rich foods to your diet. A serving of a high−fiber food generally has lower energy content than the same volume of a low−fiber food. As a result, energy intake usually decreases when people switch their consumption from low−fiber to high−fiber diets.

Increasing Your Fiber Intake

The recommended Adequate Intakes (AIs) for fiber are 38 and 25 g/day for young men and women, respectively, but the typical diet of adult Americans supplies only about 17g of dietary fiber/day.[9] According to the Dietary Guidelines, fiber is a "nutrient of public health concern." You can estimate your daily fiber intake by completing the Personal Dietary Analysis at the end of this chapter. The "Food & Nutrition Tips" feature in this section of the chapter provides tips for increasing the fiber content of diets. Eating too much fiber may interfere with the small intestine's ability to absorb certain minerals. In

Did *YOU* Know?

What Are FODMAPs?

FODMAPs (fermentable oligo-, di-, and monosaccharides and polyols) are forms of carbohydrate that the GI tract may not fully digest or absorb, especially when a person eats too much of them. When FODMAPs are in the lumen of the colon, they attract water, and the bacteria that reside in the large intestine ferment the substances for their energy needs. Side effects of the bacteria's activity often include abdominal cramps, diarrhea, bloating, and gas.

FODMAPs include fructose, lactose, and sugar alcohols such as xylitol and sorbitol. Wheat products, rye, various kinds of fruits and vegetables, beans, and high-lactose dairy foods are often excluded in low-FODMAP diets because they are rich sources of FODMAPs. Although a low-FODMAP diet can be difficult to follow for a long period, people with irritable bowel syndrome and, possibly, inflammatory bowel disease may benefit from such diets.[43]

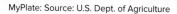

MY DIVERSE PLATE

MyPlate: Source: U.S. Dept. of Agriculture

Red Lentils

For thousands of years, people living in Mediterranean countries, the Middle East, India, and other countries of southeastern Asia have eaten lentils, a type of *legume*. Peas and beans are also legumes. Lentils, particularly green varieties, are an excellent source of fiber. Lentils also provide protein, iron, potassium, and folate. Red lentils soften quickly with cooking and can be used in stews, sauces, or dips.

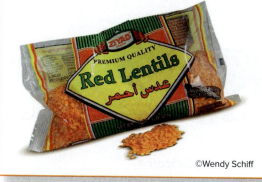

©Wendy Schiff

rare instances, consuming too much dietary fiber results in intestinal blockage, especially if fluid intake is low.

Intestinal bacteria produce gases when they metabolize fiber; therefore, registered dietitian nutritionists recommend that people adjust by gradually increasing their fiber intake. Practices that result in swallowing air, such as eating quickly; drinking carbonated beverages, especially with a straw; and chewing gum, also contribute to intestinal gas.

Food & Nutrition tips

- Read the ingredients list on the label to find out if a bread or cereal product is whole grain; whole grain or bran should be the first ingredient.

- Don't rely on the product's name or appearance. Check the ingredients. Terms such as *100% wheat, multigrain,* or *stone-ground wheat* are misleading because the product may contain little or no whole grain.

©Photodisc/Getty Images RF

- Brown rice has more fiber and flavor than white rice.

- Substitute whole-wheat pasta for regular pasta, or use half whole-wheat and half regular pasta in pasta dishes.

- Snack on pieces of fresh, frozen, or dried fruit.

- Include more nuts, beans, and seeds in your diet.

- Spread peanut or soy butter on whole-grain crackers for a fiber-filled snack.

- Add frozen, dried, or fresh fruit such as berries, raisins, or bananas instead of sugar or honey to sweeten cereal or plain yogurt.

- Add a small amount of uncooked oatmeal and wheat germ to raw ground meats when making hamburgers or meatloaf.

- Adding bran, wheat germ, and uncooked oatmeal to pancake or waffle batter also enhances the batter's fiber content.

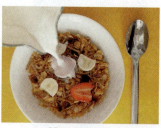

- Good dietary sources of fiber contain at least 2.5 g of fiber per serving.

©Photodisc/Getty Images RF

Concept CHECKPOINT

16. What are the signs and symptoms of type 1 and type 2 diabetes?
17. Lata wants to prevent the development of type 2 diabetes. What health-related lifestyle practices can she follow to reduce her risk of this serious metabolic disease?
18. Identify at least three signs of metabolic syndrome.
19. What is lactose intolerance?
20. List at least three ways to increase dietary fiber intake.
21. Discuss the health benefits of including dietary fiber in meals and snacks.

See Appendix G for responses.

5.8 Nutrition Matters: Glycemic Index and Glycemic Load

Learning Outcome

1 Explain the difference between the glycemic index and glycemic load.

2 Identify foods that have low or high glycemic indexes or glycemic loads.

In the early 1980s, researchers noted that the body digested carbohydrate–rich foods at different rates, and its insulin response to each food varied. Foods that contained large amounts of refined carbohydrates were digested rapidly, and the rapid flow of glucose into the bloodstream raised blood glucose and insulin levels sharply. Other carbohydrate–rich foods that had high fiber contents were digested slowly and did not cause such a dramatic increase in blood glucose and insulin levels. This observation led to the development of the dietary concepts *glycemic index* and *glycemic load*. Currently, the notion that a food's glycemic index could influence health has spurred the publication of popular diet books recommending avoiding foods with high glycemic indices, such as potatoes and bread. What is the glycemic index? Should you avoid foods that have high glycemic indices?

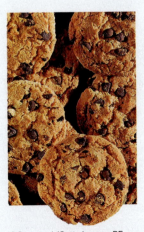
©Comstock/Getty Images RF

Blueberries: ©PhotoAlto/Getty Images RF

The glycemic index (GI) is a way of classifying foods by comparing the rise in blood glucose that occurs after eating a portion of a food that supplies 50 g of digestible carbohydrate to the rise that occurs after eating a standard source of carbohydrate, such as 50 g of glucose. A related value, the glycemic load (GL), is the grams of carbohydrate in a serving of food multiplied by the food's GI; this figure is then divided by 100. Compared to the GI, the GL may be a more realistic way of rating foods because the value indicates the relative rise in blood glucose levels after eating a *typical* serving of a carbohydrate–containing food.

Table 5.12 lists average GIs and GLs of several commonly eaten foods. Note that sucrose and other sugary foods, as well as highly refined starchy foods such as cornflakes, baked potatoes, and white rice, have high GIs (70 or more). Raw apples, carrots, spaghetti, fat–free milk, and peanuts have low to moderate GIs (less than 70). It is important to note that the GL of a food is usually lower than its GI. For example, the GI for 30 g of cornflakes is 80, but the GL value for cornflakes is only 21. Foods with low GLs have values below 15; high GL foods have values of more than 20.

Critics think the GI and GL standards have limited usefulness as a menu–planning tool because the values can vary too much. Therefore, the glycemic index and glycemic load values shown in Table 5.12 may vary significantly, depending on where the food was grown, its degree of ripeness, or the extent of its processing. Additionally, individuals often experience different blood glucose levels after they eat the same carbohydrate–rich food. Furthermore, the values reflect a single food's effect on blood glucose levels.

TABLE 5.12 Glycemic Index and Load: Average Values of Selected Foods

Food	Glycemic Index* Value	Glycemic Load** ServingSize	Value
Potato, Russet, baked	158	150 g	33
Jelly beans	114	30 g	22
White rice, medium grain, boiled	107	150 g	29
Bagel, white plain	99	70 g	24
French fries	90	150 g	21
Cola, sugar-sweetened drink	90	1 cup	16
Banana	89	120 g	16
Cornflakes cereal	80	30 g	21
Popcorn, microwave plain	79	20 g	6
Spaghetti, cooked	68	180 g	23
Orange juice	66	1 cup	12
Ice cream, vanilla, low-fat	66	50 g	7
Snickers candy bar	61	60 g	15
Apple, raw	56	120 g	6
Carrots, raw	50	80 g	2
Fat-free milk	46	1 cup	4
Peaches, canned in natural juice	43	120 g	3
Peanuts	10	50 g	0

*Compared to white bread (GI = 100); **Per serving

Source: Data from Atkinson FS et al., "International tables of glycemic index and glycemic load values: 2008," *Diabetes Care* 31(12):2281, 2008.

The effect may be reduced when the food is eaten as part of a meal that contains a mixture of macro-nutrients and fiber.

Despite the criticism directed at the use of these indices, epidemiological studies suggest an association between high GI/GL diets and serious chronic diseases.[44] As people in developing countries abandon traditional diets and eat more high GI/GL foods, they become more likely to develop obesity and type 2 diabetes, as well as cardiovascular disease and certain cancers.[45] Low GI diets may improve blood lipid levels and reduce the risk of cardiovascular disease[46] and improve HbA1c levels.[47] People with diabetes can follow a low GI or low GL diet while monitoring their total carbo-hydrate intake to control their blood glucose levels.[48]

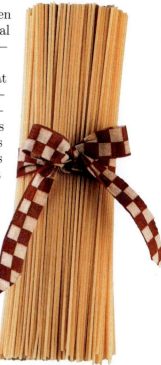
©Brand X Pictures/Getty Images RF

Concept CHECKPOINT

22. Which of these foods has the lowest glycemic index: plain, white bagel; raw apple; orange juice; or microwave popcorn?

See Appendix G for responses.

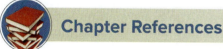

Chapter References

See Appendix H.

Stacked books: ©Stockbyte/Getty Images RF

Summary

5.1 Introducing Carbohydrates

- Carbohydrates are an important source of energy for the body. Plants use energy from the sun to make carbohydrates from water and carbon dioxide. Some of the energy is stored in the bonds that hold the carbon and hydrogen atoms together. Cells break down those bonds, releasing the energy that powers various forms of cellular work.

5.2 Simple Carbohydrates: Sugars

- The three most important dietary monosaccharides are glucose, fructose, and galactose. Glucose is a primary fuel for muscles and other cells; nervous system and red blood cells rely on glucose for energy under normal conditions. Lactose and sucrose are major dietary disaccharides.

5.3 Complex Carbohydrates

- Starch, glycogen, and most forms of dietary fiber are polysaccharides. Although fiber is not digested by humans, soluble and insoluble fiber provide important health benefits.

5.4 What Happens to Carbohydrates in the Body?

- Glucose is the primary end product of carbohydrate digestion. Hormones, particularly insulin and glucagon, maintain normal blood glucose levels. Insulin enables glucose to enter cells, where the sugar is metabolized for energy. Glucagon stimulates the liver to break down glycogen into glucose molecules and release them into the bloodstream.

5.5 Carbohydrate Consumption Patterns

- People in industrialized nations tend to eat less complex, unprocessed carbohydrates and more highly refined sugars than people living in less-developed countries. Healthy Americans should consume diets that furnish 45 to 65% of energy from carbohydrates, primarily complex carbohydrates. Refined sugar is often blamed for causing obesity, diabetes, and hyperactivity, but tooth decay is the only health problem that is clearly associated with eating carbohydrates. Many adults are lactose intolerant because they do not produce enough lactase, the intestinal enzyme needed to digest the disaccharide.

5.6 Understanding Nutrient Labeling: Carbohydrates and Fiber

- The Nutrition Facts panel provides information about total carbohydrate, total sugars, added sugars, and fiber contents of packaged foods and beverages.

5.7 Carbohydrates and Health

- Foods that contain a lot of added sugars and fats tend to be energy dense. Some nutrition scientists think high intakes of added sugars, especially in regular soft drinks, is largely responsible for Americans' rising rate of obesity.

- Diabetes mellitus is characterized by elevated blood glucose levels. Diabetes can result in cardiovascular disease, kidney failure, blindness, and lower limb amputations. There are two major types of diabetes mellitus, type 1 and type 2 diabetes. Type 2 diabetes is the more common form of the disease. People who are sedentary, have excess body fat, eat Western diets, and have a close relative with type 2 diabetes are at risk of developing this form of the disease.

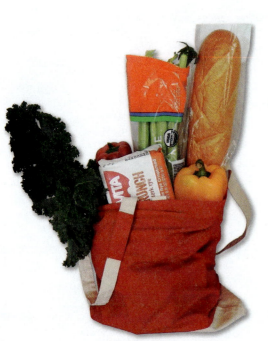

©Wendy Schiff

- Eating fiber-rich foods may reduce your risk of obesity, type 2 diabetes, cardiovascular disease, and certain intestinal tract disorders. High-fiber diets, especially those with whole grains, fruits, and vegetables, are associated with lower risk colon cancer compared to diets that contain little fiber. Additionally, foods that contain soluble fiber may improve cardiovascular health by reducing cholesterol absorption.

5.8 Nutrition Matters: Glycemic Index and Glycemic Load

- The glycemic index (GI) and glycemic load (GL) are ways of classifying certain foods by their effect on blood glucose levels. Results of some epidemiological studies suggest an association between high GI/GL diets and serious chronic diseases.

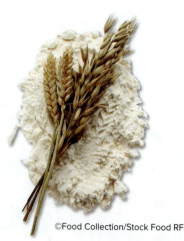

©Food Collection/Stock Food RF

Recipe for Healthy Living

Berry-Good Hot Oatmeal Cereal

This single-serving hot oatmeal with blueberries recipe is a very good source of B vitamins and fiber. For variety, substitute raisins, frozen or fresh strawberries, or raspberries for the blueberries. A serving of the cooked cereal supplies about 260 kcal, 12 g protein, 1 g fat, 50 g carbohydrate, 6 g fiber, 250 mg calcium, and 2.0 mg iron.

©C Squared Studios/Getty Images RF

INGREDIENTS:

½ cup frozen or fresh unsweetened blueberries
½ cup quick-cooking, enriched oats
¾ cup fat-free milk
1 tsp sugar
pinch of ground cinnamon (optional)

PREPARATION STEPS:

1. Place ingredients in a microwaveable bowl and stir.
2. Microwave on "high" for about 2 ½ minutes.
3. Stir and top with blueberries before eating.

Cleanup tip: After eating, soak cereal bowl in cold water before washing it.

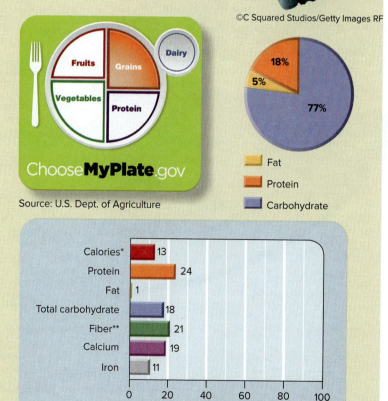

ChooseMyPlate.gov

Source: U.S. Dept. of Agriculture

18%
5%
77%

- Fat
- Protein
- Carbohydrate

Calories* — 13
Protein — 24
Fat — 1
Total carbohydrate — 18
Fiber** — 21
Calcium — 19
Iron — 11

% of DV/serving

*2000 daily total kcal
**Component of Total carbohydrate

connect Further analyze this recipe or other recipes through activities located in Connect.

Recipe box: ©C Squared Studios/Getty Images RF

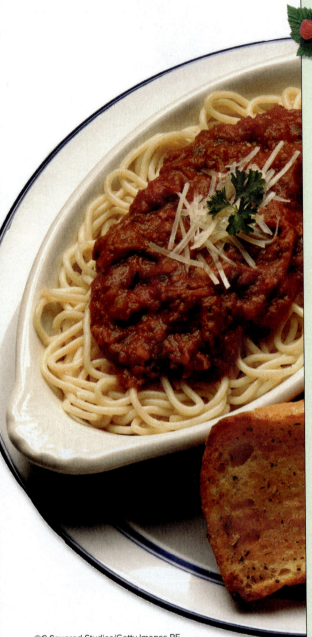

Personal Dietary Analysis

1. Refer to the 3-day food log from the "Personal Dietary Analysis" feature in Chapter 3. List the total number of kilocalories you consumed for each day of record keeping. Add the figures to obtain a total, divide the total by 3, then round the figure to the nearest whole number to obtain your average daily energy intake for the 3-day period.

Sample Calculation:

Day 1	<u>2500</u> kcal
Day 2	<u>3200</u> kcal
Day 3	<u>2750</u> kcal

Total kcal <u>**8450**</u> ÷ **3 days** = <u>**2817**</u> **kcal/day**
(average kilocalorie intake, rounded to the nearest whole number)

Your Calculation:

Day 1	_____ kcal
Day 2	_____ kcal
Day 3	_____ kcal

Total kcal _____ ÷ **3 days** = _____ **kcal/day**
(average kilocalorie intake, rounded to the nearest whole number)

2. Add the number of grams of total carbohydrate eaten each day of the period. Divide the total by 3 and round to the nearest whole number to calculate the average number of grams of total carbohydrate consumed daily.

Your Calculation:

Day 1	_____ g
Day 2	_____ g
Day 3	_____ g
Total =	_____ g

Total g _____ ÷ **3 days** = _____ **g of total carbohydrate/day**
(average, rounded to the nearest whole number)

3. Each gram of carbohydrate provides about 4 kcal; therefore, you must multiply the average number of grams of total carbohydrate obtained in step 2 by 4 to obtain the number of kcal from total carbohydrate.

Your Calculation:

_____ **g/day** × **4 kcal/g** = _____ **kcal from total carbohydrate**

4. To calculate the average daily percentage of kilocalories that carbohydrates contributed to your diet, divide the average kilocalories from total carbohydrate obtained in step 3 by the average total daily kilocalorie intake obtained in step 1; round the figure to the nearest one-hundredth. Multiply the value by 100, drop decimal point, and add the percent symbol.

Sample Calculation:

1692 kcal ÷ 2817 kcal = 0.60

0.60 × 100 = 60%

Your Calculation:

_____ kcal ÷ _____ kcal = _____

_____ × **100** = _____ %

5. On average, did you consume *at least* the RDA of 130 g of carbohydrate?
Yes _____ No _____

6. Did your average carbohydrate intake meet the recommended 45 to 65% of total
energy? Yes _____ No _____

   a. If your average carbohydrate intake was less than 130 g or below 45% of total
   calories, list five nutrient-dense, carbohydrate-rich foods you could eat that
   would boost your intake of carbohydrates.

   Foods: _____

   b. If your average carbohydrate intake was greater than 130 g or more than 65%
   of total energy, list the top five foods and beverages that contributed to your
   carbohydrate intake. _____

7. If the information is available, add the number of grams of added sugars that you
consumed each day of the 3-day period. To calculate the average number of grams
of added sugars eaten daily, divide the total number of grams by 3 and round to the
nearest whole number.

Your Calculation:

Day 1 _____ g

Day 2 _____ g

Day 3 _____ g

Total _____ g ÷ **3 days** = _____ g of added sugars/day
(average rounded to the nearest whole number)

   a. Calculate the number of kcal contributed by added sugars (each gram of sugar
   provides about 4 kcal).

   _____ g of added sugars/day × 4 kcal/g = _____ kcal

   b. Calculate the percentage of total daily kcal contributed by added sugars. (Use
   the kcal from added sugars determined in step 7a and divide the number by the
   average number of kcal/day obtained in step 1.)

   _____ kcal from added sugars ÷ _____ average daily kcal = _____ percent of total
   calories contributed by added sugars

   c. Did your intake of daily calories from added sugars meet the recommendations
   of the Dietary Guidelines (less than 10% of total calories)? _____ Yes _____No

8. Calculate your average daily intake of fiber by adding the grams of fiber consumed
over the 3-day period and dividing the total by 3.

   Day 1 _____ g

   Day 2 _____ g

   Day 3 _____ g

   Total = _____ g

Total grams _____ ÷ **3 days** = _____ g of fiber daily

a. What was your average daily fiber intake? _____ g

b. Did your average daily fiber intake meet the recommended Adequate Intakes of 38 and 25 g/day for young men and women, respectively? Yes _____ No _____

c. If your response is yes, list foods that contributed to your fiber intake.

d. If you did not meet the recommended level of fiber intake, list at least five foods that you would eat to increase your fiber intake to the recommended level.

connect Complete the Personal Dietary Analysis activity located in Connect.

Critical Thinking

1. One of your friends thinks honey is more nutritious and safer to eat than table sugar. He wants you to avoid table sugar and use only honey as a sweetener. What would you tell this person about the nutritive value and safety of honey compared to sugar?

2. Maria has diabetes, and she just found out that she is in the sixth week of pregnancy. She wants to know what she can do to increase her chances of having a problem–free pregnancy and healthy baby. What would you tell her about the importance of properly managing her blood glucose level during pregnancy?

3. How did you feel about drinking sugar–sweetened soft drinks, sports drinks, and energy drinks before reading this chapter? Has your opinion changed? If so, explain how.

4. Wyatt is a 5–year–old whose mother thinks sugar causes hyperactivity, so she forbids him from eating

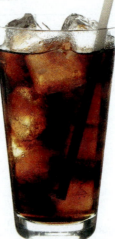
©FoodCollection/StockFood RF

sweets. When Wyatt is invited to his friends' birth–day parties, his mother gives him a small bag of apple slices to eat instead of cake and ice cream. What would you tell Wyatt's mother concerning sugar intake as a cause of hyperactivity?

5. Consider the fiber content of your diet. Do you consume enough fiber each day? If your fiber intake is adequate, what foods do you eat regularly that contribute soluble and insoluble fiber to your diet? If your fiber intake is low, list foods you would consume to increase your intake of both types of fiber.

6. Jeff experiences intestinal cramps and gas after drinking a glass of milk. He suspects that he has lactose intolerance. What steps can he take to obtain adequate nutrition without eliminating dairy foods from his diet?

Practice Test

Select the best answer.

1. Which of the following substances is a disaccharide?
   a. Maltose
   b. Starch
   c. Galactose
   d. Glycogen

2. _____ is a primary fuel for muscles and other cells.
   a. Protein
   b. Cholesterol
   c. Glucose
   d. HFCS

3. Which of the following substances is a polysaccharide?
   a. Glucose
   b. Glycogen
   c. Glucagon
   d. Galactose

4. Which of the following conditions is a common sign or symptom of untreated type 1 diabetes?
   a. Migraine headaches
   b. Obesity
   c. Diverticula
   d. Hyperglycemia

5. Dietary fiber

 a. supplies more energy, gram per gram, than fat.
 b. is not digested by the human intestinal tract.
 c. promotes tooth decay.
 d. is only in animal sources of food.

6. Insoluble fiber

 a. is in beef and pork.
 b. dissolves or swells in water.
 c. is in whole–grain products, including brown rice.
 d. increases the risk of heart disease.

7. _____ is the hormone that helps glucose to enter cells.

 a. Glucagon
 b. Insulin
 c. HFCS
 d. Maltase

8. _____ are a primary source of added sugars in American diets.

 a. Cured deli meats
 b. Sugar–sweetened soft drinks
 c. Refined cereals
 d. Canned fruits

9. Type 2 diabetes is

 a. a disease that primarily affects young children.
 b. characterized by severe hypoglycemia.
 c. often associated with excess body weight.
 d. caused by eating refined sugars.

10. Which of the following signs is associated with metabolic syndrome?

 a. Low blood pressure
 b. High fasting blood glucose
 c. Low hemoglobin
 d. High fasting HDL cholesterol

11. Which of the following conditions is clearly associated with eating certain dietary carbohydrates, especially sticky sugars?

 a. Tooth decay
 b. Type 1 diabetes
 c. Attention deficit hyperactivity disorder
 d. Hypertension

12. Which of the following substances is an intestinal enzyme that breaks down lactose?

 a. Galactose
 b. Salivary amylase
 c. Lactase
 d. Lactic acid

13. Which of the following foods is the best source of soluble fiber?

 a. Raw fruit
 b. Whole–grain oat cereal
 c. Sports drinks
 d. Cooked meat

14. Which of the following foods has a high glycemic index?

 a. Nonfat milk
 b. Cornflakes cereal
 c. Salted peanuts
 d. Raw carrots

Answers to Quiz Yourself

1. Compared to table sugar, honey is a natural and far more nutritious sweetener. **False.** (Section 5.2)

2. Ounce per ounce, sugar provides more energy than starch. **False.** (Sections 5.2 and 5.3)

3. Eating a high-fiber diet may reduce your blood cholesterol level. **True.** (Section 5.7)

4. The average American consumes 80% of his or her energy intake as refined sugars. **False.** (Section 5.5)

5. The results of clinical studies indicate that eating too much sugar makes children hyperactive. **False.** (Section 5.7)

CHAPTER 6

Fats and Other Lipids

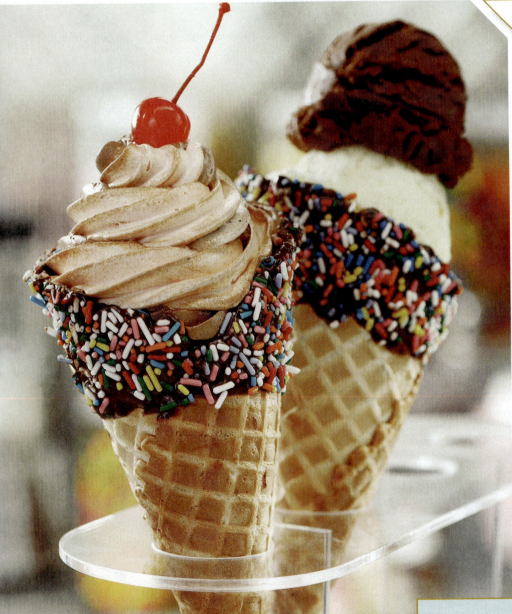

Quiz Yourself

What are trans and omega-3 fats, and which foods contain these fats? How much dietary fat is recommended? Should you avoid eating eggs because they contain cholesterol? Test your knowledge of fat and other lipids by taking the following quiz. The answers are at the end of the chapter.

1. To lose weight, use regular, stick margarine instead of butter because it has 25% fewer calories per teaspoon. _____ T _____ F

2. Egg yolks are a rich source of cholesterol. _____ T _____ F

3. Taking too many fish oil supplements may be harmful to health. _____ T _____ F

4. On average, Americans consume 60% of their calories from fat. _____ T _____ F

5. Increasing your intake of saturated fat will reduce your risk of heart disease. _____ T _____ F

connect

A wealth of proven resources are available on Connect® including SmartBook®, NutritionCalc Plus, and many other dynamic learning tools. Ask your instructor about Connect!

6.1 Introducing Lipids

Learning Outcomes

1. Identify the major kinds of lipids, including triglycerides and cholesterol.
2. List at least six functions of lipids in the body.
3. List at least three important functions of lipids in foods.

What do you think when you hear the word *fat* or *cholesterol?* Does "bad," "heart attack," or "deadly" enter your mind? If your answer is yes, are you con—cerned about the amounts and types of fat in your diet? Do you avoid eating eggs because of their cholesterol content? Does your concern have anything to do with having a family history of heart disease?

Lipids are a class of macronutrients that includes fatty acids, triglycerides (*try—glis'—er—eyeds*), phospholipids (*fos—foe—lip'—ids*), and cholesterol. In general, lipids are insoluble in water, but they are soluble in organic solvents such as alcohol and acetone. Consider what happens when you mix vinegar and olive oil to make a vinaigrette salad dressing. Vinegar is 95% water; oil is 100% lipid. Therefore, the oil does not dissolve in water to make a solution. Additionally, oil is less dense than water, so it rises to the top of the vinegar in small globules when added to vinegar. The globules join others to form an oily layer that floats on the vinegar until you shake the mixture. Shaking the ingredients mixes them temporarily. When left undisturbed, the oil and vinegar soon separate; hence the saying, "Oil and water don't mix."

You probably know fat is a major source of energy and eating too much fat can result in excess weight gain, which is unhealthy. Additionally, you may know that cholesterol is associated with heart attacks. However, you may not be aware of the many important roles that fat, cholesterol, and other lipids play in the body (Table 6.1). Lipids are crucial components of the plasma membrane that surround each human cell. In fact, a person cannot claim to be "fat free," because every cell in the body contains fat, as well as other lipids. The layer of fat under your skin (subcutaneous fat) stores energy, insulates you against cold temperatures, protects you against minor bruising, and contributes to your body's contours. In addition to storing energy, the fat deposits in your abdominal region cushion your vital organs from jarring movements and damaging blows.

In food, lipids enhance intestinal absorption of fat—soluble vitamins and phytochemicals. Dietary lipids also provide nonnutritional benefits by contribut—ing to the rich flavor, smooth texture, and appetizing aroma of foods. Whether fat is naturally in food or added to it, the nutrient often makes foods taste more appetizing. For example, if you are used to consuming whole milk that is about 3.25% fat by volume, you will recognize the difference fat makes to "mouth feel" when you drink fat—free milk that contains less than 0.5% fat.

It is not surprising that many Americans are confused about the roles of fat and cholesterol in health. The results from numerous studies conducted over the past 60 years indicate that consuming high amounts of certain lipids may increase the risk of serious health conditions, particularly cardiovascular disease (CVD), which includes heart disease and *stroke* (the loss of blood flow to a part of the brain; "brain attack").[1] On the other hand, some dietary fat is essential to good health. By reading this chapter, you will learn about the roles of lipids in your foods and body, as well as their major food sources. Additionally, you will learn how certain lipids may influence your health.

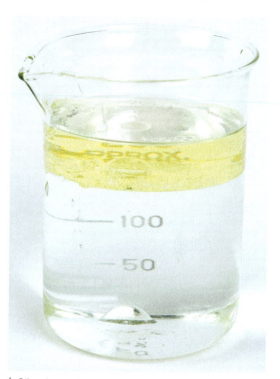
Oil and water do not mix. ©McGraw-Hill Education

TABLE 6.1 Major Functions of Lipids in the Body

Fats and certain other lipids are important for:

- providing and storing energy (fat);
- maintaining cell membranes;
- producing certain hormones;
- insulating the body against cold temperatures;
- cushioning the body against bumps and blows;
- contributing to body contours; and
- absorbing fat-soluble vitamins and phytochemicals.

lipids class of nutrients that generally do not dissolve in water

Concept CHECKPOINT

1. Although 88-year-old Rose has more body fat than is recommended, she is healthier than her much thinner 88-year-old cousin, Lily. Explain why having excess body fat can be beneficial for older adults.
2. Ingredients for a cake recipe include ½ cup of water. What would happen to the sensory quality of the baked cake if you replaced the water with the same amount of whole milk?

See Appendix G for responses.

6.2 Fatty Acids, Triglycerides, Phospholipids, and Sterols

Learning Outcomes

1 Explain the differences in the chemical structures of saturated, monounsaturated, polyunsaturated, and trans fatty acids.

2 Identify major food sources of each kind of lipid, including the essential fatty acids, phospholipids, and cholesterol.

3 Discuss the roles of essential fatty acids, phospholipids, and cholesterol in the body.

4 Discuss signs and symptoms of an essential fatty acid deficiency.

Fatty Acids

Most lipids have fatty acids in their chemical structures. Fatty acids provide energy for muscles and most other types of cells. As Figure 6.1 illustrates, a fatty acid is comprised of a **hydrocarbon chain,** a chain of carbon atoms bonded to each other and to hydrogen atoms. The first carbon in the molecule has three hydrogen atoms attached to it. Chemists call this part of the molecule the **omega** (or methyl) **end.** The last carbon in the fatty acid molecule forms an acid group.

In nature, common fatty acids have even numbers of carbon atoms. *Short—chain* fatty acids have 2 to 4 carbons; *medium—chain* fatty acids have 6 to 12 carbons; and *long—chain* fatty acids have 14 to 24 carbons. The molecules shown in Figure 6.1 contain 18 carbons; thus, they are long—chain fatty acids. Chemists identify a fatty acid by its number of carbon atoms and type of bond between carbon atoms in the hydrocarbon chain. Additionally, these factors influence how various fatty acids can affect a person's health.

Saturation

Fatty acids can be saturated or unsaturated. The carbons in the fatty acid chain shown in Figure 6.1a have single bonds between them. Note that each carbon in the chain has two hydrogen atoms attached to it. This is a **saturated fatty acid** because each carbon within the chain is saturated, that is, completely filled with hydrogen atoms.

An **unsaturated fatty acid** has two neighboring carbons within the chain that are missing two hydrogen atoms, and a double bond holds those particular carbons together (Fig. 6.1b). Unsaturated fatty acids can have one or more dou—ble bonds within the chain of carbons. The fatty acid illustrated in Figure 6.1b has only one double bond linking two carbon atoms; therefore, it is referred to as a *mono*unsaturated **fatty acid (MUFA).** The fatty acid shown in

hydrocarbon chain chain of carbon atoms bonded to each other and to hydrogen atoms

omega end first carbon of a fatty acid chain that has three hydrogen atoms attached to it

saturated fatty acid fatty acid that has each carbon atom within the chain filled with hydrogen atoms

unsaturated fatty acid fatty acid that is missing hydrogen atoms and has one or more double bonds within the carbon chain

monounsaturated fatty acid (MUFA) fatty acid that has one double bond within the carbon chain

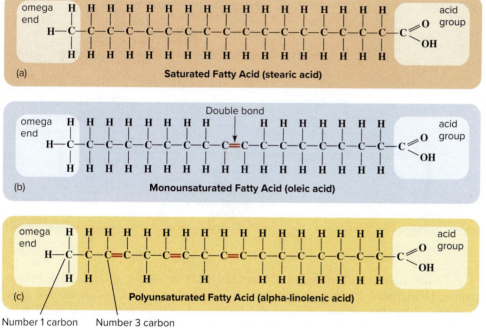

(a) **Saturated Fatty Acid (stearic acid)**

(b) **Monounsaturated Fatty Acid (oleic acid)**

(c) **Polyunsaturated Fatty Acid (alpha-linolenic acid)**

Number 1 carbon   Number 3 carbon

Figure 6.1 Fatty acids. A fatty acid is comprised of a hydrocarbon chain. The omega end contains the first carbon in the molecule; the last carbon in the molecule forms an acid group.

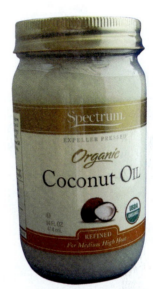

When stored at room temperature, coconut oil has the consistency of tub margarine, so it is classified as a solid fat. ©Wendy Schiff

Figure 6.1c is also unsaturated, but it has three double bonds within its hydro-carbon chain. A fatty acid that has two or more double bonds between carbons is a **polyunsaturated fatty acid (PUFA)**.

What is the difference between fats and oils? Although both substances contain fatty acids, fats are solid and most oils are liquid at room temperature. Compared to foods that contain high amounts of unsaturated fatty acids, foods that are rich sources of long-chain saturated fatty acids tend to be more solid at room temperature. A pat of butter, for example, contains more long-chain satu-rated fatty acids than a pat of margarine. Thus, butter keeps its shape better than margarine when it is not refrigerated. The "Lipids and Health: Cardiovascular Disease" section of this chapter discusses the health effects of eating diets that are rich in saturated or unsaturated fats.

Essential Fatty Acids

The body cannot make two polyunsaturated fatty acids, **alpha-linolenic** (*al'-fah lin'-o-len'-ik*) **acid** and **linoleic** (*lin'-o-lay'-ik*) **acid**. These lipids are **essential fatty acids** because they must be supplied by the diet. Alpha-linolenic acid is an **omega-3 fatty acid**. The "3" refers to the position of the first double bond that appears in the fatty acid's carbon chain, when you start counting carbons at the omega end of the molecule (see Fig. 6.1c). Cells use alpha-linolenic acid to synthesize two other omega-3 fatty acids, eicosapen-taenoic (*eye'-koss-uh-pen'-tah-ee-no'-ik*) acid (EPA) and docosahexaenoic (*doe'-koss-uh-hex'-uh-ee'-no'-ik*) acid (DHA). However, the body's ability to make EPA and DHA from alpha-linolenic acid is limited.

Linoleic acid is an *omega-6 fatty acid*. Cells can convert linoleic acid to arachidonic (*a'-rak'-ih-don'-ik*) acid (AA). The body uses EPA, DHA, and AA to make several compounds that have hormonelike functions, including *prostaglandins*. Prostaglandins produce a variety of important effects on the body, such as stimulating uterine contractions, regulating blood pressure, and promoting the immune system's inflammatory response. Figure 6.2 shows rela-tionships among the essential fatty acids.

polyunsaturated fatty acid (PUFA) fatty acid that has two or more double bonds within the carbon chain

alpha-linolenic acid an essential fatty acid

linoleic acid an essential fatty acid

essential fatty acids lipids that must be supplied by the diet

omega-3 fatty acid type of polyunsaturated fatty acid

Figure 6.2 Essential fatty acids. Alpha-linolenic acid and linoleic acid are not synthesized by the body; they must be supplied in the diet. The body uses these essential fatty acids to make DHA, EPA, and AA.

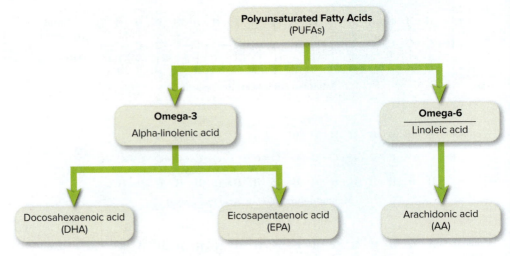

Did *YOU* Know?

People need small amounts of essential fatty acids for good health. Infants require DHA and EPA for nervous system development, and babies do not grow properly when their diets lack essential fatty acids. Other signs of essential fatty acid deficiency include scaly skin, hair loss, and poor wound healing. The Adequate Intake (AI) for alpha–linolenic acid is 1.6 g/day for men and 1.1 g/day for women. The AI for linoleic acid is 17 g/day for men and 12 g/day for women who are 19 through 50 years of age.[2] These amounts can be met by eating 2 to 3 tablespoons of vegetable fat daily, especially products made with canola and soybean oils, and meals that contain fatty fish, such as salmon and tuna, at least twice a week.

In the United States, essential fatty acid deficiency is uncommon because most Americans eat plenty of fat, especially linoleic acid. This omega–6 fatty acid is in vegetable oils often used for frying foods and making margarines and salad dressings. Additionally, whole–grain products contain linoleic acid. Certain fish are rich sources of omega–3 fatty acids ("omega–3s"), including DHA and EPA (see Table 6.6). Many Americans eat relatively small amounts of omega–3 fatty acids. The "Lipids and Health: Cardiovascular Disease" section of this chapter presents more information about essential fatty acids and their health effects.

Trans Fats

Unsaturated fatty acids usually have the two hydrogen atoms of the double–bonded carbons on the same side of the molecule. This type of structure is called a cis fatty acid. Cis fatty acids, such as oleic acid, have a "kink" or bend where the double bonds are in the carbon chain (Fig. 6.3a). A **trans fatty acid,** such as

trans fatty acid unsaturated fatty acid that has a trans double bond

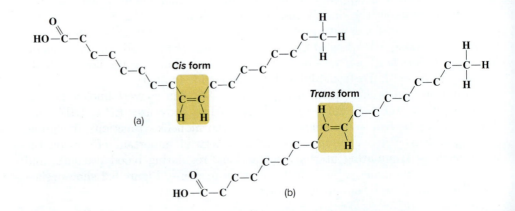

Figure 6.3 Cis and trans fatty acids. (*a*) Oleic acid is a cis fatty acid. (*b*) Elaidic acid is a trans fatty acid. For simplicity, most of the hydrogen atoms in these molecules are not shown.

elaidic acid, has the two hydrogen atoms of the double–bonded carbons on the opposite sides of the molecule (see Fig. 6.3b). Having a trans double bond enables the hydrocarbon chain to be relatively straight.

Whole milk and whole–milk products, butter, and meat naturally contain small amounts of trans fats. Although the body can use trans fatty acids for energy, these lipids are not essential, and medical researchers have not discovered any positive health effects from consuming them.[4] In the body, trans fats raise blood levels of an unhealthy form of cholesterol, which increases the risk of heart disease.[1]

Until recently, most of the trans fat in processed food (artificial trans fat) resulted from *partial hydrogenation*. **Partial hydrogenation** was a food man-ufacturing process that added hydrogen atoms to some unsaturated fatty acids in liquid vegetable oil. The partial hydrogenation process converted many of the oil's naturally occurring cis fatty acids into trans fatty acids. Oils that contained these artificial fats were called partially hydrogenated oils (PHOs). Structurally, trans fatty acids resemble saturated fatty acids and provide properties of long–chain saturated fatty acids to foods that contain them. Thus, fats that contain a high proportion of PHOs are more solid at room temperature than those with a high proportion of cis fatty acids. As a result of the partial hydrogenation pro-cess, vegetable oil could be made into vegetable shortening (a solid fat) or shaped into sticks of margarine.

In 2015, the FDA determined that PHOs posed a health risk, and the agency banned their use in foods.[5] As of July 2017, the ban will go into effect in 2018. Why did food manufacturers make products that contained PHOs? Foods made with PHOs can be stored for longer periods than foods that contain cis fatty acids. Trans fatty acids are less likely to undergo oxidation, a chemical process that alters the compound's structure. When oxidized, the fat in food becomes rancid and develops an unappetizing odor and taste. Unsaturated fatty acids that have the cis double–bond arrangement, especially polyunsaturated fatty acids, are very susceptible to oxidation.

Instead of relying on PHOs to extend the shelf life of products, manufac-turers can preserve fat and other ingredients in foods by adding antioxidants to them. Certain food additives, vitamins, and plant pigments function as antioxi-dants (see Chapter 8). The use of an artificial lipid, *interesterified (in'–ter–eh–stear'–ih–fide')* oil, to replace artificial trans fats in processed foods may also have undesirable health effects.[6] More research is needed to determine the long–term safety of consuming foods that contain interesterified oil. Processed foods that include "fully hydrogenated" or "interesterified" oil in their ingredient lists are sources of interesterified fat.

Despite the ban on PHOs, trans fat is not likely to disappear completely from Americans' diets because some foods naturally contain small amounts of this type of fat. People can learn how much trans fat is in a serving of most packaged foods by reading the ingredient list and Nutrition Facts panel that are on the product's label. According to the 2015–2020 Dietary Guidelines, Americans should keep their trans fat intake as low as possible, while eating a healthy diet.[7]

Did *YOU* Know?

Before the ban on partially hydrogenated oils, fast-food outlets relied on the trans fat for deep-fat frying menu items, such as French fries and breaded chicken. Because PHOs can no longer be used in processed or commercially prepared foods, the food industry is now relying on other oils, including high oleic oils, which are rich sources of monoun-saturated fatty acids.

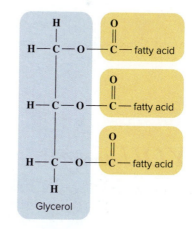

©MIXA/Alamy RF

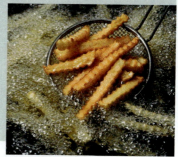

Figure 6.4 Triglyceride.

Triglycerides

A **triglyceride** has three fatty acids attached to glycerol (*glis'–er–ol*), a three–carbon compound that is often referred to as the "backbone" of the triglyceride (Fig. 6.4). Triglycerides comprise about 95% of lipids in your body and food. Triglycerides are often referred to as fats and oils. The body stores energy as triglycerides (fat).

partial hydrogenation food manufacturing process that adds some hydrogen atoms to some unsaturated fatty acids forming trans fats

triglyceride lipid that has three fatty acids attached to a three-carbon compound called glycerol

TABLE 6.2   Comparing Fats and Oils: Saturated, Monounsaturated, and Polyunsaturated Fatty Acids

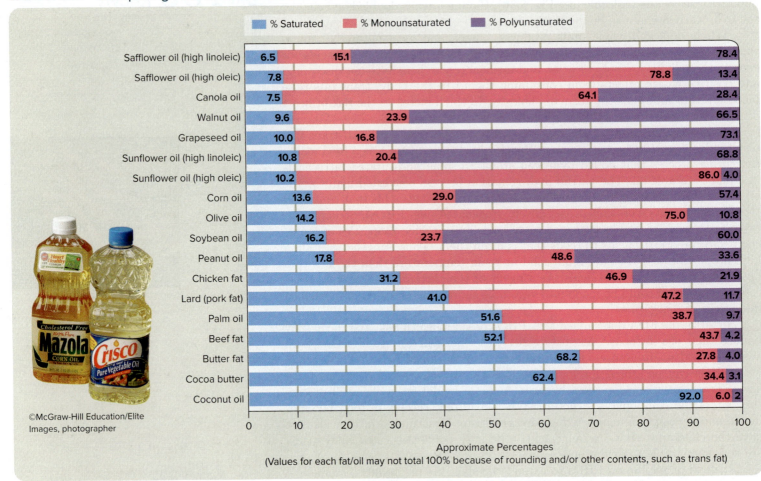

Oil/Fat	% Saturated	% Monounsaturated	% Polyunsaturated
Safflower oil (high linoleic)	6.5	15.1	78.4
Safflower oil (high oleic)	7.8	78.8	13.4
Canola oil	7.5	64.1	28.4
Walnut oil	9.6	23.9	66.5
Grapeseed oil	10.0	16.8	73.1
Sunflower oil (high linoleic)	10.8	20.4	68.8
Sunflower oil (high oleic)	10.2	86.0	4.0
Corn oil	13.6	29.0	57.4
Olive oil	14.2	75.0	10.8
Soybean oil	16.2	23.7	60.0
Peanut oil	17.8	48.6	33.6
Chicken fat	31.2	46.9	21.9
Lard (pork fat)	41.0	47.2	11.7
Palm oil	51.6	38.7	9.7
Beef fat	52.1	43.7	4.2
Butter fat	68.2	27.8	4.0
Cocoa butter	62.4	34.4	3.1
Coconut oil	92.0	6.0	2

Approximate Percentages
(Values for each fat/oil may not total 100% because of rounding and/or other contents, such as trans fat)

©McGraw-Hill Education/Elite Images, photographer

Source: Data from U.S. Department of Agriculture, Agricultural Research Service, USDA Nutrient Data Laboratory: USDA national nutrient database for standard reference, release 26, 2013.

Did *YOU* Know?

Lard is pork fat. In some parts of the United States, lard is often used to make biscuits, pie dough, and refried beans. Lard is high in saturated fat (41%), but it is not as highly saturated as butter (68%).

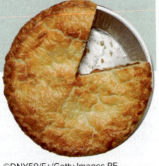

©DNY59/E+/Getty Images RF

Most triglycerides contain mixtures of unsaturated and saturated fatty acids. In a particular food, such as olives or cheese, the unsaturated and saturated fats occur in different proportions, but one type of fatty acid (saturated, mono-unsaturated, or polyunsaturated) often predominates. Table 6.2 compares the percentages of saturated, monounsaturated, and polyunsaturated fatty acids in commonly eaten fats. Note that the fat in beef and dairy products contains more saturated than unsaturated fatty acids; olive oil is a rich source of monounsaturated fatty acids; and liquid corn oil contains a greater proportion of unsaturated than saturated fatty acids. Certain animal foods, especially beef and dairy foods such as cheese, cream, and butter, contain higher percentages of saturated fatty acids than most plant fats. Exceptions are fats and oils from tropical plants such as cocoa butter, coconut oil, and palm oil. Tropical fats and oils contain more saturated than unsaturated fatty acids. Fats and oils that contain high amounts of saturated or unsaturated fatty acids are commonly called saturated fats or unsaturated fats.

Why is it important to understand the differences between saturated, unsaturated, and trans fats, and identify foods that contain high amounts of these fats? Populations that consume diets rich in saturated fat and trans fat ("unhealthy fat") have a higher risk of cardiovascular disease than populations whose diets contain more unsaturated than saturated fat.[1] Furthermore, diets that contain high amounts of unsaturated fatty acids, especially the omega−3s, may reduce the risk of CVD. The "Lipids and Health: Cardiovascular Disease" section of this chapter provides more information about this topic.

Phospholipids

A **phospholipid** is chemically similar to a triglyceride, except that one of the fatty acids is replaced by chemical groups that contain phosphorus and, often, nitrogen. Phospholipids are naturally found in plant and animal foods. **Lecithin** (*less′−uh−thin*) is the major phospholipid in food; egg yolks, liver, wheat germ, peanut butter, and soybeans are rich sources of lecithin.

Unlike triglycerides, phospholipids are partially water soluble because the phosphorus−containing portion of the molecule is **hydrophilic** (*hydro* = water; *philic* = loving); that is, it attracts water (Fig. 6.5). A phospholipid molecule also has a **hydrophobic** (*phobic* = fearing) portion that avoids watery substances and attracts oily ones. By having both hydrophilic and hydrophobic regions, a phospholipid can serve as an **emulsifier,** a substance that keeps water−soluble and water−insoluble compounds mixed together (Fig. 6.6). Manufacturers may add emulsifiers to foods to keep oily and watery ingredients from separating during storage. Processed foods, such as cheese food, salad dressing, and ice cream, often have phospholipids added as emul−sifying agents. Egg yolk, for example, naturally contains phospholipids and is used to emulsify oil and vinegar when making mayonnaise or mixing oil and milk in cake batters.

In the body, phospholipids are major structural components of cell mem−branes. Cell membranes are comprised of a double layer that is mostly phos−pholipids (Fig. 6.7). The chemical structure of the phospholipids enables the membrane to be flexible and function properly. Phospholipids are also needed for normal functioning of nerve cells, including those in the brain. Phospholipid deficiencies among adults are uncommon because the lipids are in a variety of foods and bodies of healthy adults synthesize these compounds.

Lecithin contains **choline** (*co′−leen*), a water−soluble compound that nerves use to produce the neurotransmitter *acetylcholine* (*ah−see′−till−co′−leen*). A neurotransmitter is a chemical that transmits messages between the nerve cells. The human body makes small amounts of choline, but the

phospholipid type of lipid that is chemically similar to a triglyceride, except it contains phosphorus

lecithin major phospholipid in food

hydrophilic part of a molecule that attracts water

hydrophobic part of a molecule that avoids water and attracts lipids

emulsifier substance that helps water-soluble and water-insoluble compounds mix with each other

choline water-soluble compound in lecithin

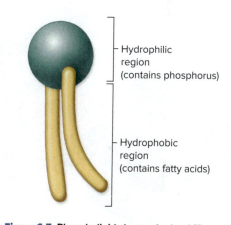

Hydrophilic region (contains phosphorus)

Hydrophobic region (contains fatty acids)

Figure 6.5 Phospholipids have a hydrophilic and a hydrophobic region.

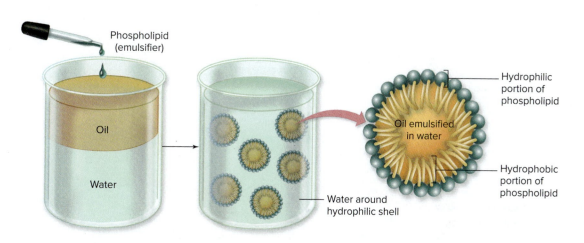

Phospholipid (emulsifier)

Oil

Water

Oil emulsified in water

Hydrophilic portion of phospholipid

Hydrophobic portion of phospholipid

Water around hydrophilic shell

Figure 6.6 **Emulsification.** Phospholipids act as emulsifiers.

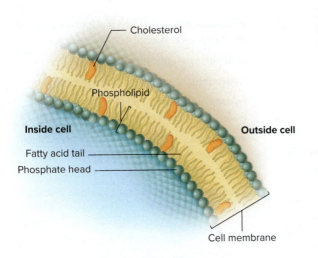

Figure 6.7 Phospholipids in cell membranes. Human cell membranes are comprised of a double layer of phospholipids. Cholesterol is embedded in the membrane.

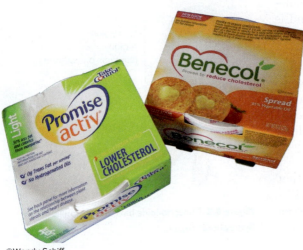

©Wendy Schiff

phospholipid is classified as a vitamin−like nutrient because deficiency symptoms can occur under certain conditions.[8] Chapter 8 provides more information about choline.

Sterols

Sterols have carbons arranged in rings, which makes them a more chemically complex type of lipid than a triglyceride or a phospholipid (Fig. 6.8). **Cholesterol** is the most well−known sterol. Many people think that cholesterol is unhealthy and foods that contain the lipid should be avoided, but it is a very important nutrient. Cholesterol is a component of every cell membrane in your body (see Fig. 6.7). Although cholesterol is not metabolized for energy, cells use the lipid to synthesize a variety of substances, including vitamin D, and steroid hormones such as estrogen and testosterone. The liver uses cholesterol to make bile, an emulsifier that facilitates lipid digestion.

Although triglycerides are widespread in foods, cholesterol is found only in animal foods. Egg yolk, liver, meat, poultry, whole milk, cheese, and ice cream are rich sources of cholesterol (Table 6.3). Even if you do not eat animal foods, your body produces cholesterol, primarily in the liver. If your body makes too much cholesterol, the excess can increase your risk of CVD.

Plant Sterols and Stanols

Plants make small amounts of substances that have chemical structures that are similar to cholesterol. These substances are *phytosterols* and *phytostanols*. Although plant sterols and stanols are not well absorbed by the human intestinal tract, these substances compete with choles−terol for absorption by the digestive tract. This competition reduces the amount of cholesterol that is absorbed. As a result, phytosterols and phytostanols are added to certain foods, beverages, and dietary supplements because they may lower elevated blood cholesterol levels, a risk factor for heart disease. Cholesterol−lowering margarine−like spreads such as Benecol® and Promise Activ® contain plant sterols and stanols. These are functional foods, because they have been developed specifically to provide beneficial health effects (see Chapter 1).

cholesterol sterol in animal foods and precursor for steroid hormones, bile, and vitamin D

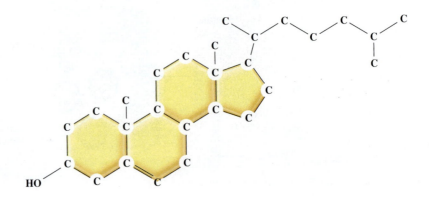

Figure 6.8 Cholesterol. Cholesterol is a complex organic molecule. For simplicity, this illustration shows only the molecule's OH group and carbon atoms.

TABLE 6.3 Approximate Cholesterol Content of Some Foods/Serving

Food	Serving Size	Cholesterol (mg)
Liver	3 oz	234
Egg	1 large	186
Egg yolk	1	186
Sardines	3 oz	121
Single-patty cheeseburger	1	111
Beef	3 oz	88
Turkey, ground	3 oz	84
Danish fruit-filled pastry	2 ½ oz	81
Shrimp	6 large, breaded and fried	80
Ham	3 oz	80
Ice cream, soft-serve	½ cup	78
Ground beef, lean (15% fat)	3 oz	77
Salmon	3 oz	75
Turkey, dark meat	3 oz	71
Egg noodles	1 cup	53
Chicken breast	3 oz	49
Hot dog	1	44
Chocolate milkshake	16 oz	43
Whole milk	1 cup	34
Cottage cheese	1 cup	32
Cheddar cheese	1 oz	30

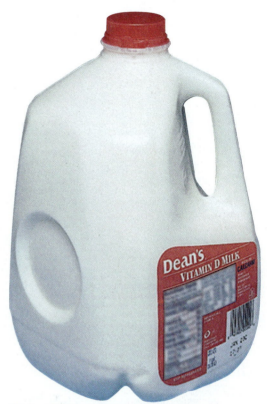

©McGraw-Hill Education/Bob Coyle, photographer

Concept CHECKPOINT

3. What are the major lipids in food and the body?
4. What is the difference between a saturated and an unsaturated fatty acid? What is the difference between a monounsaturated and a polyunsaturated fatty acid?
5. Identify at least one food that is a rich source of saturated fat, monounsaturated fat, and polyunsaturated fat.
6. Identify the two essential fatty acids.
7. How does a phospholipid differ from a triglyceride?
8. What is an omega-3 fatty acid?
9. A recipe mixes ¼ cup of oil with ¾ cup of milk. What common food could you add to keep the oil and milk emulsified?
10. Which foods contain cholesterol? List at least three functions of cholesterol in the body.

See Appendix G for responses.

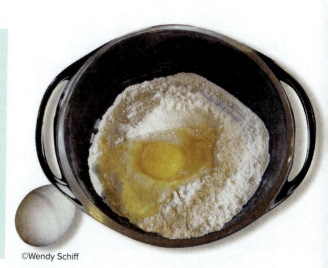

©Wendy Schiff

6.3 What Happens to Lipids in the Body?

Learning Outcomes

1 Discuss the digestion, absorption, and transport of lipids in the body.

2 Describe effects of enterohepatic circulation on cholesterol metabolism.

3 Explain the primary role of adipose cells.

Figure 6.9 summarizes some key steps in fat digestion and absorption. Triglycerides and phospholipids need to be broken down by special enzymes called **lipases** before they can be absorbed. When you eat a cheeseburger and French fries, an inactive lipase in saliva mixes with the food. As the food enters the stomach, the organ's acid environment activates the lipase, enabling some lipid breakdown to occur. The small intestine, however, is the primary site of lipid digestion.

As the fatty chyme leaves the stomach and enters your small intestine, it stimulates certain intestinal cells to release the hormone **cholecystokinin** (*kol'–e–sis'–toe–kye'–nin*) **(CCK)**. CCK signals the pancreas to secrete digestive enzymes, including *pancreatic lipase*, into the duodenum of the small intestine. **Pancreatic lipase** digests triglycerides by removing two fatty acids from each triglyceride molecule. This action converts most triglycerides into *monoglycerides*. A **monoglyceride** has a single fatty acid attached to the glycerol backbone of the molecule. Some triglycerides are completely broken down into glycerol and fatty acid molecules.

The process of digesting phospholipids is similar to that of digesting triglycerides. The enzyme *phospholipase* removes two fatty acids from a phospholipid molecule. The remaining structure contains the lipid's phosphate region (see Fig. 6.5). Cholesterol does not undergo digestion; small intestinal cells can absorb cholesterol directly from food. Glycerol, fatty acids, monoglycerides, cholesterol, and phospholipid fragments are the end products of lipid digestion.

Bile

Another function of the hormone CCK is stimulating the gallbladder to contract. This action forces some bile into the duodenum, where it mixes with chyme. Bile contains **bile salts,** compounds that enhance digestion and absorption by keeping lipids dispersed in small particles, increasing their surface area (see Fig. 6.9). As a result, pancreatic lipase gains greater access to the lipid molecules and digests them more readily. If bile is not secreted into the duodenum, lipids clump together in large fatty globules, making lipid digestion less efficient.

Bile enhances digestion by keeping fats and oils in chyme dispersed in the watery environment of the small intestine (emulsification). Bile salts have hydrophilic "heads" and hydrophobic "tails" (refer to Fig. 6.5). The tails are oriented inward, so they surround the lipid particle, while the heads face outward and toward the watery components of chyme. This action forms a **micelle** (see Fig. 6.9). As a result of micelle formation, lipids in chyme remain separated in small particles, which increases the ability of pancreatic lipase to gain access to and digest them.

What Are Lipoproteins?

Under normal conditions, the small intestine digests and absorbs nearly all of the triglycerides and phospholipids in food, but on average, only a little more than half of the dietary cholesterol is absorbed.[9] After being absorbed, short— and medium—chain fatty acids can enter the bloodstream directly. Most long—chain

Did *YOU* Know?

Monoglycerides and diglycerides may be listed as ingredients on food labels. These lipids result from the breakdown of triglycerides, and they may be added to foods during processing to improve the product's texture.

lipases enzymes that break down lipids

cholecystokinin (CCK) hormone that stimulates the gallbladder to release bile and pancreas to secrete digestive enzymes

pancreatic lipase digestive enzyme that removes two fatty acids from each triglyceride molecule

monoglyceride single fatty acid attached to a glycerol backbone

bile salts components of bile that enhance lipid digestion and absorption

micelle lipid-rich particle that is surrounded by bile salts; transports lipids to absorptive cells

fatty acids, glycerol, monoglycerides, and phospholipid fragments are reassembled into triglycerides and phospholipids within the absorptive cells of the small intes—tine. Cholesterol and the reassembled triglycerides are coated with a thin layer of protein, phospholipids, and cholesterol to form chylomicrons (see Fig. 6.9). A *chylomicron (ky'−low−my'−kron)* is a type of *lipoprotein*. **Lipoproteins** are water−soluble structures that transport lipids through the bloodstream. Chylomicrons are too large to be absorbed directly into the bloodstream. These lipoproteins must pass through the larger openings of *lacteals (lak'−te−als)*, lymphatic system vessels in each villus (see Fig. 4.29).

lipoprotein water-soluble structure that transports lipids through the bloodstream

Figure 6.9 Lipid digestion and absorption.

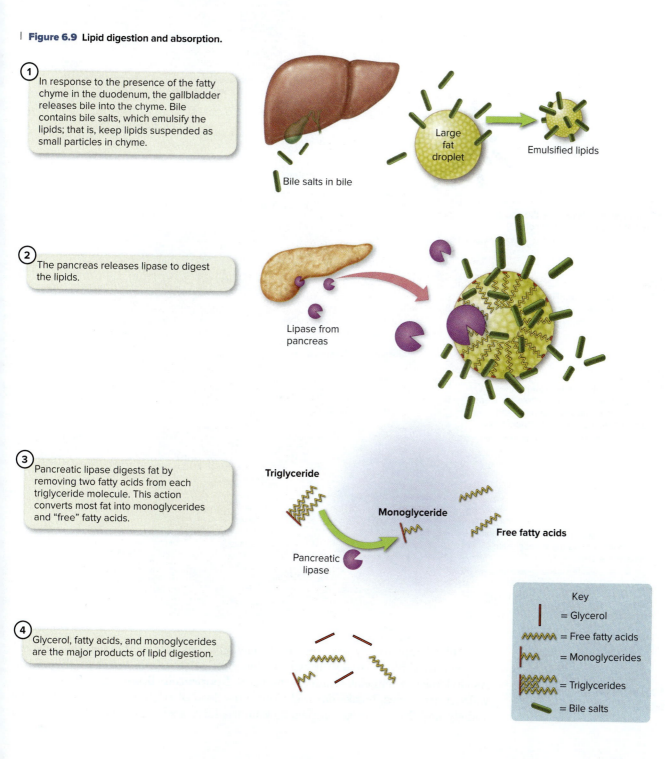

1 In response to the presence of the fatty chyme in the duodenum, the gallbladder releases bile into the chyme. Bile contains bile salts, which emulsify the lipids; that is, keep lipids suspended as small particles in chyme.

Bile salts in bile

Large fat droplet

Emulsified lipids

2 The pancreas releases lipase to digest the lipids.

Lipase from pancreas

3 Pancreatic lipase digests fat by removing two fatty acids from each triglyceride molecule. This action converts most fat into monoglycerides and "free" fatty acids.

Triglyceride

Monoglyceride

Free fatty acids

Pancreatic lipase

4 Glycerol, fatty acids, and monoglycerides are the major products of lipid digestion.

Key
| = Glycerol
= Free fatty acids
= Monoglycerides
= Triglycerides
= Bile salts

Figure 6.9 Lipid digestion and absorption. (continued)

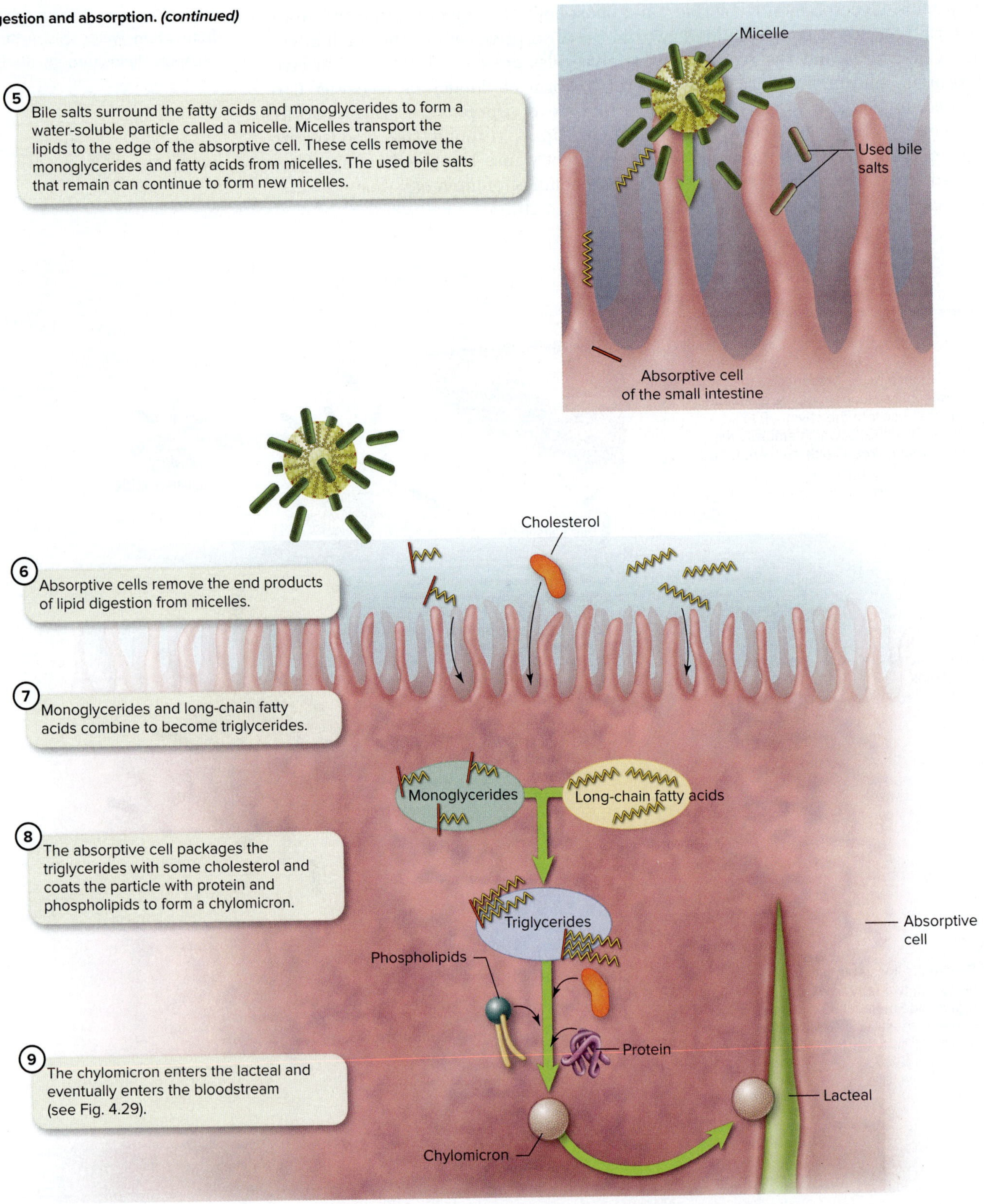

5 Bile salts surround the fatty acids and monoglycerides to form a water-soluble particle called a micelle. Micelles transport the lipids to the edge of the absorptive cell. These cells remove the monoglycerides and fatty acids from micelles. The used bile salts that remain can continue to form new micelles.

Micelle

Used bile salts

Absorptive cell of the small intestine

6 Absorptive cells remove the end products of lipid digestion from micelles.

Cholesterol

7 Monoglycerides and long-chain fatty acids combine to become triglycerides.

Monoglycerides

Long-chain fatty acids

8 The absorptive cell packages the triglycerides with some cholesterol and coats the particle with protein and phospholipids to form a chylomicron.

Triglycerides

Phospholipids

Protein

Absorptive cell

9 The chylomicron enters the lacteal and eventually enters the bloodstream (see Fig. 4.29).

Chylomicron

Lacteal

lipoprotein lipase enzyme in capillary walls that breaks down triglycerides

The lymphatic system transports chylomicrons to the thoracic duct, where they enter the bloodstream through the left subclavian vein in the chest (Fig. 6.10). As chylomicrons circulate through the body, **lipoprotein lipase,** an enzyme in the walls of capillaries, breaks down chylomicrons' load of triglycerides into fatty acids and glycerol. Nearby cells can then pick up the fatty acids and glycerol molecules to

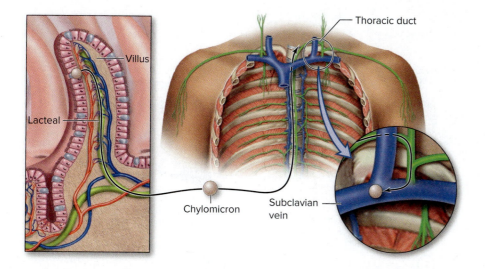

Thoracic duct

Villus

Lacteal

Chylomicron

Subclavian vein

Figure 6.10 **Journey into the general circulation.** The lymphatic system transports chylomicrons from the small intestine to the thoracic duct, where they enter the bloodstream through the left subclavian vein in the chest.

use for energy. Ten to 12 hours after a meal, most chylomicrons have been reduced to small cholesterol—rich remnants. The liver clears these remnants from the blood—stream and uses their contents to synthesize new lipids and other lipoproteins that are released into the general circulation. Figure 6.11 provides a summary of lipid digestion and absorption.

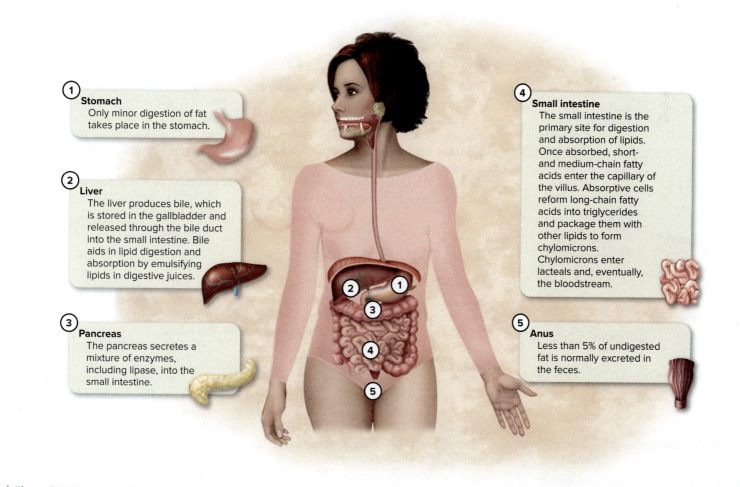

1 **Stomach**
Only minor digestion of fat takes place in the stomach.

2 **Liver**
The liver produces bile, which is stored in the gallbladder and released through the bile duct into the small intestine. Bile aids in lipid digestion and absorption by emulsifying lipids in digestive juices.

3 **Pancreas**
The pancreas secretes a mixture of enzymes, including lipase, into the small intestine.

4 **Small intestine**
The small intestine is the primary site for digestion and absorption of lipids. Once absorbed, short- and medium-chain fatty acids enter the capillary of the villus. Absorptive cells reform long-chain fatty acids into triglycerides and package them with other lipids to form chylomicrons. Chylomicrons enter lacteals and, eventually, the bloodstream.

5 **Anus**
Less than 5% of undigested fat is normally excreted in the feces.

Figure 6.11 **Summary of lipid digestion and absorption.** This illustration summarizes the basic steps of lipid digestion, absorption, transport, and elimination.

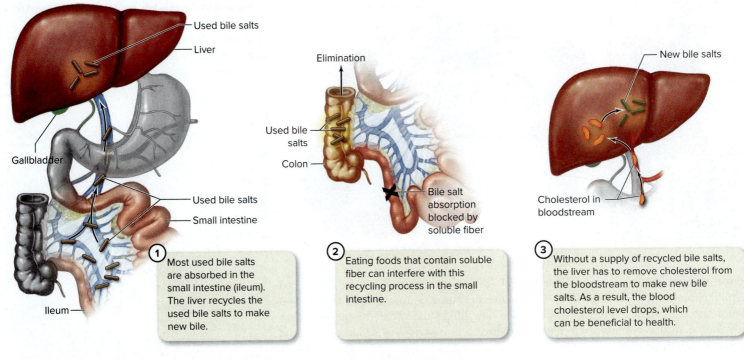

1. Most used bile salts are absorbed in the small intestine (ileum). The liver recycles the used bile salts to make new bile.

2. Eating foods that contain soluble fiber can interfere with this recycling process in the small intestine.

3. Without a supply of recycled bile salts, the liver has to remove cholesterol from the bloodstream to make new bile salts. As a result, the blood cholesterol level drops, which can be beneficial to health.

Figure 6.12 Enterohepatic circulation. Enterohepatic circulation is the process of recycling bile salts.

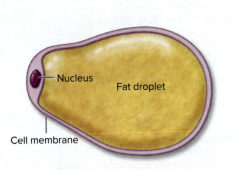

Figure 6.13 Adipose cells. A primary function of an adipose cell is storing a fat droplet.

enterohepatic circulation process that recycles cholesterol in the body

adipose cells fat cells; specialized cells that store fat

Recycling Bile Salts

Most bile salts are absorbed in the ileum, where the compounds enter the bloodstream and travel to the liver. The liver uses the bile salts to make new bile. The process of recycling bile from the intestinal tract is called **enterohepatic** (*en'−teh−roe−hih−pah'−tik*) **circulation** (Fig. 6.12). Interfering with enterohepatic circulation can reduce blood cholesterol levels because the liver must use cholesterol to make new bile salts. Plants contain substances, such as soluble fiber, that interfere with cholesterol and bile absorption (see Table 5.6 for common food sources of soluble fiber).

Using Triglycerides for Energy

Most cells can metabolize fatty acids for energy. Fat is more energy dense than carbohydrate or protein: A gram of fat supplies 9 kcal, whereas a gram of carbohydrate or protein provides only 4 kcal. Thus, a high−fat food is a more concentrated source of energy than a high−carbohydrate food. For example, you would need to eat 2½ tablespoons of sugar to obtain the amount of energy in 1 tablespoon of oil.

In many instances, your body does not need the energy from the fat in the food you have just eaten. **Adipose** (*ad'−eh−pose*) **cells,** commonly called fat cells, remove fatty acids and glycerol from circulation and reassemble them into triglycerides for storage. Most cells in your body contain triglycerides, but adipose cells are designed to store large amounts of fat (triglycerides). As illustrated in Figure 6.13, a fat droplet comprises most of an adipose cell's volume. When your body needs energy, adipose cells break down some stored triglycerides into fatty acid and glycerol molecules, and release these substances into your bloodstream. Muscle and other cells then remove the fatty acids from circulation and metabolize them. The liver clears the glycerol molecules from the bloodstream and converts them into glucose molecules that cells can also use for energy.

Eating too much fat contributes to unwanted weight gain, but consuming too much energy from protein and carbohydrates also increases body fat. Why? The body can convert excess glucose and certain amino acids into fatty acids that are used to make triglycerides. Additionally, the nonnutrient alcohol stimulates triglyceride synthesis, and excess body fat can accumulate as a result of alcohol consumption. To learn more about alcohol, read "Nutrition Matters: Drink to Your Health?" (Section 6.7). For more information about energy metabolism, see Chapter 11 and Appendix C.

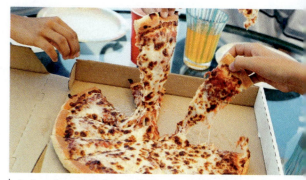

A slice of an extra-cheese, thick-crust pizza (1/10 of the pie) provides about 17 g fat, which is about 22% of the Daily Value for fat (78 g/day). ©Jacobs Stock Photography/Photodisc/Getty Images RF

Concept CHECKPOINT

11. Describe what happens to the fat in a piece of fried chicken as it undergoes digestion and absorption in a healthy person's intestinal tract. In your description, include the roles of bile, CCK, pancreatic lipase, villi, and chylomicrons.
12. Explain why high-fiber diets can reduce the concentration of cholesterol in a person's blood.
13. Why can an obese person survive starvation for a longer period than a thin person?

See Appendix G for responses.

6.4 Lipid Consumption Patterns

Learning Outcomes

1 Recall the percentage of fat in the typical American diet and the AMDR for fat.

2 Discuss Dietary Guidelines recommendations for fat and cholesterol intakes.

According to the Dietary Guidelines, people should consume diets that contain amounts of fat that are within the Acceptable Macronutrient Distribution Range (AMDR; 20 to 35% of total calories).[7] Furthermore, healthy eating patterns include rich sources of polyunsaturated and monounsaturated fatty acids, such as fish, nuts, and vegetable oils.[7] Adults should consume less than 10% of their total calories from saturated fatty acids and keep their cholesterol intake to as little as possible, while following a healthy eating pattern. Trans fat intake should also be as low as possible.

In 2013–2014, average total fat intake among adult Americans was almost 35% of total calories, and average saturated fat intake among adults was about 11% of total calories.[10] Thus, American adults consume slightly more saturated fat than the recommendation (10% of total calories). To estimate your average daily intake of total fat as well as your average daily intake of saturated fat for a 3–day period, complete the "Personal Dietary Analysis" activity at the end of this chapter.

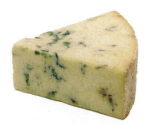

In 2015, Americans consumed over 35 pounds of cheese per person. Source: USDA, Economic Research Service: *Per capita consumption of selected cheese varieties since 1995 (in pounds per person).* https://www.ers.usda.gov/data-products/dairy-data/ ©Pixtal/age fotostock RF

Concept CHECKPOINT

14. On average, fat contributes about ___ % of the energy in an adult American's diet.
15. What is the AMDR for fat?
16. According to the Dietary Guidelines, what is the recommendation for saturated fat intake (percentage of total calories)?

See Appendix G for responses.

6.5 Understanding Nutritional Labeling: Lipids

Learning Outcomes

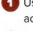 Use the Nutrition Facts panel to determine amounts of total fat and various types of fatty acids in a serving of a packaged food.

2 Compare total fat and saturated fat contents of packaged foods.

Consumers can determine how much total fat, saturated fat, trans fat, and choles-terol are in most packaged food products by reading the Nutrition Facts panel. As you can see in Figure 6.14, grams of total fat in one serving of the food (3 flatbreads) are shown, and under it, the number of grams of saturated fat and trans fat. The panel indicates that there are 3 g of total fat in each serving, and of that amount, 1 g is saturated fat. According to the panel, there are 0 g of trans fat in a serving. If a serving of food has less than 0.5 g of a specific type of fat, the amount can be reported as 0 g. By reading the list of ingredients, consumers can learn which fats and oils provided the fat in this product.

Food manufacturers are not required to indicate amounts of monounsatu-rated and polyunsaturated fat in products. However, the amount of cholesterol in a serving of the food must be listed. In this example, there is no cholesterol in the serving.

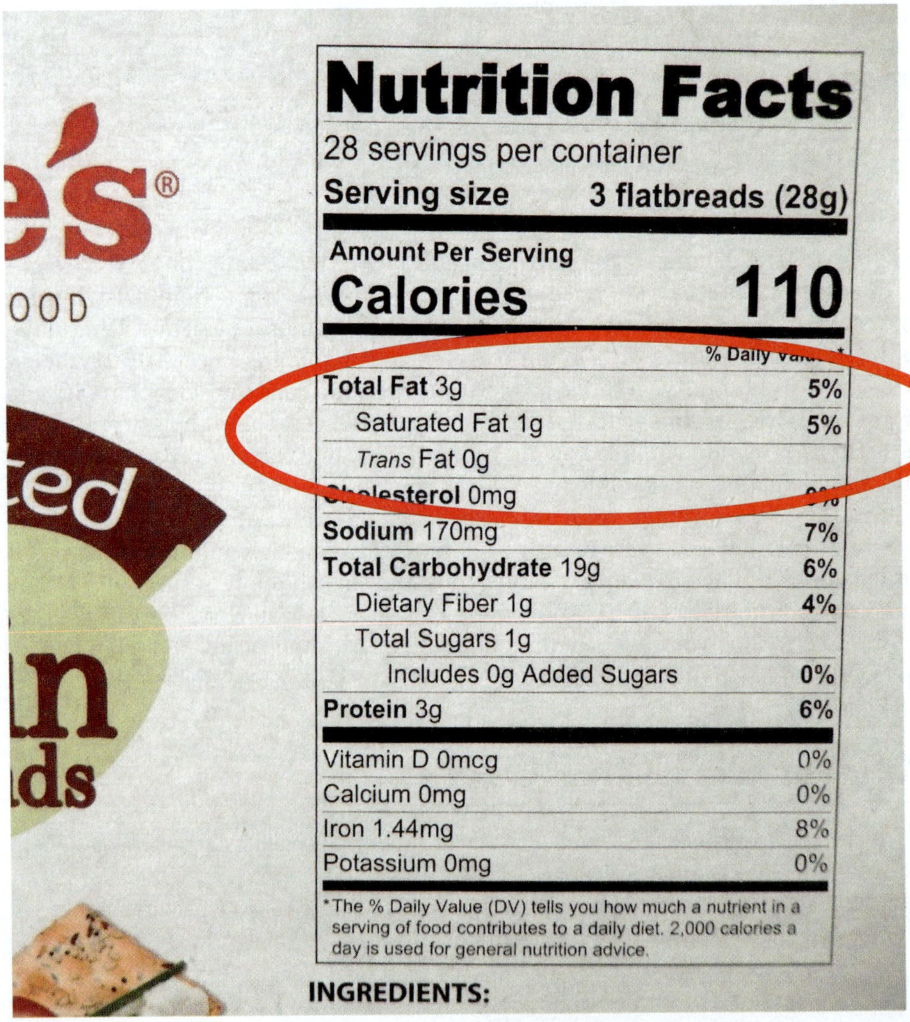

Figure 6.14 New Nutrition Facts panel
©Wendy Schiff

Nutrition Facts

28 servings per container

Serving size	3 flatbreads (28g)

Amount Per Serving

Calories   110

% Daily Value*

Total Fat 3g	5%
Saturated Fat 1g	5%
Trans Fat 0g	
Cholesterol 0mg	0%
Sodium 170mg	7%
Total Carbohydrate 19g	6%
Dietary Fiber 1g	4%
Total Sugars 1g	
Includes 0g Added Sugars	0%
Protein 3g	6%
Vitamin D 0mcg	0%
Calcium 0mg	0%
Iron 1.44mg	8%
Potassium 0mg	0%

*The % Daily Value (DV) tells you how much a nutrient in a serving of food contributes to a daily diet. 2,000 calories a day is used for general nutrition advice.

INGREDIENTS:

Concept CHECKPOINT

17. According to the Nutrition Facts panel, a serving of potato chips supplies 150 kcal, and there are 9 g of total fat in the serving of chips. Calculate the number of kcal from fat in a serving of the chips.

See Appendix G for responses.

6.6 Lipids and Health: Cardiovascular Disease

Learning Outcomes

1 Explain the process of atherosclerosis.

2 List at least three modifiable risk factors and three nonmodifiable risk factors for atherosclerosis.

3 Distinguish HDL cholesterol from LDL cholesterol.

4 Discuss dietary and other lifestyle actions that can reduce the risk of atherosclerosis.

Cardiovascular disease (CVD) includes diseases of the heart and blood vessels. Heart disease (**coronary artery disease, or CAD**) and stroke, the most common forms of CVD, are among the top five leading causes of death in the United States (see Figure 1.2). In 2015, heart disease and strokes were responsible for about 30% of deaths in the United States.[11]

From Atherosclerosis to Cardiovascular Disease

Most cases of heart disease and stroke result from **atherosclerosis** (*athero* = lipid containing; *sclerosis* [*skleh−ro'−sis*] = hardening), a chronic process that negatively affects the functioning of arteries. Normal arteries have a smooth lining (Fig. 6.15.1). When something in the bloodstream, such as excess cholesterol or

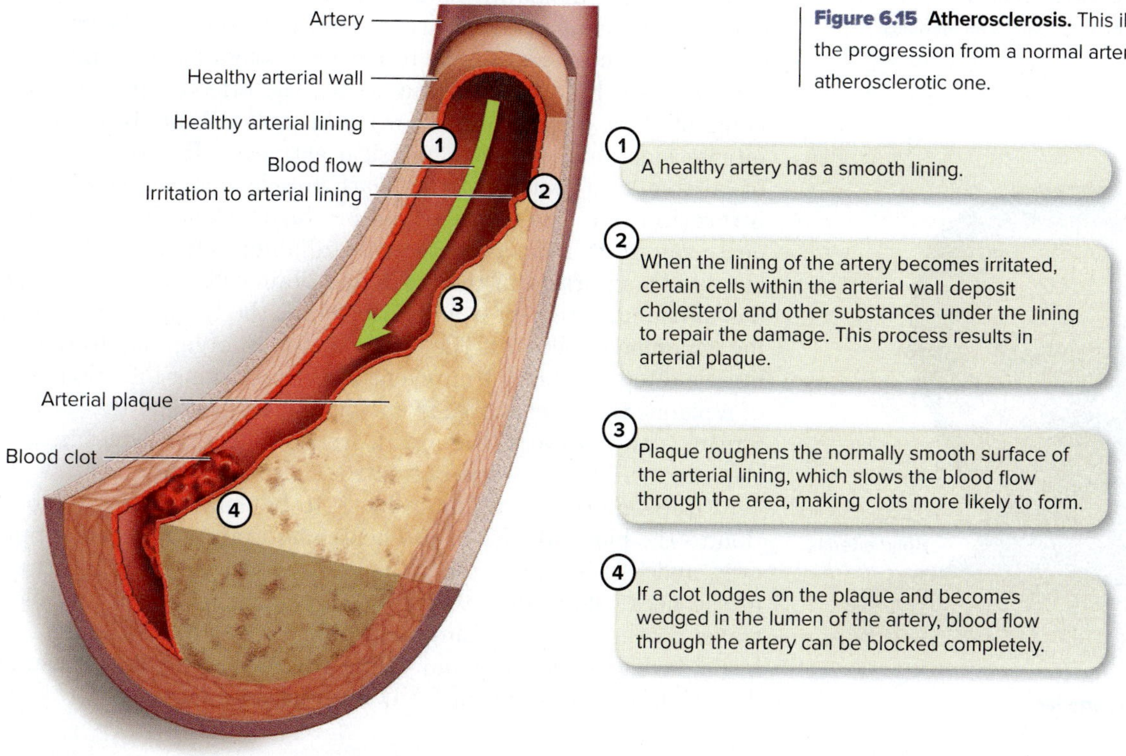

cardiovascular disease (CVD) group of diseases that affect the heart and blood vessels

coronary artery disease (CAD) a major form of CVD

atherosclerosis long-term disease process in which plaques build up inside arterial walls

Artery
Healthy arterial wall
Healthy arterial lining
Blood flow
Irritation to arterial lining
Arterial plaque
Blood clot

Figure 6.15 Atherosclerosis. This illustration depicts the progression from a normal arterial lining to an atherosclerotic one.

1 A healthy artery has a smooth lining.

2 When the lining of the artery becomes irritated, certain cells within the arterial wall deposit cholesterol and other substances under the lining to repair the damage. This process results in arterial plaque.

3 Plaque roughens the normally smooth surface of the arterial lining, which slows the blood flow through the area, making clots more likely to form.

4 If a clot lodges on the plaque and becomes wedged in the lumen of the artery, blood flow through the artery can be blocked completely.

Figure 6.16 **Healthy and atherosclerotic arteries.** Note the differences between the cross section of a healthy artery (*a*) and that of an artery nearly completely blocked as a result of atherosclerosis (*b*).
Healthy artery: ©McGraw-Hill Education/Al Telser, photographer; Clogged artery: ©Image Source/Getty Images RF

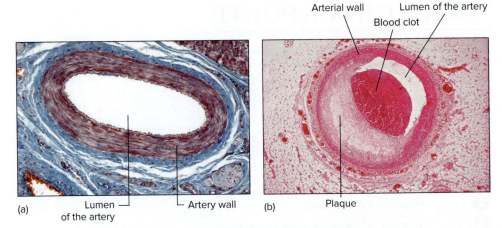

(a) Lumen of the artery — Artery wall
(b) Arterial wall — Lumen of the artery — Blood clot — Plaque

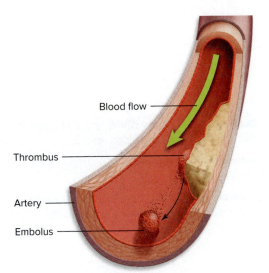

Figure 6.17 **Embolus formation.** A thrombus or part of a plaque that breaks free from where it formed and travels through the bloodstream is an embolus.

Blood flow
Thrombus
Artery
Embolus

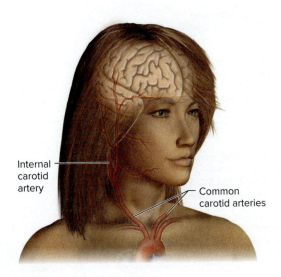

Internal carotid artery
Common carotid arteries

Figure 6.18 **Carotid arteries.**

glucose, compounds from cigarette smoke, or certain bacteria, irritates the lining of an artery, a cascade of events begins that results in atherosclerosis. The body's immune system responds to the irritation by producing inflammation within the artery. Inflammation can stimulate healing, but the process can also trigger certain cells within the arterial wall to deposit cholesterol under the artery's lining. As a result, **arterial plaque** forms (Fig. 6.15.2). In addition to cholesterol, arterial plaques contain fat, components of dead cells, and calcium. Plaque interferes with circulation in the affected area of the artery because it narrows and may even block the opening through which blood flows (*lumen*). Furthermore, plaque roughens the normally smooth surface that lines the artery. The rough lining slows blood flow in the area and makes clots more likely to form (Fig. 6.15.3). If a plaque ruptures (tears open), repairing the damage also involves clot formation, and such blood clots can be life threatening (Fig. 6.15.4). Figure 6.16 shows cross sections of a healthy artery and one that is almost completely blocked by plaque.

Blood must be able to clot, especially when blood vessels have been injured; otherwise, a person could bleed to death from a minor bruise. In some instances, however, clots form too readily at the injury site. A **thrombus** is a fixed bunch of clots that remains in place and disrupts blood flow. If a thrombus partially closes off the lumen of an artery that nourishes the heart, the affected section of the heart muscle is unable to receive enough oxygen and nutrients to function properly (see Fig. 6.16b). As a result, the affected person typically experiences bouts of chest pain, especially when his or her heart beats faster, such as during intense emotional states or physical activities. If a thrombus completely blocks blood flow to a section of the heart muscle, the muscle dies and a **myocardial infarction** (*my'–eh–card'–e–al in–farc'–shun*) (heart attack) occurs. Sudden death can result from a severe myocardial infarction. A stroke can happen when a clot blocks an artery in the brain and brain cells that are nourished by the vessel die. When an artery to a limb is blocked, the tissue in the extremity dies, causing gangrene to occur. If the affected area is large, amputation of the gangrenous limb is often necessary to prevent life–threatening infection. A thrombus or part of a plaque that breaks free from where it formed and travels through the bloodstream is an **embolus** (Fig. 6.17). An embolus that lodges in an artery can create the same serious consequences as a stationary thrombus.

Certain arteries are more likely to be damaged by atherosclerosis; in addition to the blood vessels of the heart and brain, the blood supply in the kidneys, eyes, and legs is vulnerable. When atherosclerosis occurs in the *carotid arteries* in the neck, blood flow to the brain can be decreased and clots can form that travel to the brain, causing a stroke (Fig. 6.18). Although atherosclerosis can begin during adolescence and young adulthood, the disease usually does not produce signs or symptoms of CVD until decades later.

Arteriosclerosis

In addition to interfering with blood flow, plaques reduce the flexibility of arteries, causing **arteriosclerosis** (*arterio* = artery), a condition commonly called "hardening of the arteries." Arteriosclerosis contributes to the development of **hypertension,** a chronic condition characterized by abnormally high blood pressure levels that persist even when the person is relaxed. Hypertension is a major risk factor for atherosclerosis and heart disease. The heart of a person with hypertension must work harder to circulate blood through abnormally stiff arteries. Furthermore, elevated blood pressure can cause hardened arteries to tear or burst, causing serious bleeding problems and even sudden death, depending on the artery's size and location.

Lipoproteins and Atherosclerosis

Lipoproteins transport cholesterol and triglycerides in the bloodstream, so these structures play major roles in the development of atherosclerosis. In addition to chylomicrons, the body makes three major types of lipoprotein (Fig. 6.19). Each type carries different proportions of protein, cholesterol, triglycerides, and phospholipids.

The protein content of a lipoprotein contributes to its density. A chylomicron, for example, is the largest and least dense kind of lipoprotein. Compared to the other types of lipoproteins, chylomicrons carry much more fat and very little protein. **High–density lipoprotein (HDL)** is the smallest and densest kind of lipoprotein because it transports more protein and less lipids than the other lipoproteins. HDL conveys lipids away from tissues and to the liver, where they can be processed and eliminated (Fig. 6.20). Thus, the cholesterol carried by HDL (HDL cholesterol) is often called "good" cholesterol because it does not contribute to plaque formation.

Low–density lipoprotein (LDL) transports more cholesterol than HDL in the bloodstream. LDL is needed to transport lipids to tissues, where the nutrients are used to make cell structures and vital compounds (see Fig. 6.20b). The cholesterol carried by LDL (LDL cholesterol) is often referred to as "bad" cholesterol because LDL conveys the lipid to tissues, including cells in the arterial

arterial plaque lipid-filled deposits that form under the lining of certain arteries

thrombus fixed bunch of clots that remains in place

myocardial infarction heart attack

embolus thrombus or part of a plaque that breaks free and travels through the bloodstream

arteriosclerosis condition that results from atherosclerosis and is characterized by loss of arterial flexibility

hypertension abnormally high blood pressure levels that persist

high-density lipoprotein (HDL) lipoprotein that transports cholesterol away from tissues and to the liver, where it can be eliminated

low-density lipoprotein (LDL) lipoprotein that carries cholesterol into tissues

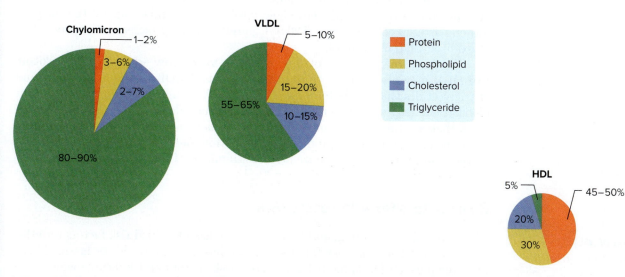

| Figure 6.19 **Major lipoproteins.** The composition of a lipoprotein contributes to its size and density.

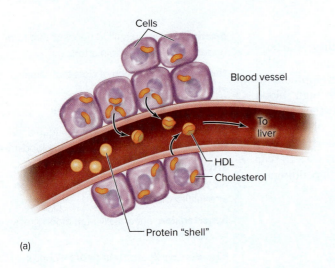

(a)

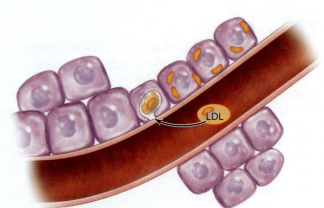

(b)

Figure 6.20 HDL, LDL, and oxidized LDL. Lipoproteins transport lipids in the bloodstream. (*a*) The liver releases protein "shells" into the bloodstream that pick up cholesterol and other lipids from cells. When filled with lipids, the shells are called high-density lipoprotein (HDL). (*b*) LDL transports cholesterol and other lipids to tissues. (*c*) Oxidized LDL cholesterol is harmful because it is taken up by arterial cells that form plaque.

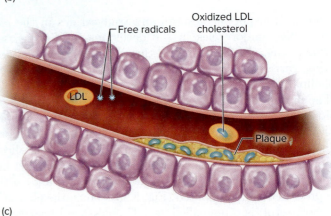

(c)

walls that make atherosclerotic plaques. However, there are different types of LDL, and not all forms of the lipoprotein are unhealthy.

Some LDLs are smaller and denser than others. People with high levels of small, dense LDLs are more likely to develop atherosclerosis than are people with low levels of these particular LDLs.[12] Additionally, chemically unstable substances ("free radicals") can damage LDL, especially small, dense LDLs. The damage results in oxidized LDL cholesterol, which is taken up by the plaque—forming arterial cells (see Fig. 6.20c). Cigarette smoking increases the production of oxidized LDL cholesterol.[13]

A third major class of lipoproteins, **very—low—density lipoprotein (VLDL),** may also contribute to atherosclerosis. VLDL carries a larger amount of triglycerides than cholesterol (see Fig. 6.19). A high level of triglycerides in the bloodstream may stimulate the production of small, dense LDL—cholesterol particles that are prone to becoming oxidized. When the oxidized particles bind to the walls of arteries, they promote inflammation and atherosclerosis.[14] Excessive alcohol and refined carbohydrate intakes stimulate VLDL production in the liver.

Risk Factors for Atherosclerosis

The National Heart, Lung, and Blood Institute has identified risk factors for atherosclerosis.[15] The more risk factors a person has, the greater his or her likelihood of developing CVD. Table 6.4 lists major risk factors and indicates which ones are nonmodifiable or modifiable. A nonmodifiable risk factor cannot be changed.

very-low-density lipoprotein (VLDL) lipoprotein that carries much of the triglycerides in the bloodstream

TABLE 6.4 Atherosclerosis: Major Risk Factors

Nonmodifiable Risk Factors
Family history of CVD
Increasing age

Modifiable Risk Factors
Unhealthy diet
Hypertension
Pre-diabetes or diabetes
Elevated blood cholesterol (especially LDL cholesterol)
Excess body fat
Physical inactivity
Tobacco use or exposure to tobacco smoke
Sleep apnea (a breathing disorder)

Nonmodifiable Risk Factors

Advancing age is a major risk factor for CVD. The risk of atherosclerosis increases for men after age 45 and for women after age 55. Having a family history of CVD also influences one's risk of the disease. A person's risk increases when he or she has a father or brother who was diagnosed with CVD before 55 years of age. Furthermore, one's risk increases when he or she has a mother or sister who was diagnosed with CVD before 65 years of age. Characteristics such as age and family history of CVD cannot be modified, but controlling other risk factors, such as smoking and hypertension, can reduce the risk of atherosclerosis.

Genetics and CVD Genetics (family history) is a major risk factor for atherosclerosis and CVD. A person's genes, for example, may code for various physical conditions that increase risk of heart disease, such as hypertension and diabetes. Additionally, genes may influence the way in which the circulatory and immune systems respond to diet. Thus, some people may be protected against the development of atherosclerosis, whereas other persons with similar diets develop serious arterial plaques early in life and die prematurely of CVD as a result.

Until recently, much of the research examining the role of diet in the development of atherosclerosis focused on the association between lipids and CVD. Nevertheless, some people with no apparent CVD risk factors still had heart attacks, strokes, and related blood vessel diseases. In many cases, affected individuals were under 40 years of age. This puzzling observation led to the discovery that the amino acid **homocysteine** (*ho'−mo−sis'−teen*) may be associated with CVD. Amino acids are the chemical units that comprise proteins. Although homocysteine is an amino acid, the substance is not found in human proteins, and higher−than−normal blood levels of homocysteine can be toxic. High blood levels of homocysteine may injure arterial walls and contribute to atherosclerosis. A few people have a genetic abnormality that causes the amino acid to accumulate in their bloodstream. These individuals have a higher risk of premature CVD than persons who do not have the genetic defect. Cells use two vitamins, B−6 and folate, to convert homocysteine into safer compounds. Deficiencies of certain B vitamins can also cause homocysteine levels to become elevated. Some medical experts think an elevated blood homocysteine level may be a "marker" in blood that indicates a person has CVD. Nevertheless, more studies are needed to determine whether elevated blood homocysteine plays a role in the development of CVD among the general population.

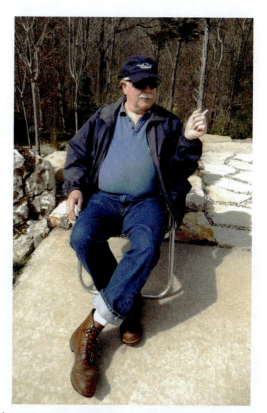

Major risk factors for CVD include advanced age, tobacco use, excess body fat, and physical inactivity.
©Wendy Schiff

homocysteine amino acid that may play a role in the development of atherosclerosis

Did *YOU* Know?

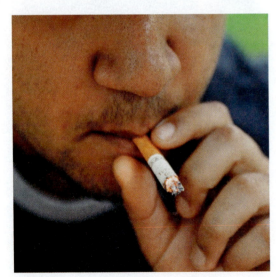

Smoking is a major risk factor for atherosclerosis. Furthermore, smoking exposes nonsmokers to cigarette smoke, which is also a risk factor for heart disease. If you smoke, simply improving your diet is unlikely to reduce your risk of heart disease; therefore, make every effort to quit using tobacco products. ©McGraw-Hill Education/Gary He, photographer

Modifiable Risk Factors

Several major risk factors for atherosclerosis involve lifestyle choices that can be modified. Hypertension, diabetes, excess body fat, and elevated blood cholesterol are modifiable risk factors that can be influenced by diet and exercise. Many people, for example, can reduce their chances of developing atherosclerosis by avoiding tobacco use, limiting their intake of saturated fat, exercising regularly, and maintaining a healthy body weight.

Nearly one in three adult Americans has hypertension, chronically elevated blood pressure.[16] Hypertension is often referred to as a "silent disease" because people with the condition frequently feel healthy and do not have obvious symptoms that indicate trouble within their circulatory system. The condition, however, is quite serious because it damages arterial walls and increases the risk of stroke, heart failure, and kidney disease. High intakes of sodium are associated with increased risk of hypertension. Chapter 9 presents information about hypertension, including healthy blood pressure values (see Table 9.10). Chapter 9 also discusses ways to reduce the likelihood of developing the condition.

Diabetes is another modifiable risk factor for atherosclerosis. Adults who have diabetes are two to four times more likely to develop heart disease or have a stroke than adults without diabetes.[17] Chapter 5 discusses diabetes in detail. Excess body fat, especially in the abdominal region, increases the risk of type 2 diabetes and hypertension; Chapter 10 focuses on sensible ways to lose body fat. Physical inactivity also contributes to excess body fat. Chapter 11 provides suggestions for becoming more physically active. Elevated blood lipids, particularly certain lipoproteins, are a risk factor for atherosclerosis. The "Reducing the Risk of Atherosclerosis: Dietary Changes" section of this chapter presents ways people can modify their diets to reduce their chances of developing atherosclerosis.

Tobacco use is another major risk factor for atherosclerosis that is modifiable. Compared to nonsmokers, smokers have two to four times the likelihood of developing heart disease and having a stroke.[18] Smokers expose other people in their environment to secondhand smoke, which is a combination of the smoke from the burning end of a cigarette and the exhaled air of the person who is smoking. Exposure to secondhand smoke is a risk factor for heart disease.[19] If you smoke, simply improving your diet is unlikely to reduce your risk of atherosclerosis; therefore, if you smoke, make every effort to quit using tobacco products. If you do not smoke, avoid breathing secondhand smoke.

Emotional stress, particularly anger, also plays a role in the development of atherosclerosis.[15] Although individuals respond to stress differently, chronic stress generally causes physical changes in the body that can damage arteries and contribute to atherosclerosis. Furthermore, people who are "stressed out" may make unhealthy food choices, drink too much alcohol, and get inadequate exercise.

It is important to understand that a risk factor is not the same as a *cause* of disease. AIDS, for example, is caused by human immunodeficiency virus (HIV); a person cannot develop AIDS without being infected with HIV. Atherosclerosis, however, is an extremely complex disease process. In most cases, no single cause for the condition can be identified. Instead, having one or more risk factors increases a person's chances of developing the condition.

Assessing the Risk of Atherosclerosis

You may not be able to prevent having a heart attack or stroke some day, but there is plenty of scientific evidence that suggests you can forestall CVD and live a longer, more satisfying life by reducing or eliminating modifiable risk factors for atherosclerosis. Diet, for example, influences the likelihood of atherosclerosis and is highly modifiable.

Medical Testing

To determine your risk of atherosclerosis, it is a good idea to have regular medi-cal checkups in which a physician checks your blood pressure and listens to blood flow in your carotid arteries to assess whether the arteries are becoming blocked (see Fig. 6.18). The physician may request a lipoprotein profile to assess your total serum cholesterol level as well as serum HDL cholesterol, LDL cholesterol, and triglyceride levels. Although this textbook generally refers to "blood cho-lesterol" or "blood lipids," the amount of lipids in serum or plasma rather than whole blood is usually measured. Serum is the liquid portion of blood; plasma is similar to serum except that it contains clotting factors.

Table 6.5 presents classifications for healthy and unhealthy fasting blood lipid levels. The "desirable" (low risk) range for total cholesterol is less than 200 mg/dl. In 2013–2014, American adults had an average total blood choles-terol level of 189 mg/dl.[20] About 12% of adults have blood cholesterol levels that were 240 mg/dl or higher, which placed them at high risk of cardiovas-cular disease.[21]

Do you know what your fasting blood cholesterol level is? Even if it is below 200 mg/dl, you may still have a high risk of atherosclerosis. Why? Although knowing the concentration of cholesterol carried by all lipoproteins is important, the amounts of certain lipoproteins in your blood, particularly LDL and HDL, are more critical risk factors. As mentioned earlier, LDL carries cholesterol to cells and HDL transports cholesterol away from cells.

Did *YOU* Know?

Blood lipoprotein levels increase after consuming foods and most beverages, and the levels can remain elevated for a few hours. To obtain accurate information about a person's usual blood lipoprotein level, the individual should be in a fasting state. Thus, a person should fast (avoid eat-ing or drinking anything except plain water) for 12 hours before having blood drawn for a lipo-protein profile.

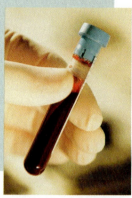

©Comstock/PunchStock RF

TABLE 6.5 Classification of Fasting Blood Lipid Levels (According to Risk of CVD)

Total Cholesterol (mg/dl)	Classification
< 200	Low risk
200 to 239	Borderline high risk
≥ 240	High risk
LDL Cholesterol (mg/dl)	**Classification**
< 100	Very low risk
100 to 129	Low risk
130 to 159	Borderline high risk
160 to 189	High risk
≥ 190	Very high risk
HDL Cholesterol (mg/dl)	**Classification**
< 40 (for men); < 50 (for women)	High risk
≥ 60	Low risk
Triglycerides (mg/dl)	**Classification**
< 150	Low risk
150 to 199	Borderline high risk
≥ 200	High risk

Source of data: National Institutes of Health, National Heart, Lung, and Blood Institute: *ATP III guidelines at-a-glance quick desk reference*. 2001. https://www.nhlbi.nih.gov/files/docs/guidelines/atglance.pdf Accessed: July 29, 2017.

People with a high ratio of total cholesterol to HDL cholesterol usually have too much LDL cholesterol in their blood and an increased risk of heart disease and stroke. A healthy ratio of total cholesterol to HDL cholesterol is less than 3.5:1; the lower the ratio, the lower the risk of CVD.[22] To calculate your risk of having a heart attack during the next 10 years, use the risk assessment tool at http://static.heart.org/riskcalc/app/index.html#!/baseline-risk.

Someday, scientists may be able to locate genes that are involved in the process of atherosclerosis and develop a blood test that identifies biological markers produced by the abnormal genes. Thus, young people could undergo testing to determine their risk of atherosclerosis well before the signs and symptoms of the condition appeared. Until then, it is wise to have regular health checkups that include blood pressure and lipid measurements (*lipoprotein profile*). Ask your physician for a copy of the laboratory results, and keep them along with others in your personal "medical file" for future reference.

C-reactive Protein   Chronic inflammation is involved in the development of CVD. The liver responds to certain kinds of inflammation by producing and releasing **high-sensitivity C-reactive protein (hs-CRP)** into the bloodstream. People with high levels of hs-CRP are more likely to develop CVD.[23] Thus, elevated hs-CRP may be a marker for atherosclerosis, like homocysteine. If you have a family history of premature CVD, consider having your homocysteine and hs-CRP levels measured.

Coronary Calcium   Cigarette smoking is significantly associated with the formation of *coronary calcium*, calcium deposits in arteries of the heart.[24] High amounts of coronary calcium are associated with increased risk of atherosclerosis. Computerized tomography (CT) scans, special computerized images that show the body's internal structures, can detect coronary calcium deposits. A CT scan, however, involves exposure to ionizing radiation, so physicians generally reserve its use for other diagnostic purposes.

Reducing the Risk of Atherosclerosis: Dietary Changes

Specific recommendations for consumption of various types of fat are primarily based on the results of epidemiological studies that examined the effects of dietary lipids on blood lipids and risk of CVD. Populations that consume diets rich in saturated fats generally have higher rates of heart disease than populations that eat less saturated fat. Saturated fat alters the structure of liver cell membranes so they no longer function properly. As a result, the liver removes less cholesterol from the bloodstream.[25] Most saturated fatty acids increase blood cholesterol levels by raising concentrations of both LDL and HDL cholesterol. Trans fats also raise blood cholesterol levels. However, trans fats raise LDL cholesterol while reducing beneficial HDL cholesterol levels.[25]

Monounsaturated fatty acids generally lower LDL cholesterol without reducing HDL cholesterol levels. Foods rich in monounsaturated fat include peanuts and peanut oil, canola oil, olives and olive oil, almonds, and avocados.

Diets containing high amounts of polyunsaturated fatty acids, particularly omega-3 fats, may reduce blood levels of total cholesterol and LDL cholesterol. In some individuals, however, polyunsaturated fat also reduces beneficial HDL cholesterol. Nevertheless, polyunsaturated fatty acids tend to be beneficial because they do not promote atherosclerosis. Foods rich in polyunsaturated fat include corn, soybean, and cottonseed oils, as well as some types of sunflower and safflower seed oils (see Table 6.2).

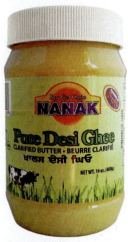

MY DIVERSE PLATE

MyPlate: Source: U.S. Dept. of Agriculture

Ghee (Indian Clarified Butter)

Ghee is a solid fat that is used for cooking, primarily in India. Traditionally, ghee was made from the milk of a type of buffalo that was native to India and Pakistan, but milk from other animals can be used. To make ghee, butter is heated until its water content evaporates completely and the solids (primarily lactose and some proteins) brown and sink to the bottom. After heating, the fat is strained to remove the solids. Scientists are exploring whether certain lipids in ghee have antioxidant activity in cells.

©Wendy Schiff

As mentioned earlier, the Dietary Guidelines recommend limiting saturated fat intake to less than 10% of total energy intake by replacing foods that are rich sources of saturated fat with foods that contain high amounts of unsaturated fat. People should limit their trans fat intake as much as possible.

What About Omega-3 and Omega-6 Fats?

The typical American diet provides far more omega–6 foods than foods that contain omega–3 fatty acids.[1] The primary omega–6 fatty acid, linoleic acid, increases inflammation and blood clotting. Some inflammation is necessary because it attracts immune system cells to disease–causing microorganisms that have entered the body. Inflammation, however, can also damage the inside of arteries. Clotting is also an important function of blood, but excess blood clotting can increase the risk of strokes, heart attacks, and other serious blood vessel disorders. The role of omega–6 fats in preventing or contributing to the development of heart disease is controversial among medical experts.[1] Thus, more research is needed to clarify the pros and cons of following diets that contain high amounts of these particular fatty acids.

Eating foods that supply omega–3 fatty acids may reduce the risk of heart disease and stroke.[1] The body incorporates omega–3 fatty acids into cell mem–branes and uses these lipids to make compounds that can reduce inflammation, serum triglycerides, and blood clotting. Table 6.6 lists foods that are sources of omega–3 fatty acids, including several species of fish. Certain fatty fish are rich sources of DHA and EPA, long–chain omega–3 fatty acids.

Alpha–linolenic acid is an omega–3 fatty acid that the body can convert to DHA and EPA (see Figure 6.2). Flaxseeds, soybeans, and walnuts are good sources of alpha–linolenic acid. As mentioned earlier, the body can only make small amounts of DHA and EPA from alpha–linolenic acid. Therefore, it is important to include other sources of these long–chain fatty acids in your diet.

To obtain beneficial long–chain omega–3 fatty acids such as DHA, the Dietary Guidelines recommend that Americans eat at least 8 ounces of various seafood a week.[7] Because large species of fish can contain high amounts of the toxic compound *methylmercury*, young children, pregnant and breastfeeding women, and women who are likely to become pregnant should not eat certain kinds of fish, including shark, king mackerel, marlin, and swordfish.[7] Shrimp, canned light tuna, salmon, pollock, and catfish are low in methylmercury. According to the Dietary Guidelines, women who are pregnant or breastfeeding can safely consume up to 12 ounces of low–mercury fish and shellfish weekly (see Chapter 3). The "Recipe for Healthy Living" feature of this chapter has an easy recipe made with salmon.

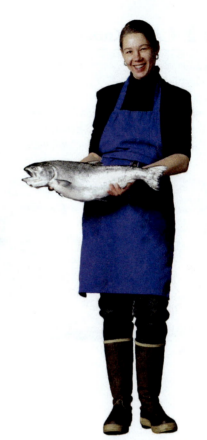

Salmon is a rich source of omega-3 fatty acids, including DHA and EPA. ©Adam Crowley/Getty Images RF

TABLE 6.6 Food Sources of Omega-3 Fats

Fish/Shellfish
Herring, salmon, sablefish, anchovies, tuna, bluefish, sardines, catfish, striped bass, mackerel, trout, halibut, pollock, flounder, shrimp, mussels, crab
Oils
Flaxseed, walnut, canola, soybean
Nuts and Seeds
Walnuts, flaxseeds
Other
Algae

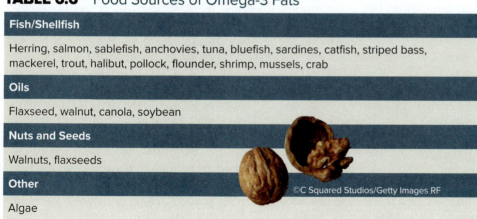

©C Squared Studios/Getty Images RF

Did *YOU* Know?

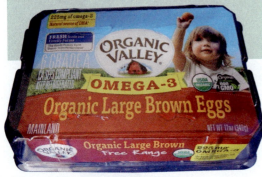

©Wendy Schiff

What if you do not like to eat fish? Taking supplements that contain omega−3s may reduce inflammation and the risk of deadly forms of heart disease.[1] Omega−3 supplements seem to be safe, but these fatty acids may interfere with normal blood clotting.[26] As a result, taking too many omega−3 supplements may increase your risk of stroke. It is important to note that fish liver oil supplements are not the same as fish oil or omega−3 supplements. Fish liver oils, such as cod liver oil, are rich sources of vitamins A and D. These vitamins are toxic when taken in large amounts. Check with your physician before you embark on a cam−paign to increase omega−3 fatty acids in your diet. The "Food & Nutrition Tips" that follows provides some ideas for increasing your intake of omega−3 fatty acids from dietary sources.

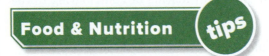

- Eat seafood, especially fatty fish, two times a week. Before cooking, marinate fresh fish in olive or canola oil that has been seasoned with a small amount of garlic, pepper, and lemon juice. The light coating of oil on fish can help keep the food from drying out during cooking.

- Bake, grill, or broil fish.

- Add tuna to salads, or mix tuna with a little olive oil and spread on toast.

- If you don't want the flavor of olive oil in a food, use canola oil, soybean oil, or liquid margarines made from these oils for frying or sautéing.

- Sprinkle chopped walnuts on salads, yogurt, or cereal, or simply eat the nuts as a snack.

Should People Avoid Eggs?

Eggs are a relatively economical source of protein and many micronutrients. However, egg yolks are the most concentrated source of cholesterol in the typi−cal American diet. The yolk of a large egg contains 5 grams of fat and about 190 mg of cholesterol. To reduce their cholesterol consumption, many Americans eat fewer fresh eggs than in the past. Whole eggs, however, are often hidden in commonly eaten foods such as salad dressings, noodles, frozen custards, sauces, and baked goods.

Does eating egg yolks increase the risk of atherosclerosis? For the gen−eral population, egg consumption does not increase the risk of cardiovascular disease.[27] In general, the cholesterol in food does not have as much effect on blood cholesterol levels of healthy people as the saturated fat does. Why? In a healthy person, the liver produces less cholesterol when large amounts of cholesterol are eaten. On the other hand, eating large amounts of saturated fat increases the liver's cholesterol production. Because foods that are high in cholesterol are often rich sources of saturated fat, dietary cholesterol was blamed for raising blood cholesterol levels. Egg yolks, however, have almost twice as much unsaturated fat as saturated fat.

Egg whites have no fat or cholesterol. For those who must limit their cho−lesterol intake, egg whites can often be used in recipes that call for whole eggs. Products that substitute for whole eggs are available in supermarkets. The Food & Nutrition Tips features in this section provide practical steps to reduce the amount of solid fat, added sugars, and salt in foods.

©Wendy Schiff

Food & Nutrition tips

This table provides suggestions for common ingredient substitutions for recipes and indicates how the changes can improve the nutritional quality of the products.

Recipe Includes	Substitution	Nutritional Benefits
Butter or margarine (baked products)	Replace with the same amount of applesauce Replace each 1 cup of fat with ½ cup mashed cooked carrots, sweet potato, or squash	Reduces calories and unhealthy fats and adds some fiber, phytochemicals, and vitamins
Cream	Replace with equal amount of whole milk or half-and-half	Reduces calories and unhealthy fat
Cream cheese (regular)	Replace with equal amount of fat-free or reduced-fat ("Neufchatel") cream cheese	Reduces calories and unhealthy fat
Cheese (full fat)	Replace with equal amount of low-fat or nonfat cheese *Note: Do not replace with nonfat cheese in cooked dishes because the cheese does not melt properly.*	Reduces calories and unhealthy fat
Whole or 2% milk	Replace with equal amount of low-fat or fat-free milk	Reduces calories and unhealthy fat
Evaporated milk	Use fat-free evaporated milk	Reduces calories and unhealthy fat
Condensed milk	Use fat-free evaporated milk *Note: Product will not be as sweet.*	Reduces calories, unhealthy fat, and added sugars
Sour cream	Replace with fat-free or low-fat sour cream Replace with plain, fat-free yogurt	Reduces calories and unhealthy fat
Egg	Replace each whole egg with 2 egg whites or ¼ cup egg substitute	Reduces cholesterol
Vegetable oil	Reduce amount by 25% Replace each 1 cup of oil with 3/4 cup mashed cooked carrots, sweet potato, pumpkin, or squash in baked products	Reduces calories and fat and adds fiber, vitamins, and phytochemicals
Sugar (white, brown, and syrups)	Reduce the amount of sugar by 25–50% Use a sugar substitute that is appropriate for baked products (check labels)	Reduces calories and added sugars
Salt	Reduce the amount by 50-75% Season with fresh herbs or ground herb products that have no added salt	Reduces sodium

Did *YOU* Know?

About 80% of stick margarine is fat—the same percentage of fat as in butter. A pat of stick margarine (approximately a teaspoon) also supplies about the same amount of energy as a pat of butter—35 kcal.

©McGraw-Hill Education/Ken Cavanagh, photographer

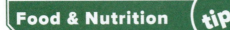

Food & Nutrition tips

- Eat fewer commercially prepared baked goods, snack foods, and fried fast-food items.

- Purchase brands of microwave popcorn that have little added fat. Buy plain popcorn, and to pop the kernels, use a small amount of hot oil in a covered saucepan or use a hot-air machine.

- Commercial frostings are high in fat. Remove most of the frosting from a serving of cake before eating it. (Frosting is primarily sugar and fat, which are empty calories.) You can make your own frosting by mixing soft margarine or smooth peanut butter with a little milk, powdered sugar, and vanilla flavoring.

MY DIVERSE PLATE

MyPlate: Source: U.S. Dept. of Agriculture

Pico de Gallo

Pico de gallo (*pee'-ko-dee-guy'-yo*) is a Mexican salsa made with fresh ingredients, including chopped tomatoes, onions, hot peppers (such as serrano and jalapeño), fresh cilantro leaves, lime juice, and a dash of salt. The salsa is eaten as a dip for tortilla chips or served on a variety of foods, including scrambled eggs, burritos, and grilled poultry, fish, or meat. A one-half cup serving of the salsa provides 20 kcal, almost no fat, and 1 g of fiber.

©Wendy Schiff

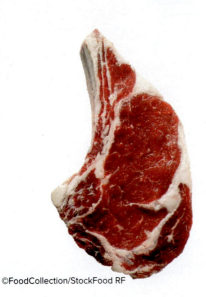

©FoodCollection/StockFood RF

Will Weight Loss and Exercise Help?

Excess body fat, especially around the midsection of the body, is associated with unhealthy LDL cholesterol and triglyceride levels. Physical inactivity and excess energy consumption contribute to unwanted weight gain. Performing moderate-intensity physical activity nearly every day and balancing energy intake with energy expenditure each day can help people achieve and maintain healthy body weights. Taking such steps can also reduce elevated LDL cholesterol and triglyceride levels.

Food Selection and Preparation

You can change your food selection and preparation practices to reduce the amount of unhealthy fat in your diet. Fatty meats such as rib steaks are often more tender and expensive than leaner cuts such as chuck roasts. Certain cooking methods, however, can increase the tenderness of lean cuts of meat. Moist cooking methods, such as pot roasting or tightly covering the baking dish with foil, help tenderize meats without adding fat. In addition to using a moist cooking method, reduce the oven temperature from 350°F to less than 325°F. The meat will take longer to cook, but it is less likely to toughen and dry out. After cooking, avoid eating the visible fat that remains. For example, trim away much of the fat from the meat and do not use pan drippings to make sauces or gravies. Steaming meats and vegetables is a cooking method that does not require adding fat during preparation. Stir-frying pieces of raw vegetables, meat, fish, shellfish, and poultry in small amounts of hot vegetable oil cooks them quickly and preserves micronutrients. Additionally, when you brown ground beef in a pan, drain much of the fat before you add other ingredients to the meat. Dipping raw foods in batter and deep-fat frying them adds considerable amounts of fat to your diet because breading serves as a sponge that soaks up oil. If you prepare breaded fried foods, place the items on paper towels after cooking them to soak up as much excess fat as possible. Some people think the breading is the "best part" of a fried food, but removing some or all of the breading before eating the item can reduce your overall fat intake. Although it is easy to peel greasy breading from fried fish, much of the fat that you eat is hidden in foods and beverages. For example, do you drink 2% milk? Fat comprises only 2% of the milk's volume, but the lipid contributes 37% of the beverage's calories. Fat-free milk actually contains less than 0.5% fat by volume, and fat contributes essentially no energy to the beverage.

What about the fat content of the cream cheese, margarine, or butter that you spread on a piece of toast? About 90% of the calories in cream cheese and about 100% of the calories in butter are from fat. Vegetable oils are almost 100% fat, so fat contributes all the energy in most salad dressings. Fried foods, chips, and salad dressings are high in fat; bacon, sausage, hot dogs, luncheon meats, and hard cheeses are also fatty foods. Nuts, including peanuts and almonds, have high fat contents, but they generally contain high amounts of healthy monounsaturated fats.

Instead of striving to eliminate all fatty foods from your diet, try reducing your intake of them, especially rich sources of saturated fats. For example, if you drink 2% or whole milk, switch to 1% or fat–free milk. Nearly all the lipids in fat–free milk have been removed; that is why it tastes watery to people who are not accustomed to drinking it. Except for energy and lipid content, the nutritional value of fat–free milk is basically the same as that of whole and 2% milks. The "Food & Nutrition Tips" feature in this section provides more practical suggestions for reducing your saturated fat intake.

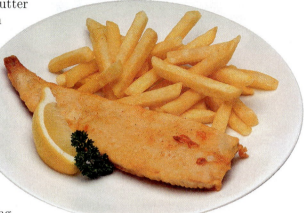

©Ingram Publishing/Alamy RF

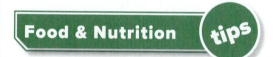

Food & Nutrition tips

- Reduce your intake of solid fats.

- Purchase lean meats and trim visible fat from meat before cooking. Before eating cooked meat, trim and discard any remaining visible fat.

- Try replacing some fatty foods with reduced-fat or fat-free alternatives. For example, substitute plain, fat-free yogurt in recipes that call for sour cream. Place a spoonful of the yogurt, instead of butter or sour cream, on a baked potato.

- Because most nuts are rich sources of healthy unsaturated fats, replace foods that contain saturated fat with nuts. For example, use peanut or soy nut butters instead of cheese or luncheon meat in sandwiches. Some nut butters contain added sugars, so read the Nutrition Facts panel and ingredients list before selecting these products.

- Replace some or all of the solid fat in recipes for baked goods with vegetable oil or unsweetened applesauce. In general, 1 cup of applesauce can replace 1 cup of fat.

- Pretzels, air-popped popcorn, and most fruits and vegetables are low fat and generally more nutrient-dense than chips, cookies, pastries, and candy bars.

- Patronize fast-food restaurants that offer low-saturated fat menu items such as salads without added cheese and meat, baked or broiled chicken and fish, low-fat yogurt, and bean burritos.

- Use less salad dressing on salads. When in restaurants, order salad dressings "on the side" so you can control the amount that is added.

- When following recipes, replace butter with vegetable oils (canola, peanut, or corn oil, for example). Reduce the amount of fat in the recipe by about 20% (butter is 80% fat; oil is 100% fat).

Did *YOU* Know?

Garlic, onions, and chives are sources of sulfur-containing compounds, such as allicin, that have antioxidant properties. Fresh garlic and garlic supplements have been promoted to lower blood cholesterol levels. However, there is a lack of strong scientific support for consuming fresh garlic or garlic supplements to reduce elevated blood cholesterol.[28] Furthermore, taking dietary supplements that contain garlic may interfere with blood's ability to form clots, which can increase one's risk of bleeding.

©C Squared Studios/Getty Images RF

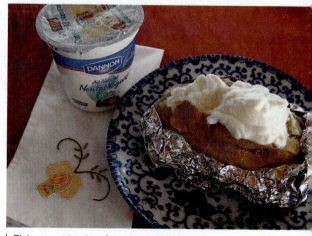

Plain yogurt is a low-fat substitute for sour cream.
Potato: ©Wendy Schiff

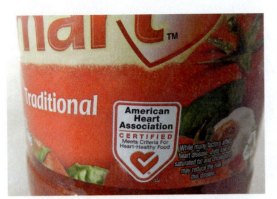

This product's label displays the American Heart Association's heart-healthy symbol next to a diet-related health claim. ©Wendy Schiff

Did *YOU* Know?

Eggs with brown shells are not more nutritious than eggs with white shells; the color of an eggshell is determined by the breed of hen that laid it. Also, grading does not reflect the nutritional content of an egg. When cracked open and placed on a plate, the membrane of a "AA" grade egg tends to hold the yolk and white together better than membranes of lower-grade eggs.

©Pixtal/age fotostock RF

Other Dietary Modifications

In addition to modifying your fat intake, you can reduce your risk of CVD by making other dietary changes. Eating foods that are rich sources of fiber, particularly soluble fiber (see Chapter 5), can reduce LDL cholesterol levels without lowering beneficial HDL cholesterol levels.

Consuming high amounts of sucrose or fructose can result in elevated blood triglyceride levels. The body can convert excess fructose into triglycerides. If your triglyceride level is too high (> 150 mg/dl), consider cutting back on your intake of refined carbohydrates by eating less candy and pastries and drinking fewer sugar-sweetened soft drinks.

Drinking small amounts of alcohol (1 to 2 drinks/day) can raise beneficial HDL cholesterol levels. Consuming too much alcohol, however, contributes to hypertension and damages every organ of the body. Furthermore, excess alcohol consumption has devastating effects on society, as well as on personal safety and relationships. If you consume several alcoholic beverages regularly, consider reducing your intake to no more than one serving per day. Section 6.7 discusses alcohol metabolism and the drug's effects on health.

Registered dietitian nutritionists often promote the traditional Mediterranean diet for healthy eating as well as reducing elevated blood lipid levels and the risk of CVD. The Mediterranean diet (see Fig. 3.19) recommends eating more fish and seafood, and smaller amounts of red meat; using heart-healthy unsaturated fatty acids; engaging in regular physical activity; and drinking a glass of wine daily. This diet also emphasizes phytochemical-rich fruits, vegetables, beans, and nuts.

Hypertension is a major risk factor for CVD. Dietary Approaches to Stop Hypertension ("the DASH diet") is a healthy dietary pattern that promotes fruits and vegetables, low-fat dairy products, whole-grain foods, tree nuts, seeds, fish, poultry, and legumes to reduce blood pressure. (*Legumes* include peanuts, split peas, and soybeans.) Unlike the typical American diet ("Western diet"), the DASH diet is high in fiber and low in saturated fat, cholesterol, and refined carbohydrates, such as added sugars. Additionally, the standard DASH diet recommends limiting sodium intake to less than 2300 mg/day. Table 6.7 summarizes ways certain actions, such as dietary manipulations and other therapeutic lifestyle changes, may alter a person's blood lipid levels.

What If Lifestyle Changes Do Not Work?

Some people are unable to lower their risk of CVD significantly by making dietary changes, exercising regularly, and losing excess body fat. If your blood lipids are too high and the levels have remained elevated even after you have made these lifestyle modifications, it is important to discuss additional treatment options with your physician. Millions of Americans take a class of prescription drugs called *statins* to reduce their elevated blood lipid levels. Statins interfere with the liver's metabolism of cholesterol, effectively reducing LDL cholesterol and triglyceride levels as a result. Statins are relatively safe when taken as directed.[29]

TABLE 6.7   Ways to Lower Your Risk of CVD

Action	Potential Benefits
Increase physical activity level	Raises HDL levels
Lose excess body fat	Lowers elevated triglycerides, blood pressure, and risk of type 2 diabetes; may increase HDL
Quit smoking	May raise HDL and lower LDL levels
Make specific dietary changes:	
Reduce intake of saturated fats and avoid trans fats	Raises HDL and lowers LDL
Replace saturated fats with polyunsaturated and monounsaturated fats	Lowers LDL
Include some omega-3 and omega-6 fats	Reduces triglycerides; may raise HDL and reduce blood pressure
Replace butter with olive oil or spread made from plant sterols/stanols	Reduces LDL
Eat more whole-grain, fiber-rich foods, especially those containing soluble fiber	Reduces total cholesterol and LDL without altering HDL
Consume foods that contain antioxidant nutrients and certain phytochemicals, such as red grapes and red wine (see Table 1.3). Dietary supplements of these compounds are not recommended.	Reduces risk of heart disease, but the mechanism is unclear
Reduce added sugar and excessive alcohol intake	Lowers triglyceride levels
Limit sodium intake; adopt DASH diet	Lowers elevated blood pressure

Concept CHECKPOINT

18. Define *atherosclerosis, arteriosclerosis, arterial plaque, thrombus,* and *embolus.* Discuss the series of physiological changes that occur in arteries and contribute to the development of CVD.

19. List three kinds of fish that often contain high amounts of methylmercury.

20. List at least two major risk factors for atherosclerosis that are nonmodifiable and at least five that are modifiable.

21. Bernard's HDL cholesterol level is 62 mg/dl. Based on this information, does Bernard have a high risk or low risk of CVD? Explain your answer.

22. What is "hs-CRP"? What can you learn about your risk of heart disease and stroke from having a lipoprotein profile performed on your blood?

23. Suggest at least four ways people can reduce their intakes of saturated and trans fats and increase their intakes of unsaturated fats.

24. What is a statin?

See Appendix G for responses.

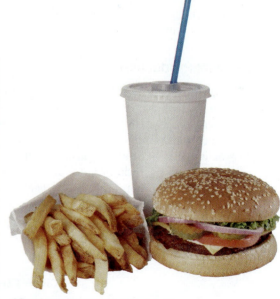

©Ryan McVay/Stockbyte/Getty Images RF

6.7 Nutrition Matters: Drink to Your Health?

Learning Outcomes

1 Identify amounts of beer, wine, and distilled spirits in a standard drink.

2 Classify people who drink alcohol according to their usual pattern of consumption.

3 Identify factors that affect alcohol metabolism.

4 Discuss alcohol's effects on health.

What do beer, wine, vodka, whiskey, sake (*sak′−e*), koumiss (*koo′−mis*), and kefir (*keh−feer′*) have in common? These beverages contain *ethanol*, a two−carbon compound that chemists classify as an alcohol. Alcohols such as etha−nol, glycerol, and cholesterol are organic molecules that have one or more *hydroxyl (OH)* groups in their chemical structures (Fig. 6.21). This textbook refers to ethanol sim−ply as "alcohol."

Offering wine in religious ceremonies, toasting the bride and groom with champagne at a wedding, or bar−hopping with friends on their 21st birthdays—for many Americans, alcohol consumption is a part of celebrating religious rites and life's milestones. When consumed in moderation, alcoholic beverages can make social situations more enjoyable. Many people, however, experience serious problems as a result of their drinking habits. This section focuses on alcohol metabolism, as well as the chemical's effects on the body.

Alcohol Production

Throughout the world, people have been producing and drinking alcoholic beverages for thousands of years. The chemical process that results in alcohol is not complicated and occurs naturally. The process requires certain microbes, warm conditions, and a source of simple sugars. Although some types of bacteria produce alcohol, commercial alcoholic beverage production relies on *yeast*, one−celled fungi (*fun′−ji*) that break down (*ferment*) simple sugars in the absence of oxygen to obtain energy and the metabolic waste product, alcohol. Grains, fruit, and potatoes—just about anything that contains simple sugars—will ferment under the proper conditions. Yeast will even ferment lactose in milk.

Alcohol is soluble in water, and alcoholic beverages gen−erally contain a considerable amount of water. Beers are typically 3 to 6% alcohol, wines contain about 8 to 14% alcohol, and malt liquors are about 7% alcohol by volume. Alcohol is poisonous (*toxic*), and yeast die when the con−centration of alcohol in the fermenting solution reaches 14 to 16%. The distilling process increases the alcohol con−centration of an alcoholic beverage. Distilled spirits (hard liquors) such as whiskey, bourbon, and vodka are generally 40 to 50% alcohol. You can determine the percentage of alcohol in hard liquor by dividing the "proof" declaration on the label by two. Tequila, for example, is "80 proof," or 40% alcohol.

Although each gram of alcohol provides 7 kcal, alcohol is not a nutrient; it is a mind−altering drug that is often clas−sified as a food. Beer and wine contain simple carbohydrates and small amounts of certain minerals and B vitamins. Dis−tilled spirits have essentially no nutritional value other than water. Mixing distilled spirits with juices, cocktail mixes,

$$CH_3 — CH_2 — OH$$

Ethanol

Figure 6.21 Ethanol. Ethanol is a simple two-carbon compound.

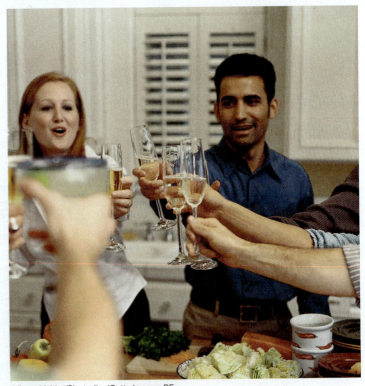

TABLE 6.8 Approximate Alcohol, Carbohydrate, and Energy Contents of Alcoholic Beverages*

Beverage	Amount (fl oz)	Kcal	Alcohol (g)	Carbohydrates (g)
Beer				
Regular	12.0	139	13	11
Lite	12.0	103	11	5
Table Wines	5.0	114	14	5
Distilled Spirits				
Gin, rum, vodka, whiskey	1.5	96	14	0

* Protein and fat contribute little or nothing to the caloric content.

Source: U.S. Department of Agriculture.

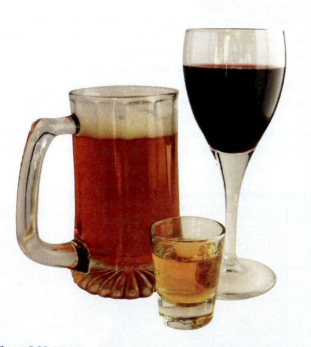

Figure 6.22 What's a standard drink? A standard drink is approximately 12 ounces of beer, 1½ ounces of liquor, or 5 ounces of wine.
©Wendy Schiff

or other flavorings increases the alcoholic beverage's energy content and may add some nutrients, particularly simple sugars, depending on the ingredients in the mixer. Table 6.8 indicates the grams of alcohol and carbohydrates in certain alcoholic drinks, as well as their caloric content. A standard drink (approximately 12 ounces of beer, 5 ounces of wine, or 1½ ounces of liquor) contains 13 to 14 grams of alcohol (Fig. 6.22).

How the Body Processes Alcohol

Alcohol requires no digestion and readily passes through the tissues lining the inside of the mouth, esophagus, stomach, and small intestine. When alcohol is consumed with meals, food delays its absorption from the stomach and slows the rate at which the drug enters the bloodstream. To reduce alcohol's harmful effects, the body detoxifies the simple chemical by converting it into less damaging compounds. Detoxification begins in the stomach, where the enzyme gastric alcohol dehydrogenase metabolizes up to 20% of the alcohol. Most of the remaining alcohol passes through the small intestinal wall and circulates to the liver, the primary site for metabolizing alcohol. Since alcohol is a poison, the liver shifts its metabolic focus from macronutrient metabolism to alcohol detoxification when the compound enters its tissues.

The liver relies on two biochemical pathways to metabolize alcohol. When relatively low doses are consumed, the enzyme alcohol dehydrogenase converts most of the alcohol to acetaldehyde, a substance that is more toxic than alcohol. Another enzyme, aldehyde dehydrogenase, reacts with acetaldehyde to form acetate, which can also be harmful. Acetate, however, can be metabolized to carbon dioxide (CO_2) and water (H_2O), or the molecule can be used to synthesize fatty acids and cholesterol (Fig. 6.23).

If a person consumes excessive amounts of alcohol such as during a drinking binge, the alcohol overwhelms the liver's ability to metabolize the drug using the dehydrogenase pathway. When this occurs, the second method of processing alcohol, the microsomal ethanol oxidizing system (MEOS), takes over. Unlike the alcohol dehydrogenase pathway, MEOS wastes energy in the form of body heat that dissipates into the environment. Thus, alcoholics typically gain little weight from their energy intake when alcohol supplies most of their energy.

Factors That Influence Alcohol Metabolism You may have noticed that a few of your friends who drink can "hold their liquor" better than others. Why are some people able to drink more alcohol at one time than others? Several factors account for the variability. In addition to the amount and timing of alcohol consumption, personal characteristics such as sex, body size and composition, age, and prior drinking history affect the body's detoxification rate. For example, a healthy person who weighs 154 pounds (70 kg) metabolizes about 1 alcoholic drink per hour. Drinking caffeinated beverages, exercising, or taking vitamins does not increase this rate. To sober up, the drinker must stop consuming alcohol and give his or her liver time to metabolize the drug.

Alcohol is not stored in the body. Until the liver can detoxify the toxic chemical, it circulates in the bloodstream and diffuses into the watery fluids within and surrounding cells. The lungs and perspiration eliminate some of

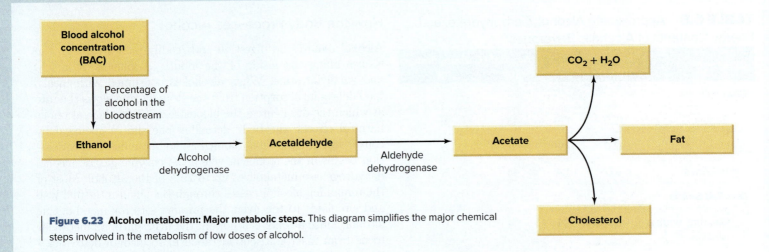

Figure 6.23 Alcohol metabolism: Major metabolic steps. This diagram simplifies the major chemical steps involved in the metabolism of low doses of alcohol.

the alcohol; that's why you can smell alcohol when you're around someone who's been drinking. The kidneys also filter some of the drug from the bloodstream and elimi— nate it in urine. To determine whether someone is legally intoxicated as a result of drinking alcohol, law enforce— ment officials use special devices to analyze the alcohol in blood, urine, or expired air to estimate the person's **blood alcohol concentration (BAC)**. BAC is reported as a

blood alcohol concentration (BAC) percentage of alcohol in the bloodstream

percentage that indicates the amount of alcohol in the blood. In the United States, a BAC of 0.08% is the legal limit for intoxication for automobile operators who are 21 years of age or older.

Men and women have different physical responses to alcohol. Women tend to become more impaired than men do after drinking the same amount of alcohol, even when dif— ferences in body weight are taken into account (Fig. 6.24). The reasons for these sexual differences are unclear, but they probably involve physiological factors including body size and composition. The average man is larger than the average woman, and larger people can often drink more alcohol without showing ill effects than smaller individuals

Figure 6.24 Alcohol consumption and approximate BAC. This table shows the relationship between the number of alcoholic drinks consumed on an empty stomach per hour and BACs for healthy men and women. For example, a 170-pound man will have his BAC reach 0.05% after he has three drinks, whereas a 140-pound woman will have her BAC reach 0.05% after drinking only two drinks. However, alcohol's effects on individuals can vary. In the United States and Canada, a person is legally intoxicated when his or her BAC is 0.08% or higher (2017).

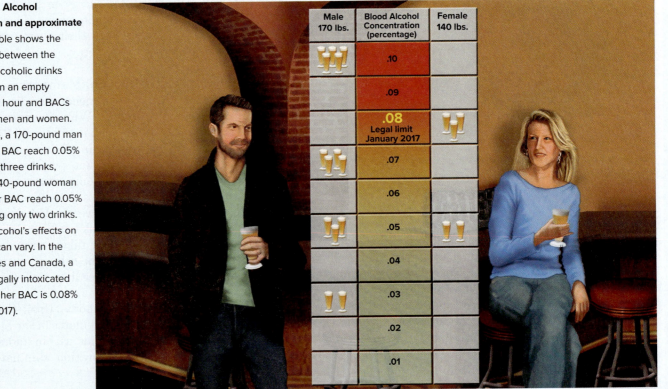

because they have bigger livers that detoxify more alcohol at a time. Additionally, a healthy 150–pound man typically has more body water than a healthy 150–pound woman. After the man drinks a beer, the alcohol diffuses out of his bloodstream and into the water compartments of his body. The woman's body has less water, so more alcohol remains in her bloodstream after she drinks a beer. As a result, her BAC rises faster, and she becomes more intoxicated after drinking the same amount of alcohol per hour as her male counterpart. Compared to men who drink heavily, women have a higher risk of serious health problems, especially damage to their liver, brain, and heart, when they abuse the same amounts of alcohol.[30]

Prior alcohol exposure also influences the rate of alcohol metabolism. People who drink regularly develop tolerance. Tolerance occurs as the levels of liver enzymes needed to metabolize alcohol increase, and as a result, the rate of alcohol metabolism increases. Consequently, the regular drinker needs to consume more alcohol at a time to achieve the same mind–altering effects as a person who drinks infrequently. Tolerance can lead to alcohol dependence (alcoholism).

Classifying Drinkers

In 2015, almost 52% of Americans who were 12 years of age or older reported being current alcohol drinkers during the 30 days prior to the survey.[31] Almost one–quarter of the current drinkers engaged in binge drinking at least once, and 6.5% of current drinkers drank heavily during this period.

What is "moderate drinking" or "binge drinking"? Although there is no universally accepted definition for "light," "moderate," or "heavy" drinking, medical practitioners and alcohol researchers often follow the classification guidelines listed in Table 6.9. Binge drinking is a form of heavy drinking, but the definition of binge drinking often differs according to sex. According to the Centers for Disease Control and Prevention, binge drinking is defined as having four or more drinks

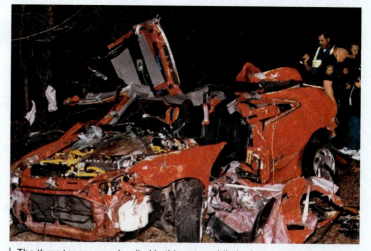

The three teenagers who died in this automobile had consumed alcohol before the accident. Source: Centers for Disease Control and Prevention/Gwinnett County Police Department

during an occasion (about 2 hours) for females and five or more drinks during an occasion for males.[32] Regardless of their backgrounds, binge drinking is a common practice among Americans.

Alcohol Use Disorder

A "problem drinker" experiences problems at home, work, and school that are associated with his or her drinking habits. According the experts with the National Institutes of Health, a person with a severe drinking problem has an alcohol use disorder (AUD).[33] In 2015, about 6% of Americans who were 18 years of age or older had an AUD. Both problem drinkers and people with AUD (alcoholism) engage in behaviors that place themselves and others in danger, such as drinking and driving.

A person who is *dependent* on alcohol (an alcoholic) has an uncontrollable need to drink; is unable to limit his or her alcohol consumption; suffers withdrawal symptoms, such as shakiness and anxiety, when alcohol is unavailable after a period of heavy drinking; and experiences *tolerance* to the drug. Tolerance develops over time as the drinker's body becomes better able to metabolize the alcohol. As a result, the person with AUD needs to consume more of the drug to obtain the same effects that he or she experienced prior to becoming dependent. Table 6.10 lists possible signs of alcohol use disorder.

Alcohol and Health

Alcohol is a central nervous system depressant. Mild alcohol intoxication often produces pleasant sensations and relaxed inhibitions. Consuming large amounts, however, depresses normal motor functioning, including breathing, and death can result. Alcohol use is often involved in motor vehicle accidents, falls, and drownings, as well

TABLE 6.9 Classifying Drinkers

Classification of Drinker	Amount of Alcohol Consumed (Standard Drinks)	
	Males	**Females**
Moderate	Up to 2 drinks/day	Up to 1 drink/day
Heavy	15 or more drinks/week	8 or more drinks/week
Binge	5 or more drinks/occasion (about 2 hours)	4 or more drinks/occasion (about 2 hours)

Source: Centers for Disease Control and Prevention, Alcohol & Public Health: "Frequently asked questions." Updated June 8, 2017. https://www.cdc.gov/alcohol/faqs.htm Accessed: July 29, 2017.

TABLE 6.10 Signs of Alcohol Abuse

Check all of the boxes that apply.

☐ Had times when you drank more than you intended?
☐ Wanted to reduce or stop drinking, or you tried to, but you couldn't?
☐ Had a strong need or urge to drink?
☐ Felt that drinking or its aftereffects interfered with your ability to take care of your personal responsibilities, do your job, or keep up with school work?
☐ Continued to drink even though it was causing trouble with your family or friends?
☐ Gotten into situations while or after drinking that increased your chances of being harmed, such as driving, swimming, using machinery, walking in a dangerous area, or having unsafe sex?
☐ Continued to drink even though it was making you feel depressed or anxious, or your drinking was causing other health problems?
☐ Continued to drink even after having a memory blackout?
☐ Found that when the effects of alcohol were wearing off, you had withdrawal symptoms, such as trouble sleeping, shakiness, irritability, anxiety, depression, restlessness, nausea, or sweating?

If you checked one or more of these boxes, your alcohol use may already be a concern for you and others. Consider seeking professional help.

Adapted from: National Institutes of Health, National Institute of Alcohol Abuse and Alcoholism: *Alcohol use disorder.* ND. http://www.niaaa.nih.gov/alcohol-health/overview-alcohol-consumption/alcohol-use-disorders Accessed: July 29, 2017.

as acts of violence and abuse. An estimated 88,000 Americans die each year as a result of excessive alcohol use.[34] Thousands of other people suffer physical injuries and have damaged interpersonal relationships related to excess alcohol consumption.

The potentially harmful physiological effects of abusing the drug vary from person to person, primarily because of differences in overall health, drinking habits, and genetic background. Alcohol affects every cell in the body, and when consumed in excess, the drug damages every system in the body, particularly the gastrointestinal, nervous, and cardiovascular systems. Figure 6.25 summarizes major damaging physiological effects of alcohol.

Alcohol and the Gastrointestinal Tract If you have consumed distilled spirits without adding mixers, you probably felt a burning sensation as the alcohol entered your throat and stomach. This sensation is an indication of alcohol's irritating effects on the lining of your gastrointestinal tract. Not surprisingly, chronic drinking contributes to intestinal ulcer formation, particularly in the

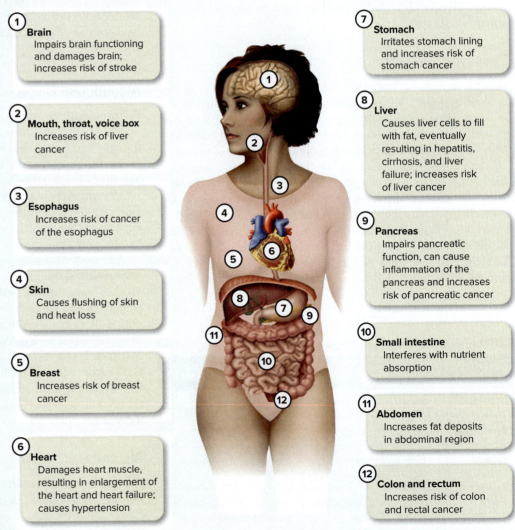

1 Brain
Impairs brain functioning and damages brain; increases risk of stroke

2 Mouth, throat, voice box
Increases risk of liver cancer

3 Esophagus
Increases risk of cancer of the esophagus

4 Skin
Causes flushing of skin and heat loss

5 Breast
Increases risk of breast cancer

6 Heart
Damages heart muscle, resulting in enlargement of the heart and heart failure; causes hypertension

7 Stomach
Irritates stomach lining and increases risk of stomach cancer

8 Liver
Causes liver cells to fill with fat, eventually resulting in hepatitis, cirrhosis, and liver failure; increases risk of liver cancer

9 Pancreas
Impairs pancreatic function, can cause inflammation of the pancreas and increases risk of pancreatic cancer

10 Small intestine
Interferes with nutrient absorption

11 Abdomen
Increases fat deposits in abdominal region

12 Colon and rectum
Increases risk of colon and rectal cancer

Figure 6.25 Some of alcohol's effects on the body. Chronic alcohol abuse seriously damages several organs and increases the risk of various cancers.

esophagus and stomach. An ulcer is a sore. Intestinal ulcers can cause chronic bleeding and may penetrate through the intestinal wall. When this occurs, intestinal contents leak into the abdominal cavity, causing serious and often deadly infections. Although the reasons are unclear, chronic alcohol consumption increases the risk of *alcoholic pancreatitis*, a painful and sometimes fatal condition characterized by inflammation and destruction of the pancreas.

People who consume alcohol have an increased risk of cancers of the digestive system. Such cancers include mouth, throat, esophagus, liver, colon, and rectal cancers.[35]

Alcohol and the Brain Alcohol's effects on the central nervous system, especially the brain, appear within a few minutes of having a drink. Alcohol acts as a depressant, slowing the transmission of messages between nerve cells (neurons). At low BACs (< 0.06%), the drinker is relaxed and less inhibited socially as regions of the brain that control decision making and reasoning ability are depressed. If the person continues to drink and his or her BAC increases to between 0.08 and 0.15%, the person loses control over voluntary muscles, particularly muscles that move the lips, eyes, and limbs. As a result, the drinker's speech is slurred, his or her eyes have difficulty focusing on objects, and the person's ability to drive or operate any heavy equipment is seriously compromised. When the drinker's BAC reaches 0.25% or higher, his or her brain is unable to process information. Higher BACs usually result in loss of consciousness ("passing out"). Moreover, coma and even death can occur as the brain loses control over lung and heart functioning. Table 6.11 lists BAC levels and typical nervous system effects that can occur at each level.

Alcohol can disrupt the ability of neurons in the brain to transmit messages. Long-term consumption of excessive amounts of alcohol can cause the neurons to shrink, and the brain develops other structural abnormalities. Confusion and memory loss are common signs of the extensive brain damage that occurs in a chronic heavy drinker.

Alcohol Poisoning As a college student, you may have observed binge drinking or engaged in the practice. In 2015, Americans who were 21 to 25 years of age were more likely to binge drink than Americans in other age groups.[31] Youthful binge drinking is a serious public health concern because the behavior is often associated with driving while drunk. Furthermore, the practice may increase a person's later risk of alcoholism and can result in death.

Binge drinking has become an expected "rite of passage" for American youth celebrating their 21st birthday. The practice of trying to consume 21 drinks quickly while celebrating "power hour" ("21 for 21") can have deadly consequences. On March 15, 2004, Jason Reinhardt was celebrating his 21st birthday with friends in a bar. Jason rapidly drank 16 shots of alcohol. Although he managed to return to his friends' house and go to bed, his lifeless body was discovered a few hours later. The young man's blood alcohol concentration was 0.361, well within the deadly range (see Table 6.11). What makes binge drinking so dangerous?

Binge drinking increases a person's BAC rapidly and to a point at which signs of alcohol poisoning occur. An individual suffering from alcohol poisoning is confused, "passes out" and cannot be aroused (comatose), breathes slowly and irregularly, and has pale or bluish skin. Alcohol poisoning

TABLE 6.11 Typical Effects of Alcohol at Various BAC Levels (Adults)

Blood Alcohol Concentration	Physiological and Psychological Effects
0.02	Some loss of good judgment, altered mood, relaxation
0.05	Reduced inhibitions, resulting in exaggerated emotional and behavioral responses to situations Impaired judgment, good mood
0.08	Loss of balance, slower-than-normal reaction time, impaired reasoning ability and memory Reduced ability to control one's behavior
0.10	Major impairment of hearing, vision, and muscular coordination Slurred speech and obvious delayed reaction time
0.15	Poor muscular control, vomiting, loss of balance
0.20	Cannot walk without help, mental confusion May pass out
0.25 or above	Loss of consciousness, coma, possible death from respiratory arrest (breathing stops)

Adapted from: Centers for Disease Control and Prevention, Injury Prevention and Control, Motor Vehicle Safety: *Impaired driving: Get the facts*: BAC *Effects*. Page last updated: January 26, 2017. http://www.cdc.gov/MotorVehicleSafety/Impaired_Driving/impaired-drv_factsheet.html; University of Notre Dame, McDonald Center for Student Well-Being: *Blood alcohol concentration*. ND. http://mcwell.nd.edu/your-well-being/physical-well-being/alcohol/blood-alcohol-concentration/. Accessed: January 26, 2017.

can cause the heartbeat to slow down and the lungs to stop functioning, resulting in death. Additionally, if a comatose person vomits, his or her stomach contents can enter the lungs, causing the person to choke to death. Jason died in his sleep from alcohol poisoning. His breathing rate slowed, his heartbeat became irregular, and his organs gradually shut down while he slept. Thus, it is important to recognize that alcohol poisoning is a life–threatening condition. If you suspect someone has consumed a deadly amount of alcohol, do not waste time trying to estimate how many drinks that person has drunk; call 911 immediately.

Alcohol and the Liver In addition to harming the brain, alcohol can damage the liver. Some acetaldehyde that forms when alcohol is metabolized enters the complex series of biochemical pathways that eventually produce carbon diox–ide, water, and ATP, the primary energy storage molecule for cells. The liver, however, also uses acetaldehyde to make fatty acids for synthesizing triglycerides (see Fig. 6.23). Even after a single bout of heavy drinking, fat accumulates in liver cells and causes a condition called "fatty liver." Fatty liver may be reversible; if the affected person avoids alcohol for an extended period, the liver metabolizes the fat, and the organ eventually heals itself. If the person continues to drink, the buildup of fat destroys his or her liver cells, and tough scar tissue replaces them. This irreversible condition is called *liver cirrhosis* or hardening of the liver (Fig. 6.26). Alco-holics are prone to develop *hepatitis*, inflammation of the liver. Hepatitis increases the risk of liver cancer.

The scarred regions of an alcoholic's liver have no func–tion other than holding the organ together. Under normal conditions, a healthy liver can regenerate sections of itself,

but when destruction of liver cells is extensive, the organ begins to fail. In this situation, the affected person will die unless he or she undergoes liver transplantation. Chronic alcohol abuse is a major cause of liver failure among adult Americans.

Alcohol and the Cardiovascular System Consuming light to moderate amounts of alcohol raises HDL cholesterol levels and decreases platelet stickiness.[36] Platelets are cell fragments involved in the blood–clotting process. Reduc-ing the likelihood of blood clot formation lowers the risk of heart attack and certain types of strokes.

Some medical researchers think drinking beer and red wine is healthier than consuming white wines or spirits. Although the alcohol in beer is the same as that in wine and distilled spirits, red wine and beer have higher levels of certain antioxidants and B vitamins than other alcoholic beverages, which may explain their health benefits. Pur-ple grape juice, which is used to make red wine, contains the same antioxidants as the wine and appears to protect against heart disease as well. The role of moderate alco-hol consumption in coronary artery disease prevention is controversial. Drinking small amounts of alcohol seems to reduce the risk of heart disease, but consuming moderate to excessive amounts is associated with increased risks of hypertension, stroke, heart failure, and weight gain.[36] More research is needed to determine if alcohol alone or other compounds present in certain alcoholic beverages provide beneficial effects on heart health when consumed.

Alcohol and Cancer As mentioned earlier, alcohol increases the risk of oral cavity, esophageal, stomach, liver, pancreatic, and colorectal cancer. Heavy drinkers who smoke tobacco products have a much greater risk of developing cancers of the oral cavity and esophagus than people who drink less and do not smoke. Furthermore, women who con-sume one or more drinks daily have a higher risk of breast cancer than women who avoid alcohol or drink less than one standard drink per day.

Alcohol and Interactions with Other Drugs People who drink alcohol while taking other drugs, including prescrip-tion medications and over–the–counter remedies, need to recognize that alcohol's harmful effects may be amplified by the medications. Additionally, alcohol may interact with other drugs, causing serious side effects that do not occur when a drug is consumed alone. For example, combining alcohol with products that contain the pain–reliever acet-aminophen can cause severe liver damage and even death.

Effects of Alcohol on Nutritional Status When con-sumed in moderation, alcohol stimulates the appetite. Alcohol, however, lowers blood glucose levels and raises blood triglycerides. Chronic, excessive alcohol intake can have adverse effects on the drinker's nutritional intake and

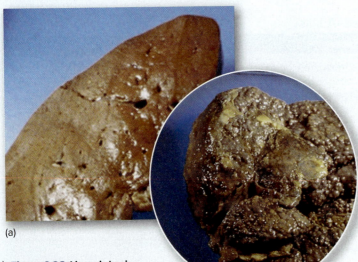

(a)

(b)

Figure 6.26 Liver cirrhosis.
The photograph on the left (*a*) shows a normal liver; the one on the right (*b*) shows a liver damaged by alcoholic cirrhosis.
©Arthur Glauberman/Science Source

status. Many alcoholics consume a considerable portion of their energy as alcohol, which often displaces nutrient—dense foods from their diets and increases their risk of malnutrition. The excess alcohol damages the liver and interferes with the absorption, metabolism, and storage of various micronutrients. Consuming too much alcohol may also increase the excretion of certain minerals, particularly minerals magnesium and zinc.[37]

Poor diets contribute to deficiencies of vitamin A, vitamin C, and the B vitamins thiamin and folate among alcoholics. It is not unusual for chronic alcoholics to become thiamin deficient and develop *Wernicke—Korsakoff syndrome*, a brain disorder characterized by mental confusion, memory loss, and uncoordinated muscular movements. The person with this condition typically staggers when trying to walk. Taking thiamin supplements can resolve some signs of the syndrome, but the person must avoid drinking alcohol while being treated.

Although chronic alcohol abuse is associated with an increased risk of bone loss and fractures, light to moderate alcohol drinkers tend to have stronger bones and lower risk of fractures than nondrinkers, especially among women who are past child bearing age.[38] More research, however, is needed to determine the effects of alcohol on bone health.

Alcohol and Body Water Billboard and commercial advertisements for alcoholic beverages often show sweaty, physically active young adults gulping down beer or liquor to relieve their thirst. These ads are misleading. Alcohol is not a good thirst quencher because it is a diuretic that suppresses the production of antidiuretic hormone (ADH) by the pituitary gland. Without ADH's action, the kidneys produce more urine, and the body loses water and certain vitamins and minerals along with it. If a dehydrated drinker consumes even more alcohol to relieve thirst, this response only increases his or her water losses. Drinking water and other nonalcoholic drinks is the best way to keep the body well hydrated.

Fetal Alcohol Spectrum Disorders When a pregnant woman drinks alcohol, her embryo/fetus also "drinks" alcohol because the drug passes freely from the mother's bloodstream into the embryo/fetus's bloodstream. Alcohol is most devastating when it affects an embryo because organs develop during the first 2 months after conception. Unfortunately, many women are not aware that they are pregnant during this early stage of their child's prenatal (before birth) development, and they may drink socially or binge drink. Alcohol is toxic to cells, including rapidly dividing embryonic cells. An infant born with a *fetal alcohol spectrum disorder* (*FASD*) has some degree of developmental abnormalities as a result of its mother's consumption of alcohol during pregnancy. *Fetal alcohol syndrome* (*FAS*) is a devastating form of FASD. A child with FAS is born with certain facial and heart defects, as well as extensive, irreversible damage to its

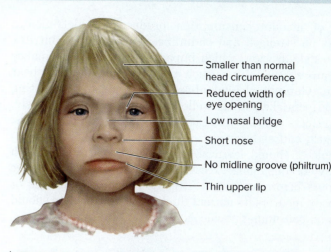

- Smaller than normal head circumference
- Reduced width of eye opening
- Low nasal bridge
- Short nose
- No midline groove (philtrum)
- Thin upper lip

Figure 6.27 Fetal alcohol syndrome. Physical deformities and developmental delays are characteristics of fetal alcohol syndrome (FAS), a type of fetal alcohol spectrum disorder.

nervous system that causes intellectual disability (Fig. 6.27). Children with FAS also experience delayed and abnormal physical development.

The amount of alcohol that can be safely consumed by a pregnant woman has not been determined. Therefore, if you or someone you know is trying to conceive or is pregnant, you or that person should "play it safe" and avoid alcohol. The risks are too high to justify even one drink. Table 6.12 identifies people, including pregnant women, who should not drink alcohol.

Alcohol and Physical Performance

Although some athletes may think consuming a small amount of alcohol before a competitive event might help relieve anxiety, alcohol reduces eye—hand coordination and slows reaction times even when BACs are relatively low (0.02 to 0.05%). Studies indicate conflicting findings concerning the effects of low to moderate amounts of alcohol on strength and endurance. In some instances, low to moderate intakes of alcohol reduce endurance and have negative effects on strength, but in other cases, this

TABLE 6.12 Who Should Avoid Alcohol?

Women who suspect they are pregnant, know they are pregnant, or are trying to become pregnant
People who plan to drive or use heavy machinery
People taking certain over-the-counter or prescription medications
People with medical conditions that alcohol can aggravate
Recovering alcoholics
People younger than 21 years of age

Source: Adapted from National Institute on Alcohol Abuse and Alcoholism: *Drinking levels defined*. ND. https://www.niaaa.nih.gov/alcohol-health/overview-alcohol-consumption/moderate-binge-drinking Accessed: July 29, 2017.

level of alcohol consumption produces no detrimental effects on strength and endurance. Alcohol can contribute to dehydration, which impairs muscular performance and causes heat injuries such as heat exhaustion and heat stroke. Chronic alcohol abuse causes muscular wasting that affects skeletal as well as heart muscle. Obviously, such effects will have negative effects on muscular mass, strength, and endurance.

Athletes should learn about alcohol's effects on health and avoid consuming excess alcohol, especially during the 48 hours before an event. After exercise, and until his or her body recovers its normal fluid status, the athlete should focus on consuming nonalcoholic beverages.

Where to Get Help for Problem Drinking or an Alcohol Use Disorder

If you think you are abusing alcohol or are dependent on the drug, seek help from your personal physician. For information about alcohol abuse, you can contact the National Drug and Alcohol Treatment Referral Routing Service at 1–800–662–HELP. You can also visit the websites of Alcoholics Anonymous (www.aa.org), the Substance Abuse and Mental Health Services Administration (http://www.samhsa.gov), or Al–Anon/Alateen (www.al–anon.alateen.org).

Concept CHECKPOINT

25. Summarize the effects of alcohol on the body, including the liver.
26. What is BAC? What is the legal limit for BAC in the United States?
27. Samuel drinks three 12-ounce cans of beer daily. Based on this information, is Samuel a moderate, heavy, or binge drinker?

See Appendix G for responses.

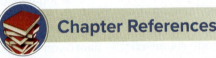

Chapter References

See Appendix H.

Summary

6.1 Introducing Lipids

- Lipids are needed for energy, proper growth and development, nerve functioning, maintenance of healthy skin and hair, and the production of bile and several hormones. Major lipids are triglycerides, phospholipids, and sterols. In addition to being a source of fuel, body fat contributes to body contours, insulates the body against cold temperatures, and protects against damaging blows.

6.2 Fatty Acids, Triglycerides, Phospholipids, and Sterols

- Triglycerides, an important fuel for the body, comprise most of the lipid content of your food and body. Lipids can be sources of the essential fatty acids. Furthermore, the fat in food enhances absorption of fat-soluble vitamins and phytochemicals. Dietary lipids also contribute to the appealing flavor, texture, and aroma of foods. Although consuming some lipids is essential for health, high amounts may increase your risk of serious health conditions, including obesity, certain cancers, and CVD.

- Most lipids have fatty acids in their chemical structures. Fatty acids can be saturated or unsaturated, and unsaturated fatty acids can be either monounsaturated or polyunsaturated. The body cannot synthesize the omega-6 fatty acid linoleic acid or the omega-3 fatty acid alpha-linolenic acid; these essential fatty acids must be supplied by the diet. The typical American diet provides omega-6 fat than omega-3 fat. Fatty fish, canola and soybean oils, walnuts, and flaxseed are sources of the omega-3 fats.

- Trans fatty acid molecules have a different configuration than cis fatty acid molecules. This difference enables fats that contain a high proportion of trans fatty acids to be more solid at room temperature than fats with a high proportion of cis fatty acids. Partial hydrogenation partially hardens the oil so that it can be made into shortening or shaped into sticks of margarine. Diets that contain high amounts of trans fats are associated with an increased risk of heart disease and stroke. Partially hydrogenated oils have been banned as food additives.

- A triglyceride has three fatty acids attached to glycerol. Triglycerides comprise about 95% of lipids in the body and in food. Triglycerides usually contain mixtures of unsaturated and saturated fatty acids, but one type of fatty acid (saturated, monounsaturated, or polyunsaturated) tends to predominate. In general, animal fats contain higher percentages of saturated fatty acids than plant fats. Important exceptions are highly saturated cocoa butter, coconut oil, and palm oil.

- Phospholipids have both hydrophilic and hydrophobic regions, and as a result, they are partially soluble in water and can serve as emulsifiers. Phospholipids are the major structural component of cell membranes and are needed for proper functioning of nerve cells, including those in the brain. Lecithin is the major phospholipid in food; egg yolks, liver, wheat germ, peanut butter, and soybeans are rich sources of this compound.

- The sterol cholesterol is a component of every cell membrane. Cells use cholesterol to make a variety of substances, including vitamin D, bile, and steroid hormones such as estrogen and testosterone. Cholesterol is found only in animal foods. Plants synthesize sterols and stanols that are not well absorbed by humans. Plant sterols and stanols, however, may be beneficial to health because they interfere with cholesterol absorption.

6.3 What Happens to Lipids in the Body?

- The triglycerides and phospholipids in food undergo digestion primarily in the upper part of the small intestine. Cholesterol is not broken down and is absorbed through the intestinal wall. Before leaving the small intestine, triglycerides, cholesterol, and other lipids are coated with a layer that contains protein to form chylomicrons. Chylomicrons enter the lymphatic system of the small intestine and eventually reach the bloodstream. The liver uses lipids to make various lipoproteins, substances that transport lipids in the bloodstream. Enterohepatic circulation enables the liver to recycle bile salts to make new bile.

- Triglycerides and carbohydrates are major sources of cellular energy. If energy is not needed, adipose cells remove fatty acids and glycerol from circulation and use them to synthesize triglycerides for storage. When energy is needed, adipose cells break down some stored triglycerides and release glycerol and fatty acids into the bloodstream.

6.4 Lipid Consumption Patterns

- Fat contributes about 35% of Americans' average daily energy intake. According to the Dietary Guidelines, fat should comprise 20 to 35% of total energy intake; the AMDR for fat is 20 to 35% of total calories.

6.5 Understanding Nutritional Labeling: Lipids

- Consumers can use nutrient labels to determine how much total fat, saturated fat, and trans fat are in packaged food.

6.6 Lipids and Health: Cardiovascular Disease

- CVD affects the heart and blood vessels. In the United States, heart disease is the leading cause of death. Atherosclerosis

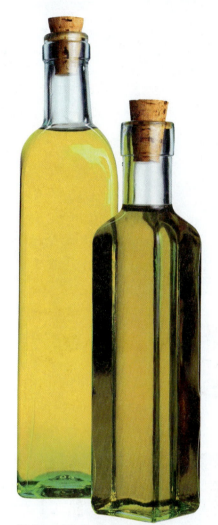
©C Squared Studios/Getty Images RF

©Brand X Pictures/Getty Images RF

is a long-term process that can result in CVD. Numerous risk factors are associated with atherosclerosis; some risk factors are nonmodifiable, but many are related to lifestyle practices that can be altered. Smoking cigarettes, eating certain fats, and being physically inactive are lifestyle practices that increase a person's risk of atherosclerosis and CVD.

- Blood lipid levels can have a major influence on the risk of atherosclerosis. Having high blood levels of HDL cholesterol is healthier than having high LDL cholesterol levels because elevated LDL cholesterol contributes to atherosclerosis, whereas elevated HDL cholesterol reduces the risk of this condition.

- Exercising and replacing saturated and trans fats with unsaturated fats may reduce LDL levels and increase HDL levels. On the other hand, physical inactivity and eating high amounts of saturated fat may raise LDL and blood triglyceride levels, increasing one's risk of atherosclerosis. Healthy people, however, generally do not experience an increase in their blood cholesterol levels when they eat cholesterol in foods.

- Although oils, fatty spreads, and salad dressings are obvious sources of dietary fat, much of the fat we eat is not visible. Saturated fat contributes much of the calories in fatty meats, luncheon meats, sausage, hot dogs, hard cheeses, and whole milk. If people make dietary modifications, lose excess weight, and exercise regularly, and their blood lipid levels still remain elevated, they should discuss additional treatment options with their physicians. Millions of Americans take prescription statin medications to reduce their elevated blood lipid levels.

6.7 Nutrition Matters: Drink to Your Health?

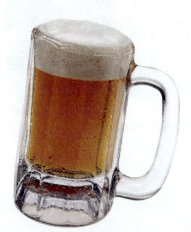
©Brand X Pictures/Getty Images RF

- Alcohol (ethanol) is a water-soluble, two-carbon compound that is toxic to cells. Beers are typically 3 to 6% alcohol, and wines contain about 8 to 14% alcohol by volume. Each gram of alcohol provides 7 kcal, but alcohol is not a nutrient; it is a mind-altering drug. A standard drink (approximately 12 ounces of beer, 5 ounces of wine, or 1½ ounces of liquor) contains 13 to 14 grams of alcohol.

- Alcohol requires no digestion and readily passes through the tissues lining the inside of the mouth, esophagus, stomach, and small intestine. The body detoxifies alcohol by converting the chemical into less damaging compounds. Until the liver has had enough time to metabolize all the alcohol that has been consumed, the amount of the drug that remains circulates in the bloodstream. In the United States, a blood alcohol concentration of 0.08% is the legal limit for intoxication for automobile operators who are 21 years of age or older (2017). Binge drinking is a major public health problem in the United States.

- Although drinking some alcohol raises HDL, excessive amounts of the drug damages every system in the body, particularly the gastrointestinal, nervous, and cardiovascular systems. Alcohol has especially devastating effects on an embryo. Infants born with fetal alcohol syndrome (FAS) have certain facial and heart defects, as well as extensive, irreversible damage to their nervous systems that causes intellectual disability. Therefore, pregnant women should not drink alcohol.

Recipe for Healthy Living

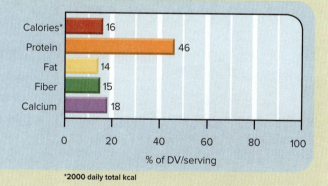
©Wendy Schiff

Salmon Salad Sandwiches

Are you tired of eating burgers? Try something different that's easy to prepare and a rich source of omega-3 fatty acids: salmon salad sandwiches. You can use canned salmon or leftover baked salmon to make the salad. This recipe makes enough salad for two sandwiches. Each sandwich provides approximately 312 kcal, 11 g fat, 23 g protein, 4.2 g fiber, and 230 mg calcium.

INGREDIENTS:

1 cup canned or cooked salmon
2 Tbsp pickle relish
2 Tbsp minced (finely chopped) sweet onion
2 Tbsp lite mayonnaise
4 slices whole-wheat bread
1 slice fresh tomato (optional)
1 piece leaf lettuce (optional)

PREPARATION STEPS:

1. If using canned salmon, drain fluid from salmon. In a bowl, break up salmon with a fork, including the small bones. Add other ingredients to the salmon and mix until well blended.

2. Toast slices of whole-wheat bread.

3. Spread ½ cup of salad on one slice of the toasted bread. Add a fresh tomato slice and/or piece of leaf lettuce, if desired.

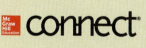

Further analyze this recipe or other recipes through activities located in Connect.

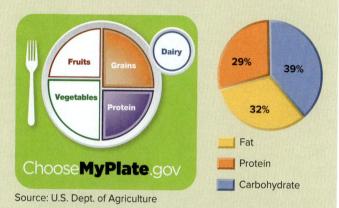

ChooseMyPlate.gov

Source: U.S. Dept. of Agriculture

- 39% Carbohydrate
- 32% Fat
- 29% Protein

Fat
Protein
Carbohydrate

	% of DV/serving
Calories*	16
Protein	46
Fat	14
Fiber	15
Calcium	18

0   20   40   60   80   100

*2000 daily total kcal

Personal Dietary Analysis

1. Refer to the 3-day food log from the "Personal Dietary Analysis" feature in Chapter 3. List the total number of kilocalories you consumed for each day of record keeping. Add the figures to obtain a total, divide the total by 3, then round the figure to the nearest whole number to obtain your average daily energy intake for the 3-day period.

Sample Calculation:

Day 1	<u>2000</u> kcal
Day 2	<u>1700</u> kcal
Day 3	<u>2350</u> kcal

Total kcal **<u>6050</u> ÷ 3 days = <u>2017</u> kcal/day**
(average kilocalorie intake, rounded to the nearest whole number)

Your Calculation:

Day 1	_____ kcal
Day 2	_____ kcal
Day 3	_____ kcal

Total kcal _____ ÷ **3 days** = _____ **kcal/day**
(average kilocalorie intake, rounded to the nearest whole number)

2. Add the number of grams of fat eaten each day of the period. Divide the total by 3 and round to the nearest whole number to calculate the average number of grams of fat consumed daily.

Sample Calculation:

Day 1	<u>50</u> g
Day 2	<u>57</u> g
Day 3	<u>42</u> g
Total =	<u>149</u> g

Total grams **<u>149</u> ÷ 3 days = 50 g/day (average)**

Your Calculation:

Day 1	_____ g
Day 2	_____ g
Day 3	_____ g
Total =	_____ g

Total grams _____ ÷ **3 days** = _____ **g of fat/day**
(average, rounded to the nearest whole number)

3. Each gram of fat provides about 9 kcal; therefore, you must multiply the average number of grams of fat that you ate daily (step 2) by 9 to obtain the average number of kilocalories from fat.

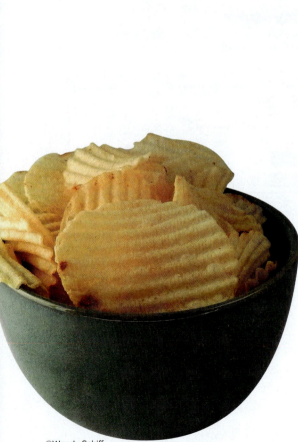
©Wendy Schiff

Sample Calculation:

<u>50</u> g/day × 9 kcal/g = <u>450</u> kcal from fat

Your Calculation:

_____ g/day × 9 kcal/g = _____ kcal from fat

4. To calculate the average percentage of calories that fat contributed to your diet, divide the average number of calories from fat obtained in step 3 by the average total daily calorie intake obtained in step 1 and round to the nearest one-hundredth. Multiply the value by 100, drop the decimal point, and add the percent symbol.

Sample Calculation:

<u>450</u> kcal ÷ <u>2017</u> kcal = 0.22

0.22 × 100 = <u>22</u>%

Your Calculation:

_____ kcal ÷ _____ kcal = _____

_____ × 100 = _____ %

5. Did your average daily fat intake meet the U.S. Dietary Guidelines recommended 20 to 35% of total energy?

Yes _____ No _____

6. If your average fat intake was more than 35% of your total energy intake, which foods contributed to your intake of fats?

Foods: _____

7. Review the log of your 3-day food intake. Calculate your average daily intake of saturated fat by adding the grams of saturated fat consumed over the 3-day period and dividing the total by 3.

Your Calculation:

Day 1 _____ g

Day 2 _____ g

Day 3 _____ g

Total = _____ g

Total g _____ ÷ **3 days** = _____ **g of saturated fat daily**

a. What was your average daily saturated fat intake? _____ g

b. Was your average daily intake less than the Dietary Guidelines recommended limit for an adult (less than 10% of total calories)? _____ Yes _____ No

c. If your average saturated fat intake was greater than the recommended limit, list foods that contributed to your intake. _____

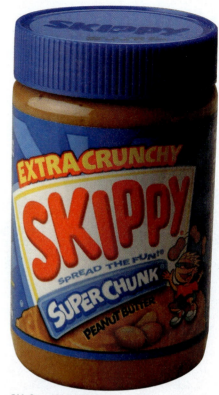

©McGraw-Hill Education/Elite Images, photographer

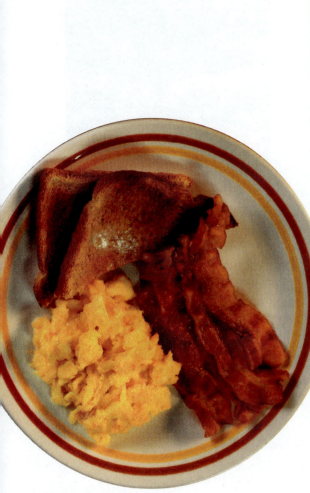

©Spike Mafford/Getty Images RF

Using Nutrient Labels: Fats

1. Remove the labels from two different packaged foods that contain fat. Using information from each of the product's Nutrition Facts panel, answer the following questions.

a. Name of product #1 _____

Name of product #2 _____

b. How many kcal are in one serving of each food?

Product 1 _____ kcal
Product 2 _____ kcal

c. How many grams of fat, saturated fat, and trans fat are in a serving?

Product 1

_____ grams of total fat

_____ grams of saturated fat

_____ grams of trans fat

Product 2

_____ grams of total fat

_____ grams of saturated fat

_____ grams of trans fat

d. Calculate the percentage of total kcal/serving that are from saturated fat. First, multiply the number of grams of saturated fat by 9 (number of kcal per gram of fat). Then, divide the number of kcal contributed by saturated fat by the total number of kcal per serving. (The Nutrition Label uses the term "Calories" for kcal.) To obtain the percentage, move the decimal point two places to the right, remove the decimal point, and insert % symbol.

Product 1 _____ grams of saturated fat × 9 kcal = _____ kcal of saturated fat/serving

_____ % total kcal/serving contributed by saturated fat

Product 2 _____ grams of saturated fat × 9 kcal = _____ kcal of saturated fat/serving

_____ % total kcal/serving contributed by saturated fat

e. Read the list of ingredients for each product. If the food contains saturated fat and trans fat, identify ingredients that contributed saturated fat or trans fat to the product.

Saturated fat ingredients in Product 1 _____

_____

Trans fat ingredients in Product 1 _____

_____

Saturated fat ingredients in Product 2 _____

_____

Trans fat ingredients in Product 2 _____

_____

connect Complete the Personal Dietary Analysis activity located in Connect.

Assessment: Evaluating Your Solid Fat Intake

Do You Consume:	Rarely or Never	1 to 2 Times/ Week	3 to 5 Times/ Week	Daily
1. Bacon, hot dogs, sausage, salami, bologna, or other fatty luncheon meat?	0	1	2	3
2. Whole milk?	0	1	2	3
3. 2% milk?	0	1	2	3
4. Ice cream or milkshakes?	0	1	2	3
5. Sour cream or cream cheese?	0	1	2	3
6. Fatty cuts of pork or beef?	0	1	2	3
7. Hard cheeses, such as cheddar or Swiss?	0	1	2	3
8. Butter?	0	1	2	3
9. Stick margarine?	0	1	2	3
10. Gravy, cheese sauce, or cream-based sauce?	0	1	2	3
11. Buttered popcorn or "rinds"?	0	1	2	3
12. Biscuits, croissants, doughnuts, Danish pastries, pies, cakes, or cookies?	0	1	2	3
13. Products made with lard?	0	1	2	3
14. Cream in your coffee or tea?	0	1	2	3
15. Pizza?	0	1	2	3
16. Creamed soups such as cream of potato soup or New England clam chowder?	0	1	2	3
TOTAL	_____	_____	_____	_____

Scoring: Add points in each column and then add those figures together. (The higher the total points, the higher your solid fat intake.)

My "Solid Fat Score" is _____

If your score is 30 or more: Your solid fat intake is probably too high. Note which of these fatty foods you eat more than three times per week. Consider reducing your intake of these items and replacing them with foods that do not contain solid fat.

©Brand X Pictures/Getty Images RF

Critical Thinking

1. Calculate your risk of having a heart attack by completing the American Heart Association's Heart Attack Risk Calculator at https://www.heart.org/gglRisk/main_en_US.html. Based on your results, should you be concerned about your risk of CVD? If you are concerned, discuss steps you can take to reduce your risk of atherosclerosis and CVD.

2. Do you avoid fried foods and look for "lite" and "fat-reduced" foods when shopping for groceries? If your answer is no, explain why not.

3. Plan a meal that supplies 20 to 35% of energy from fat. The meal should include foods from the major food groups and provide 700 to 900 kcal.

4. Recently, your friend Paul's 50-year-old grandfather had a mild heart attack. Paul is very concerned about his risk for having a heart attack. What would you tell him?

5. Develop a blog for college students that describes atherosclerosis and the role that personal choices (lifestyles) play in the development of the disease.

6. If you drink alcohol, consider filling out the checklist shown in Table 6.10. According to this assessment, do you have a problem with your alcohol consumption habits? If your answer is yes, what can you do to obtain help?

Practice Test

Select the best answer.

1. Fats in foods
   a. add taste and contribute to "mouth feel."
   b. are digested and absorbed in the stomach.
   c. carry water-soluble nutrients.
   d. need to be eliminated to have a healthful diet.

2. Solid fats generally have a high proportion of _____ fatty acids.
   a. unsaturated
   b. saturated
   c. polyunsaturated
   d. monounsaturated

3. A saturated fatty acid has
   a. one double bond within the hydrocarbon chain.
   b. two double bonds within the hydrocarbon chain.
   c. no double bonds within the hydrocarbon chain.
   d. three or more double bonds within the hydrocarbon chain.

4. Which of the following statements is true?
   a. Certain fish are rich sources of omega-3 fatty acids.
   b. Omega-3 fatty acids increase the risk of cardiovascular disease.
   c. Trans fats are rich sources of omega-3 fatty acids.
   d. The human body converts dietary fiber into omega-3 fatty acids.

5. Trans fatty acids are
   a. naturally in many foods.
   b. a by-product of the hydrogenation process.
   c. essential to good health.
   d. found primarily in fatty fish.

6. Phospholipids
   a. do not have fatty acids in their chemical structures.
   b. lack glycerol in their chemical structures.
   c. do not occur naturally.
   d. are partially water-soluble.

7. Cholesterol is
   a. metabolized for energy.
   b. found only in animal foods.
   c. not made by the human body.
   d. harmful to health.

8. The primary site of triglyceride digestion and absorption is the
   a. stomach.
   b. liver.
   c. small intestine.
   d. gallbladder.

9. Lipoproteins

   a. are water—insoluble.
   b. transport lipids in the bloodstream.
   c. contain glucose.
   d. are toxic to cells.

10. Modifiable risk factors for atherosclerosis include

    a. family history.
    b. age.
    c. tobacco use.
    d. racial/ethnic background.

11. Homocysteine is a(n)

    a. form of folate.
    b. lipid that lowers blood pressure.
    c. possible marker for cardiovascular disease.
    d. essential amino acid.

12. Alcohol metabolism is not influenced by a person's

    a. sex.
    b. level of caffeine consumption.
    c. prior history of alcohol use.
    d. body size and composition.

13. After her college graduation party, Jade's BAC was 0.16%. This level is _____ times the legal limit.

    a. 2
    b. 4
    c. 3
    d. 5

14. Brita was a binge drinker during the first 3 months of her pregnancy. Her baby was born with FAS. Which of the following conditions is a sign of FAS?

    a. Chronic vomiting
    b. Iron deficiency anemia
    c. Bleeding gums
    d. Thin upper lip

ANSWERS TO Quiz Yourself

1. To lose weight, use regular, stick margarine instead of butter because it has 25% fewer calories per teaspoon. **False.** (Section 6.6)

2. Egg yolks are a rich source of cholesterol. **True.** (Section 6.6)

3. Taking too many fish oil supplements may be harmful to health. **True.** (Section 6.6)

4. On average, Americans consume 60% of their energy from fat. **False.** (Section 6.4)

5. Increasing your intake of saturated fat will reduce your risk of heart disease. **False.** (Section 6.6)

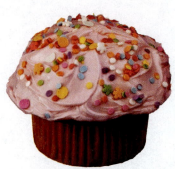

©Brand X Pictures/Getty Images RF

CHAPTER 7

Proteins

Quiz Yourself

How much protein is recommended for optimal health? Can people obtain enough protein by eating only plant foods? What happens if you eat more protein than your body needs? Before reading Chapter 7, take the following quiz to test your knowledge of protein. The answers are at the end of the chapter.

1. Animal foods such as meat and eggs are almost 100% protein. _____ T _____ F

2. Foods made from soybeans can be sources of high-quality protein. _____ T _____ F

3. Americans typically consume more protein from animal sources than from plant foods. _____ T _____ F

4. Registered dietitian nutritionists generally recommend that healthy people take amino acid supplements to increase their protein intake. _____ T _____ F

5. People can nourish their hair by using shampoo that contains protein. _____ T _____ F

Mc Graw Hill Education **connect®**

A wealth of proven resources are available on Connect® including SmartBook®, NutritionCalc Plus, and many other dynamic learning tools. Ask your instructor about Connect!

©Pixtal/age fotostock RF

7.1 What Are Proteins?

Learning Outcomes

1 List the primary function of proteins in the body.

2 Identify the basic structural unit of proteins and its components.

3 Classify an amino acid as essential or nonessential.

Since ancient times, many people have believed that eating animal foods, particularly meat, was necessary for good health and optimal physical performance. Milo of Croton, an ancient Greek Olympian wrestler with extraordinary strength, reportedly consumed about 20 pounds of meat daily. Although accounts of Milo's superhuman capacity for eating meat are unreliable, modern athletes often make protein-rich foods and protein supplements the foundation of their diets. Furthermore, it is not unusual for nonathletes to associate meat with protein and a lack of protein with poor muscular development and weak muscular strength.

Many Americans think a meal is not adequate unless it contains large portions of meat. Although it is true that meat is a rich source of protein, other foods, including eggs, milk, grains, dry beans, and lentils, are often overlooked as sources of protein. For example, the beef patty of a cheeseburger provides protein, as does the melted cheese that tops the burger and the bun that makes the sandwich convenient to eat.

Proteins are complex organic molecules that are chemically similar to lipids and carbohydrates because they contain carbon, hydrogen, and oxygen atoms. Proteins, however, contain nitrogen, the element cells need to make a wide array of important biological compounds. Plants, animals, bacteria, and even viruses contain hundreds of proteins.

Protein is an important class of nutrients, but it is not more valuable to your health than other nutrients. Nutrients work together in your body like members of a well-trained basketball team on the playing court. Making one player the star while neglecting to develop the other athletes' skills can have disastrous effects on the team's success. Similarly, overemphasizing one class of nutrients in your diet, such as protein, while ignoring other nutrients, can lead to nutritional imbalances that result in serious health problems. By reading this chapter, you will learn about the roles of proteins in your body and their major food sources. You will also learn how proteins influence your health.

Proteins in the Body

Proteins are necessary for muscle development and maintenance, but the more than 200,000 different proteins in your body have a wide variety of functions, including those shown in Table 7.1.[1] Skin, blood, nerve, bone—all cells in your body—contain proteins. Structural proteins such as *collagen* are in your cartilage, ligament, and bone tissue. *Keratin* is another structural protein; it is in your hair, nails, and skin. Contractile proteins in your muscles enable you to move, and transport proteins carry many substances in the bloodstream. Proteins are also necessary for your blood to clot properly.

Certain hormones, such as insulin and glucagon, are proteins. Hormones and neurotransmitters are chemical messengers that regulate body processes and responses, such as growth, metabolism, and hunger. *Neurotransmitters* send

proteins large, complex organic molecules made up of amino acids

TABLE 7.1 Proteins in the Body

The body uses proteins to make or function as:
New cells and many components of cells
Structures such as hair and nails
Enzymes
Lubricants
Clotting compounds
Antibodies
Compounds that help maintain fluid and pH balance
Certain hormones and neurotransmitters
Energy source (minor, under usual conditions)

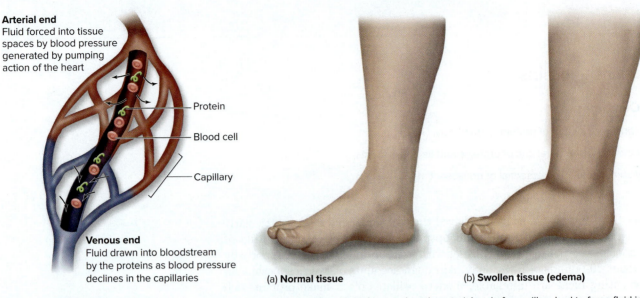

Arterial end
Fluid forced into tissue spaces by blood pressure generated by pumping action of the heart

— Protein

— Blood cell

— Capillary

Venous end
Fluid drawn into bloodstream by the proteins as blood pressure declines in the capillaries

(a) **Normal tissue**   (b) **Swollen tissue (edema)**

Figure 7.1 Normal fluid balance and edema. Under normal conditions, blood pressure is high enough at the arterial end of a capillary bed to force fluid into the tissue space that surround capillaries. At the venous end of the capillary bed, blood pressure is lower, and proteins in the bloodstream help draw fluid back into the capillaries. (*a*) As a result of the balance between blood pressure and proteins in the bloodstream, the tissues contain normal amounts of fluid. (*b*) When blood pressure is greater than the counteracting force of the proteins in the bloodstream, fluid remains in the tissues, causing edema.

signals from one nerve cell to another. Some neurotransmitters are proteins. Nearly all enzymes are proteins. Enzymes speed up the rate of (*catalyze*) chemical reactions without becoming a part of the products (see Fig. 4.8). Additionally, infection–fighting **antibodies** are proteins. Although cells can use proteins for energy, normally they metabolize very little for energy, conserving the nutrient for other important functions that carbohydrates and lipids are unable to perform.

In the bloodstream, proteins transport nutrients and oxygen. Proteins in blood, such as *albumin*, also help maintain the proper distribution of fluids in blood and body tissues (Fig. 7.1). The force of blood pressure moves watery fluid out of the bloodstream and into tissues. Blood proteins help counteract the effects of blood pressure by attracting the fluid, returning it to the bloodstream. During starvation, the level of protein in blood decreases, and as a result, some water leaks out of the bloodstream and enters spaces between cells. The resulting accumulation of fluid in tissues is called **edema** (*eh–dee'–mah*).

Proteins also help maintain **acid–base balance,** the proper pH of body fluids. To function properly, blood and tissue fluids need to maintain a pH of 7.35 to 7.45, which is slightly basic.[1] (To review the concept of pH, see Chapter 4.) Metabolic processes can produce acidic or basic by–products. If a particular body fluid becomes too acidic or too basic, cells can have difficulty functioning and may die. A **buffer** can protect the pH of a solution. Proteins can act as buffers, because they have acidic and basic components. For example, if cells form an excess of hydrogen ions (H^+), the pH of tissues decreases. To help restore the pH level to within the normal range, the basic portions of protein molecules bind to the excess H^+, neutralizing the excess ions and raising the pH.

Amino Acids

Proteins are comprised of smaller chemical units called **amino acids.** The human body contains proteins made from 20 different amino acids (see Appendix D). To understand how the body uses amino acids, it is necessary to learn some basic chemistry that relates to these compounds.

antibodies infection-fighting proteins

edema accumulation of fluid in tissues

acid-base balance maintaining the proper pH of body fluids

buffer substance that can protect the pH of a solution

amino acids nitrogen-containing chemical units that comprise proteins

Each amino acid has a carbon atom that anchors a hydrogen atom and three different groups of atoms: the **amino** or **nitrogen—containing group,** the **R group,** and the **acid group.** The chemical structure of the amino acid alanine shown in Figure 7.2 indicates these three groups. Note that the nitrogen atom is in the amino group. The R group varies with each type of amino acid, so it identifies the molecule as a particular amino acid, such as *serine* or *lysine*. When the nitrogen—containing group is removed, the R group, acid group, and anchoring carbon atom form the "carbon skeleton" of an amino acid (see Fig. 7.2). The carbon skeleton is an important component of an amino acid because the body can convert the carbon skeletons of certain amino acids to glucose and use the simple sugar for energy.

Classifying Amino Acids

Traditionally, nutritionists classify amino acids as either nonessential or essential according to the body's ability to make them. A healthy human body can make 11 of the 20 amino acids that are in its proteins. These compounds are the **nonessential amino acids.** The remaining nine amino acids are **essential amino acids** that must be supplied by foods because the body cannot synthesize them or make enough to meet its needs. Sometimes, nonessential and essential amino acids are referred to as "dispensable" and "indispensable" amino acids, respectively. Table 7.2 lists amino acids according to their classification as essential and nonessential.

Several nonessential amino acids are "conditionally essential," which means they become essential in certain situations. For example, cells can make cysteine from methionine and serine. If a person's methionine and serine intake is inadequate, his or her body cannot make enough cysteine to meet its needs, and dietary sources of the amino acid are necessary.

Figure 7.2 Amino acid: Basic chemical structure.

TABLE 7.2 Amino Acids in Human Proteins

Essential		Nonessential	
Histidine	Threonine	Alanine	Cysteine*
Isoleucine	Tryptophan	Aspartic acid	Glutamine*
Leucine	Valine	Asparagine	Glycine*
Lysine		Glutamic acid	Proline*
Methionine		Serine	Tyrosine*
Phenylalanine		Arginine*	

* Under certain conditions, this amino acid can become essential.

Concept CHECKPOINT

1. What is the chemical unit that makes up a protein?
2. List at least four different functions of proteins in the body.
3. Identify the three groups of atoms that make up a typical amino acid.
4. What is the "carbon skeleton" of an amino acid?
5. How many different kinds of amino acids are needed to make human proteins? How many of these amino acids are essential?

See Appendix G for responses.

Did *YOU* Know?

Taurine is a nonessential, sulfur-containing amino acid that human cells do not use to make proteins. The amino acid, however, has many functions in the body. Humans need taurine to form components of bile, and the amino acid acts as an antioxidant, lowers blood pressure, and reduces inflammation. The human liver can make small amounts of taurine, but the amino acid is a dietary essential for cats and foxes.[2]

Taurine may be added to energy drinks as an "energy-booster," and athletes often consume taurine-caffeine–containing energy drinks in an effort to boost their endurance and performance. There is, however, a lack of scientific evidence supporting the notion that the taurine in these products provides additional performance-related benefits beyond those of the caffeine ingredient. At present, taurine in doses of up to 10 g/day appears to have low toxicity.[2]

©Wendy Schiff

amino or **nitrogen-containing group** portion of an amino acid that contains nitrogen

R group part of amino acid that identifies the molecule as a particular amino acid

acid group acid portion of a compound

nonessential amino acids group of amino acids that the body can make

essential amino acids amino acids the body cannot make or make enough to meet its needs

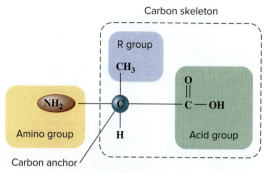

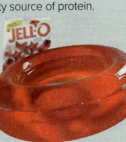
7.2 Proteins in Foods

Learning Outcomes

1 Explain the difference between a high-quality protein and a low-quality protein.

2 Identify foods that are rich sources of high-quality proteins.

3 List at least three amino acids that are often "limiting amino acids" in plant foods.

People often associate animal foods with protein, but beans, nuts, seeds, grains, and certain vegetables are good sources of protein, too. In fact, nearly all foods contain protein, but no naturally occurring food is 100% protein. Protein comprises only about 20 to 30% of the weight of a piece of beef; 25% of the weight of drained, water–packed tuna fish; and only 12% of an egg's weight. Nevertheless, animal foods generally provide higher amounts of protein than similar quantities of plant foods. A 3–ounce serving of broiled lean ground beef supplies 23 g of protein; a 3–ounce serving of steamed broccoli or cooked carrots provides only about 1 g of protein. In general, most plant foods provide less than 3 g of protein per ounce. Table 7.3 lists some commonly eaten foods and their approximate protein content per serving.

TABLE 7.3 Approximate Protein Content of Some Commonly Eaten Foods/Portion

Food	Serving Size	Protein g/serving
Chicken, breast, roasted, meat only	4 oz	34
Ham, lean, cooked	4 oz	30
Hamburger, 80% lean, broiled	4 oz	29
Pepperoni pizza, regular crust, 14″ pie	2 slices (200 g)	25
Tuna, canned, water-packed, drained	4 oz	22
Miso (soybean product)	½ cup	16
Lasagna with meat sauce	8 oz	15
Cottage cheese, 2% low-fat	4 oz	13
Milk, fat-free	1 cup	8
Peanut butter	2 Tbsp	8
Tofu, regular	½ cup	8
Bagel, plain	1 (3 ½″ diam)	7
American processed cheese	1 oz	7
Baked beans, vegetarian	½ cup	6
Egg, hard cooked	1	6
Vanilla ice cream	1 cup	4
White rice	1 cup	4
Peas, green	½ cup	4
Banana	1	1

Soup: ©FoodCollection/StockFood RF; Pea pods: ©Mitch Hrdlicka/Getty Images RF; Baked beans: ©telliott4/Getty Images RF; Ham: ©Brand X Pictures/Getty Images RF; Tofu on plate and Pizza: ©C Squared Studios/Getty Images RF; Bagels: ©Getty Images RF

Certain parts of plants contain more protein than other parts. Seeds, tree nuts, and legumes supply more protein per serving than servings of fruit or the edible leaves, roots, flowers, and stems of vegetables. Tree nuts include walnuts, cashews, and almonds; **legumes** are plants that produce pods that have a single row of seeds, such as soybeans, peas, peanuts, lentils, and beans (Fig. 7.3). A 3–ounce serving of almonds, dry–roasted peanuts, or sunflower seed kernels supplies about 20 g of protein. Many seeds and nuts, however, pack a lot of calories from fat. Snack on just 3 ounces of almonds, dry–roasted peanuts, or sunflower seed kernels, and you will add almost 500 kcal to your diet!

Mature peas, lentils, and most kinds of beans contain more protein and complex carbohydrate than fat. Eating a 3–ounce serving of vegetarian baked beans, for example, adds about 4 g of protein, 14 g of carbohydrate, and less than 1 g of fat to your diet. Although soybeans contain more fat than carbohydrate, soy fat is high in unsaturated fatty acids. The health benefits of unsaturated fatty acids are discussed in Chapter 6.

Figure 7.3 Legumes. Legumes, such as these soybeans, are plants that produce pods that have a single row of seeds.
Bowl of soybeans: ©Spencer Jones/Photodisc/Getty Images RF; Soybean pods: ©C Squared Studios/Getty Images RF

Protein Quality

Foods differ not only in the amount of protein they contain but also in their protein quality. A **high–quality (complete) protein** contains all essential amino acids in amounts that support protein deposition in muscles and other tissues, as well as a young child's growth.[3] High–quality proteins are well digested and absorbed by the body. Meat, fish, poultry, eggs, and milk and milk products contain high–quality proteins. Egg protein generally rates very high for protein quality because it is easy to digest and has a pattern of essential amino acids that closely resembles that needed by humans.

A **low–quality (incomplete) protein** lacks one or more of the essential amino acids or contains inadequate amounts of these nutrients. Furthermore, the human digestive tract does not digest low–quality protein sources as efficiently as foods containing high–quality protein. The essential amino acids that are in relatively low amounts are referred to as *limiting* amino acids because they reduce the protein's ability to support growth, repair, and maintenance of tissues. In most instances, tryptophan, threonine, lysine, and the sulfur–containing amino acids methionine and cysteine are the limiting amino acids in foods.[4]

Most plant foods are not sources of high–quality proteins. *Quinoa (keen'–wa)* and soy protein are exceptions. Quinoa is botanically related to sugar beets and spinach, but the quality and amount of protein in quinoa seeds are superior to those of many cereal grains.[5] Cooked quinoa is often used as a cereal (see "Recipe for Healthy Living" at the end of this chapter). The quality of soy protein is comparable to that of most animal proteins.[6] Processed soybeans are used to make a variety of nutritious foods, including soy milk, infant formula, and meat substitutes. Furthermore, eating foods made from soybeans may reduce the risk of chronic diseases, such as certain cancers.[6] More research, however, is needed to determine the long–term health benefits of eating diets that contain soy products.

Understanding the concept of protein quality is important. Regardless of how much protein is eaten, a child will fail to grow properly if his or her diet lacks essential amino acids. The "Vegetarianism" section of this chapter explains how you can obtain these and other essential nutrients by eating only plant foods.

legumes plants that produce pods with a single row of seeds

high-quality (complete) protein protein that contains all essential amino acids in amounts that support the deposition of protein in tissues and the growth of a young person

low-quality (incomplete) protein protein that lacks or has inadequate amounts of one or more of the essential amino acids

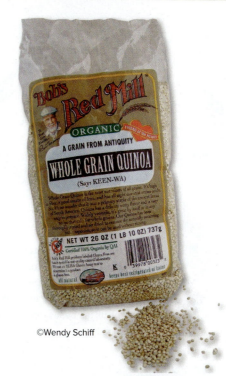

©Wendy Schiff

Concept CHECKPOINT

7.3 What Happens to Proteins in the Body?

Learning Outcomes

1 Explain how cells make proteins.

2 Describe what happens to excess amino acids in the body.

3 Explain what happens to proteins as they undergo digestion and absorption in the human digestive tract.

4 Explain the concept of nitrogen balance, and identify conditions in which the body is in a state of positive or negative nitrogen balance.

5 Calculate a person's RDA for protein based on his or her body weight.

peptide bond chemical attraction that connects two amino acids together

polypeptide protein comprised of two or more amino acids

peptides small chains of amino acids

gene portion of DNA

In a television crime series, police in a major city are investigating what could be a homicide. A man has been reported missing by his parents, who suspect foul play and their daughter–in–law's involvement in their son's disappearance. While knocking on the door of the missing man's house, police notice some dried blood on the front porch. The man's wife, who lives in the house, tells police that the blood is from her injured dog. How can police know she is telling the truth? The blood holds important clues. Every organism synthesizes proteins— including those in blood—that are unique. Samples of the blood can be analyzed to determine whether it contains proteins from a dog or another animal, such as a human. We will leave it to your imagination to finish this story, but we will examine a real–life story: how human cells make proteins.

How the Body Uses Amino Acids to Synthesize Proteins

Your body makes proteins by following information coded in your DNA, or deoxyribonucleic ($de-ox'-e-rye'-bow-new-klay'-ik$) acid, the hereditary material in a cell's nucleus. To make proteins, cells assemble the 20 amino acids in specific sequences according to the information provided by DNA. To under–stand this process, imagine proteins as various chains made from 20 different amino acid "beads." Figure 7.4 illustrates some of these beads and how they can be assembled into chains. Note that each bead has two metal wires that are used to link it with another bead. To make a copy of a particular beaded chain, you would follow directions for connecting the beads in a specific order and length by hooking the metal wires of each bead together. Consider the vast variety of beaded chains comprised of different bead sequences and chain lengths that you could make from just 20 different beads.

In living things, the beaded chains are proteins that contain amino acids. An amino acid can connect to another amino acid by a **peptide bond,** a chemi–cal attraction between the acid group of one amino acid and the amino group of another amino acid (Fig. 7.5). A **polypeptide** forms when two or more amino

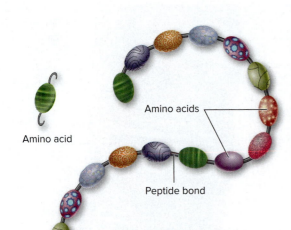

Amino acids

Amino acid

Peptide bond

Figure 7.4 **Amino acids form proteins.** Each type of bead represents a specific amino acid in human proteins. The "hook" that connects the beads represents a peptide bond.

acids join to form a chain (see Fig. 7.4). **Peptides** are small chains of amino acids that usually contain fewer than 15 amino acids. Dipeptides and tripeptides are compounds that consist of two and three amino acids, respectively. Most naturally occurring proteins are polypeptides comprised of 50 or more amino acids.

Figure 7.6 summarizes the basic steps of protein synthesis. Protein synthesis begins with DNA in the cell's nucleus. DNA is a twisted, two–stranded molecule referred to as a double helix. To begin the process, a section of the DNA double helix unwinds, exposing a gene. A **gene** is a portion of DNA that contains infor–mation concerning the order of amino acids that comprise a specific protein. *Mes–senger ribonucleic acid (mRNA)*, a compound that is chemically similar to DNA, is formed by *transcription* (see Fig. 7.6). The actual production of a protein occurs in the cytoplasm, so mRNA leaves the nucleus and moves to ribosomes—the protein–manufacturing sites in the cytoplasm. Ribosomes translate the gene's coded instructions for adding amino acids to the polypeptide chain. During this translation process, *transfer ribonucleic acid (tRNA)* conveys specific amino acids, one at a time, to the ribosomes. At the ribosomes, the amino acid from tRNA is added to the last amino acid, causing the peptide chain to grow longer. After the mRNA is read completely, the ribosome releases the polypeptide, and then the new protein gener–ally undergoes further processing at other sites within the cytoplasm.

Diets that contain low–quality protein can result in poor growth, slowed recov–ery from illness, and even death. These situations occur because protein synthesis

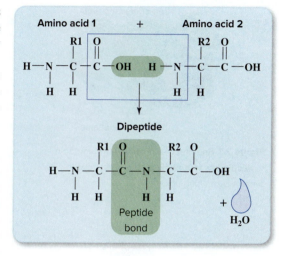

Figure 7.5 Peptide bond. A dipeptide forms when two amino acids bond and a molecule of water is released in the process.

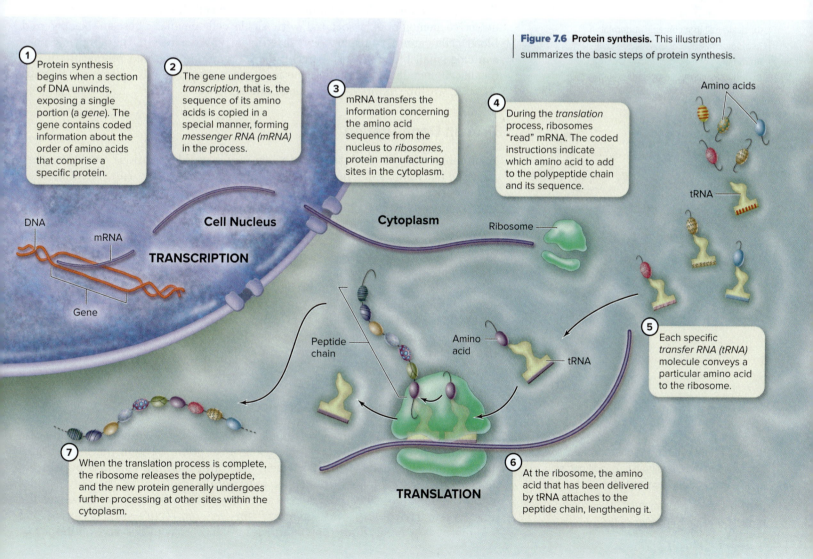

Figure 7.6 Protein synthesis. This illustration summarizes the basic steps of protein synthesis.

1 Protein synthesis begins when a section of DNA unwinds, exposing a single portion (a *gene*). The gene contains coded information about the order of amino acids that comprise a specific protein.

2 The gene undergoes *transcription,* that is, the sequence of its amino acids is copied in a special manner, forming *messenger RNA (mRNA)* in the process.

3 mRNA transfers the information concerning the amino acid sequence from the nucleus to *ribosomes,* protein manufacturing sites in the cytoplasm.

4 During the *translation* process, ribosomes "read" mRNA. The coded instructions indicate which amino acid to add to the polypeptide chain and its sequence.

5 Each specific *transfer RNA (tRNA)* molecule conveys a particular amino acid to the ribosome.

6 At the ribosome, the amino acid that has been delivered by tRNA attaches to the peptide chain, lengthening it.

7 When the translation process is complete, the ribosome releases the polypeptide, and the new protein generally undergoes further processing at other sites within the cytoplasm.

DNA

mRNA

Cell Nucleus

TRANSCRIPTION

Gene

Cytoplasm

Ribosome

Amino acids

tRNA

Peptide chain

Amino acid

tRNA

TRANSLATION

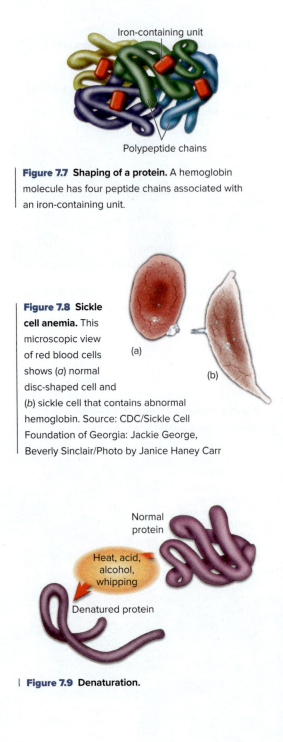

Figure 7.7 Shaping of a protein. A hemoglobin molecule has four peptide chains associated with an iron-containing unit.

Iron-containing unit

Polypeptide chains

Figure 7.8 Sickle cell anemia. This microscopic view of red blood cells shows (*a*) normal disc-shaped cell and (*b*) sickle cell that contains abnormal hemoglobin. Source: CDC/Sickle Cell Foundation of Georgia: Jackie George, Beverly Sinclair/Photo by Janice Haney Carr

(a)

(b)

Normal protein

Heat, acid, alcohol, whipping

Denatured protein

Figure 7.9 Denaturation.

in cells cannot proceed when the supply or "pool" of amino acids does not have one or more of the essential amino acids needed for constructing the polypeptide chain. When this happens, production of the protein stops. The partially made polypeptide chain is dismantled, and its amino acids are returned to the pool.

When assembly of the new protein has been completed, the polypeptide acid chain coils and folds into a three−dimensional shape that is characteristic of that particular protein. In some instances, more than one polypeptide chain curls around each other to form large protein complexes. For example, hemoglobin, a protein in red blood cells, is comprised of four polypeptide chains coiled together (Fig. 7.7). The shape of a protein is important because it influences the com−pound's activity in the body.

Occasionally, the wrong amino acid is introduced into the amino acid chain during the protein synthesis process. Cells usually check for such errors and replace the amino acid with the correct one. If the DNA code is faulty, however, the wrong amino acid will be inserted into the chain consistently, forming an abnormal polypeptide. Such errors often cause genetic defects that have dev−astating, even deadly, effects on the organism. *Sickle cell anemia*, for exam−ple, is an inherited disease characterized by abnormal hemoglobin. Cells in red bone marrow synthesize hemoglobin by following DNA instructions concerning proper amino acid sequencing. If the DNA codes for the insertion of the wrong amino acid in two of hemoglobin's four polypeptide chains, the resulting protein is defective and does not function correctly. Figure 7.8a shows a red blood cell that contains normal hemoglobin; the red blood cell shown in Figure 7.8b has the defective hemoglobin associated with sickle cell anemia. Crescent−shaped red blood cells cannot transport oxygen efficiently. As a result, the abnormal cells can clog small blood vessels, causing pain, organ damage, and premature death. Sickle cell anemia is a common genetic disorder that generally affects people with African, Caribbean, or Mediterranean ancestry.

Protein Denaturation

A protein undergoes **denaturation** when it is exposed to various conditions that alter the macronutrient's natural folded and coiled shape (Fig. 7.9). We often cook protein−rich foods to make them more digestible and safe to eat, but heat also causes the proteins in foods to unfold. The protein in raw egg white, for example, is almost clear and has a jellylike consistency. When you cook egg white, it becomes white and firm as its proteins become denatured. Other treatments often used during food preparation also denature proteins, including whipping or exposing them to alcohol or acid. Wine, for example, is often used in marinades because the alcohol it contains denatures proteins in meat, helping tenderize it. Adding acidic lemon juice to milk denatures ("curdles") the proteins in milk. In your stomach, hydrochloric acid denatures food proteins, making them easier to digest. Dena−turation does not "kill" a protein (because proteins are not living), but the process usually permanently alters the protein's shape and functions. Once an egg white has been cooked or milk has curdled, the food cannot return to its original state.

Protein Digestion and Absorption

When you eat oatmeal mixed with milk for breakfast, the large proteins in these foods must be digested before undergoing absorption. Protein digestion begins in the stomach, where hydrochloric acid denatures food proteins and **pepsin,** an enzyme, digests proteins into smaller polypeptides. Soon after the polypeptides enter the small intestine, the pancreas secretes protein−splitting enzymes, includ−ing trypsin (*trip'−sin*) and chymotrypsin (*ki'−mo−trip'−sin*). *Trypsin* and *chymotrypsin* break down polypeptides into shorter peptides and amino acids.

denaturation altering a protein's natural shape and function by exposing it to conditions such as heat, acids, and physical agitation

pepsin gastric enzyme that breaks down proteins into smaller polypeptides

Enzymes released by the absorptive cells of the small intestine break down most of the shortened peptides into dipeptides, tripeptides, and individual amino acids. Within the absorptive cells, di– and tripeptides are broken down into amino acids. Thus, amino acids are the end products of protein digestion. After being absorbed, the amino acids enter the hepatic portal vein and travel to the liver, where they may enter the general circulation.

By the time cells obtain amino acids from blood, they cannot distinguish the ones that were originally in oat proteins from those that were in milk proteins. The cells, however, now have all the amino acids they need to make human proteins. Protein digestion and absorption is very efficient: Very little dietary protein escapes digestion and is eliminated in feces. Figure 7.10 summarizes protein digestion and absorption.

Protein Turnover

Not all protein must be supplied by the diet. **Protein turnover,** the process of breaking down old or unneeded proteins into their component amino acids and recycling them to make new proteins, occurs constantly within cells. Amino acids that are not incorporated into proteins become part of a small amino acid pool, a readily available supply of amino acids that cells can use for future protein synthesis. The amino acid pool is an *endogenous*, or internal, source of nitrogen. The body obtains about two–thirds of its amino acid supply from endogenous sources and the remainder from *exogenous* (dietary) sources.

Did *YOU* Know?

Despite information provided in commercials or advertisements, you cannot "feed" your hair, nails, or skin by using shampoos, conditioners, or lotions containing proteins or other nutrients. Hair, nails, and the outermost layer of skin are not living. By eating a nutritious diet, you will provide your body with the nutrients it needs to make healthy hair, nails, and skin.

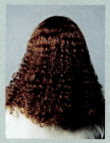

©McGraw-Hill Education/Joe DeGrandis, photographer

protein turnover cellular process of breaking down proteins and recycling their amino acids

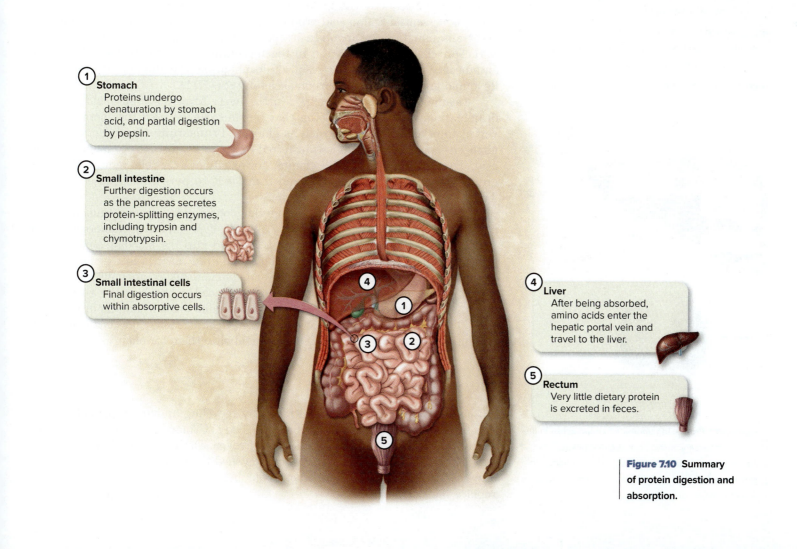

Figure 7.10 Summary of protein digestion and absorption.

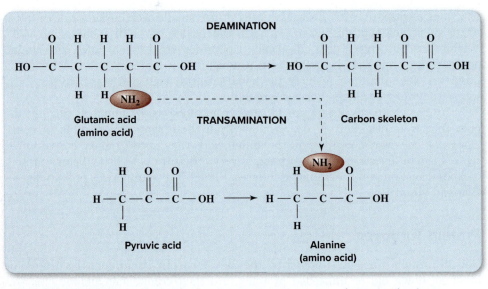

Figure 7.11 Deamination and transamination. Deamination is the process of removing the nitrogen-containing group from an unneeded amino acid. Transamination occurs when the nitrogen-containing group is transferred to another substance to make an amino acid.

Transamination and Deamination

A healthy human body can make 11 of the 20 amino acids. The liver is the main site of nonessential amino acid production. Chemical reactions called deamination and transamination are involved in the synthesis of amino acids. **Deamination** is the process of removing the nitrogen−containing group (usually NH_2) from an unneeded amino acid. As a result of deamination, the amino acid that gives up its amino group becomes a carbon skeleton (Fig. 7.11).

Deamination occurs primarily in the liver. After an amino acid undergoes deamination, the carbon skeleton that remains can be used for energy or con−verted to other compounds, such as glucose. **Transamination** occurs when the nitrogen−containing group is transferred to another substance to make an amino acid. To make the amino acid alanine, for example, liver cells remove the amino group (NH_2) from glutamic acid and transfer it to pyruvic acid (see Fig. 7.11). Transamination reactions are reversible.

Liver cells remove excess NH_2 from the bloodstream, forming ammonia (NH_3), a highly poisonous waste product (Fig. 7.12). The liver can use the ammonia to make **urea,** a metabolic waste product that is released into the bloodstream. The kid−neys filter urea, small amounts of ammonia, and *creatinine* (a nitrogen−containing waste produced by muscles) from blood and eliminate the compounds in urine.

If you consume more protein than you need, what happens to the extra amino acids? The body does not store excess amino acids in muscle or other tis−sues. The unnecessary amino acids undergo deamination, and cells convert the carbon skeletons into glucose or fat, or metabolize them for energy (see Fig. 7.12).

Nitrogen Balance

Although your body conserves nitrogen by recycling amino acids, each day you lose some protein and nitrogen from your body. Urinary elimination of urea and creatinine accounts for most of the lost nitrogen. Daily nitrogen losses also occur as your nails and hair grow, and when you shed the outermost layer of your skin and cells from your intestinal tract. Your body uses amino acids from foods to replace the lost nitrogen.

deamination removal of the nitrogen-containing group from an amino acid

transamination transfer of the nitrogen-containing group from an unneeded amino acid to a carbon skeleton to form an amino acid

urea waste product of amino acid metabolism

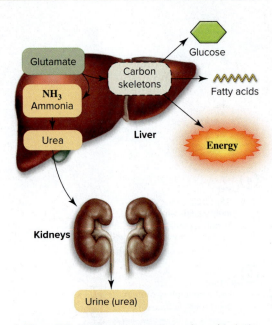

Figure 7.12 Processing unneeded amino acids. In the liver, unnecessary amino acids are deaminated, and the remaining carbon skeletons can be converted to glucose or fat, used to make nonessential amino acids, or metabolized for energy.

Normally, an adult's body maintains its protein content by maintaining **nitrogen balance (equilibrium),** that is, balancing nitrogen intake and protein turnover with losses. During certain stages of life or physical conditions, however, nitrogen intake and retention do not equal nitrogen losses. When the body is in a state of **positive nitrogen balance,** it retains more nitrogen than it loses as proteins are added to various tissues. In this case, a person must eat more protein to satisfy the increased need for the nutrient. Positive balance occurs during periods of rapid growth such as pregnancy, infancy, and puberty, and when people are recovering from illness or injury. Hormones such as insulin, growth hormone, and testosterone stimulate positive nitrogen balance. Performing weight (resistance) training also leads to nitrogen retention.[7] When the body is in a state of **negative nitrogen balance,** the body loses more nitrogen than it retains and protein intake is less than what the body needs. Negative balance occurs during starvation, serious illnesses, and severe injuries. Recovery from the illness or injury results in positive nitrogen balance until nitrogen equilibrium is restored. Figure 7.13 illustrates the concept of nitrogen balance and lists conditions that result in positive and negative nitrogen balance.

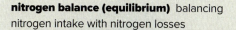

nitrogen balance (equilibrium) balancing nitrogen intake with nitrogen losses

positive nitrogen balance state in which the body retains more nitrogen than it loses

negative nitrogen balance state in which the body loses more nitrogen than it retains

How Much Protein Do You Need?

The Estimated Average Requirement (EAR) for protein is 0.66 g of protein/kg of body weight.[4] The EAR for protein increases during pregnancy, breastfeeding, periods of rapid growth, and recovery from serious illnesses, blood losses, and burns. Recall from Chapter 3 that scientists use EARs to establish Recommended Dietary Allowances (RDAs). A healthy adult's RDA for protein is 0.8 g/kg of body weight. By reviewing DRI tables (Appendix I), you will note that the RDAs for protein vary during certain ages and conditions.

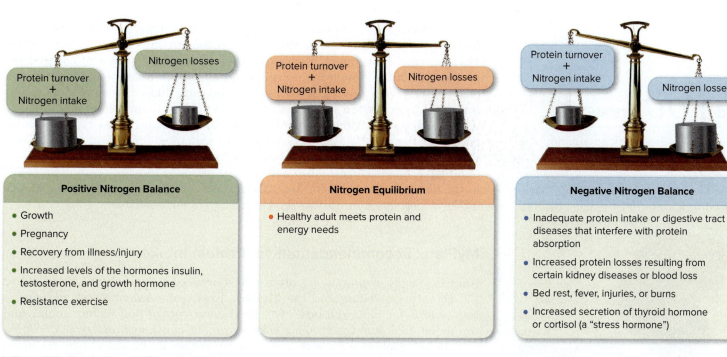

Positive Nitrogen Balance

- Growth
- Pregnancy
- Recovery from illness/injury
- Increased levels of the hormones insulin, testosterone, and growth hormone
- Resistance exercise

Nitrogen Equilibrium

- Healthy adult meets protein and energy needs

Negative Nitrogen Balance

- Inadequate protein intake or digestive tract diseases that interfere with protein absorption
- Increased protein losses resulting from certain kidney diseases or blood loss
- Bed rest, fever, injuries, or burns
- Increased secretion of thyroid hormone or cortisol (a "stress hormone")

Figure 7.13 Nitrogen balance. This diagram illustrates the concept of nitrogen balance and lists conditions that result in positive and negative nitrogen balance. Note that nitrogen balance occurs when nitrogen intake plus turnover equals nitrogen losses.

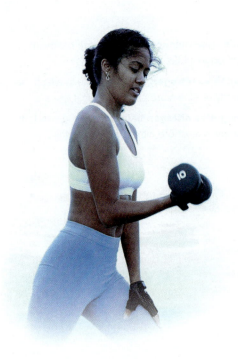

Resistance exercise can result in positive nitrogen balance.
©liquidllibrary/Getty Images RF

To determine your RDA for protein, multiply your weight in kilograms by 0.8 grams. If you are underweight or overweight, use a healthy weight for your height when making this calculation (see the body mass index chart in Chapter 10). For example, a healthy man who is 5−feet, 10−inches tall and weighs 75 kilograms (his weight in pounds divided by 2.2) should consume 60 grams of protein daily (75 kg × 0.8 g) to meet his RDA for the nutrient. The "Personal Dietary Analysis" at the end of this chapter can help you estimate your daily protein intake.

Concept CHECKPOINT

9. Explain the basic steps involved in protein synthesis.

10. Define *denaturation*, *deamination*, and *transamination*.

11. Describe conditions that can cause the body to be in negative nitrogen balance. Describe conditions in which the body is in positive nitrogen balance.

12. A healthy young woman weighs 143 pounds. Calculate her RDA for protein.

13. Explain what happens to proteins in beans as they undergo digestion and absorption in the human digestive tract.

See Appendix G for responses.

7.4 Protein Consumption Patterns

Learning Outcomes

1 Compare the percentage of calories that protein contributes in the typical American diet to the AMDR for protein.

2 Identify foods groups that contribute most of the protein in the typical American diet.

In 2013–2014, protein comprised 15.6% of adult Americans' average energy intake for a day.[8] For healthy adults, this level of consumption is within the Acceptable Macronutrient Distribution Range (AMDR), which is 10 to 35% of energy from protein.[4] In 2010, Americans generally ate about the same percentage of total daily calories from protein as they did in the early 1900s.[9] Americans, however, consumed more protein from meat, fish, and poultry than from grains. In 1909, grain products contributed approximately 37% of Americans' typical protein intake. At that time, meat, fish, and poultry accounted for 31% of the protein in the American diet. In 2010, grain products supplied only 20% of Americans' pro−tein intake, whereas meat, fish, and poultry provided most of the protein (43%) in the diet (Fig. 7.14).[9] As of May 2017, newer data concerning the population's intake of proteins from various food sources were not available.

MyPlate: Recommendations for Protein Intake

Animal sources of protein are often rich sources of saturated fat. According to the Dietary Guidelines and the MyPlate food plan, Americans should choose lean or low−fat meat and poultry.[10] The leanest cuts of beef include round, and top round, loin, and top sirloin steaks, as well as chuck and arm roasts.

Before cooking a piece of beef, you can reduce its fat content by trimming the visible fat away from the meat. When buying ground beef, consider choosing "extra lean" products. The label on a package of extra lean ground beef should state that the meat is at least 95% lean. When cooked, extra lean ground beef can

Did *YOU* Know?

Humans use nearly every part of an animal for food. "Meat" is muscle tissue; "tripe" is from the stomach of cattle; "prairie or Rocky Mountain oysters," "lamb or calf fries," and *huevos del toro* are testicles of male sheep or cattle; and "sweetbreads" are the thymus glands of calves and lambs. In some cultures, people even consume the tongues, brains, and blood of certain animals.

©Wendy Schiff

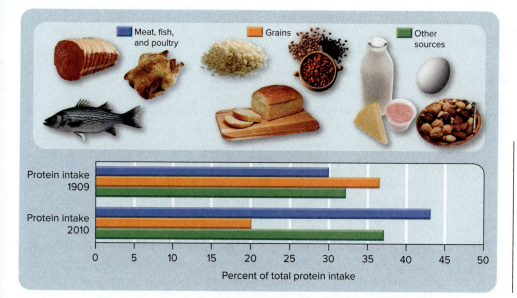

Figure 7.14 Protein consumption patterns. In 2010, Americans ate more protein from meat, fish, and poultry than they did in the early 1900s.

Roast: ©Ryan McVay/Stockbyte/Getty Images RF; Fish: ©Davies & Starr/Photodisc/Getty Images RF; Chicken: ©Louis Hiemstra/ Getty Images RF; Rice: ©McGraw-Hill Education/Jacques Cornell, photographer; Bread and Nuts: ©C Squared Studios/ Getty Images RF; Beans: ©Brand X Pictures/Getty Images RF; Dairy foods: ©Stockbyte/Getty Images RF; Egg: ©Siede Preis/ Getty Images RF

taste "dry." You can improve the taste of the beef by adding a small amount of "heart healthy" olive oil to the raw meat before shaping it into hamburger pat—ties. The leanest cuts of pork include pork loin, tenderloin, and center loin.

You can choose lean turkey, roast beef, or low—fat luncheon meats for sandwiches, instead of processed meat products. Processed meat products, such as ham, bacon, sausage, frankfurters, and bologna and salami, generally contain a lot of saturated fat, and they also have high amounts of added sodium. Excessive sodium intakes are associated with increased risk of hypertension. If you decide to purchase processed meats, check the Nutrition Facts panels on products' labels to compare fat as well as sodium contents.

The MyPlate plan also recommends varying your protein choices. For exam—ple, consider eating fish that are rich sources of beneficial omega—3 fatty acids, such as salmon, trout, and herring. You can also replace main menu items that contain meat with dishes made with dry beans, split peas, or foods made from soybeans. Additionally, consider snacking on nuts, such as peanuts, almonds, cashews, walnuts, and pecans, instead of pieces of meat or cheese.

Concept CHECKPOINT

14. What is the AMDR for adult protein intake?

15. Describe how Americans' food sources of protein have changed since the early 1900s.

16. Consider your usual food choices. Using the recommendations of the MyPlate food guide, discuss ways you can reduce your intake of protein from animal foods.

See Appendix G for responses.

Ham, bacon, sausage, frankfurters, and deli meats generally contain high amounts of saturated fat and sodium. Source: Scott Bauer/ARS/USDA

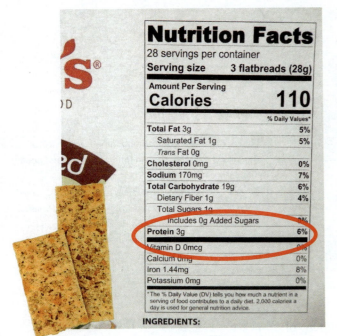

7.5 Understanding Nutritional Labeling: Protein

Learning Outcomes

1 Explain how to use the Nutrition Facts panel to determine the grams of protein in a serving of a packaged food.

2 Explain how you can use the ingredient list on a food label to determine the quality of the protein in the product.

You can determine how much protein is in a packaged food product by reading the Nutrition Facts panel on the label. As you can see in Figure 7.15, one serving of these crackers contains 3 g of protein. The FDA does not require food manufacturers to include information about the % Daily Value for protein when the food is intended for adult consumption. However, the manufacturer has to display the %DV for protein when the label has a claim about the product's protein contents. Most Americans consume plenty of protein, so protein intake is not a public health concern. The Daily Value for protein (adults) is 50 g. The panel does not provide information about a product's protein quality, but you can judge from the list of ingredients.

Concept CHECKPOINT

17. According to the Nutrition Facts panel on a food package, a serving of the food supplies 5 g of protein. Using the information provided in this section, calculate the %DV of protein for the product.

See Appendix G for responses.

7.6 Proteins: Economical Considerations

Learning Outcomes

1 Describe ways people can reduce the amount of meat in their diet without sacrificing protein quality.

2 Explain how using mixtures of foods with complementary proteins can help reduce animal protein intake.

If you are like most Americans, your daily protein intake is higher than the RDA. Furthermore, animal foods contribute the largest share of the protein in your diet. In fact, animal foods, including eggs and milk products, supply almost two-thirds of the protein in the American diet.[9] Some of these foods, however, are among the most expensive items on our grocery lists, and you may be able to reduce your food costs if you eat less of them. Furthermore, you may reap substantial health benefits by reducing your animal protein intake and increasing your consumption of plant foods.

Animal foods are among the best dietary sources of essential amino acids, so is it safe to eat less animal protein? Yes! One way you can lower your intake is to include only one animal source of protein in a meal and reduce its serving size. For example, if your breakfast is a 6-ounce slice of ham with two large fried eggs, you are obtaining over 400 kcal and 42 g of high−quality protein. That is enough protein in one meal to meet the RDA for a person who weighs 116 pounds. Instead of eating such a large serving of ham with the fried eggs, have 3 ounces of ham without the eggs, or skip the ham and eat just the eggs. Two fried eggs supply over 12 g of high−quality protein and only 190 kcal.

An easy way to reduce your meat consumption is to replace meat with other high−quality protein sources. Eggs, milk, cheese, and yogurt are animal sources of high−quality protein that you can substitute for meat, fish, or poultry items in your diet. For example, simply have a cheese sandwich instead of eating a submarine sandwich made with various luncheon meats and cheeses. If you are interested in eating less fat, a serving of low−fat cottage cheese or low−fat yogurt makes a protein−rich substitute for the "sub" or cheese sandwich.

Another way to reduce the amount of animal food in your diet and your food costs is to make meals that contain less animal protein and more plant protein. Many commonly eaten menu items provide the proper amounts and mixtures of essential amino acids without relying heavily on animal products. Throughout the world, people with limited access to meat and other animal foods rely heavily on recipes that combine small amounts of animal protein with larger portions of certain plant proteins. Proteins in animal foods contain enough essential amino acids to extend or "beef up" the lower−quality plant proteins in dried peas, mature beans, cereals, and other grain products. Pasta made from white flour, for example, contains cereal (wheat) proteins that have limiting amounts of lysine. By mixing large amounts of cooked pasta with smaller amounts of lysine−rich meat, seafood, chicken, or cheese, the proteins in the animal foods enhance the quality of the wheat proteins. As a result, the body can use the amino acids in pasta for growth, repair, and maintenance of tissues.

Pancakes, waffles, crepes, and cornflakes with milk are examples of break−fast foods that extend egg and milk proteins with large amounts of cereal pro−teins. Many popular Asian dishes mix small amounts of chicken, beef, or seafood with large portions of rice; Italian dishes often combine pasta with small amounts of cheese or meat sauce. Serving meals that extend the high−quality protein in animal foods is an economical way to feed large numbers of people. For example, you can use 1 pound of ground meat to make a single hamburger for each of your four friends. However, you will have enough chili con carne to feed six or more friends if you combine that pound of ground meat with three cans of kidney beans and a couple of large cans of tomatoes. The ground meat has plenty of cysteine and methionine, the essential amino acids that are low in kidney beans. By mixing plant and animal sources of protein together in chili con carne, the beef protein extends the quality of the protein in the kidney beans. Although the chili recipe calls for adding tomatoes to the meat and beans, tomatoes are botanically classified as fruit, so they add very little protein to the dish. (Imagine eating chili con carne without tomatoes!) If you want to extend the chili even more, add cooked macaroni to the mixture. Macaroni is made from wheat, so it contains cereal proteins that are enhanced by the proteins in the meat and beans. For more practical ways to "stretch" your food dollars without sacrificing the nutritional quality of your diet, read the "Nutrition Matters" at the end of this chapter.

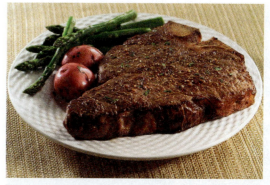
Animal foods are among the most expensive items on our grocery lists. ©Getty Images RF

Food & Nutrition tips

Commercially canned beans often have considerable amounts of salt added to them. Consider purchasing canned or frozen beans that have little or no added salt. Dried beans do not have salt added to them, but they take a long time to cook, unless you soak them for several hours before cooking. The soaking process softens the beans, reducing cooking time and making them more digestible and less likely to contribute to intestinal gas.

Combining Complementary Proteins

Although it is not necessary to consume all essential amino acids during a meal for the body to utilize them for growth, certain plant−based recipes ensure that these compounds are consumed during a day. **Complementary combinations**

complementary combinations mixing certain plant foods to provide all essential amino acids without adding animal protein

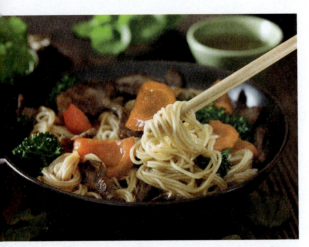

Traditional Asian dishes, such as beef stir-fry, combine small amounts of animal protein with larger amounts of cereal and vegetable proteins. ©cobraphotography/Shutterstock RF

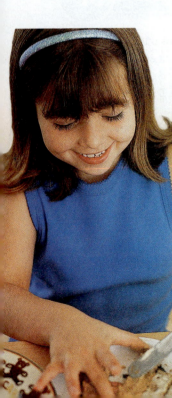

Peanut butter on bread provides complementary plant proteins. ©Daniel Pangbourne/Photodisc/Getty Images RF

are mixtures of certain plant foods that provide all essential amino acids without adding animal proteins. However, to make dishes that contain complementary amino acid combinations, you must know which plant foods are good protein sources and which essential amino acids are limiting or low in those plant foods. Most plant foods are poor sources of one or more essential amino acids, particularly tryptophan, threonine, lysine, and methionine. Split peas, for example, are good sources of lysine, but they contain low amounts of tryptophan and methionine. Cereal grains such as wheat, rice, and corn are good sources of tryptophan and methionine, but they tend to be low in lysine. Wheat germ, however, is a rich source of lysine. Legumes are low in methionine. Seeds such as sesame and sunflower seeds are generally low in lysine. Walnuts, cashews, almonds, and other tree nuts also contain low amounts of lysine. Although most fruits and some kinds of vegetables are poor sources of protein, they add appealing colors and textures as well as vitamins, minerals, and phytochemicals to plant–based meals.

Many cultures have traditional foods that combine complementary plant proteins. For example, a peanut butter sandwich combines two foods that supply complementary plant proteins. Peanuts are a fair source of lysine. Bread contains some methionine, but the grain product is very low in lysine. Serving the two foods together as a peanut butter sandwich provides adequate amounts of these essential amino acids. Table 7.4 lists some other foods that are examples of complementary protein combinations. When menu planning, you can combine a variety of legumes, grains, tree nuts, and seeds with vegetables to prepare dishes that provide adequate mixtures of the essential amino acids. Figure 7.16 shows three categories of plant proteins (legumes, grains, and tree nuts and seeds) that make complementary combinations when legumes are mixed with grains, seeds, and/or tree nuts.

Not every mixture of plant foods creates a complementary combination. For example, making a fruit salad by combining apples, grapes, and oranges will not provide a complementary mixture of essential amino acids. Fruits are nutritious foods, but they are generally poor sources of protein. Combining Boston, iceberg, and romaine varieties of lettuce with carrots and onions makes a tasty salad, but simply mixing leafy greens with other vegetables does not make a complementary combination because vegetables have small amounts of protein that tend to contain low amounts of essential amino acids. However, adding sunflower seed kernels, kidney or black beans, cashews, and bread cubes to the salad boosts the amount of protein and provides a complete mix of amino acids. To increase the

TABLE 7.4 Complementary Protein Dishes

Red beans and rice
Peanut or soy nut butter on bagel, sprinkled with wheat germ
Hummus (mashed chickpeas/garbanzo beans) with sesame seeds
Hummus on whole-grain pita bread
Black beans and cornmeal tortilla
Split pea soup with toasted whole-wheat bread
Meatless kidney bean chili with macaroni
Cornmeal tortilla with black bean salsa
Peanut butter on whole-grain crackers, sprinkled with wheat germ
Tofu with brown rice and cashews

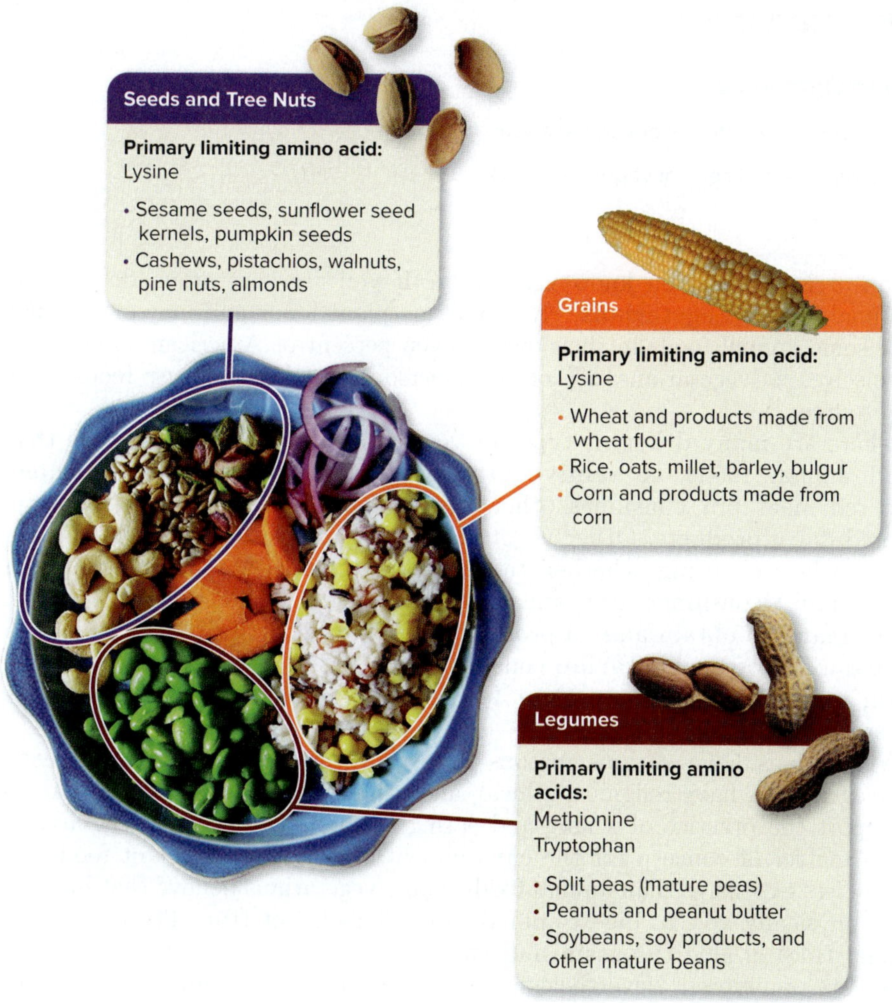

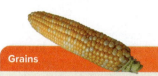

Seeds and Tree Nuts

Primary limiting amino acid:
Lysine

• Sesame seeds, sunflower seed kernels, pumpkin seeds
• Cashews, pistachios, walnuts, pine nuts, almonds

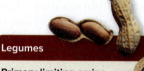

Grains

Primary limiting amino acid:
Lysine

• Wheat and products made from wheat flour
• Rice, oats, millet, barley, bulgur
• Corn and products made from corn

Legumes

Primary limiting amino acids:
Methionine
Tryptophan

• Split peas (mature peas)
• Peanuts and peanut butter
• Soybeans, soy products, and other mature beans

Figure 7.16 Complementary combinations. To ensure an adequate mix of amino acids, combine legumes with grains, seeds, and/or tree nuts.

Plate of foods and Corn: ©Wendy Schiff; Pistachios and Peanuts: ©C Squared Studios/Getty Images RF

essential amino acid content of the salad even further, you can add a small amount of hard–cooked egg, shredded cheese, or bits of *tofu*, a soybean product, to it. If you are interested in trying foods made from soybeans, the "Food & Nutrition Tips" feature on this page provides information about some of the more popular foods made from soybeans.

Food & Nutrition tips

The following information describes popular soybean foods and tips for how to use them in menu planning.

• Plain tofu has little flavor, so it can be added to a variety of foods, including stir-fried vegetables and scrambled eggs.

• Tempeh is a fermented soybean and grain mixture that can substitute for meat in sandwiches and casseroles.

• Soy nuts are roasted soybeans that are often eaten as a snack. Ground soy nuts form a spread that is used like peanut butter.

• Soy milk is made from crushed soybeans. Soy milk is usually fortified with calcium and vitamins A, D, B-12, and riboflavin. Regular soy milk can substitute for cow's milk as a beverage or in recipes. Soy milk cheeses and yogurt are also available.

• Texturized soy protein (TSP) is made from soybean flour. A TSP product that resembles ground beef can be used to replace half or all of the ground beef in meatloaf, meatball, chili, taco, or meat sauce recipes.

• Soy protein concentrate is a high-protein, high-fiber refined soybean product that is used to boost the protein content of foods.

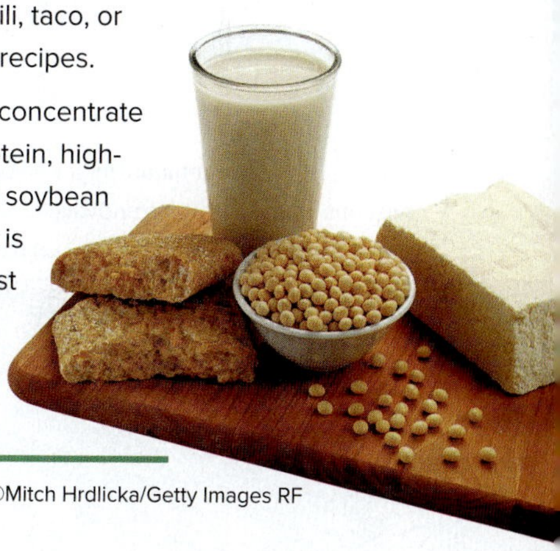

©Mitch Hrdlicka/Getty Images RF

Concept CHECKPOINT

18. Give examples of common foods that are high-quality substitutes for meat and foods that extend a source of high-quality protein.

19. Does a recipe that combines apples and oranges with peanuts provide a complementary mixture of proteins? Explain why or why not.

20. A recipe mixes cereals made from wheat, rice, and corn. What plant foods could you add to this combination of cereals to make the recipe a source of high-quality protein?

See Appendix G for responses.

7.7 Vegetarianism

Learning Outcomes

 1 Describe different forms of vegetarianism.

2 Discuss pros and cons of vegetarian diets.

vegetarians people who eat plant-based diets

semivegetarian (or flexitarian) vegetarian who eats animal products, except red meat

lactovegetarian vegetarian who consumes milk and milk products for animal protein

ovovegetarian vegetarian who eats eggs for animal protein

lactoovovegetarian vegetarian who consumes milk products and eggs for animal protein

vegan vegetarian who eats only plant foods

Are you or is anyone you know vegetarian? If you are vegetarian, do you eat any animal foods? **Vegetarians** rely heavily on plant foods and may or may not include some animal foods in their diets. Seven percent of American adults refer to themselves as vegetarians; 2% of these persons avoid eating any foods from animal sources.[11]

There are many different types of vegetarian diets, including some that contain animal foods. A **semivegetarian** (or **flexitarian**), for example, avoids red meat but consumes other animal foods, including fish, poultry, eggs, and dairy products. Other vegetarians have more restrictive diets, particularly when choosing whether to eat animal foods. A **lactovegetarian** (*lacto* = milk) consumes milk and milk products, including yogurt, cheese, and ice cream, to obtain animal protein. An **ovovegetarian** (*ovo* = egg) eats eggs, and a **lactoovovegetarian** consumes milk products and eggs. A **vegan,** or total vegetarian, eats only plant foods. Table 7.5 lists types of vegetarian diets.

Vegetarians have various reasons for eating few or no animal products. Many vegetarians have religious, ethical, and other philosophical beliefs that do not support the practice of killing and eating animals. For others, vegetarianism is a matter of concern for the environment and economics; plant foods are generally less expensive than animal foods. Some vegetarians believe that humans are not physically able to digest animal foods. This is not true. The omnivore's intestinal tract is able to obtain nutrients from both plants and animals, and humans are omnivores. Nevertheless, eating more plant than animal sources of protein may provide important health benefits.

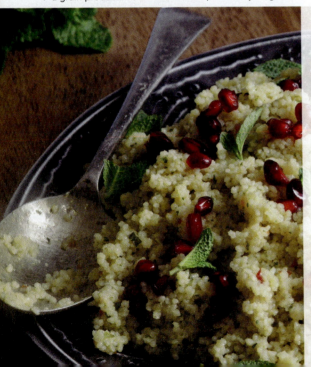

A vegan, or total vegetarian, might enjoy this dish: couscous with vegetables and chickpeas. Couscous is a grain product. ©martinturzak/iStockphoto/Getty Images RF

TABLE 7.5 Types of Vegetarian Diets

Type of Vegetarian Diet	Animal Foods Included
Semivegetarian (flexitarian)	All except red meats
Lactovegetarian	Milk and milk products No animal flesh or eggs
Ovovegetarian	Eggs but no other animal foods
Lactoovovegetarian	Milk and milk products and eggs but no other animal foods
Vegan	No animal foods
Fruitarian	No animal foods (nuts and seeds only)
Macrobiotic	No animal foods (will eat organically grown whole grains, fruits and vegetables, and soups made with vegetables, seaweed, grains, beans, and miso)

Is Vegetarianism a Healthy Lifestyle?

Vegetarian diets are often lower in saturated fat and energy than "Western" diets that contain animal foods, particularly plenty of red meat. Compared to people who eat meat, vegetarians tend to have a lower risk of obesity, type 2 diabetes, hypertension, and certain cancers.[12] Furthermore, vegans tend to be leaner than nonvegans. It is difficult, however, to pinpoint diet as responsible for vegetarians' health status. Why? Vegetarians often adopt other healthy lifestyle practices, such as exercising regularly; practicing relaxation activities, such as meditation; and avoiding tobacco products and excess alcohol.

Compared to the typical American diet, vegetarian diets provide more fiber, soy protein, folate (a B vitamin), beta–carotene (a phytochemical that the body can convert to vitamin A), vitamins E and C, and the minerals potassium and magnesium.[13] Furthermore, vegetarian diets often supply less saturated fat and cholesterol than diets that include animal foods.

Poorly planned, plant–based diets may not contain enough vitamins B–12 and D, minerals iron and calcium, and omega–3 fatty acids to meet a person's nutritional needs.[12] Plant foods contain little or no vitamin B–12, and there are few dietary sources of vitamin D other than fortified cow's milk. Furthermore, mineral nutrients such as calcium and iron are more available from animal than from plant foods. Plants often contain phytochemicals that interfere with the body's absorption of minerals, particularly iron, zinc, and calcium. Recall from Chapter 6 that the body is unable to make much DHA and EPA from alpha–linolenic acid, an essential omega–3 fatty acid.

Vegetarians who do not consume fish may need to obtain DHA and EPA by eating certain algae or taking dietary supplements that contain the algae. Vegans can obtain vitamin B–12, vitamin D, iron, zinc, and several other micronutrients by consuming fortified foods such many brands of ready–to–eat cereal, soy and rice beverages, and Red Star® vegetarian nutritional yeast. Vegetarians can also take a daily multiple vitamin/mineral supplement to provide dietary "insurance."

Humans digest animal proteins to a greater extent than plant proteins.[14] Therefore, vegetarians may need to increase their protein intakes. Total vegetarians, including vegan athletes, can obtain adequate amounts of the essential amino acids by eating quinoa, processed soybean products, and foods that combine complementary plant proteins.

In general, plant foods have low energy density: They add bulk to the diet without adding a lot of calories. Children have higher protein and energy needs per pound of body weight than adults. Because plant foods add bulk to the diet, vegan children are likely to eat far less food than adult vegans because they become full sooner during meals. Thus, very young vegans may be unable to eat enough plant foods to meet their protein, micronutrient, and energy needs.

Therefore, it is very important for parents or other caretakers to plan nutritionally adequate diets for vegetarian children and monitor the youngsters' growth rates.

Vegan women who breastfeed their infants may produce milk that is deficient in vitamin B–12, particularly if the mothers' diets lack the vitamin. These infants of vegan mothers have a high risk of developing severe developmental delays associated with neurological damage, especially when breast milk is their only source of vitamin B–12.[15] Pregnant vegan women should consult with their physicians about the need to take a vitamin B–12 supplement to reduce the likelihood of having a baby who is deficient in this nutrient. Additionally, vegan mothers who breastfeed their infants may need to provide the babies with a source of vitamin B–12 as well. Table 7.6 summarizes the nutritional advantages and possible nutritional disadvantages of vegetarian diets.

MY DIVERSE PLATE

MyPlate: Source: U.S. Dept. of Agriculture

Miso

Miso, a seasoning paste made from fermented soybeans, is a staple of traditional Japanese diets. Miso is added to soup (misoshiru) and vegetables. Two tablespoons of miso supply about 70 kcal, 4 g protein, 2 g fat, and 1280 mg sodium. Although miso adds flavor to foods, the paste is very salty; therefore, it should be used in small amounts.

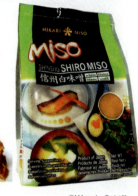

©Wendy Schiff

Did *YOU* Know?

There is nothing inherently "bad" about eating small portions of red meat. Red meat is a good source of zinc and iron, minerals that are often less bioavailable from plant foods.

TABLE 7.6 Vegetarian Diets: Nutritional Aspects

Advantages	Possible Disadvantages
High in: Vitamins C, E, and folate	**Low in:** Vitamins B-12 and D
Beta-carotene	Iron, zinc, and calcium
Fiber	Omega-3 fatty acids
Magnesium and potassium	Certain essential amino acids (children)
Low in: Fat (saturated)	Energy (children)
Cholesterol	

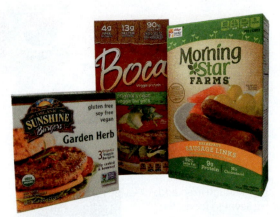

Commercially prepared vegetarian foods, such as these products, are often available in the frozen food section of supermarkets. ©Wendy Schiff

Switching from the typical Western diet to vegetarianism can be a healthy practice for teens; vegetarian youth often eat more fruits and vegetables and less fat than their nonvegetarian peers. On the other hand, female vegetarian teenagers may have a higher risk of unhealthy weight control practices and eating disorders, such as *anorexia nervosa*, than young people who eat meat.[16] Anorexia nervosa ("anorexia") is a serious psychological disorder that can result in starvation and suicide. The Chapter 10 "Nutrition Matters" provides more information about anorexia nervosa and other eating disorders.

Meatless Menu Planning

Many common menu items can be converted into vegetarian foods by removing the meat, fish, or poultry. For example, pizza and lasagna can be prepared without meat and still provide plenty of protein from the cheese as well as the crust or pasta. Stir—fried foods can also be a reliable source of protein without adding meat, fish, or poultry. To stir—fry, heat a small amount of peanut or canola oil in a frying pan and add cooked rice and pieces of raw vegetables. While the mixture is heating, add a beaten egg to it and stir so the egg cooks thoroughly. Before serving the dish, sprinkle cashews or sunflower seed kernels over the hot rice and vegetable mixture. Table 7.7 presents more meatless menu suggestions.

Commercially prepared vegetarian foods that substitute for meat, fish, and poultry items are often available in the frozen food section of supermarkets. These vegetarian products can look and taste like their nonvegetarian counterparts, but they generally do not contain cholesterol and may be lower in saturated fat. Such foods include soy—based sausage patties or links, soy hot dogs, "veggie" burgers, and soy "crumbles" that look like bits of cooked ground beef. Asian restaurants usually offer vegetarian dishes. Some "Western—style" restaurants offer vegetarian menu items, or their cooks can modify menu items by substituting meatless sauces, omitting meat from stir—fries, and adding vegetables or pasta in place of meat.

With careful planning, vegetarians can overcome the nutritional limitations of a plant—based diet and consume adequate diets. If you are interested in learning more specific details about vegetarian cookery and menu planning, contact a registered dietitian nutritionist (RDN) or university extension nutritionist in your area. The MyPlate website also offers suggestions for planning nutritionally adequate meatless meals. For more information, visit https://www.choosemyplate.gov/tips—vegetarians.

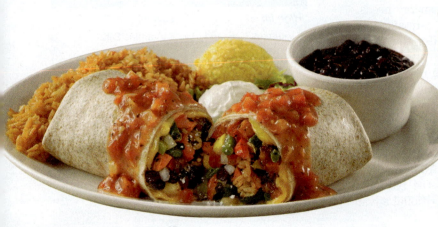

©John E. Kelly/Getty Images RF

TABLE 7.7 Meatless Menu Ideas

- Cooked pasta with marinara sauce and grated Parmesan or part-skim mozzarella cheese

- Vegetable lasagna with layers of cheese, thinly sliced zucchini, mushrooms, and bell peppers

- Vegetable stir-fry with bits of tofu and cheese

- Grilled vegetable kabobs served over cooked rice and black beans

- Black or red bean burritos

- Red bean and corn tacos

Concept CHECKPOINT

21. Describe how the diets of semivegetarians differ from other vegetarian diets.
22. Identify nutrients that are most likely lacking in a vegan's diet.
23. Explain why vegans must be careful when planning vegan meals for children.

See Appendix G for responses.

7.8 Protein Adequacy

Learning Outcomes

1 Discuss potential health problems that may occur with excessive protein intake.

2 Explain why protein-energy malnutrition is a serious nutritional state, especially for young children.

If some protein is necessary for proper growth and good health, can eating extra amounts of the nutrient make you *extra* healthy or physically fit? Intuitively, the idea of eating more protein to improve your health seems logical, but protein is no different from the other nutrients. If your diet contains adequate amounts of protein, then eating "more is not better."

In many parts of the world, the lack of foods containing high–quality proteins is a serious problem, particularly for young children. Protein deficiency interferes with a child's normal growth and development, and contributes to many childhood deaths. The following sections examine protein malnutrition.

Excessive Protein Intake

Heart disease and cancer are the leading causes of death in developed countries, including the United States. In these nations, the typical Western diet that contains high amounts of red or processed meats is associated with increased risk of certain chronic diseases, particularly heart disease[17] and colorectal cancer.[18,19] Consumption of red meat and processed meats, such as sausage, may increase the risk of pan–creatic cancer;[20] processed, smoked, and/or salted meats or fish increase the risk of stomach cancer.[21] More research, however, is needed to clarify the role of high–protein diets in the risk of certain cancers.

High–protein diets are generally not recommended for healthy people. Excess intakes of dietary protein may lead to higher–than–normal urinary losses of calcium. However, scientists do not agree on whether the loss of calcium con–tributes to poor bone health.[22,23]

Protein–rich foods from animals, especially liver, eggs, meat, and certain fish, are rich sources of **purines**, nitrogen–containing chemicals that comprise genetic material, including DNA. The liver breaks down purines to form uric acid. Healthy kidneys remove uric acid from the bloodstream and excrete the waste product in urine. A diet that is high in animal proteins may increase the level of uric acid in the bloodstream and urine. *Gout* is a type of arthritis that can develop in people who have elevated blood levels of uric acid. The condi–tion is characterized by the buildup of uric acid crystals in joints, especially in the foot and big toe. Medication is used to treat gout. Having an excess of uric acid in urine can contribute to the formation of kidney stones. Thus, people who have a history of kidney stones, have kidney disease, or are at risk of kidney disease should check with their physician before eating a high–protein diet.[24]

MY DIVERSE PLATE

MyPlate: Source: U.S. Dept. of Agriculture

Locusts

In parts of Africa, Cambodia, and the Philippines, many people eat locusts, especially when the insects are plentiful. Popular ways to cook locusts include removing the wings and legs before frying with seasonings or placing locusts on skewers and roasting them over hot embers. The legs and wings are removed from the grilled insects before they are cooked or eaten. Over 60% of the dry weight of a locust is protein, so the insect is an excellent source of the macronutrient.

Source: Food and Agricultural Organization, http://www.fao.org/ag/locusts/en/info/info/faq/.

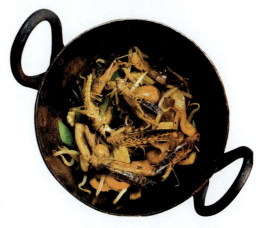

©IT Stock/Alamy RF

purines nitrogen-containing chemicals in genetic material

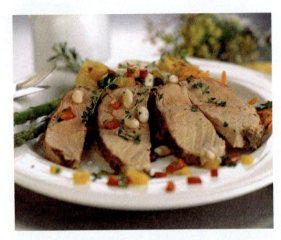

Some weight-loss diets promote large servings of protein-rich foods. ©Ingram Publishing/SuperStock RF

Excess amino acid or protein intake can lead to dehydration, because the kidneys need more water to dilute and eliminate the toxic waste products of amino acid metabolism in urine. Dehydration is a potentially life−threatening condition in which the body's water level is too low. People with liver or kidney diseases may need to avoid protein−rich diets and amino acid supplements because metabolizing the excess amino acids is a burden to their bodies.

What About High-Protein Weight-Loss Diets?

Certain popular weight−loss diets, such as the Atkins, Protein Power, and Paleo diets, promote high intakes of protein. While following high−protein diets to lose weight, people often report decreased feelings of hunger and increased sense of fullness (satiety) after meals. High−protein diets that limit total calorie intake appear to promote the loss of excess body fat and have other beneficial effects on health. Such diets, however, are often difficult for people to maintain for long periods.[25] Chapter 10 provides information about the safety and effectiveness of various popular weight−loss diets.

What About Protein or Amino Acid Supplements?

For thousands of years, humans have obtained amino acids by eating plants and animals. The use of amino acid and protein supplements as sources of the nutrient is a relatively recent development, and little is known about the long−term safety of using these products. Chapter 11 provides more information about protein needs of physically active people and examines the evidence concerning the value and safety of using certain foods and dietary supplements to enhance physical performance.

Protein Deficiency

Although food insecurity exists in the United States, protein deficiency is uncommon. (See the Chapter 1 "Nutrition Matters" for information about food insecurity.) People suffering from alcoholism, anorexia nervosa, or certain intestinal tract disorders are at risk of protein undernutrition. People with low incomes, especially those who are elderly, are also at risk of protein deficiency. Many elderly Americans have limited incomes and must make difficult choices concerning their expenses. If you were old, chronically ill, and on a low fixed income, what would you think was more important: purchasing nutritious foods or costly prescription medications that control your serious health problems?

Protein Energy Malnutrition

protein-energy malnutrition (PEM) condition that results from diets that provide inadequate amounts of protein and energy

As mentioned in Chapter 1, the lack of food is often widespread in poor nations in which populations endure frequent famine resulting from crop failures, political unrest, or civil wars. In these countries, **protein−energy malnutrition (PEM)** affects people whose diets lack sufficient protein as well as energy. The failure to consume nourishing food also results in vitamin and mineral deficiencies.

When food is limited, it is often more difficult for children to obtain nutritionally adequate diets than for adults to do so. Why? Adults may be able to consume enough plant proteins to meet their protein and energy needs, but children have smaller stomachs and higher energy and protein needs per pound of body weight than adults. They are unable to eat enough plant foods to meet their relatively high protein and other nutrient requirements.

In children, being underweight is often a sign of PEM. According to the World Health Organization (WHO), 50 million children were underweight throughout the world in 2014.[26] Children whose diets lack sufficient protein and energy do not grow and are very weak, irritable, and vulnerable to dehydration and infections, such as measles, that can kill them. If these children survive, their growth may be permanently stunted and their intelligence may be lower than normal because undernutrition during early childhood can cause permanent brain damage.

Forms of PEM At one time, nutrition experts thought there were only two types of PEM, **kwashiorkor** and **marasmus.** The distinctions between these conditions, however, are often blurred because protein deficiency is unlikely when a person's energy intake is adequate. Nevertheless, registered dietitian nutritionists generally consider *kwashiorkor, marasmic kwashiorkor,* and *marasmus* as forms of PEM.

Kwashiorkor (*qwash'−e−or'−kor*) primarily occurs in developing countries where mothers commonly breast-feed their infants until they give birth to another child. The older youngster, who is usually a toddler, is fairly healthy until abruptly weaned from his or her mother's milk to make way for the younger sibling. Although the toddler may obtain adequate energy by consuming a traditional diet of cereal grains, the diet lacks enough complete protein to meet the youngster's high needs, and he or she soon develops signs of protein deficiency. Children affected by kwashiorkor have stunted growth (see Fig. 1.15); unnaturally blond, sparse, and brittle hair; and patches of skin that have lost their normal coloration. Children with kwashiorkor have some subcutaneous (under the skin) fat and swollen cheeks, arms, legs, and bellies that make them look well fed, but their appearance is misleading. An important function of certain proteins in blood is to maintain proper fluid balance within cells and blood vessels, as well as between cells. During starvation, levels of these proteins decline, resulting in edema, which can make the protein−deficient child look plump and over−fed instead of thin and undernourished. In many cases, the child suffering from kwashiorkor does not obtain enough energy and eventually develops marasmic kwashiorkor, a condition characterized by edema and wasting (Fig. 7.17). *Wasting* is the loss of organ and muscle proteins as the body tears down these tissues to obtain amino acids for energy metabolism.

Severe PEM causes extreme weight loss and a condition called marasmus (*mah−raz'−mus*), which is commonly referred to as starvation (Fig. 7.18). Obvious

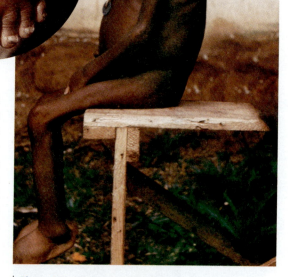

Figure 7.17 Marasmic kwashiorkor. This Nigerian child is suffering from marasmic kwashiorkor. Note the edema in the child's abdomen and feet. The inset photo shows "pitting" edema—swollen tissues that become deformed when pressed with a finger. These photos were taken during the Nigerian civil war that occurred in the late 1960s. Source: Centers for Disease Control and Prevention/Dr. Lyle Conrad

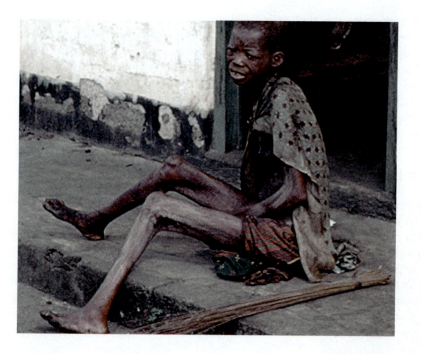

kwashiorkor form of undernutrition that results from consuming adequate energy and insufficient high-quality protein

marasmus starvation

Figure 7.18 Severe protein-energy malnutrition. This photo of a Nigerian person suffering from marasmus was taken during the civil war that occurred in the late 1960s. Source: Centers for Disease Control and Prevention/Dr. Lyle Conrad

signs of marasmus are weakness and wasting. The marasmic person is so thin that his or her ribs, hips, and spine are visible through the skin. People suffering from marasmus avoid physical activity to conserve energy, and they are often irritable. If marasmus is not treated with a nutritious diet, death results.

Concept CHECKPOINT

24. In the United States, which groups of people are most likely to suffer from protein-energy malnutrition?

25. Why is protein-energy malnutrition a devastating condition for young children?

26. Police bring a 2-year-old child into a hospital; the child is so underweight, his bones are visible through the skin. The police report indicates the child was severely neglected by his parents. According to this information, is this child suffering from kwashiorkor, severe protein-energy malnutrition, or sickle cell anemia? Choose one of these conditions and explain why you selected it.

See Appendix G for responses.

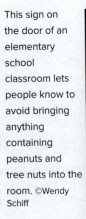

This sign on the door of an elementary school classroom lets people know to avoid bringing anything containing peanuts and tree nuts into the room. ©Wendy Schiff

7.9 Food Allergies, Celiac Disease, and PKU

Learning Outcomes

1 Explain the cause of a food allergy, identity foods that are most likely to cause food allergies in vulnerable people, and list three common signs or symptoms of a food allergy.

2 Explain what causes celiac disease, identify foods that a person with celiac disease must avoid, and list three common signs or symptoms of the disease.

3 Explain the cause of phenylketonuria, and discuss how the condition is treated.

4 Distinguish between nutrigenetics and nutrigenomics.

Did *YOU* Know?

According to conventional wisdom, babies who have siblings or parents with peanut allergy should not eat products made with peanuts because the peanuts will trigger allergic responses in the infants. In 2015, however, findings of a study indicated that feeding young infants peanut-containing foods *reduces* the likelihood that the babies will develop peanut allergies later in childhood.[27] Thus, caregivers may contribute to the development of peanut allergy by not introducing peanuts into the diets of infants. The results of this study are changing how the medical profession views food allergy prevention, not just for peanuts, but also for tree nuts, eggs, fish, wheat, and other foods that are considered highly allergenic.

There is no question that cells need amino acids to function properly. In some instances, however, certain amino acids or proteins cause havoc in the body, resulting in serious health problems and even death. The following sections take a closer look at three protein—related conditions that affect the lives of millions of Americans. By following special diets, people with these conditions can live normal and productive lives. This section also includes information about *nutritional genomics*, the science that explores ways genes interact with dietary choices and the environment.

What Is a Food Allergy?

Have you ever experienced an allergic reaction after eating certain foods or drinks? A food allergy is an inflammatory response that results when the body's immune system reacts inappropriately to one or more harmless substances (*allergens*) in the food. In most instances, the allergen is a protein. People with food allergies may experience swelling of their lips and tongue as they eat the food or soon after they swallow it. If the allergen in the food that is eaten does not undergo dena—turation by stomach acid, the molecule enters the small intestine. Immune system cells in the small intestine may recognize the food protein as a foreign substance and try to protect the body by mounting a defensive response. In other instances, the cells of the small intestine absorb the food allergen, and the body's immune system reacts to it. As a result of the immune response, the person who is allergic to that food experiences typical signs and symptoms.

Common signs and symptoms of food allergies include *hives*, red raised bumps that usually appear on the skin; swollen or itchy lips; skin flushing; a scaly skin rash (eczema); difficulty swallowing; wheezing and difficulty breath—ing; and abdominal pain, vomiting, and diarrhea. Allergic reactions generally occur within 30 minutes to a couple of hours after eating the offending food. In severe cases, sensitive people who are exposed to food allergens can develop *anaphylactic shock*, a serious drop in blood pressure that affects the whole body. Anaphylaxis (*an—a—pha—lax'—is*) can be fatal, unless emergency treatment is provided. Genetics play a major role in the risk of food allergies; people who have family histories of allergies to foods are more likely to develop these conditions.

Although any food protein has the potential to cause an allergic reac—tion in a susceptible person, the most allergenic proteins are in cow's milk, eggs, peanuts and other nuts, wheat, soybeans, fish, and shellfish. Allergic responses to nonprotein food dyes or other food additives such as *sulfites* can also occur. Sulfites are a group of sulfur—containing compounds that result from the metabolism of certain amino acids. Sulfites can be found naturally in foods, but the compounds are often added to wines, potatoes, and shrimp as a preserva—tive. People who suffer from asthma often develop breathing difficulties after consuming food treated with sulfites. Other sulfite—sensitive people report skin flushing (redness and warmth), hives, difficulty swallowing, vomiting, diarrhea, and dizziness after consuming foods that contain the compounds.

In the United States, approximately 5% of children and 4% of adults suffer from food allergies.[28] Since 1997, the prevalence of food allergies among children under 18 years of age has been increasing in the United States. Children with food allergies are more likely than other children to experience other allergies and asthma. As they mature, children often "outgrow" allergies to wheat, milk, soy, and eggs.[29] On the other hand, allergies to peanuts, tree nuts, fish, and shellfish tend to persist into adulthood.

Accurate diagnosis of a food allergy should be undertaken by an immunol—ogist, a physician who specializes in the diagnosis and treatment of allergies. Skin testing is a reliable way to identify allergens. Although hair analysis, cytotoxic or electrodermal testing, and kinesiology are promoted by alternative medical prac—titioners to diagnose allergies, these are unproven diagnostic methods.

Treatment of food allergies involves strict avoidance of the offending foods. Parents or caregivers of young children with food allergies should read food labels carefully to check for allergens listed among ingredients. Additionally, they should educate teachers and other adults who associate with the allergic child about the importance of not exposing the youngster to specific foods. In 2004, the U.S. Congress passed the Food Allergen Labeling and Consumer Protection Act, which required food manufacturers to identify potentially allergenic ingredients, such as soy, milk, and peanuts, on product labels (Fig. 7.19).

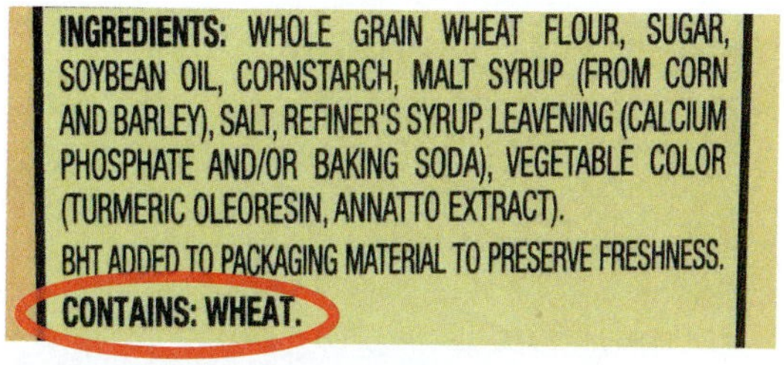

INGREDIENTS: WHOLE GRAIN WHEAT FLOUR, SUGAR, SOYBEAN OIL, CORNSTARCH, MALT SYRUP (FROM CORN AND BARLEY), SALT, REFINER'S SYRUP, LEAVENING (CALCIUM PHOSPHATE AND/OR BAKING SODA), VEGETABLE COLOR (TURMERIC OLEORESIN, ANNATTO EXTRACT).
BHT ADDED TO PACKAGING MATERIAL TO PRESERVE FRESHNESS.
CONTAINS: WHEAT.

Figure 7.19 Allergen labeling.
©Wendy Schiff

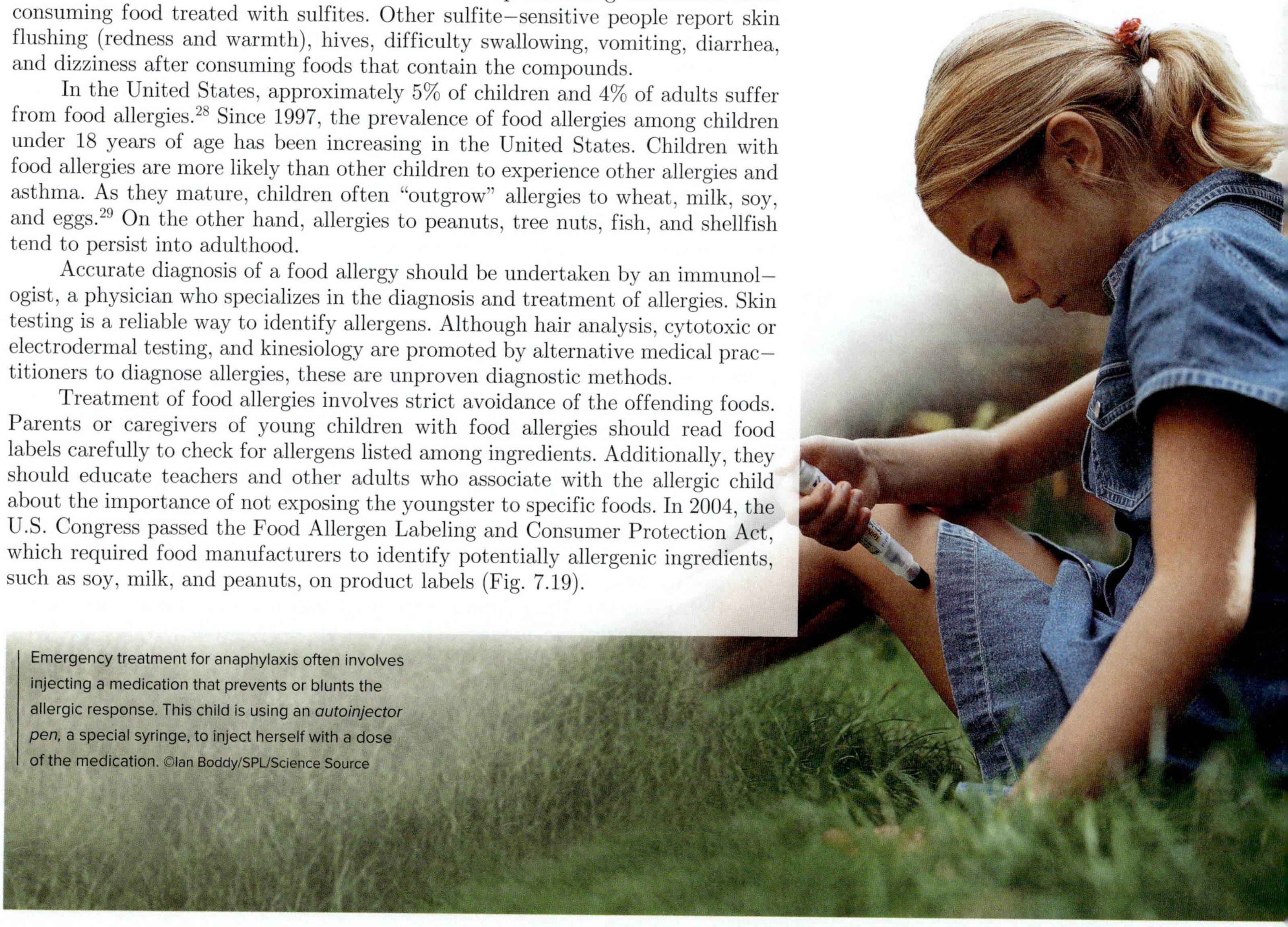

Emergency treatment for anaphylaxis often involves injecting a medication that prevents or blunts the allergic response. This child is using an *autoinjector pen,* a special syringe, to inject herself with a dose of the medication. ©Ian Boddy/SPL/Science Source

Did *YOU* Know?

Celiac disease is not the same as a condition called *gluten sensitivity*. People who have gluten sensitivity also develop health problems when they eat foods that contain gluten, but their small intestine is not damaged. Some symptoms of gluten sensitivity, particularly tiredness and abdominal pain, are similar to those of celiac disease. Therefore, it is important for people who think they cannot eat foods that contain gluten to undergo medical testing to determine whether they actually have celiac disease. Regardless of whether a person has gluten sensitivity or celiac disease, the treatment is the same—avoiding gluten.

TABLE 7.8 Gluten-Free Diet

People with celiac disease should avoid foods that contain:
wheat, including wheat, enriched, durum, graham, and semolina flours; farina, wheat bran, wheat germ, cracked wheat, wheat protein
barley
rye
triticale
Unless contaminated with any of the above foods, products that contain the following ingredients are generally safe to eat for people with celiac disease:
arrowroot, buckwheat, cassava, corn, flax, oats (small amounts), millet, nuts, quinoa, rice, sorghum, soy, tapioca

What Is Celiac Disease?

Celiac (see'—lee—ak) disease is a common inherited condition that results in poor absorption of nutrients (malabsorption) from the small intestine. People with the disease cannot tolerate foods that contain gluten, a group of related proteins in wheat, barley, and rye. Gluten provides the chewy texture and stiff structure of breads and other baked products made from wheat, barley, and rye. After a person with celiac disease eats foods or is exposed to substances that contain gluten, a component of the protein stimulates the body to mount an immune response in the small intestine that inflames or destroys villi. (Villi are the tiny, fingerlike projections of small intestine that absorb nutrients [see Fig. 4.29].) Even though the affected person's food intake may be nutritionally adequate, malnutrition results because his or her intestinal tract lacks healthy villi.

The signs and symptoms of celiac disease vary from person to person but usually include abdominal bloating, chronic diarrhea, and weight loss. Children with this condition also experience poor growth due to nutrient malabsorption and protein malnutrition. Some people have no obvious signs or symptoms of the disease, despite the damage occurring to their small intestines. Serious health problems such as anemia (a blood disorder), osteoporosis (weak bones), infertility, liver disease, and intestinal cancer can result from untreated celiac disease.

In the United States, as many as 1 in 141 people has celiac disease, but most of them are not aware that they have the disease.[30] Although the tendency to develop the disease is probably inherited, environmental factors often play a role by triggering the condition. A serious viral infection or severe emotional stress, for example, may activate the disorder in a genetically susceptible person.

No single medical test is effective in determining whether a person has celiac disease. However, blood testing and intestinal biopsies are often used to diagnose the condition. The biopsy involves removing tiny pieces of tissue from the small intestine. The tissue samples undergo microscopic examination to evaluate the condition of the villi. The presence of damaged villi can help confirm the diagnosis of celiac disease.

There is no cure for celiac disease, but persons with the condition can achieve and maintain good health by following a special gluten–free diet very carefully. Many supermarkets have a special section with a variety of gluten–free foods. Table 7.8 lists foods that must be avoided by people with celiac disease as well as those that are safe for them to consume. Although people with the condition can eat corn, rice, and soy products, these foods may be contaminated with gluten if they are processed in factories that also manufacture wheat products. Because gluten may be used to make medications, dietary supplements, and lipsticks, people with celiac disease should read ingredient lists to determine whether such "hidden" sources of gluten are present. The U.S. Food and Drug Administration (FDA) has rules for the use of the claim "gluten–free" on product labels (see http://www.fda.gov/forconsumers/consumerupdates/ucm363069.htm).

Katie Adams was diagnosed with celiac disease when she was in college. The first "Real People, Real Stories" feature in this section introduces Katie and describes how she manages her diet to avoid signs, symptoms, and complications of celiac disease.

REAL PEOPLE | REAL STORIES

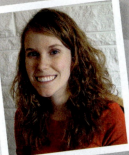

Katie Adams

When Katie Adams was an American college student, she had the opportunity to attend England's renowned Cambridge University during her junior year. Within a few months after Katie began her studies in England, she began to experience frequent bouts of abdominal pain not long after eating. Making matters even worse, she suffered from nearly constant diarrhea. Although her weight was at a healthy level when she first went to England, she began to lose pounds despite eating adequate amounts of food.

Eventually, Katie reached the point at which she could no longer ignore her health problems. While at Cambridge, she was examined by a physician who thought her signs and symptoms were the result of celiac disease. Although Katie was unfamiliar with the disease, she decided to forgo being tested for the condition until she returned to the United States.

After coming home from England, Katie underwent specialized testing by a physician who diagnoses and treats conditions affecting the intestinal tract. This testing detected the presence of antibodies to proteins in gluten. She also underwent an endoscopic examination of her upper gastrointestinal tract. This exam enabled the gastroenterologist to see the condition of her small intestine and remove a small part of the damaged tissue to view under a microscope. As a result of these definitive tests, Katie was diagnosed with celiac disease. The only treatment for celiac disease is complete avoidance of gluten-containing foods.

Eating out is especially difficult for people with celiac disease because of restaurants' widespread inclusion of breads, rolls, pasta, and desserts made from wheat flour in menus. Katie learned how to locate the few restaurants in her community that cater to people with celiac disease by having kitchens that are dedicated to gluten-free food preparation.

Today, Katie maintains her good health by continuing to avoid gluten. Although her diet is very restrictive, she knows from experience that if she "cheats" by eating even a small amount of food that contains gluten, she'll get sick again. After such occasions, she returns to following a gluten-free diet, and within several days, her intestinal tract heals itself.

According to Katie, people who are unfamiliar with celiac disease should take the condition seriously and accommodate the special dietary needs of people who have the disease. For example, if you invite someone with celiac disease to share a meal or snack with you, wash your hands after you prepare foods that contain gluten and don't offer those foods to the person. Additionally, prepare some gluten-free foods for your guest who has celiac disease to eat safely. She says, "It's discouraging when people think I'm simply a 'picky eater' and just making life hard for them. The more people who understand celiac disease, the easier my life becomes!"

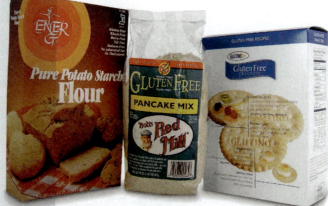

Gluten-free foods. ©Wendy Schiff

What Is PKU?

Phenylketonuria (*fen'–il–keet'–n–your'–e–ah*) or PKU is a rare genetic metabolic disorder that affects about 1 in 10,000 to 1 in 15,000 infants in the United States.[31] PKU usually occurs when cells are unable to produce an enzyme that converts the essential amino acid phenylalanine (*fen–il–al'–ah–neen*) to other compounds. As a result, phenylalanine or its toxic by–products build up in tissues and damage cells, including nerve cells in the brain. If PKU is not diag– nosed and treated within a few weeks of birth, the affected infant can develop intellectual disability within the first year of life.

In the United States, all states require newborns to undergo blood test– ing for PKU and several other treatable inherited diseases.[32] Infants who have PKU are generally given special formulas that lack phenylalanine. Phenylalanine is essential for growth and development; therefore, young children can consume a small amount of the amino acid. As the children grow and mature, fruits, vegetables, and special low–protein foods can be added to their formula diet. However, children and adults with the disorder need to avoid foods that are rich sources of phenylalanine, such as nuts, milk products, eggs, meats, and other animal foods. Additionally, people with PKU should not consume diet soft drinks and other foods and beverages containing the alternative sweetener aspartame, because the sweetener is a source of phenylalanine (see Chapter 5 for information about aspartame).

Throughout their lives, individuals with PKU may need to follow the restrictive diet, especially if they cannot take medication that helps their body metabolize phenylalanine. Furthermore, people with the disorder need to undergo frequent blood tests to make sure they are maintaining a healthy concentration of phenylalanine in their bodies. Monitoring blood phenylala– nine is especially important during pregnancy. An expectant woman who has PKU must carefully control her phenylalanine level to avoid exposing her embryo/fetus to excessive amounts of the amino acid. If she fails to control the concentration of phenylalanine in her blood, she can give birth to a baby with severe birth defects, including a smaller–than–normal brain. The second "Real People, Real Stories" in this section features Dallas Clasen, a college student who has PKU.

What Is Nutritional Genomics?

nutritional genomics science that investigates the complex interactions among gene functioning, dietary choices, and the environment

nutrigenetics study of how a person's genetic makeup affects the way his or her body responds to food

nutrigenomics study of how nutrients and other food components can affect one's genetic expression

Human DNA has approximately 23,000 genes that code for protein synthesis ("the human genome").[33] **Nutritional genomics** is a relatively new science that inves– tigates the complex interactions among gene functioning, dietary choices, and the environment. Such interactions influence a person's health status. Nutritional genomics includes **nutrigenetics,** the study of how a person's genetic makeup affects the way his or her body responds to food. For example, people who are genetically vulnerable to develop celiac disease are healthy until they consume foods that contain gluten. Nutritional genomics also involves **nutrigenomics,** the study of how nutrients and other food components can affect a person's *genetic expression*. Gene expression results in protein synthesis. As mentioned earlier, newborns with a particular genetic defect develop PKU when they con– sume amounts of phenylalanine that are harmless to babies who do not have the defect. By providing a diet that is low in phenylalanine to newborns with PKU, the infants develop normally.

REAL PEOPLE | REAL STORIES

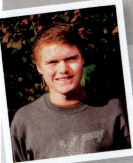

Dallas Clasen

Dallas Clasen is majoring in engineering at the University of Wisconsin-Platteville. In addition to keeping up with his coursework, he runs cross country at school and participates in triathlons. Like most college students, Dallas is very busy, but unlike most students, he has to pay very close attention to his diet. Dallas was born with a rare inherited metabolic disorder, an inborn-error of metabolism called phenylketonuria (PKU).

A few days after birth, Dallas underwent standard newborn blood testing. The results of the test indicated that the level of phenylalanine in his blood was about 40 times higher than the normal amount, a sign of PKU. To avoid developing severe brain damage and other physiological effects of PKU, Dallas was cared for by a physician who specializes in treating children with the disorder. The primary treatment for PKU is a low-phenylalanine diet.

Most foods that are rich sources of protein, especially high-quality animal proteins, contain more phenylalanine than people with PKU can tolerate. Thus, from the time Dallas was a week old, he has consumed a formula that does not contain the amino acid. In addition to the formula, Dallas can eat limited amounts of grain products and most fruits and vegetables. He also consumes special low-phenylalanine foods that resemble "regular" foods but are not available in supermarkets. As part of Dallas's college meal plan, he has access to the special foods through the university's food service.

Foods that are eaten away from home can present problems for people with PKU. When at a restaurant, Dallas usually orders French fries or "sub" sandwiches that are made with vegetables but do not contain any cheese or meat. Instead of drinking milk, Dallas drinks his special formula or sports drinks that do not contain the nonnutritive sweetener aspartame (see Chapter 5). He is so accustomed to his special diet, he thinks meat looks "gross." In addition to following the special diet, Dallas takes Kuvan®, a prescription medication that stimulates the enzyme that converts phenylalanine to tyrosine. He takes 14 capsules after breakfast with apple juice. The medication does not help everyone with PKU, but it allows Dallas to consume more foods that contain phenylalanine. "I can eat double the amount of the amino acid," Dallas says. To determine whether his special diet and medication are working, each week Dallas pricks his finger and allows a few drops of blood to soak into a special paper. Then he sends the paper to a laboratory that checks the level of phenylalanine in his blood.

In the past, children with PKU were often allowed to eat regular foods after they were about 6 years of age. However, the importance of continuing the low-phenylalanine diet became evident when many of the children experienced learning and behavioral problems as they matured. Dallas is aware of the consequences that can occur if he does not limit his phenylalanine intake, and he accepts the need to follow the special diet for the rest of his life. "Being on a strict diet has not only made me disciplined, it has taught me to do whatever is needed to always take good care of myself," says Dallas. "I have learned that we are all different, anyway. So, accept who you are!"

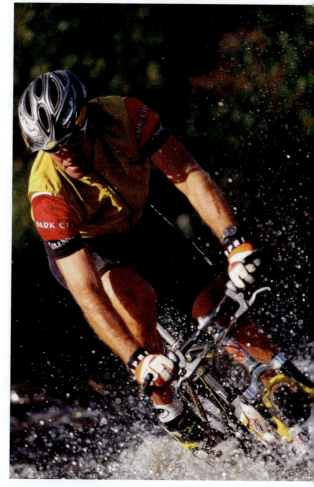

©Ingram Publishing RF

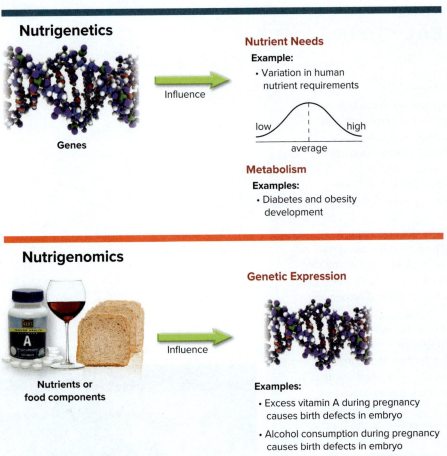

Nutrigenetics

Genes

Influence →

Nutrient Needs

Example:
• Variation in human nutrient requirements

low   high
         average

Metabolism

Examples:
• Diabetes and obesity development

Nutrigenomics

Nutrients or food components

Influence →

Genetic Expression

Examples:
• Excess vitamin A during pregnancy causes birth defects in embryo
• Alcohol consumption during pregnancy causes birth defects in embryo
• Food allergies and intolerances in vulnerable persons

Figure 7.20 **Nutritional genomics.**
DNA and DNA: ©Digital Vision/Getty Images RF; Vitamin bottle: ©McGraw-Hill Education/John Flournoy, photographer; Glass of wine: ©FoodCollection/StockFood RF; Bread: ©Ingram Publishing RF

Nutritional genomics may explain why special diets or dietary supplements can have different effects on the health of different individuals (Fig. 7.20). A young man, for example, may develop kidney stones while taking a daily dietary supplement that contains 1000 mg vitamin C. However, another man who is the same age and takes the same amount of vitamin C each day does not form kidney stones. Thus, the effectiveness of a specific diet, dietary supplement, medication, or lifestyle intervention may largely depend on one's genes. In the future, physicians may be able to consider such individual differences to provide more personalized treatments and preventive measures.

Genetic Testing Kits

Several biotechnology companies sell at-home genetic test kits for individuals to collect a small amount of saliva and mail the saliva sample to the company for genetic analysis. As a result of the saliva analysis, the company develops an "optimal health" plan based on the person's genetic makeup. Consumers, however, are encouraged to use caution when considering purchasing at-home genetic testing kits because the industry of nutrigenetic testing is not well regulated.[34] People who are interested in having genetic testing should consult their physician.

Concept CHECKPOINT

27. List three common signs or symptoms of food allergy and celiac disease.
28. Discuss what parents of infants with PKU can do to help their children grow and develop normally.
29. Explain how nutritional genomics may be used to improve a person's health.

See Appendix G for responses.

7.10 Nutrition Matters: Stretching Your Food Dollars

Learning Outcomes

1 Discuss practical ways to save money when purchasing food.

2 Compare similar foods to determine the most economical product.

Are you concerned about the high cost of food? If you are, how can you lower your food costs without sacrificing proper nutrition? You can trim food costs, and preserve and even improve the nutritional quality of your diet, by analyzing your food buying practices and making a few changes. This section focuses on ways you can eat well for less. Please note that the pricing of products reflects retail food prices during the summer of 2016 in a major Midwestern city, but you should find them useful for comparing current prices where you live.

Where and What You Buy

Where you buy foods and beverages and what you decide to purchase are major factors in determining your overall food expenditures. If you frequently purchase meals and snacks from vending machines, convenience stores, fast–food outlets, and other restaurants, you may be spending too much on such "convenience" foods. In general, the less time you spend preparing food, the more money you will spend by having someone at a commercial outlet prepare the food for you. Even if a fast–food restaurant hamburger seems like a bargain because it is "only $1.00," you are likely paying a premium for the French fries and soft drink that you purchase to accompany the sandwich. From a nutrition standpoint, fast foods are often energy dense—high in saturated fat and added sugars—and low in micronutrients (except sodium), fiber, and phytochemicals.

You probably already know that supermarkets have the same snack foods and staple items (bread and milk) as convenience stores and usually offer these foods at lower prices. Furthermore, supermarkets have a much larger selection of foods, particularly more nutrient–dense raw or less processed foods, than convenience stores. It may be easier to stop at a convenience store and load up on foods while you load up on gas than to shop in a supermarket. However, you pay extra for the convenience, and your diet may suffer as a result of poor food choices.

A good way to save money is to buy foods in large quantities at "bulk" food stores or at smaller, "no frills," cash–only grocery stores. Although shopping at these places can reduce your food costs, food choices are usually more limited than the selection in supermarkets. It is important to recognize that buying food in bulk is a bargain only if you can use the item before it spoils.

How to Shop Wisely in Supermarkets To lower your food costs, plan your meals and snacks before you shop for food. Prepare a shopping list to help avoid needless or impulse purchases and having to return to the store to buy forgotten items. Keep the grocery list in a convenient place, such as on the refrigerator, and jot down items as they become depleted.

When shopping for groceries, you will need to compare *unit costs* of similar food products. A "unit" of a packaged food item is usually indicated in ounces, pounds, cups, or other serving sizes. Food packages and containers are available in different sizes and hold different amounts of food, which can make comparing costs of similar foods difficult. Using a small calculator to compare prices can be helpful. For example, a box of one brand of shredded wheat cereal contains 15.0 ounces of cereal and costs $3.89; a box of a different brand of shredded wheat that contains 11.5 ounces of cereal costs $3.69. Which box contains cereal that is lower in cost? To answer this question, determine the unit price of the cereal in each box by dividing the cost of the entire package by the number of units of food it contains.

©Comstock/Stockbyte/Getty Images RF

Box #1

$3.89 entire box ÷ 15.0 ounces = approximately $.26/ounce

Box #2

$3.69 entire box ÷ 11.5 ounces = approximately $.32/ounce

In this situation, the larger box of cereal is a better buy, even though it costs more than the smaller box. Some supermarkets indicate unit prices on shelf tags, but the tags may be difficult to read or confusing.

Blueberries: ©PhotoAlto/Getty Images RF

Supermarkets offer a wide variety of prepared foods, including deli items, frozen entrées, fresh cut–up fruit packaged in single–serving plastic bags or cups, and rotisserie chicken. Although these "fast foods" are convenient, food processing and packaging add to the cost of food. Such foods may contain unhealthy amounts of salt, solid fat, or sugar. To save money and improve your diet, rely less on prepared foods and more on "slow foods"—foods that require some of your time and effort to prepare. Figure 7.21 uses various forms of chicken to illustrate this point. A 2.5–lb rotisserie–cooked chicken costs $3.50/lb, but you can save money by purchasing a whole chicken ($2.69/lb) and cooking it yourself. Instead of buying raw, skinless, boneless chicken breasts ($6.19/lb), buy raw split chicken breasts that have the bones and skin ($1.99/lb). Remove the skin and bones after the chicken breasts are cooked. You can use the cooked chicken immediately, freeze the meat in containers for a future meal, or chill the meat before chopping it to make chicken salad.

Eating more fruits and vegetables is the natural way to add micronutrients, fiber, and phytochemicals to your diet. Many supermarkets offer fresh fruit and vegetables that have been trimmed, cut up, and packed into containers. Before you reach for one of these items, compare its price with that of its raw counterpart. For example, a 2.2–oz, single–serving package of sliced apples sells for $1.25, and a pound of raw apples is priced at $1.99. In this case, buying the raw apples and slicing them yourself is a money–saving practice. To make this determination,

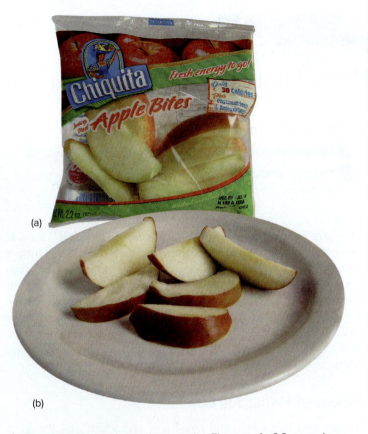

(a)

(b)

Figure 7.22 Comparing apples to apples. The cost of a 2.2–oz package of apple slices (*a*) is almost five times the cost of the same amount of fresh, bulk, sliced raw apples (*b*).
©Wendy Schiff

you will need to calculate the unit price of each product (Fig. 7.22). An ounce of the packaged apples costs about 57 cents ($1.25 divided by 2.2 oz/package). A pound of raw apples equals 16 ounces, so an ounce of these apples costs about 12 cents ($1.99 divided by 16). Thus, the prepackaged sliced apples cost almost five times more than the bulk raw apples.

Produce that is grown in the United States is usually less expensive when it is in season and more plentiful. For example, berries are plentiful in the spring and early summer, tomatoes and melons in late summer, and apples in the fall. "Fresh" produce that is shipped long distances to supermarket suppliers is often picked before its peak ripeness. As a result, the fruits and vegetables may not taste as good or be as nutritious as locally grown produce. Produce, for example, loses some of its vitamin C content when it is bruised or becomes wilted. Therefore, consider buying fresh produce, for example, directly from local farmers, if possible. Although you still need to compare prices of farmers' market items with those of fresh produce sold in supermarkets, you may be able to find reasonably priced produce that is grown within 100 miles of your home at farmers' markets. Buying produce from local farmers helps support your community's economy, too.

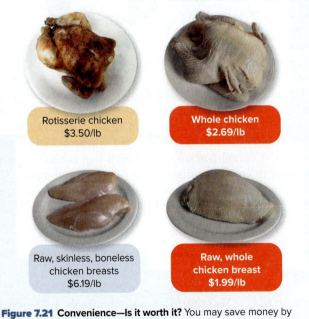

Rotisserie chicken
$3.50/lb

Whole chicken
$2.69/lb

Raw, skinless, boneless chicken breasts
$6.19/lb

Raw, whole chicken breast
$1.99/lb

Figure 7.21 Convenience—Is it worth it? You may save money by purchasing a raw whole chicken and cutting it into parts or a whole chicken breast and removing the skin and bones.

Roast chicken, Whole raw chicken, Raw skinless chicken and Raw chicken breast: ©Wendy Schiff

An alternative to buying produce directly from growers is to purchase frozen or canned fruits and vegetables. These products are often less expensive than their fresh counterparts. Furthermore, produce that is destined to be frozen is generally harvested when ripe and frozen immediately, maximizing much of its vitamin content and fresh flavor.

The following practices can help you save money while shopping for food.

- Use unit pricing to compare costs of similar packaged products.
- Be wary of appealing offers that are not bargains. For example, items marked "3 for $1.00" or "10 for $10.00" can be confusing to consumers. It is important to understand that you do not need to buy the entire quantity. For example, if a store offers 3 kiwifruits for a dollar, and you cannot use 3 of them, buy one for 34 cents. That price is still a bargain compared to buying kiwifruits that are "2 for $1.00." Also, beware of offers such as "10 oranges for $10." Paying $1 for an orange is not a bargain! The same store may be selling a bag of 10 oranges for $5. At that price, each orange costs only 50 cents.
- Package sizes can be misleading, so ignore the size of a package and compare net weights of package contents to determine the best value.
- Compare the unit price of organic foods and similar conventionally produced items. If an organic food item is more expensive, consider purchasing the conventional product instead.
- Compare unit prices of preportioned snack foods such as chips or cookies in 100–Calorie packages with prices of the typical, larger package–size products. Such preportioned snacks may be convenient and helpful if you are trying to control your calorie intake, but they are usually more costly per ounce than the same foods purchased in larger packages. Furthermore, people may eat more of the preportioned snack foods, because they think they are lower in calories than the same items packed in larger containers. Make your own preproportioned snacks. For example, buy a large package of oatmeal cookies and place two–cookie portions into reusable storage bags. When you want a snack, eat the two cookies.
- Use coupons when purchasing brand–name items. However, be aware that many stores offer similar products, often referred to as "store brands," that are less expensive than the brand–name items. Although store brand items do not have name recognition, these products are usually just as nutritious as their corresponding brand–name items.

- Limit your carbonated soft drink, commercially prepared coffee, energy drink, and bottled water purchases. When you are thirsty, locate the nearest water fountain and have a drink for free!
- Check "sell by," "best if used by," or "use by" dates on packages of perishable foods such as eggs and dairy products. Compared to canned and frozen foods, perishable foods lose their appealing sensory qualities, such as fresh taste and appearance, more rapidly during storage. The "sell by" date informs store employees about the length of time the product should be displayed for sale. Obviously, it is best to buy foods before the sell–by date. The "best if used by" or "use by" dates indicate the last day to use the product before it loses its best flavor and other sensory qualities. The date does not indicate the last day to purchase the food because of safety concerns.[35] Also, read food product labels for storage information. Many products must be refrigerated after opening to delay spoilage. Chapter 12 provides more information about proper food storage practices.
- Have at least one vegetarian meal a week.
- Red meats are among the most expensive protein sources, so have more meals in which chicken, turkey, or fish is the main source of animal protein.
- Canned fish can be a less expensive choice than fresh fish because there is less waste (skin and large bones).
- Remember that any food product is not a good buy if the item spoils before you can use it.

For more ways to save money on food, read the "Food & Nutrition Tips" at the end of this section.

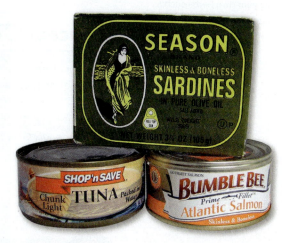

Canned fish, such as tuna, salmon, and sardines, can be a less expensive choice than meat or fresh fish. ©Wendy Schiff

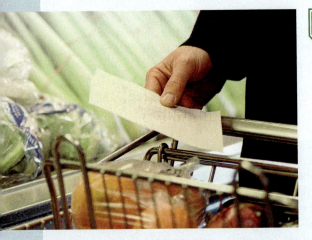

Prepare a shopping list to help avoid needless or impluse purchases. ©Rob Melynchuk/Getty Images RF

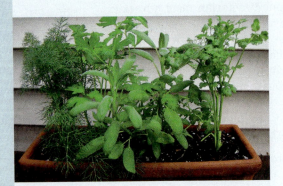

For fresh seasonings, grow your own herbs such as basil, oregano, parsley, and thyme. ©Wendy Schiff

Food & Nutrition tips

- Foods that contain a lot of empty calories often look more appealing when your stomach is empty. To reduce the likelihood of buying such foods on impulse, avoid shopping for groceries when you are hungry.

- Be wary of buying food items that are displayed near or along checkout aisles. They are usually energy-dense foods that are not nutrient dense, such as candy bars, energy drinks, and baked goods.

- Many perishable foods, such as shredded cheese and fluid fat-free milk, can be frozen.

- If you drink coffee, buy a small coffeemaker, a can of ground coffee, and coffee filters to make the beverage. Consider carrying a small thermos of coffee in your backpack. It is much less expensive to make a cup of your own coffee than to buy one from a coffeehouse.

- Canned beans are often sold in large cans that may be cheaper per ounce than beans in smaller cans. If the larger-sized product is less expensive, buy it. After opening the large can of beans, remove the amount needed for the meal, and freeze the remainder in an air-tight container for a future meal.

- For fresh seasonings, grow your own herbs. Basil, oregano, parsley, cilantro, and thyme grow well in flower pots placed in a sunny area. Snip leaves as needed for recipes, while keeping the rest of the plants intact. Snipping off some leaves stimulates the plant to grow more leaves.

- Share potluck dinners with friends. Plan the menu and ask your friends to bring certain items, such as vegetable or fruit salads and whole-grain rolls or breads. Inexpensive entrees (the main food items on the menu) include spaghetti and meat sauce, chicken burritos, vegetarian chili, tuna and noodle casserole, and tacos made with canned tuna fish.

Concept CHECKPOINT

30. List at least five ways to save money while shopping for food.

31. You can purchase a 3.5-pound bag of frozen sliced peaches for $7.99 or 3.5 pounds of fresh peaches for $2.49 per pound. Considering your situation, which is the more economical way to buy peaches? Explain why.

See Appendix G for responses.

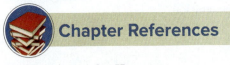

Chapter References

See Appendix H.

Stacked books: ©Stockbyte/Getty Images RF

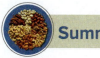 **Summary**

7.1 What Are Proteins?

- Proteins are organic compounds that contain nitrogen, the element cells need to make a wide array of important biological compounds with structural or metabolic functions in the body. Additionally, a relatively small amount of protein contributes to the body's energy needs.

- Proteins are comprised of amino acids. The typical amino acid has nitrogen-containing or amino, acid, and R groups. The diet must supply nine of the amino acids (essential amino acids), because the body cannot make them or make enough of them to meet its needs. Under normal conditions, cells can synthesize the remaining amino acids if the raw materials are available.

7.2 Proteins in Foods

- A high-quality or complete protein contains all essential amino acids in amounts that support growth in children. Most animal proteins are high quality. A low-quality or incomplete protein lacks or contains inadequate amounts of one or more of the essential amino acids.

- Tryptophan, threonine, lysine, methionine, and cysteine are often the limiting amino acids in foods.

7.3 What Happens to Proteins in the Body?

- Human proteins are comprised of 20 different amino acids arranged in various combinations. Cells produce proteins by linking amino acids together in specific sequences that are dictated by instructions coded in DNA. Faulty DNA results in the wrong amino acids being inserted into peptide chains, causing genetic defects. If an essential amino acid is not available when protein synthesis occurs, proteins in muscles and organs can provide the essential amino acids. Otherwise, protein synthesis halts, and the amino acids in the unfinished peptide are removed and returned to the amino acid pool. Excess amino acids are metabolized for energy or converted into body fat.

- Protein turnover is the process of breaking down old or unneeded proteins into their component amino acids and recycling them to make new proteins. The body conserves nitrogen by recycling amino acids, but each day, it loses some protein and nitrogen. In positive nitrogen balance, the body retains more nitrogen than it loses; in negative nitrogen balance, the body loses more nitrogen than it retains.

- The protein requirement increases during pregnancy, breastfeeding, periods of growth, and recovery from serious illnesses, blood losses, and burns. The adult RDA for protein is 0.8 g/kg of body weight.

- Protein digestion begins in the stomach, where hydrochloric acid denatures food proteins and pepsin breaks proteins into polypeptides. In the small intestine, enzymes secreted by the pancreas and absorptive cells digest polypeptides primarily into di- and tripeptides. The absorptive cells convert the peptides into amino acids. The end products of protein digestion, amino acids, travel to the liver. The liver uses the amino acids or releases them into the general circulation.

7.4 Protein Consumption Patterns

- The AMDR for adults is 10 to 35% of energy intake from protein. Total protein consumption as a percentage of daily calories has

©Keith Ovregaard/Cole Group/Getty Images RF

Nuts: ©C Squared Studios/Getty Images RF

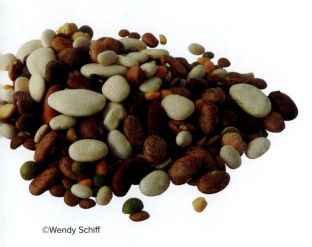

©Wendy Schiff

remained about the same since the early twentieth century, but Americans now eat more animal protein. People can reduce their intake of animal protein without sacrificing the protein quality of their diets.

7.5 Understanding Nutritional Labeling

- The Nutrition Facts panel on a packaged food product label provides information concerning the amount of protein in a serving of the food.

7.6 Proteins: Economical Considerations

- The average American consumes more protein than the RDA for the nutrient.

- In general, meat, fish, poultry, eggs, milk, and milk products contain high-quality proteins. When compared to animal foods, most plant foods provide low-quality protein. Quinoa and foods made from processed soybeans are good plant sources of essential amino acids.

7.7 Vegetarianism

- Vegetarian diets are based on plant foods and limit animal foods to some extent. Although vegetarians are generally healthier than people who eat Western diets, it is difficult to pinpoint diet as responsible for vegetarians' better health. If not properly planned, plant-based diets may not contain enough energy, high-quality protein, omega-3 fatty acids, vitamins B-12 and D, and iron and calcium to meet a person's nutritional needs, especially children's needs.

7.8 Protein Adequacy

- High-protein diets are generally not recommended for healthy individuals.

- PEM affects people whose diets lack sufficient protein as well as energy; children are more likely to be affected by PEM than adults. In impoverished developing countries, PEM is a major cause of childhood deaths.

7.9 Food Allergies, Celiac Disease, and PKU

- A food allergy is an inflammatory response that occurs when the body's immune system reacts inappropriately to an allergen. Accurate diagnosis of a food allergy should be undertaken by an immunologist. Treatment involves avoidance of foods that contain the allergens.

- Celiac disease is an inherited condition that causes malabsorption of nutrients. People with the disease cannot eat foods that contain gluten because the body's response to the protein damages villi in the small intestine. There is no cure for celiac disease, but people with the condition can be healthy as long as they avoid gluten-containing foods.

- Phenylketonuria (PKU) is a rare genetic metabolic disorder that occurs when cells cannot produce an enzyme that converts phenylalanine to other compounds. If PKU is not detected in early infancy, phenylalanine and its toxic by-products build up and damage tissues, including nerve cells in the brain. Treatment involves a special diet that contains limited amounts of phenylalanine and, in some cases, medication.

7.10 Nutrition Matters: Stretching Your Food Dollars

- In general, the less time a person spends preparing food, the more money he or she will spend by having someone else prepare the food. Convenience foods are often energy dense—high in solid fat and added sugar. A good way to save money is to buy foods in large quantities at "bulk" food stores, but buying food in bulk is a bargain only if the items can be used before they spoil.

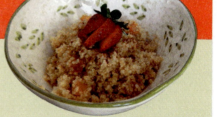

Recipe for Healthy Living

Apricot Quinoa

The ancient Incas of South America cultivated quinoa and relied on the protein-rich vegetable as a dietary staple. Today, cooked quinoa is often added to vegetable salads or served as an accompaniment to chicken or pork. This quinoa recipe makes about two ½-cup servings. Each serving provides about 250 kcal, 7 g protein, 3 g fat, 6 g fiber, 3 mg iron, 2 mg zinc, and 57 mcg folate.

Cooked quinoa: ©Wendy Schiff

INGREDIENTS:

- 1 ⅓ cups water
- ½ cup quinoa
- ⅓ cup dried apricots, chopped
- ¼ tsp ground cinnamon
- 1 Tbsp maple syrup

PREPARATION STEPS:

1. Add water to a small saucepan and bring to a boil. Add quinoa to boiling water.

2. Cover saucepan and cook quinoa over medium heat until all the water is absorbed (about 12–15 minutes).

3. Remove from heat; fluff quinoa with fork; and stir chopped apricots into the quinoa.

4. Place quinoa into a bowl, drizzle with maple syrup, and sprinkle cinnamon on the quinoa.

5. If desired, garnish with fresh fruit. Serve warm.

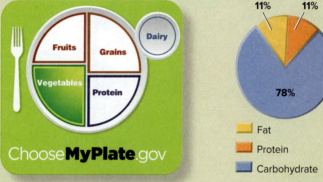

ChooseMyPlate.gov

Source: U.S. Dept. of Agriculture

- Fat — 11%
- Protein — 11%
- Carbohydrate — 78%

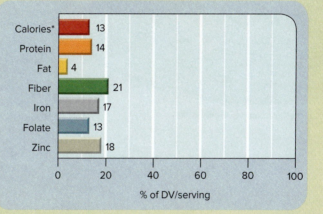

	% of DV/serving
Calories*	13
Protein	14
Fat	4
Fiber	21
Iron	17
Folate	13
Zinc	18

*2000 daily total kcal

connect Further analyze this recipe or other recipes through activities located in Connect.

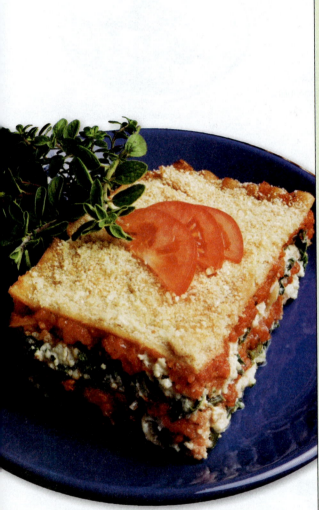

©Michael Lamotte/Cole Group/Getty Images RF

Personal Dietary Analysis

1. Refer to the 3-day food log from the "Personal Dietary Analysis" feature in Chapter 3. Calculate your average protein intake by adding the grams of protein eaten each day, dividing the total by 3, and rounding the figure to the nearest whole number.

Sample Calculation:

Day 1	<u>76</u> g
Day 2	<u>55</u> g
Day 3	<u>103</u> g
Total grams	**<u>234</u> g ÷ 3 days = <u>78</u> g of protein/day**

Your Calculation:

Day 1	_____ g
Day 2	_____ g
Day 3	_____ g
Total grams	_____ ÷ **3 days** = _____ **g/day**

My average daily protein intake was _____ g.

2. The RDA for protein is based on body weight. Using the RDA of 0.8 g of protein/kg of body weight, calculate the amount of protein that you need to consume daily to meet the recommendation. To determine your body weight in kilograms, divide your weight (pounds) by 2.2, then multiply this number by 0.8 to obtain your RDA for protein. Then round the figure to the nearest whole number.

My weight in pounds _____ ÷ 2.2 = _____ kg

My weight in kg _____ × 0.8 = _____ g

My RDA for protein = _____ g

   a. Did your average intake of protein meet or exceed your RDA level that was calculated in step 1? _____ yes _____ no

   b. If your answer to 2a is yes, which foods contributed the most to your protein intake?

3. Review the log of your 3-day food intake. Calculate the average number of kilocalories that protein contributed to your diet each day during the 3-day period.

   a. Each gram of protein provides about 4 kcal; therefore, you must multiply the average number of grams of protein obtained in step 1 by 4 kcal to obtain the average number of kcal from protein.

Sample Calculation:

78 g/day × 4 kcal/g = 312 kcal from protein

Your Calculation:

_____ g/day × 4 kcal/g = _____ average number of kcal from protein

4. Determine your average energy intake over the 3-day period by adding the kilocalories for each day and dividing the sum by 3, and round to the nearest whole number.

Sample Calculation:

Day 1	2500 kcal
Day 2	3200 kcal
Day 3	2750 kcal
Total kcal	**8450** ÷ 3 days = **2817** kcal/day (average caloric intake)

Your Calculation:

Day 1	_____ kcal
Day 2	_____ kcal
Day 3	_____ kcal
Total kcal	_____ ÷ 3 days = _____ kcal/day (average)

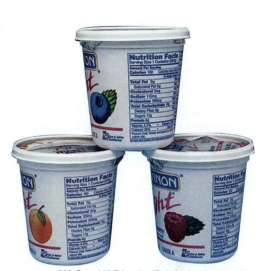

©McGraw-Hill Education/Bob Coyle, photographer

5. Determine the average percentage of energy that protein contributed to your diet by dividing the average kilocalories from protein obtained in step 3 by the average total daily energy intake obtained in step 4. Then round this figure to the nearest one-hundredth. Multiply this value by 100 (move the decimal point two places to the right, drop the decimal point, and add a percent symbol).

Sample Calculation:

312 kcal from protein ÷ 2817 kcal intake = 0.11 (rounded)

0.11 × 100 = 11%

Your Calculation:

_____ kcal from protein ÷ _____ kcal intake = _____

_____ × 100 = _____ %

6. Did your average intake of protein meet the recommendation of 10 to 35% of total calories? If your average protein intake was below 10%, list at least five foods you could eat that would boost your intake.

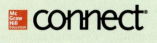 Complete the Personal Dietary Analysis activity located in Connect.

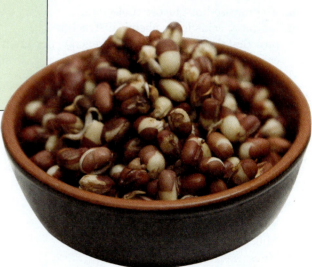

©Image Source/Glow Images RF

Critical Thinking

1. Have you used or are you currently using protein or amino acid supplements? _____ yes _____ no

   If you answered yes, explain why you use these supplements.

2. Are you a vegetarian? If so, describe your dietary practices (for example, vegan, lactoovovegetarian, or semi-vegetarian), and explain why you decided to become vegetarian. If you are not a vegetarian, explain why you would or would not consider this lifestyle.

3. Plan a day's meals and snacks for a healthy 132–pound (60 kg) adult lactoovovegetarian female who is not pregnant or breastfeeding. The menu should contain all essential amino acids but contain no animal foods other than eggs and foods from the dairy group. Your meal plan can range from 1800 to 2200 kcal, and it should include foods from the major food groups and follow the recommendations of the U.S. Department of Agriculture's MyPlate food guide.

4. Using only plant foods, plan a day's meals and snacks for a healthy 154–pound (70 kg) adult vegan male. The menu should supply at least 2200 kcal, follow the recommendations of MyPlate, and include foods from the major food groups (except for the dairy group, unless calcium–fortified soy milk is used).

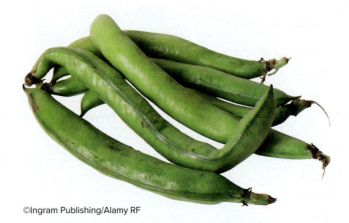

©Ingram Publishing/Alamy RF

5. A recipe for bean salad has the following main ingredients:

   1 cup kidney beans
   1 cup green beans
   1 cup butter beans
   1 cup black beans
   1 ½ cups wine vinegar
   ⅓ cup canola oil
   ¼ cup chopped onion

   Explain why this recipe is not a complementary mixture of plant proteins. What plant foods could you add to the recipe to make it a complementary mixture?

Practice Test

Select the best answer.

1. A protein

   a. is comprised of glucose molecules.
   b. has fatty acids in its chemical structure.
   c. provides the same amount of energy per gram as a carbohydrate.
   d. is a complex inorganic molecule.

2. Which of the following statements is false?

   a. Certain hormones are proteins.
   b. Nearly all enzymes are proteins.
   c. Proteins are part of triglycerides.
   d. The body uses amino acids to make antibodies.

3. Which of the following foods generally provide the least amount of protein per serving?

   a. Fruits
   b. Milk
   c. Nuts
   d. Seeds

4. Which of the following foods is not a source of complete protein?

   a. Peanut butter
   b. Cheese
   c. Fish
   d. Eggs

5. In cells, _____ controls the assembly of amino acids into proteins.

   a. PEU
   b. DNA
   c. IOM
   d. ATP

6. _____ is the process of removing nitrogen from an amino acid.

   a. Transamination
   b. Denaturation
   c. Hydrogenation
   d. Deamination

7. Which of the following physical states is characterized by positive nitrogen balance?

   a. Starvation
   b. Illness
   c. Puberty
   d. Marasmus

8. What is the RDA for protein of a healthy adult woman who weighs 62 kg?

   a. 49.6 g
   b. 59.6 g
   c. 69.6 g
   d. 79.6 g

9. Which of the following foods is a source of complementary protein?

   a. Trail mix made with cashews, raisins, almonds, honey, and dried banana flakes
   b. Mashed chickpeas spread on pita bread
   c. Leafy greens salad topped with peanuts
   d. Whole–wheat bread with an apricot spread

10. Which of the following foods is a source of high–quality protein that a vegan would eat?

    a. Quinoa
    b. Yogurt
    c. Brown rice
    d. Sweet potatoes

11. A sign of marasmus is

    a. increased muscle growth.
    b. rapid weight gain.
    c. diabetes.
    d. wasting.

12. People with celiac disease should

    a. take amino acid supplements.
    b. limit their protein intake to 20 g per day.
    c. avoid foods that contain gluten.
    d. eliminate protein from plant sources.

13. Which of the following tips is a recommended way to reduce food costs?

    a. Buying food in bulk, if it can be used before spoiling
    b. Purchasing preportioned, packaged foods
    c. Shopping at convenience stores, if the stores are within 5 miles of your home
    d. Eating at fast–food outlets at least three times a week

Answers to Quiz Yourself

1. Animal foods such as meat and eggs are almost 100% protein. **False.** (Section 7.2)

2. Foods made from soybeans can be sources of high-quality protein. **True.** (Section 7.2)

3. Americans typically consume more protein from animal sources than from plant foods. **True.** (Section 7.6)

4. Registered dietitian nutritionists generally recommend that healthy people take amino acid supplements to increase their protein intake. **False.** (Section 7.8)

5. People can nourish their hair by using shampoo that contains protein. **False.** (Section 7.3)

©Photodisc/Getty Images RF

CHAPTER 8

Vitamins

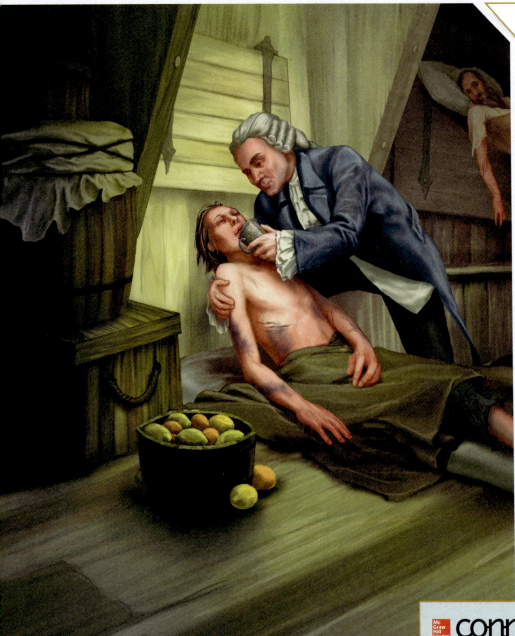

Quiz Yourself

Can vitamins give you more energy or reduce your chances of developing heart disease or cancer? Which cooking methods can increase the loss of vitamins from foods? Which vitamins are added to cereal grains during enrichment? Test your knowledge of vitamins by taking the following quiz. The answers are at the end of the chapter.

1. Natural vitamins are better for you because they have more biological activity than synthetic vitamins.
_____ T _____ F

2. Certain vitamins are toxic.
_____ T _____ F

3. Vitamin E is an antioxidant.
_____ T _____ F

4. Vitamins are a source of "quick" energy.
_____ T _____ F

5. According to scientific research, taking large doses of vitamin C daily prevents the common cold. _____ T _____ F

Mc Graw Hill Education connect®

A wealth of proven resources are available on Connect® including SmartBook®, NutritionCalc Plus, and many other dynamic learning tools. Ask your instructor about Connect!

8.1 Vitamins: Basic Concepts

Learning Outcomes

1. Explain why all vitamins have been discovered.
2. Define *vitamin,* and explain how scientists determine whether a substance is a vitamin.
3. Classify vitamins according to whether they are fat soluble or water soluble.
4. Discuss ways to conserve the vitamin content of foods or increase vitamin bioavailability.
5. Explain the function of an antioxidant.
6. Define *enrichment* and *fortification.*

For centuries, taking lengthy ocean voyages was a dangerous venture, not just because of the threat of severe storms and pillaging pirates but also because of a terrifying and deadly disease called **scurvy.** The first signs and symptoms of scurvy—fatigue and *petechiae (peh−tee'−key−eye)*, pinpoint hemorrhages under the skin—occurred about 20 to 40 days after setting sail. As the disease progressed, the affected person's skin bruised easily; gums swelled, became spongy, and bled after being barely touched; teeth loosened and fell out. Wounds healed slowly or remained open sores. Not surprisingly, the person suffering from scurvy also became irritable and depressed. A particularly devastating sign of the disease was the opening up of old scars, exposing wounds that could become infected. Scurvy victims eventually died, generally from infections, brain hemorrhages, or heart complications.

In 1753, British physician James Lind published an article describing an experiment he had performed on 12 sailors suffering from scurvy. Lind divided the sick sailors into six pairs, and each pair received a different treatment. The six treatments were cider, vinegar, sulfuric acid, seawater, nutmeg, or oranges and lemons. Lind observed that the pair of sailors given the citrus fruit were the only ones to recover from scurvy. By today's standards, Lind's experiment was primitive, but as a result of his testing, Lind found the cure for scurvy: eating oranges and lemons. Eventually, food rations for British sailors included lemon juice to prevent the disease. The sailors earned the nickname "limeys" because at that time, people often referred to citrus fruits collectively as "limes."

Today, we know that scurvy results from a deficiency of vitamin C and that citrus fruits are among the richest dietary sources of the vitamin. Although Lind is often credited with having discovered the cure for scurvy, he did not suspect the disease resulted from the lack of something in the typical seafarer's diet. At that time, scientists were unaware that food contained vitamins. Lind thought scurvy was a digestive system disorder that could be treated with substances associated with warm climates.[1] In his experiment, Lind happened to administer citrus fruits to a pair of the sailors with scurvy because these fruits were associated with such climates.

In 1911, Polish chemist Casimir Funk discovered a substance in an extract made from rice bran that he thought would cure the disease beriberi. Funk called

scurvy vitamin C–deficiency disease

Lemon and Orange: ©C Squared Studios/Getty Images RF

the compound a "vitamine" (*vita* = necessary for life; *amine* = a type of nitrogen-containing substance) because of its chemical structure. The term *vitamine* was later modified to *vitamin*, when scientists determined that there were several kinds of these substances in foods and not all were amines. By the end of the 20th century, scientists had added riboflavin, niacin, biotin, B−6, B−12, pantothenic acid, folate, ascorbic acid, A, D, E, and K to the list of vitamins. Humans also require choline, especially during *prenatal* (before birth) development. Like vitamin D, the body can make choline, but under certain conditions, the body does not synthesize enough to meet its needs. Choline is considered to be a *vitamin−like* essential nutrient.

It is unlikely that any vitamins still need to be discovered. Why? Babies grow and thrive on infant formulas, synthetic liquid diets containing vitamins and other nutrients known to be essential for health. Additionally, very ill people who cannot eat solid food can be kept alive for years on liquid synthetic feedings that contain all known nutrients, including vitamins. If a vitamin remained undiscovered, infants and people who are unable to consume solid foods would not be able to survive on formula diets.

This chapter presents information about the 13 vitamins and choline, including physiological roles and major food sources. By reading this chapter, you will learn what can happen to the body when consumption of certain vitamins is too small or too great. Many Americans take vitamin supplements to prevent disease; the "Vitamins as Medicines" section of this chapter examines current scientific evidence concerning the usefulness of taking megadoses of certain vitamins. Recall from Chapter 1 that a megadose is an amount of a vitamin or mineral that greatly exceeds the recommended amount.

What Is a Vitamin?

vitamin complex organic molecule that regulates certain metabolic processes

What is a vitamin? A **vitamin** is a complex organic compound that regulates certain metabolic processes in the body. A vitamin meets the following criteria:

- The body cannot synthesize the compound or make enough to maintain good health.

- The compound naturally occurs in commonly eaten foods.

- Signs and symptoms of a health problem (*deficiency disorder*) eventually occur when the substance is missing from the diet.

- Good health is restored, if the deficiency disorder is treated early by supplying the missing substance.

Although vitamins are organic molecules in foods, they are distinctly different from carbohydrates, fats, and proteins. Foods generally contain much smaller amounts of vitamins than of macronutrients. A slice of whole−wheat bread, for example, weighs 28 grams. Of that weight, only about 0.005% (1.48 mg) is comprised of vitamins; carbohydrate, water, protein, fat, and minerals make up the remaining weight of the bread. Furthermore, the body requires vitamins in milligram or microgram amounts, but it needs grams of macronutrients.

In the past, amounts of most vitamins in foods, particularly fat−soluble vitamins, were often expressed in *International Units* (*IUs*). Today, IUs have largely been replaced by more precise milligram or microgram measures. One microgram of vitamin D, for example, equals 40 IUs of the vitamin. Food composition tables and the information panels on food and supplement labels often still list IU values for fat−soluble vitamins.

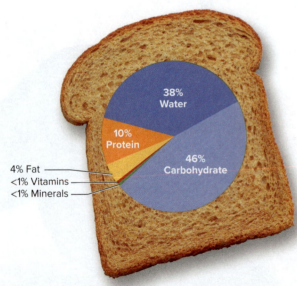

38% Water

10% Protein

46% Carbohydrate

4% Fat
<1% Vitamins
<1% Minerals

A slice of bread weighs about 1 ounce (28 g). Vitamins comprise only about 0.005% (1.48 mg) of the weight of the bread. ©Jules Frazier/Getty Images RF

Classifying Vitamins

Vitamins A, D, E, and K are **fat—soluble vitamins.** These vitamins are in the lipid portions of foods and tend to associate with lipids in the body. Thiamin, riboflavin, niacin, vitamin B—6, pantothenic acid, folate, biotin, vitamin B—12 (collectively known as the B vitamins), and vitamin C are **water—soluble vitamins.** Water—soluble vitamins dissolve in the watery components of food and the body. (Choline is also water soluble.) Table 8.1 presents the vitamins and provides some other names that may be used to identify them.

Why is it important to know the difference between fat— and water—soluble vitamins? The body generally has more difficulty eliminating excess fat—soluble vitamins because these nutrients do not dissolve in watery substances such as urine. As a result, the body stores extra fat—soluble vitamins, primarily in the liver and in body fat. Over time, these vitamins can accumulate and cause toxicity, especially vitamins A and D. On the other hand, the body stores only limited amounts of most water—soluble vitamins; vitamin B—12 is an exception. Furthermore, kidneys can filter excesses of water—soluble vitamins from the bloodstream and eliminate them in urine. Thus, water—soluble vitamins are generally not as toxic as fat—soluble vitamins.

Roles of Vitamins

Vitamins play numerous roles in the body, and each of these micronutrients generally has more than one function (Fig. 8.1). Some vitamins, such as vitamin D, act as hormones; other vitamins, such as thiamin, riboflavin, and niacin, are parts of special molecules that enzymes need to function. In general, vitamins regulate a variety of body processes, including those involved in cell division and development as well as the growth and maintenance of tissues.

Advertisements for vitamins often promote the notion that the micronutrients can "give" you energy. Vitamins, however, are not a source of energy because cells do not metabolize them for energy. Although the body does not use vitamins directly for energy, many vitamins participate in the chemical reactions that release energy from glucose, fatty acids, and amino acids. The diagram in Appendix E presents a simplified view of energy metabolism and indicates vitamins that are involved in the various steps of the process.

Most vitamins have more than one chemical form that functions in the body. For example, *retinol*, *retinal*, and *retinoic acid* are chemically related types of vitamin A that have roles in the body. Additionally, some vitamins have precursors (*provitamins* or *previtamins*) that do not function as vitamins until the body converts them into active forms. For example, the plant pigment beta—carotene is a provitamin for vitamin A, and vitamin D_3 is a previtamin for vitamin D.

What Is an Antioxidant?

When many biochemical reactions take place, the compounds participating in the reactions lose or gain electrons. When an atom or molecule gains one or more electrons, it has been *reduced*. When an atom or molecule loses one or more electrons, it has been *oxidized*. An **oxidizing agent** is a substance that removes electrons from atoms or molecules. An oxidation reaction can form a **radical** (commonly referred to as a "free radical"), a substance with an unpaired electron. Radicals are highly reactive (chemically unstable), and they remove electrons from more stable molecules, such as proteins, fatty acids, and DNA (Fig. 8.2). As a result, radicals can damage or destroy these molecules. If the loss of electrons is uncontrolled, a chain reaction can occur in which excessive oxidation takes place and affects many cells. Many medical researchers suspect excess oxidation is responsible for promoting

TABLE 8.1 Classifying Vitamins

Fat-Soluble Vitamins
A (retinol)
D
E (alpha-tocopherol, other tocopherols)
K

Water-Soluble Vitamins
Thiamin (thiamine, B-1)
Riboflavin (B-2)
Niacin (B-3, nicotinamide, nicotinic acid)
B-6 (pyridoxine)
B-12 (cobalamin, cobalamine)
Biotin (H)
Pantothenic acid (B-5)
Folate (folic acid)
C (ascorbic acid)

Vitamin-Like
Choline

fat-soluble vitamins vitamins A, D, E, and K

water-soluble vitamins thiamin, riboflavin, niacin, vitamin B-6, pantothenic acid, folate, biotin, vitamin B-12, and vitamin C

oxidizing agent substance that removes electrons from atoms or molecules

radical substance with an unpaired electron

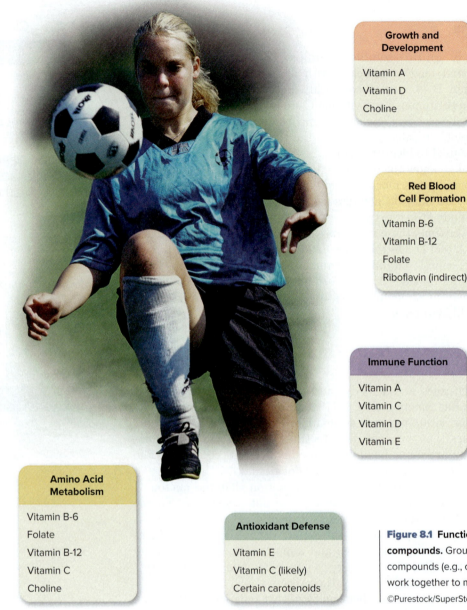

Bone Health

Vitamin A
Vitamin D
Vitamin K
Vitamin C

Energy Metabolism

Thiamin
Riboflavin
Niacin
Pantothenic acid
Biotin
Vitamin B-12
Vitamin B-6

Blood Clotting

Vitamin K

Amino Acid Metabolism

Vitamin B-6
Folate
Vitamin B-12
Vitamin C
Choline

Growth and Development

Vitamin A
Vitamin D
Choline

Red Blood Cell Formation

Vitamin B-6
Vitamin B-12
Folate
Riboflavin (indirect)

Immune Function

Vitamin A
Vitamin C
Vitamin D
Vitamin E

Antioxidant Defense

Vitamin E
Vitamin C (likely)
Certain carotenoids

Figure 8.1 Functions of vitamins and related compounds. Groups of vitamins and related compounds (e.g., choline and certain carotenoids) work together to maintain good health.
©Purestock/SuperStock RF

chemical changes in cells that ultimately lead to heart attack, stroke, cancer, Alzheimer's disease, and even the aging process.

Some radical formation in the body is necessary and provides some benefits.[2] Radicals, for example, stimulate normal cell growth and division. Additionally, white blood cells generate radicals as part of their activities that destroy infectious agents. Under normal conditions, cells regulate oxidation reactions by using anti—oxidants such as vitamin E. **Antioxidants** protect cells by giving up electrons to radicals. When the chemically unstable substance accepts an electron, it can form a more stable structure that does not pull electrons away from other compounds. By sacrificing electrons, antioxidants protect molecules such as polyunsaturated fatty acids in the membrane or DNA in the nucleus from being oxidized (Fig. 8.3).

Sources of Vitamins

antioxidants substances that gives up electrons to radicals to protect cells

Plants, animals, fungi, and even bacteria supply natural forms of vitamins in our diets. In addition to foods, vitamin supplements are another source of these micro—nutrients. Although chemists can synthesize vitamins, certain types of bacteria

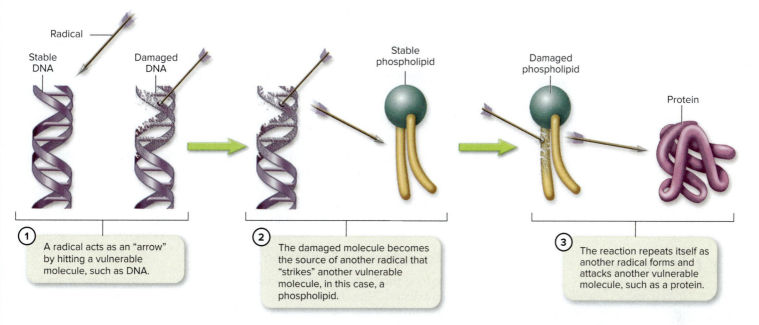

1. A radical acts as an "arrow" by hitting a vulnerable molecule, such as DNA.

2. The damaged molecule becomes the source of another radical that "strikes" another vulnerable molecule, in this case, a phospholipid.

3. The reaction repeats itself as another radical forms and attacks another vulnerable molecule, such as a protein.

Figure 8.2 What is a radical? A radical is a highly reactive substance because it has an unpaired electron. Radicals remove electrons from more stable molecules, such as DNA in the cell's nucleus.

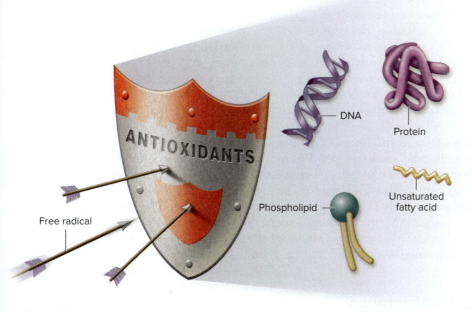

Figure 8.3 Antioxidant action. Antioxidants can protect the cell's plasma membrane and DNA from radicals.

Did *YOU* Know?

Rancidity results when fat in food, particularly the unsaturated fat, undergoes oxidation. Rancid fat makes the food smell and taste bad, and people usually refuse to eat it. To inhibit oxidation of fatty acids and increase a food's shelf life, manufacturers add antioxidants such as BHT and BHA to the food during production.

and algae produce vitamins. These organisms can be grown in laboratory settings for the purpose of "harvesting" their vitamins to use in supplement production.

Regardless of whether a particular vitamin is naturally in foods or syn—thesized in a laboratory, it generally has the same chemical structure and works equally well in the body—but there are exceptions. The natural form of vitamin E has more **biological activity,** that is, it produces more effects in the body, than synthetic vitamin E. On the other hand, *synthetic folic acid,* the type of folate that is added to flour and many ready—to—eat and cooked cereals, has almost twice the biological activity as the natural form of the vitamin.

biological activity describes vitamin's degree of potency or effects in the body

Many adult Americans take multivitamin supplements that contain two or more vitamins and may also supply one or more minerals (*multivitamin/mineral supplement*). According to data collected in the 2007–2010 National Health and Examination Survey, 32% of adults reported regular use of a multivitamin/mineral supplement.[3] Such products are often marketed as "one–a–days" or for a particular target audience, such as men, people with diabetes, athletes, or older adults.

It is not necessary to consume 100% of every vitamin each day. If you are healthy and usually follow a nutritionally adequate diet, your cells should contain a supply of vitamins that can last for several days and possibly even years, depending on the vitamin. Furthermore, bacteria that reside in your lower intestinal tract produce certain vitamins, particularly biotin and vitamin K, and you can absorb these micronutrients to some extent. Additionally, your body can synthesize vitamin D and niacin under certain conditions.

Vitamin Enrichment and Fortification

When raw food products undergo processing, they often lose considerable amounts of micronutrients. Manufacturers can enrich the foods with micronutrients to restore their original nutrient contents. In the United States, many manufacturers of grain products choose to enrich their products. The federally regulated grain enrichment program specifies amounts of four B vitamins (thiamin, riboflavin, niacin, and folic acid) and the mineral iron that the manufacturers must add to their refined wheat flour and certain other milled grain products. Grain enrichment helps protect Americans from developing the deficiency diseases associated with the lack of these nutrients. However, grain enrichment does not replace the vitamin E, vitamin B–6, potassium, magnesium, several other micronutrients, and fiber that were naturally in the unrefined grains. This is the major reason registered dietitian nutritionists and other nutrition experts promote regular consumption of whole–grain products, such as whole–wheat bread and brown rice.

Fortification involves the addition during manufacturing of one or more vitamins (and/or other nutrients) to a wide array of commonly eaten foods. The vitamins that are added may or may not be in the food naturally. For example, milk is often fortified with vitamins A and D, and many ready–to–eat cereals have additional vitamins baked into or sprayed on them before packaging. In the United States, fortification and enrichment of foods have improved vitamin intakes of Americans. However, some food manufacturers add vitamins to foods and beverages, particularly flavored drinks, that would otherwise be considered sources of empty calories. Many nutrition experts are concerned that by substituting such human–made products for more natural foods and beverages, Americans may consume excessive amounts of a few vitamins while reducing their intake of others.

Vitamin Absorption

The small intestine is the primary site of vitamin absorption. However, the intestine does not absorb 100% of the vitamins in food. Vitamin absorption tends to increase when the body's needs for the micronutrients are also higher than usual. The body's requirements for vitamins generally increase during periods of growth, such as infancy and adolescence, and during pregnancy and breastfeeding.

Fat–soluble vitamins are chemically similar to lipids, and the vitamins are in fatty portions of food. Thus, processes that normally occur during fat digestion facilitate the absorption of fat–soluble vitamins. For example, bile enhances lipid as well as fat–soluble vitamin absorption. In the small intestine, the presence of fat stimulates the secretion of a hormone that causes the gallbladder to release bile. Therefore, adding a small amount of fat to low–fat foods, such as

Did *YOU* Know?

Riboflavin is naturally yellow. If you take a dietary supplement that contains high amounts of riboflavin, your kidneys will excrete the excess, and you may notice the bright yellow color of your urine.

tossing raw vegetables with some salad dressing, adding a pat of soft margarine to steamed carrots, or stir—frying green beans in peanut oil, can enhance the intestinal tract's ability to absorb the fat—soluble vitamins in these foods. To review lipid digestion, see Chapter 6.

Diseases or conditions that affect the GI tract can reduce vitamin absorp— tion and result in deficiencies of these micronutrients. People with the inherited disease *cystic fibrosis (sis'—tik fie—broe'—sis)* are unable to digest fat properly because the disease causes blockages to form in ducts that convey pancreatic enzymes to the small intestine. As a result, cystic fibrosis reduces fat absorption, and people with the disease often develop deficiencies of fat—soluble vitamins. People who are unable to absorb vitamins may need to take large oral doses of vitamin supplements just to enable small amounts of the vitamins to be absorbed. In other cases, physicians inject vitamins into their patients' bodies, completely bypassing the need for the intestine to absorb the micronutrients.

Vitamin Deficiency and Toxicity Disorders

A diet that contains adequate amounts of a wide variety of foods, including minimally processed fruits, vegetables, and whole—grain breads and cereals, can help supply the vitamin needs of most healthy people. Vitamin deficiency disor— ders generally result from inadequate diets or conditions that increase the body's requirements for vitamins, such as reduced intestinal absorption or higher— than—normal excretion of the micronutrients. Today, severe vitamin deficiencies are uncommon in the United States, thanks in part to modern food preservation practices, food enrichment and fortification, and the year—round, widespread availability of fresh fruits and vegetables from other countries. Many Americans, however, consume considerably less than recommended amounts of certain vita— mins, particularly E, D, and the vitamin—like compound choline.[4]

A few segments of the population have a high risk of vitamin deficiencies. These vulnerable people include alcoholics, older adults, and patients who are hospitalized for lengthy periods. Additionally, people who have anorexia nervosa, intestinal conditions that interfere with vitamin absorption, or rare metabolic defects that increase their vitamin requirements are more likely to develop vita— min deficiency disorders than people who do not have these conditions.

If your usual diet is nutritionally adequate but you occasionally have low intakes of vitamins, you are unlikely to develop vitamin deficiency diseases because your cells store these micronutrients to some extent. The likelihood of developing a deficiency disease increases when a person's diet consistently lacks the vitamin. When this happens, the person's body stores or tissue levels of the vitamin become depleted, and the signs and symptoms of the nutrient's deficiency disease begin to occur. A person, for example, can become vitamin C–deficient after about a month of consuming a diet that provides little or no vitamin C.[5]

If you are considering taking vitamin supplements or are taking them already, you need to recognize that more is not necessarily better. When cells are saturated with a vitamin, they contain all they need and cannot accept additional amounts of the micronutrient. When this situation occurs, continuing to take the vitamin can produce a toxicity disorder because exposure to the excess micronu— trient or its by—products can damage cells.

Do you need to be concerned about developing a vitamin toxicity disorder? Probably not, unless you are taking excessive amounts (megadoses) of vitamin supplements or consuming large amounts of vitamin—fortified foods regularly. In their natural states, most commonly eaten foods do not contain toxic levels of vitamins. Taking a "one–a–day" type of multivitamin supplement regularly is unlikely to cause toxic effects in adults because these products usually contain less than two times the Daily Values of each micronutrient component.

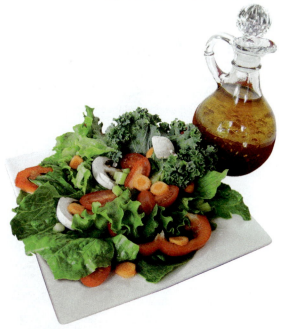

©Wendy Schiff

Did *YOU* Know?

A plant's vitamin content is largely determined by its genetic makeup; growing conditions, including soil composition and sunlight exposure; and maturity when harvested.

Did *YOU* Know?

Have you ever wondered why a freshly peeled apple, eggplant, potato, or banana eventually turns brown? Damaged plant cells release an enzyme that results in the production of brown pigments when it is exposed to air. The action of this enzyme can be reduced by sprinkling salt or sugar on cut pieces of raw food; coating the pieces with an acidic solution, such as lemon juice; or covering them with airtight plastic wrap and chilling the food. Because heat destroys the enzyme, the unappetizing discoloring won't occur if you cook the fruit or vegetable immediately after peeling.

©Photodisc/Getty Images RF

A farmers' market can be a source of locally grown fresh produce during the growing season.
Source: USDA Photo by Bill Tarpening

Preserving the Vitamin Content of Foods

Regardless of whether you pick fruits and vegetables from your own garden or buy them from a farmers' market or supermarket, many kinds of produce, especially berries and leafy vegetables, are highly perishable. Therefore, these foods should be eaten as soon as they are harvested or purchased to ensure maximum vitamin retention. In many instances, unpackaged ("bulk") fresh fruits or vegetables that are sold in supermarkets do not have dates indicating when they should be used, and consumers have no way of knowing when the produce was harvested.

Fresh fruits and vegetables can lose substantial amounts of vitamins as a result of improper handling or lengthy storage conditions. Therefore, select fresh produce carefully when buying it in grocery stores. Avoid produce that is bruised, wilted, or shriveled, or shows signs of decay such as mold. If you are uncertain how to choose ripe fruits and vegetables, ask the person who manages the produce section of the store for advice.

Some vitamins, such as niacin and D, resist destruction by usual food storage conditions or preparation methods. Other vitamins—particularly vitamin C, thiamin, and folate—are easily destroyed or lost by improper food storage and cooking methods. Fresh produce is more likely to retain its natural vitamin content when stored at temperatures near freezing, in high humidity, and away from air. Therefore, you should keep most fresh fruits and vegetables in plastic packaging and chilled until you are ready to use them. Tomatoes, bananas, and garlic should be stored at room temperature. Although precut, packaged salad greens and other vegetables may be convenient to use, they are highly perishable and should be used soon after purchasing.

Exposure to excessive heat, alkaline substances, light, and air can destroy certain vitamins, especially vitamin C. To reduce such losses, trim, peel, and cut raw fruits and vegetables just before eating or serving them. The darker leaves of vegetable greens generally contain more vitamins than the inner, paler color leaves or stems. Therefore, lightly trim away the outer leaves of lettuce and cabbage, and keep edible peels intact; just remove rotten or shriveled parts.

Water-soluble vitamins can leach out of food and dissolve in the cooking water, which is often discarded. By cooking vegetables in small amounts of water and reusing that water for soups or sauces, you are likely to consume those water-soluble nutrients. When preparing produce for cooking, cut the food into large pieces to reduce the amount of surface area that will be exposed to heat, water, and other conditions that can increase vitamin losses. Whenever possible, cook fruits and vegetables in their skins, and if the skins are edible, eat them, too.

Quick cooking methods that involve little contact between produce and water, such as microwaving, steaming, and stir-frying, can conserve much of the vitamin content of the food. According to the Food and Drug Administration (FDA), microwave cooking does not reduce the nutrient content of foods any more than do conventional cooking methods.[6] Microwave cooking may help conserve more vitamins in food because the method cooks quickly and without the need to add much water.

To steam vegetables, place them in a steamer basket that fits inside a pot, add enough water to touch the bottom of the basket, cover the pot, and then heat the water until it boils (Fig. 8.4). As the steam gently cooks the vegetables, add more water, if necessary. To stir-fry vegetables, heat a small amount of oil in a wok or pan that has deep sides, add small pieces of fresh vegetables, and stir the mixture, lightly coating the vegetables with oil (Fig. 8.5). Stir—fried vegetables should be cooked until they are barely tender to retain their nutrients as well as appealing textures, flavors, and colors. The "Recipe for Healthy Living" feature of this chapter has a recipe for stir—fried vegetables.

Are fresh fruits and raw vegetables better sources of vitamins than canned or frozen versions? Sometimes they are. During the canning process, the heating of food can cause the destruction of certain vitamins. However, produce that is frozen immediately after being harvested and then properly stored can be just as nutritious as fresh produce. Frozen fruits and vegetables are often economical alternatives to fresh produce, but they need to be cooked without thawing to conserve much of their vitamin content. The thawing process causes some of the water that was naturally in the produce to drip out, taking water—soluble vitamins with it. If this water is discarded, vitamins in the fluid are lost. The following "Food & Nutrition Tips" provides practical ways to preserve the vitamin content of food.

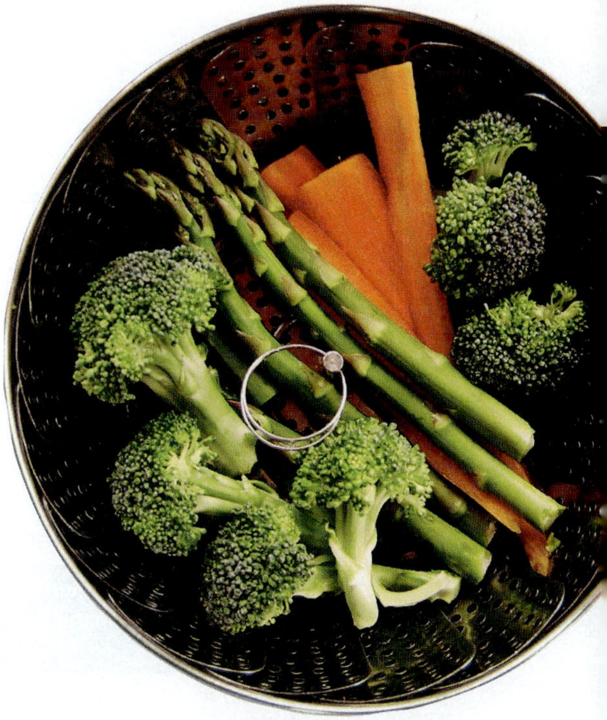

Food & Nutrition tips

- Eat fresh fruits and vegetables along with their edible peels or skins whenever possible.

- Cook fresh vegetables by microwaving, steaming, or stir-frying. Vegetables generally have high water content; therefore, add no water or just a small amount when microwaving vegetables.

- Do not overcook vegetables and minimize reheating because prolonged heating reduces vitamin content.

- Do not add margarine or butter to vegetables during cooking because fat-soluble vitamins and phytochemicals may enter the fat and be discarded when the fat is drained before serving. Fat in foods can enhance the body's absorption of fat-soluble vitamins; therefore, you can add some fat, such as olive oil or soft margarine, to vegetables after they are cooked.

- Store canned foods in a cool place. Canned foods can vary in the amount of nutrients they contain, largely because of differences in storage times and temperatures. If the can has been on the shelf for an extended period of time, the food's vitamin content may have deteriorated, and its taste and texture may be less than desirable. To get maximal nutritive value from canned vegetables, drain the liquid that is packed with the food and use it as a base for soups, sauces, or gravies. If the liquid is too salty, discard it.

Figure 8.4 **Conserving vitamins.** Steaming vegetables can conserve much of the vitamin content of the produce. ©Wendy Schiff

Concept CHECKPOINT

1. List at least three criteria used to designate a substance as a vitamin.
2. List three factors that distinguish vitamins from macronutrients.
3. Define the following terms: *provitamin, antioxidant,* and *radical.*
4. List the vitamins that must be added to refined grains to enrich them, according to the government's grain enrichment program.
5. Discuss at least five ways to preserve the vitamin content of fruits and vegetables during food preparation and storage.

See Appendix G for responses.

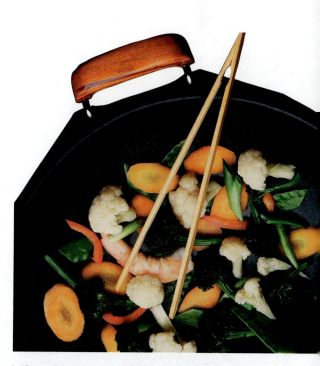

Figure 8.5 **Conserving vitamins.** Stir-frying conserves vitamins by cooking vegetables quickly without adding water. ©Ed Carey/Cole Group/Getty Images RF

8.2 Fat-Soluble Vitamins

Learning Outcomes

 1 List the four fat-soluble vitamins, and identify good dietary sources of each fat-soluble vitamin (or provitamin).

2 Discuss major functions of each fat-soluble vitamin.

3 Identify health problems associated with excesses and deficiencies of fat-soluble vitamins.

This section focuses on fat–soluble vitamins. Table 8.2 presents a summary of general information about all fat–soluble vitamins. Unless otherwise noted, RDA/AI values are for adults 19 to 50 years of age, excluding pregnant or breastfeed–ing women. Figure 8.6 indicates food groups of MyPlate that are good sources of fat–soluble vitamins.

TABLE 8.2   Summary of Fat-Soluble Vitamins

Vitamin	Major Functions in the Body	Adult RDA/AI (adult RDA = bold)	Major Dietary Sources	Major Deficiency Signs and Symptoms	Major Toxicity Signs and Symptoms
Vitamin A (preformed and provitamin A)	Normal vision and reproduction, cellular growth, and immune system function	**700–900 mcg RAE**	Preformed: liver, milk, fortified cereals Provitamin: yellow-orange and dark green fruits and vegetables	Night blindness, xerophthalmia, poor growth, dry skin, reduced immune system functioning	**Adult Upper Limit (UL) = 3,000 mcg/day** Nausea and vomiting, headaches, bone pain and fractures, hair loss, liver damage, interference with vitamin K absorption
Vitamin D	Absorption of calcium and phosphorus, maintenance of normal blood calcium, calcification of bone, maintenance of immune function	**15–20 mcg**	Vitamin D–fortified milk, fortified cereals, fish liver oils, fatty fish	Rickets in children, osteomalacia in adults: soft bones, depressed growth, and reduced immune system functioning	**Adult UL = 100 mcg/day** Poor growth, calcium deposits in soft tissues
Vitamin E	Antioxidant, maintenance of nervous and immune system functions	**15 mg** (alpha-tocopherol)	Vegetable oils and products made from these oils, certain fruits and vegetables, nuts and seeds, fortified cereals	Loss of muscular coordination, nerve damage, reduced immune system function	**Adult UL = 1000 mg/day** Excessive bleeding as a result of interfering with vitamin K metabolism
Vitamin K	Production of active blood-clotting factors	**90–120 mcg**	Green leafy vegetables, canola and soybean oils, and products made from these oils	Excessive bleeding	**Adult UL = undetermined** Unknown

Oil: ©McGraw-Hill Education/Jacques Cornell, photographer; Milk with orange and broccoli: ©McGraw-Hill Education/Ken Karp, photographer; Broccoli and Kale: ©Stockbyte/Getty Images RF; Salmon: ©C Squared Studios/Getty Images RF

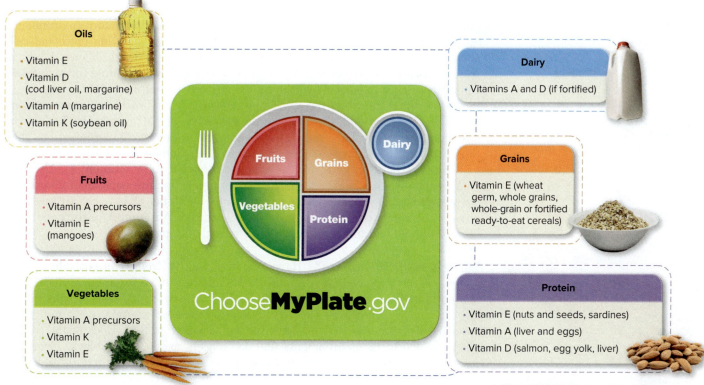

Oils
• Vitamin E
• Vitamin D
(cod liver oil, margarine)
• Vitamin A (margarine)
• Vitamin K (soybean oil)

Fruits
• Vitamin A precursors
• Vitamin E
(mangoes)

Vegetables
• Vitamin A precursors
• Vitamin K
• Vitamin E

Dairy
• Vitamins A and D (if fortified)

Grains
• Vitamin E (wheat
germ, whole grains,
whole-grain or fortified
ready-to-eat cereals)

Protein
• Vitamin E (nuts and seeds, sardines)
• Vitamin A (liver and eggs)
• Vitamin D (salmon, egg yolk, liver)

Figure 8.6 MyPlate and fat-soluble vitamins. This illustration highlights MyPlate food groups that are generally good sources of fat-soluble vitamins.
Source: U.S. Dept. of Agriculture
Oil: ©D. Hurst/Alamy RF; Mango and Cereal: ©Stockbyte/Getty Images RF; Carrots: ©Comstock/Getty Images RF; Milk: ©Judith Collins/Alamy RF; Almonds: ©Ingram Publishing/SuperStock RF

Vitamin A

Do you associate vitamin A with eating carrots and good vision? It is true that vitamin A is involved in the visual process and carrots contain vitamin A pre-cursors. However, vitamin A can multitask: It has numerous functions in the body. Furthermore, carrots are not the only source of vitamin A precursors; many fruits and vegetables are rich sources of these compounds.

Vitamin A is actually a family of compounds that includes retinol. **Retinol (preformed vitamin A)** is the most active form of the vitamin in the body. Although retinol and the other forms of vitamin A are only in animal foods, plants contain hundreds of yellow–orange pigments called **carotenoids.** A few carotenoids are vitamin A precursors because the body can use them to make some retinol. Amounts of vitamin A in food are often reported as micrograms of retinol activity equivalents (RAE). One RAE is approximately 1 mcg of retinol.

All cells in the body need vitamin A to develop and function properly. Vitamin A participates in the processes of cell production, growth and development, function, and maintenance. For example, the vitamin is necessary for the production, maturation, and maintenance of **epithelial cells,** cells that form protective tissues that line the body, including skin and linings of the digestive, respiratory, and reproductive tracts (Fig. 8.7). Certain epithelial cells secrete *mucus*, a sticky

retinol (preformed vitamin A) most active form of vitamin A in the body

carotenoids yellow-orange pigments in fruits and vegetables

epithelial cells cells that form protective tissues that line the body

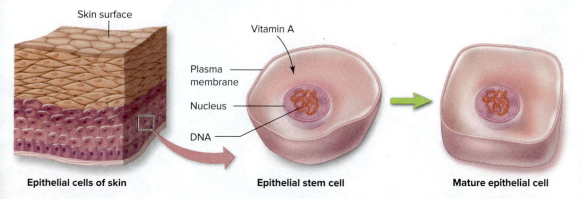

Skin surface

Vitamin A

Plasma membrane

Nucleus

DNA

Epithelial cells of skin   **Epithelial stem cell**   **Mature epithelial cell**

Figure 8.7 Vitamin A and epithelial cells. Vitamin A is necessary for epithelial stem (unspecialized) cells to differentiate and mature properly.

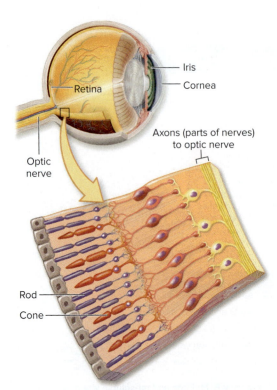

Figure 8.8 **Vitamin A and vision.** The retina, the light-sensitive area inside each eye, contains *rods* and *cones,* specialized nerve cells that are essential for vision.

fluid that keeps the tissue moist and forms a barrier against many environmen-tal pollutants and infectious agents. When the mucus-secreting epithelial cells do not have vitamin A, they deteriorate and no longer produce mucus. A lack of vitamin A can also reduce fertility, because the vitamin is required for maintain-ing the epithelial cells that line the reproductive tracts of men and women.

Vitamin A plays a role in regulating the activity of the immune system. Recall from Chapter 4 that the immune system helps protect the body from infections. Thus, vitamin A–deficient people are at greater risk of infections than those with adequate levels of the vitamin in their bodies.

Normal bone growth and development also require vitamin A. Although your bones do not appear to change their shape, they are constantly remodeled by processes that involve tearing down and rebuilding the tissues to meet the physical demands that you place on them each day. Vitamin A participates with other vitamins and minerals in the bone remodeling process.

What Is Night Blindness? Have you ever walked from a brightly lit theater lobby into the darkened movie auditorium and felt blinded for a few seconds? This is a normal visual response to the sudden and dramatic reduction in light inten-sity. The *retina*, the light–sensitive area inside each eye, contains *rods* and *cones,* specialized nerve cells that are essential for vision (Fig. 8.8). Rods enable you to adapt to poorly lit environments and see objects as shades of black. Cones are responsible for color vision and function in well–lit environments. Rods and cones need vitamin A, particularly retinol, to function properly.

Food & Nutrition tip

When preparing salads or other dishes, do not discard the edible dark green leaves of lettuce, cabbage, or broccoli. These darkly pigmented parts of the plants contribute more provitamin A carotenoids to your diet than the lighter-colored parts. Use them in salads or on sandwiches. In addition to carotenoids, many fruits and vegetables contain hundreds of other phytochemicals that may benefit your health. To obtain a variety of these compounds, include colorful vegetables and fruits in your meals and snacks.

Fruits and vegetables generally are good sources of antioxidants, including carotenoids such as beta-carotene and lycopene.
©C Squared Studios/Getty Images RF

Figure 8.9 illustrates the visual cycle involving rods. Rods remove retinol from the bloodstream and convert it to retinal. In dark conditions, retinal binds to a protein called *opsin* to form **rhodopsin** (*visual purple*). Rhodopsin is necessary for vision in dim light. When you are in a dark environment and exposed to a small amount of light, such as moonlight, the light strikes your rods, activating rhodopsin. Activation alters the shape of the retinal portion of rhodopsin and bleaches the compound. This process causes retinal to split away, reforming opsin. The transformation of rhodopsin to opsin stimulates the rod to send a nervous impulse to the brain that signals the visual processing areas to interpret what is seen. After splitting away from opsin, retinal can bind to the protein, forming rhodopsin again.

As a result of the visual process shown in Figure 8.9, some retinal is destroyed. To replace the retinal, rods remove some retinol (vitamin A) from the bloodstream and convert it to retinal. *Night blindness*, the inability to see in dim light, occurs if retinol is unavailable. Night blindness is an early sign of vitamin A deficiency. Although cone cells also need vitamin A to function, the inability to see certain colors (color blindness) is not the result of a vitamin A deficiency.

Food Sources of Vitamin A

Animal foods such as liver, butter, fish liver oils, and eggs are good sources of preformed vitamin A. Some foods are fortified with the vitamin during processing. Vitamin A–fortified milk, yogurt, margarine, and cereals are important sources of

rhodopsin vitamin A–containing protein that is needed for vision in dim light

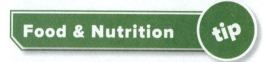
Food & Nutrition tip

Be wary of claims that taking vitamin A supplements will improve your vision so you will not need to wear eyeglasses or contact lenses. Vitamin A deficiency does not cause the kinds of visual defects that are correctable with glasses or contacts. Furthermore, large doses of vitamin A are toxic.

©Vincenzo Lombardo/Getty Images RF

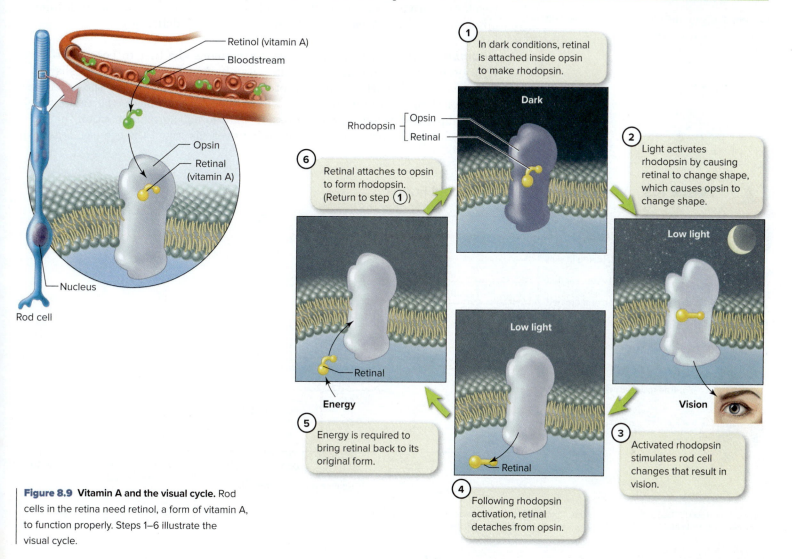

Figure 8.9 Vitamin A and the visual cycle. Rod cells in the retina need retinol, a form of vitamin A, to function properly. Steps 1–6 illustrate the visual cycle.

Did YOU Know?

beta-carotene carotenoid that the body can convert to vitamin A

keratin tough protein found in hair, nails, and the outermost layers of skin

the nutrient for Americans. Carrots, spinach and other leafy greens, pumpkin, sweet potatoes, broccoli, mangoes, and cantaloupe are rich sources of **beta—carotene,** a carotenoid that the body can convert to vitamin A. However, the body obtains only 1 mcg of retinol from every 12 mcg of beta—carotene in a food.

In addition to beta—carotene, common carotenoids include lutein (*loo'—tee—en*), zeaxanthin (*zee—ah—zan'—thin*), and lycopene (*lie'—ko—peen*). Green, leafy vegetables, such as spinach and kale, have high concentrations of lutein and zeaxanthin. Tomato juice and other tomato products, including pizza sauce, contain considerable amounts of lycopene. Although lutein, zeaxanthin, and lycopene are carotenoids, the body does not convert them to vitamin A. Nevertheless, these plant pigments may function as beneficial antioxidants in the human body.

Darkly pigmented fruits and vegetables usually contain more beta—carotene and other provitamin A carotenoids than lightly colored produce. For example, carrots, sweet potatoes, mangoes, and peaches contain more beta—carotene than celery, white potatoes, apples, and bananas. Dark green fruits and vegetables also contain carotenoids, but their green pigment *chlorophyll* contents hide the yellow—orange pigments. Table 8.3 lists some foods that are sources of vitamin A and its precursors.

Dietary Adequacy

For adults, the RDA for vitamin A is 700 to 900 mcg RAE. Deficiencies of the vitamin are rare in the United States.[7] Preschool children who do not eat enough vegetables, urban poor, older adults, and people with severe alcoholism, fat malabsorption, or liver diseases are at risk for vitamin A deficiency.

Vitamin A Deficiency Epithelial cells are among the first to become affected by a deficiency of vitamin A. In skin, vitamin A–deficient epithelial cells produce too much **keratin,** a tough protein found in hair, nails, and the outermost layers of skin. Keratin accumulates within the skin and makes the tissue rough and bumpy. Keratin also forms in tissues that do not normally contain the protein, such as the *cornea*, the clear covering over the iris of the eye (see Fig. 8.8).

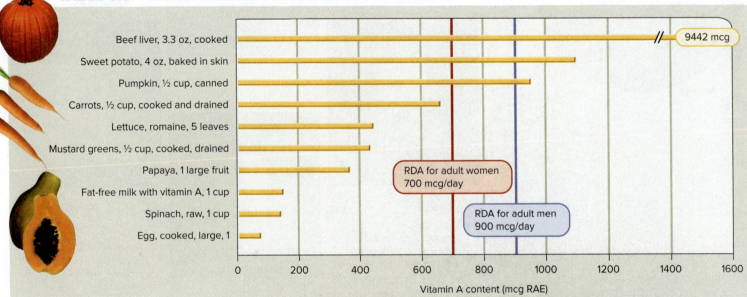

TABLE 8.3 Vitamin A Content of Selected Foods

Food	Vitamin A content (mcg RAE)
Beef liver, 3.3 oz, cooked	9442 mcg
Sweet potato, 4 oz, baked in skin	~1100
Pumpkin, ½ cup, canned	~950
Carrots, ½ cup, cooked and drained	~670
Lettuce, romaine, 5 leaves	~440
Mustard greens, ½ cup, cooked, drained	~430
Papaya, 1 large fruit	~370
Fat-free milk with vitamin A, 1 cup	~150
Spinach, raw, 1 cup	~140
Egg, cooked, large, 1	~80

RDA for adult women 700 mcg/day
RDA for adult men 900 mcg/day

Source: Data from U.S. Department of Agriculture, Agricultural Research Service: *USDA national nutrient database for standard reference,* Release 26, 2013.
Pumpkin: ©Ingram Publishing/Alamy RF; Carrots: ©PhotoAlto/SuperStock RF; Papaya: ©Brand X Pictures/Getty Images RF

The cornea enables light to enter the eye. The epithelial cells that line the inner eyelids secrete mucus that helps keep the cornea moist and clean. In a person suffering from chronic vitamin A deficiency, these cells accumulate keratin, and the white of the eye develops "foamy" areas (Fig. 8.10). Eventually, the epithelial cells harden and stop producing mucus. This condition is called **xerophthalmia** (*zir−op−thal'−me−a*) or "dry eye." Corneas affected by xerophthalmia can be damaged easily by dirt and bacteria. Unless a person with xerophthalmia receives vitamin A, the condition eventually leads to blindness.

Each year, thousands of children in developing nations, especially in Africa and Southeast Asia, become blind because of severe vitamin A deficiency.[8] Vitamin deficiency also reduces the effectiveness of the immune system, and many children suffering from vitamin A deficiency die from infections such as measles. In countries where vitamin A deficiency is widespread, public health efforts are being taken to reduce the prevalence of the condition. Such efforts include educating people about the need to eat regionally grown foods that are rich in beta−carotene and giving vitamin A injections periodically to vulnerable populations. In some countries, governments encourage food manufacturers to fortify commonly eaten foods, such as sugar and margarine, with vitamin A.

Vitamin−A deficient women are more likely to die during pregnancy than pregnant women who are not lacking the vitamin.[7] Furthermore, infants who are born to vitamin A–deficient women are more likely to die than babies born to healthy women. However, pregnant women should not take vitamin A supplements to prevent birth defects without consulting with their physicians. When taken during pregnancy, excess vitamin A is a **teratogen,** an agent that causes birth defects.

Vitamin A Toxicity The UL for vitamin A intake is 3000 mcg/day for adults. Excessive consumption of vitamin A can damage the liver because the organ is the main site for vitamin A storage. Toxicity signs and symptoms include headache, nausea, vomiting, visual disturbances, hair loss, bone pain, and bone fractures.

Miscarriage and birth defects may result when excessive amounts of vitamin A are taken early in pregnancy. Women of childbearing age should limit their overall intake of vitamin A to about 100% of the Daily Value (20 mcg). In addition, women who may become pregnant or who are pregnant should restrict their intake of rich food sources of vitamin A, such as liver and fish liver oils.

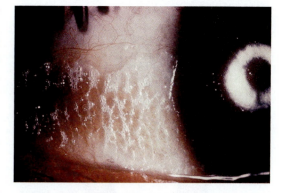

Figure 8.10 **Early sign of xerophthalmia.** Vitamin A deficiency can cause drying (the white foamy areas) of the surface of the eye. If untreated, this condition can lead to blindness. Source: Centers for Disease Control and Prevention

xerophthalmia condition affecting the eyes that results from vitamin A deficiency

teratogen agent that causes birth defects

carotenemia yellowing of the skin that results from excess beta-carotene in the body

Did *YOU* Know?

In the early 1900s, teams of explorers raced to discover and explore the North and South Poles. Starvation was a major risk of embarking on such expeditions. Some explorers learned survival techniques from the Inuits, an Eskimo population who inhabit the Arctic region of North America. The Inuits warned the explorers to avoid eating polar bear and seal livers because severe illness and death could result. Unfortunately, many Western explorers did not know that their sled dogs were also not safe for human consumption.

From 1911 to 1913, Douglas Mawson and Xavier Mertz were on an ill-fated expedition to explore an area near the South Pole. As the two men struggled to return to their winter base camp, they had to eat their sled dogs, particularly the animals' livers, to avoid starvation. Both men suffered terribly from the diet; Mertz did not survive. Over 50 years later, scientists determined that sled dogs can accumulate large amounts of vitamin A in their livers without showing ill effects. However, eating just a few ounces of sled dog liver can be toxic for humans.

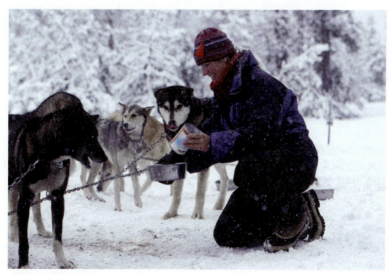

©Ingram Publishing/SuperStock RF

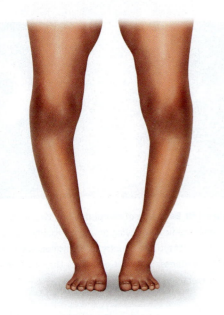

Figure 8.11 **Rickets.** A child suffering from rickets has soft bones that do not grow properly. The youngster's leg bones bow under the weight of carrying the upper part of the body.

rickets vitamin D deficiency disorder in children

Carotenemia (*kar'−et−eh−ne'−me−ah*), a condition characterized by yellowing of the skin, can result from eating too much beta−carotene−rich produce or taking too many beta−carotene supplements.[7] This condition occasionally develops in infants who eat a lot of baby foods that contain carrots, apricots, winter squash, or green beans. In most instances, carotenemia is harmless. The skin's natural color eventually returns to normal when the carotenoid−rich foods are no longer eaten.

Physicians may prescribe medications derived from vitamin A, such as isotretinoin, to treat severe acne and other skin disorders. Although these medications are less toxic than natural vitamin A, ingesting excessive amounts can produce harmful symptoms. Furthermore, vitamin A derivatives can cause miscarriage or severe birth defects in the offspring of women who use them during pregnancy. Therefore, women of childbearing age should avoid pregnancy while using these medications.

Vitamin D

By the 1700s, some people in parts of northern Europe had learned that exposing children to sunlight or giving the youngsters fish liver oil could prevent or treat **rickets.** Children with rickets have bones that are soft and can become misshapen. Leg bones, for example, bow under the weight of carrying the upper part of the body (Fig. 8.11). Additionally, the affected child's joints, rib cage, and hips (pelvis) become deformed, and the child may complain of muscle pain. In 1922, scientists discovered a fat−soluble factor in cod liver oil that was needed for proper bone health and preventing rickets. The scientists thought the factor that cured rickets was a vitamin, and they named the substance *vitamin D*. The fat−soluble factor in cod liver oil is still considered a vitamin because rickets can be prevented and treated by taking vitamin D supplements or eating vitamin D–rich foods. However, vitamin D is actually a hormone.

The body can make vitamin D after skin cells are exposed to the sun's ultraviolet radiation (*UVB*, in particular), which explains why the nutrient is often called the "sunshine vitamin." The radiation converts a substance in skin that is derived from cholesterol into a previtamin (*vitamin D_3*). Vitamin D_3 circulates to the liver, where the substance is converted to the inactive compound *25−OH vitamin D*. Eventually, the kidneys convert 25−OH vitamin D into the active hormone we call "vitamin D" (Fig. 8.12). Certain foods and dietary supplements are also sources of vitamin D_3. The kidneys convert the vitamin D_3 from these sources into the active form of the vitamin.

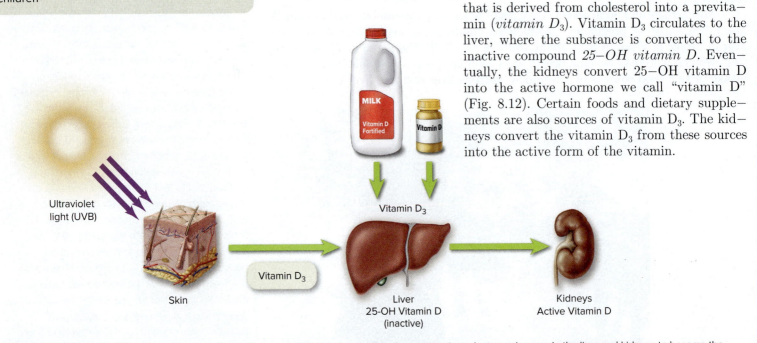

Ultraviolet light (UVB)

Vitamin D_3

Skin

Vitamin D_3

Liver
25-OH Vitamin D
(inactive)

Kidneys
Active Vitamin D

Figure 8.12 **Vitamin D.** After skin synthesizes vitamin D_3 from a cholesterol derivative, the previtamin undergoes changes in the liver and kidneys to become the active form of the vitamin. Forms of previtamin D that are in certain foods and dietary supplements must also undergo changes in the liver and kidneys to become active vitamin D.

REAL PEOPLE | REAL STORIES

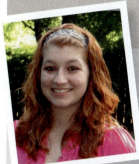
©Alicia Croker

Amanda Croker

Amanda Croker, a junior majoring in East Asian Language and Culture at the University of Kansas, routinely tried to limit her sun exposure to avoid sunburn and the possibility of skin cancer in the future. "My skin is so light," Amanda says, "I even got a sunburn in Kansas in the middle of October because I was outside for a couple hours!" She was unaware that her efforts to protect her skin were also limiting her body's ability to make vitamin D, "the sunshine vitamin."

"I'm taking a prescription dose of vitamin D because my family doctor tested my blood and found out that I didn't have enough of the vitamin in my body," Amanda says. "She told me that people need sunlight to make vitamin D, but she said she wasn't surprised that I'm deficient, since I have red hair. I told her that I try to avoid being out in the sun for more than 30 minutes because I 'crisp' when I get exposed to sun. Anyway, I don't notice that much of a difference now that I'm on the medication." Although Amanda does not "feel" different now, her bones eventually may have become soft and weak, if her doctor had not discovered that Amanda was vitamin D–deficient. Before the discovery and purification of vitamin D, children were given cod liver oil to prevent rickets, the vitamin's deficiency disease.

As a result of the treatment, Amanda's blood level of vitamin D became normal within a few weeks. Because few foods are good sources of vitamin D, she will need to take a daily supplement of the micronutrient, which is available without a prescription, for the rest of her life. By taking the supplement, she should be able to maintain a healthy blood level of the fat-soluble vitamin.

Why Is Vitamin D Necessary?

Vitamin D is necessary for the metabolism of the minerals calcium and phosphorus, and the production and maintenance of healthy bones (Fig. 8.13). Vitamin D stimulates small intestinal cells to absorb calcium and phosphorus from food. When vitamin D is lacking, the intestine absorbs only 10 to 15% of the calcium in foods; with the vitamin, intestinal absorption of dietary calcium increases to 30 to 80%.[9] Vitamin D also stimulates bone cells to form *calcium phosphate*, the major mineral compound in bone. Without adequate vitamin D, bone cells cannot deposit enough calcium and phosphorus to produce strong bones.

When blood calcium levels drop, vitamin D works with *parathyroid hormone (PTH)* to signal bones to release calcium. PTH also stimulates the kidneys to increase vitamin D production and decrease the elimination of calcium in urine. These actions help raise the level of calcium in blood to normal (Fig. 8.14). Removing too much calcium from bones can weaken them, but calcium is essential for normal heartbeat and other muscle contractions. If bones did not supply calcium for such vital functions, a person could experience serious, even fatal consequences.

Vitamin D has other roles in the body, including regulating neuromuscular and immune function and reducing inflammation.[10] Vitamin D is also involved in controlling cell growth, and as a result, the micronutrient may reduce the risk of certain cancers. However, more research is needed to clarify the vitamin's role in immune function and disease prevention.

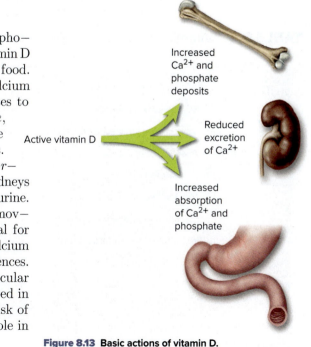

Active vitamin D

Increased Ca^{2+} and phosphate deposits

Reduced excretion of Ca^{2+}

Increased absorption of Ca^{2+} and phosphate

Figure 8.13 Basic actions of vitamin D.

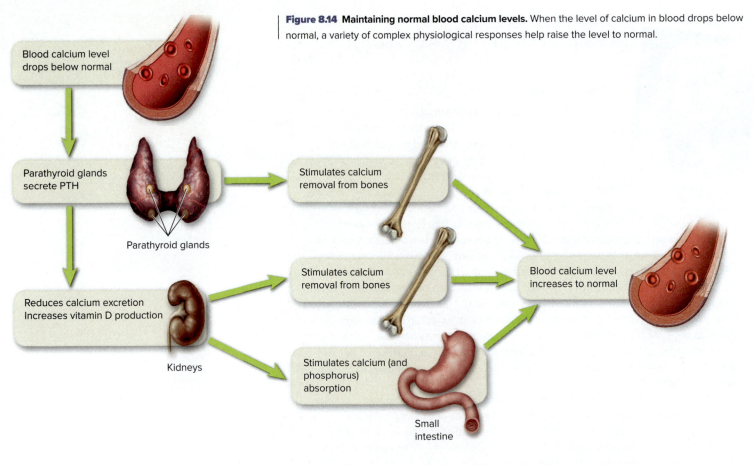

Figure 8.14 Maintaining normal blood calcium levels. When the level of calcium in blood drops below normal, a variety of complex physiological responses help raise the level to normal.

Sources of Vitamin D

Fish liver oils and fatty fish, especially salmon, herring, and catfish, are among the few foods that naturally contain previtamin forms of vitamin D. Milk is routinely fortified with vitamin D, and some brands of ready—to—eat cereals, orange juice, and margarine have the vitamin added to them as well. Table 8.4 lists some

TABLE 8.4 Vitamin D Content of Selected Foods

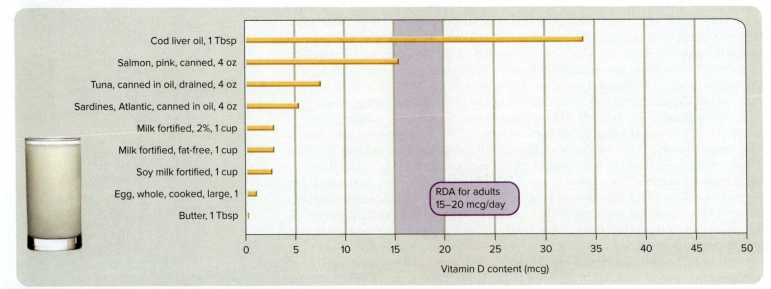

Source: Data from U.S. Department of Agriculture, Agricultural Research Service: *USDA national nutrient database for standard reference,* Release 26, 2013.
Milk ©McGraw-Hill Education/Ken Karp, photographer

food sources of vitamin D. Food composition tables often list the vitamin D content of foods in International Units; 1 mcg of vitamin D equals 40 IU.

Vitamin D and Sunlight Vitamin D is not widespread in food; therefore, your body depends on sun exposure to synthesize the vitamin. The amount of time you need to spend in the sun to form adequate amounts of vitamin D depends primarily on your location, the time of day and year, and your age and skin color. If you live south of about the 33rd parallel in the United States and you are outdoors when sunlight is most intense (between 10 A.M. and 3 P.M.), you may obtain enough sun exposure to make vitamin D during most of the year.[11] In North America, the 33rd parallel extends from about Charleston, South Carolina, through Dallas, Texas, to San Diego, California (Fig. 8.15). The Earth's atmosphere blocks ultraviolet (UV) radiation. If you live north of the 33rd parallel, the angle of the winter sun is such that the sun's rays must pass through more of the atmosphere than at other times of the year (Fig. 8.16). As a result, your skin may not make sufficient amounts of previtamin D during the winter, and you may not have adequate vitamin D stored in your body to last until spring. Therefore, you may need to take a supplement that contains 100% of the adult Daily Value for vitamin D (see Appendix B), especially from November through February. Clouds, shade, window glass, and air pollution are environmental factors that can also limit the amount of UV radiation that reaches your skin.

Skin contains *melanin*, the brown pigment that can reduce the skin's ability to produce vitamin D from sunlight. Darker skin contains more melanin than lighter skin. If you have dark skin, you may need to spend even more time in the sun to form adequate amounts of the vitamin. Otherwise, you should consider consuming foods that contain the vitamin or a vitamin D supplement regularly.

Although you may think tanned skin is attractive, tanning and severe sunburn increase the risk of developing wrinkles and skin cancer. UV radiation is a major risk factor for skin cancer, including melanoma, the most deadly form of skin cancer. Dermatologists often advise people to apply sunscreens consistently before going outdoors. Using a sunscreen, however, limits skin's ability to synthesize previtamin vitamin D_3. When properly applied, a sunscreen with a *sun protection factor (SPF)* of 8 or more blocks sunlight that is needed to form D_3.[10] To allow your body to make some active vitamin D, you can expose your skin to the sun for about 15 minutes *before* applying a commercial sunscreen. Concerns about the risk of skin cancer have made it difficult for scientists to develop guidelines for the amount of sunlight exposure that is necessary to optimize vitamin D synthesis.

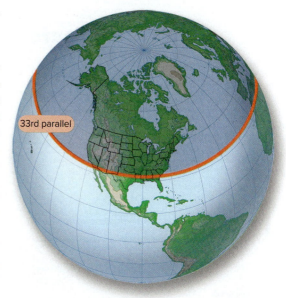

Figure 8.15 Latitude and vitamin D status. If you live in North America south of the 33rd parallel and are outdoors when sunlight is most intense during the day, you are likely to obtain enough sun exposure to synthesize vitamin D most of the year.

Did *YOU* Know?

Information provided by tanning parlors may include claims that the tanning process is safe. Nevertheless, the ultraviolet radiation emitted by tanning beds increases the risk of wrinkles and skin cancer. Therefore, the use of tanning beds should be avoided.

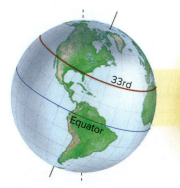
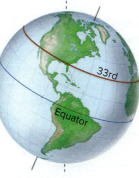

Summer solstice
(Northern Hemisphere tilts toward the sun)

Sun

Winter solstice
(Northern Hemisphere tilts away from the sun)

Figure 8.16 Seasonal variations in sunlight intensity. If you live north of the 33rd parallel, the angle of the winter sun is such that the sun's rays must pass through more of the atmosphere than at other times of the year. As a result, skin tends to form less previtamin vitamin D in the winter.

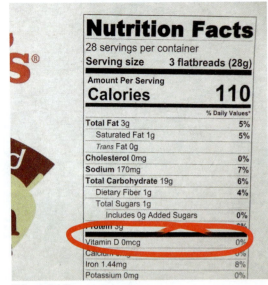

©Wendy Schiff

osteomalacia adult rickets; condition characterized by poorly mineralized (soft) bones

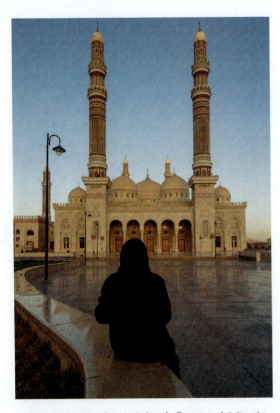

Figure 8.17 Clothing and vitamin D status. Adults who are almost fully covered during the day, such as for religious reasons, are at risk for osteomalacia.
©John Lund/Blend Images LLC RF

Dietary Adequacy

For adults under 70 years of age, the RDA for vitamin D is 15 mcg/day. Many Americans who are 2 years of age and older do not consume enough vitamin D to meet the RDA.[4] According to the Dietary Guidelines, the vitamin is a "nutrient of public health concern." Younger people, however, generally have higher blood levels of the vitamin than older adults.

In the United States, a national effort to fortify milk with vitamin D began in the 1930s, and as a result, rickets became rare in this country. Although severe rickets is uncommon, public health officials are concerned about the recent increase in the number of cases reported among infants and toddlers. Breast milk contains insufficient amounts of vitamin D to prevent rickets. Infants who are most likely to develop rickets are breastfed, and they have dark skin, minimal sunlight exposure, and little or no vitamin D intake.[10] Exposing breastfed babies to sunlight reduces their risk of the disease, but as mentioned earlier, medical experts do not know how much sun exposure is necessary. Thus, breastfed infants should consume a supplement containing 10 mcg (400 IU) of vitamin D per day soon after birth. The adult form of rickets is called **osteomalacia** (*ahs'−tee−o−mah−lay'−she−a*). The bones of people with osteomalacia have normal amounts of *collagen*, the protein that provides structure for the skeleton, but they contain less−than−normal amounts of calcium. The bones are soft and weak, and break easily as a result. Muscle weakness is also a symptom of osteomalacia.

Adults who are confined indoors or almost fully covered during the day, such as for religious reasons, are at risk for osteomalacia (Fig. 8.17).[10] Osteomalacia is a risk for adults who have kidney, liver, or intestinal diseases because these conditions may reduce both vitamin D production and calcium absorption. Exposing skin to sunlight, eating vitamin D–rich foods, or taking vitamin D supplements can help adults avoid vitamin D deficiency and osteomalacia.

As a person ages, production of vitamin D_3 in skin declines and conversion of the previtamin to active vitamin D in kidneys also decreases. As a result of these age−related changes, older adults are more likely to develop vitamin D deficiency than younger persons. Older adults are also at risk for bone fractures. An analysis of several studies indicated older adults who took 700 to 800 IUs of vitamin D per day had a lower risk of hip fractures than elderly persons who took 400 IUs of vitamin D per day. Thus, people over 50 years of age may benefit from using a daily vitamin D supplement.[12]

Although *osteoporosis* is usually associated with inadequate calcium intakes, a long−term vitamin D deficiency contributes to the condition because calcium absorption is reduced.[10] The calcium section of Chapter 9 provides more information about osteoporosis.

Vitamin D Toxicity The body stores vitamin D. Long−term ingestion of vitamin D supplements that supply 10,000 to 40,000 IU/day can accumulate in the body and produce toxicity.[10] When excess vitamin D is consumed, the small intestine absorbs too much calcium from foods, and the mineral is deposited in soft tissues, including the kidneys, heart, and blood vessels. The calcium deposits can interfere with cells' ability to function, which can cause cellular death. Other signs and symptoms of vitamin D toxicity include muscular weakness, loss of appetite, diarrhea, vomiting, and mental confusion. You do not have to be concerned about your body making toxic levels of vitamin D when exposed to sunlight because skin limits its production of the previtamin, vitamin D_3.[10] The Upper Limit (UL) for vitamin D is 100 mcg/day (4000 IU/day).

Vitamin E

Vitamin E has several forms, but only the *alpha−tocopherol (al'−fah toe−koff'−e−roll)* form is used by the body.[13] **Alpha−tocopherol** (*vitamin E*) is an antioxidant that protects polyunsaturated fatty acids in cell membranes from being damaged by radicals (Fig. 8.18). Such oxidative damage may be associated with the development of atherosclerosis, the process that occurs within arteries and contributes to heart attack and stroke; cancer; and premature cellular aging and death. Other roles for vitamin E include maintaining immune system function.

Food Sources of Vitamin E

Rich food sources of vitamin E include sunflower seeds, almonds, and plant oils, especially sunflower, safflower, canola, and olive oils. Products made from vitamin E–rich plant oils, such as margarines and salad dressings, also supply the micronutrient. Other important dietary sources of the vitamin include fish, whole grains, nuts, seeds, and certain vegetables. Meats, processed grain products, and dairy products generally do not contain much vitamin E. Table 8.5 lists some common foods that are sources of the micronutrient.

Harvesting, processing, storage, and cooking methods influence the amount of vitamin E retained in food. During the milling process, most of the vitamin E that is in whole grains is lost, and it is not restored by enrichment. Furthermore, vitamin E is highly susceptible to destruction by exposure to oxygen, metals, and light, as well as high temperatures that occur when heating oil for deep−fat frying.

Dietary Adequacy

For adults, the RDA for vitamin E is 15 mg/day of alpha−tocopherol. Although many American adults do not consume recommended amounts of vitamin E, vita−min E deficiency is rare.[13] A healthy body stores the vitamin in body fat, skeletal muscle, and the liver.

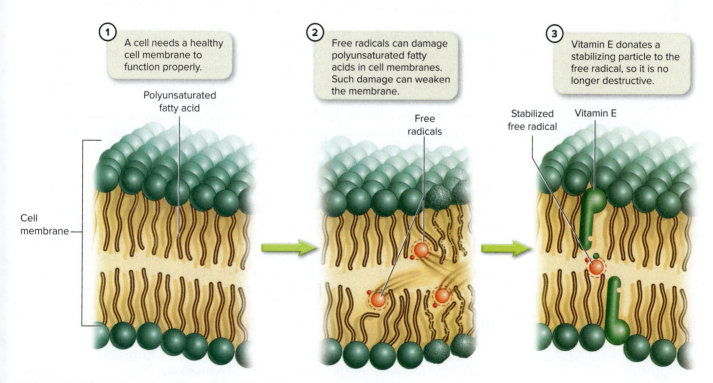

1. A cell needs a healthy cell membrane to function properly.

2. Free radicals can damage polyunsaturated fatty acids in cell membranes. Such damage can weaken the membrane.

3. Vitamin E donates a stabilizing particle to the free radical, so it is no longer destructive.

Polyunsaturated fatty acid

Free radicals

Stabilized free radical

Vitamin E

Cell membrane

Figure 8.18 Vitamin E and the cell membrane. Vitamin E protects unsaturated fatty acids in cell membranes from being damaged by radicals.

TABLE 8.5   Vitamin E Content of Selected Foods

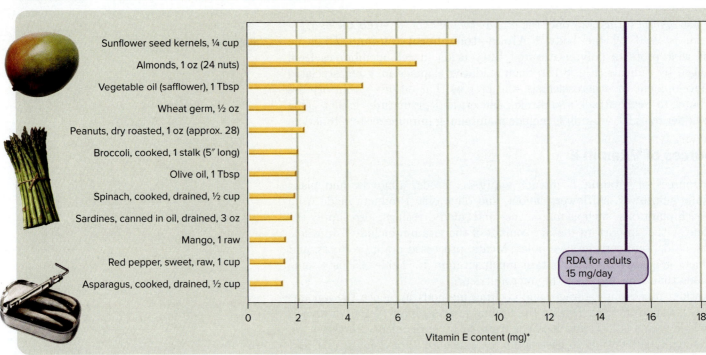

* As alpha-tocopherol.

Source: Data from U.S. Department of Agriculture, Agricultural Research Service: *USDA national nutrient database for standard reference,* Release 26, 2013.
Mango: ©Stockbyte/Getty Images RF; Asparagus and Sardines: ©Brand X Pictures/Getty Images RF

Amounts of vitamin E may be reported as a number of IUs. One mg of alpha–tocopherol is about 1.5 IU of the natural form of the vitamin. Synthetic vitamin E is used to fortify foods and produce supplements that contain the vitamin. One mg of vitamin E is equal to 2.22 IU of the synthetic form of the vitamin.[13]

Vitamin E Deficiency   People who have diseases that interfere with fat absorption may become deficient in vitamin E because dietary fat enhances intestinal absorption of the micronutrient. Vitamin E deficiency can reduce the functioning of the nervous and immune systems. Long–term vitamin E deficiency results in nerve damage, loss of neuromuscular control, and blindness.[13]

Infants who are born too early (premature infants) may have low vitamin E stores because the vitamin is transferred from mother to fetus late in pregnancy. If premature infants develop signs of vitamin E deficiency, they can be given special infant formulas and supplements that provide the vitamin.

Vitamin E Toxicity   For healthy adults, the UL for vitamin E is 1000 mg/day of alpha–tocopherol. Consuming amounts of vitamin E in foods has not been associated with any negative effects on health.[13] However, taking dietary supplements that supply excessive amounts of the vitamin may interfere with vitamin K's role in blood clotting and lead to uncontrolled bleeding (hemorrhage). Therefore, people who are taking medications that interfere with blood clotting ("blood thinners") should check with their physicians before using vitamin E supplements.

Vitamin K

In the early 1930s, Danish researcher Henrick Dam discovered a factor in alfalfa that played a role in blood clotting (coagulation). Dam named the factor vitamin "K" after *koagulation,* the Danish spelling of *coagulation.* Vitamin K is a family of compounds that includes *phylloquinone* (*fill−o−kwin'−own*) from plants and *menaquinones* (*men−eh−kwin'−owns*) in fermented foods, such as sauerkraut, cheddar cheese, natto, and miso. Natto and miso are made from fermented soybeans and are popular in Japan. Bacteria that normally live in the intestinal tract also make menaquinones, but the extent to which bacteria contribute to the body's vitamin K supply is unclear.[14]

The presence of dietary fat, bile, and pancreatic juice help vitamin K be absorbed in the small intestine. Some vitamin K is stored in the liver, and some is incorporated in lipoproteins for transport in the bloodstream. The liver also breaks down vitamin K and eliminates the vitamin's by−products by adding them to bile.

Why Is Vitamin K Necessary?

Blood contains inactive clotting factors and cell fragments called *platelets* that are necessary for blood clotting to occur. When a blood vessel is cut, blood in the injured area undergoes a complex series of steps to form a clot that stops the bleeding (Fig. 8.19). A clot is comprised of strands of the protein *fibrin* that trap blood cells, forming a mesh. The liver synthesizes several blood−clotting factors, and the organ needs vitamin K to produce four of them, including *prothrombin*, properly. When vitamin K is unavailable, the blood does not clot effectively. Some people take the prescribed medication warfarin because their blood clots too easily. Vitamin K can interfere with warfarin's "blood−thinning" activity, so people who take the medication should not consume vitamin K supplements. Additionally, these patients should try to maintain consistent dietary intakes of the vitamin each day.

Vitamin K also helps bone−building cells produce *osteocalcin*, a protein needed for normal bone mineralization. Low blood levels of vitamin K are associated with the risk of *osteoporosis*, a condition characterized by bones with low mineral density. However, more research is needed to clarify the vitamin's role in bone health.

Food Sources of Vitamin K

Major food sources of vitamin K are green leafy vegetables such as kale, turnip greens, salad greens, cabbage, and spinach; broccoli; and green beans. Other reliable sources of the vitamin are soybean and canola oils, and products made from these oils, such as salad dressing. Table 8.6 lists some foods that are sources of the vitamin. The chemical structure of vitamin K is very stable and resists being destroyed by usual cooking methods.

Figure 8.19 Vitamin K and blood clotting. When a blood vessel is cut, blood in the injured area undergoes a series of steps to form a clot that stops the bleeding. The liver needs vitamin K to make prothrombin and three other blood-clotting factors. Fibrin: ©Science Photo Library RF/Getty Images RF

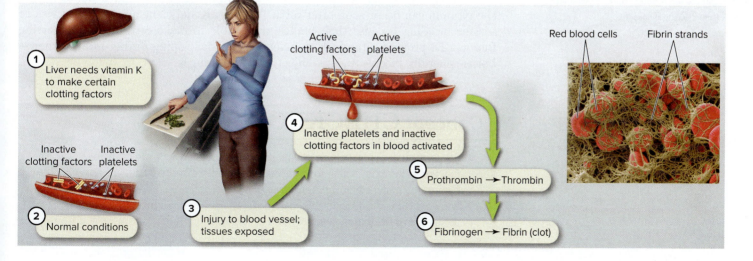

1. Liver needs vitamin K to make certain clotting factors

Inactive clotting factors   Inactive platelets

2. Normal conditions

3. Injury to blood vessel; tissues exposed

Active clotting factors   Active platelets

4. Inactive platelets and inactive clotting factors in blood activated

5. Prothrombin → Thrombin

6. Fibrinogen → Fibrin (clot)

Red blood cells   Fibrin strands

TABLE 8.6 Vitamin K Content of Selected Foods

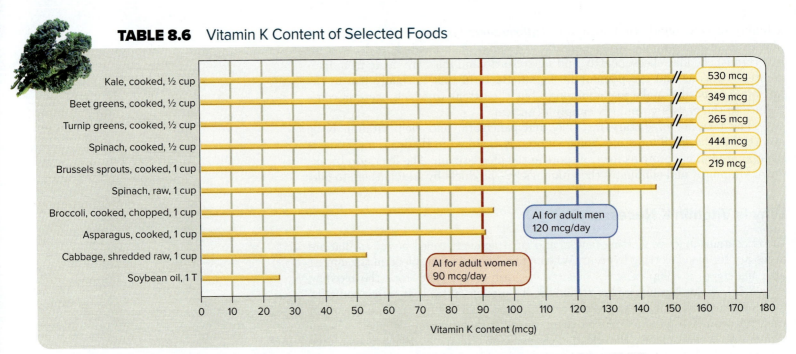

Food	Vitamin K content (mcg)
Kale, cooked, ½ cup	530 mcg
Beet greens, cooked, ½ cup	349 mcg
Turnip greens, cooked, ½ cup	265 mcg
Spinach, cooked, ½ cup	444 mcg
Brussels sprouts, cooked, 1 cup	219 mcg
Spinach, raw, 1 cup	
Broccoli, cooked, chopped, 1 cup	
Asparagus, cooked, 1 cup	
Cabbage, shredded raw, 1 cup	
Soybean oil, 1 T	

AI for adult men 120 mcg/day

AI for adult women 90 mcg/day

Vitamin K content (mcg)

Source: Data from U.S. Department of Agriculture, Agricultural Research Service: *USDA national nutrient database for standard reference,* Release 26, 2013.
Kale ©Wendy Schiff

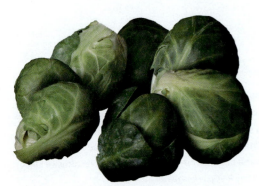

Brussels sprouts are a good source of vitamin K.
©Brand X Pictures/Getty Images RF

Dietary Adequacy

No RDAs for vitamin K have been established, but AIs for the vitamin are 120 mcg/day for men and 90 mcg/day for women. The AIs can be met easily by eating a salad that contains 1 cup of leafy vegetables and 2 tablespoons of salad dressing made with soybean oil. Ingesting amounts of natural forms of vitamin K that exceed the AIs has not been reported to be harmful to humans.

Vitamin K: Deficiency Although the body stores very little vitamin K, defi‐ciencies among adults rarely occur.[14] Vitamin K deficiency, however, can develop in people who have liver diseases or conditions that impair fat absorption, such as cystic fibrosis. Additionally, long‐term antibiotic therapy can reduce the number of bacteria in the colon that synthesize vitamin K and, as a result, might contribute to a deficiency of the nutrient. The most reliable sign of vitamin K deficiency is an increase in the time it takes for blood to clot.

Babies are generally born with low vitamin K stores, and a deficiency of the vitamin can occur soon after birth. Vitamin K–deficient infants are at risk of serious bleeding because their bodies are unable to make certain blood‐clotting factors. To prevent vitamin K deficiency from developing during infancy, new‐borns generally receive a single injection of vitamin K.

Concept CHECKPOINT

6. Prepare a table of fat-soluble vitamins. For each vitamin, indicate its major function in the body, major food sources, deficiency disorder (if it has a specific name), and major signs and symptoms of the deficiency disorder. If the vitamin is known to be toxic, also indicate major toxicity signs and symptoms. Check your table against the information provided in Table 8.2.

See Appendix G for responses.

8.3 Water-Soluble Vitamins

Learning Outcomes

1 List the water-soluble vitamins, and identify good dietary sources of each vitamin (or its precursor).

2 Discuss major functions of each water-soluble vitamin.

3 Identify health problems associated with excesses and deficiencies of water-soluble vitamins.

In the body, most water–soluble vitamins function as components of specific coenzymes. A **coenzyme** is a small, organic molecule that interacts with enzymes and, as a result, regulates a chemical reaction. To synthesize a coenzyme, cells combine one of the B vitamins with a nitrogen–containing, nonprotein compound (Fig. 8.20). When activated by the coenzyme, the enzyme enables the reaction to occur (see Fig. 8.20).

Many of the chemical reactions involved in the metabolism of carbo–hydrates, fats, and amino acids involve coenzymes that contain B vitamins. Thiamin, riboflavin, niacin, vitamin B–6, and pantothenic acid function as part of coenzymes involved in energy metabolism. Coenzymes containing these vitamins are also necessary for synthesizing glucose, amino acids, and certain lipids.

Foods contain B vitamins in their coenzyme forms. Health–food stores often sell supplements that contain coenzymes, but buying these products is a waste of money. In the small intestine, coenzymes in food or supplements are not absorbed intact. The compounds undergo digestion to release their B vitamin components. The small intestine absorbs many of the B vitamins that were in foods and supplements, and the micronutrients eventually enter the general cir–culation. Cells then remove the free vitamins from the bloodstream and use them to rebuild coenzymes.

This section of the chapter focuses on the water–soluble vitamins: thiamin, riboflavin, niacin, B–6, folate, B–12, biotin, pantothenic acid, and C; as well as the vitamin–like nutrient choline. Table 8.7 provides a summary of general information about all the water–soluble vitamins and choline. Figure 8.21 indi–cates food groups that are good sources of water–soluble vitamins.

Thiamin

In the body, thiamin is used to make a coenzyme that participates in chemical reactions involved in the release of energy from carbohydrates. Additionally, the thiamin–containing coenzyme plays a role in the metabolism of certain amino acids, and the coenzyme may be necessary for the synthesis of neurotransmitters. A neurotransmitter is a chemical produced by a nerve cell that enables the cell to communicate to other nerve cells.

Food Sources of Thiamin

Foods that contribute thiamin to American diets include whole–grain and enriched breads and cereals, pork, legumes, and orange juice. Brewer's yeast is a rich source of thiamin, but most Americans do not eat the product. Table 8.8 lists some common foods that are good sources of thiamin. Overcooking and cooking food in alkaline solutions, such as water to which some baking soda has been added to brighten the color of green vegetables, can destroy thiamin.

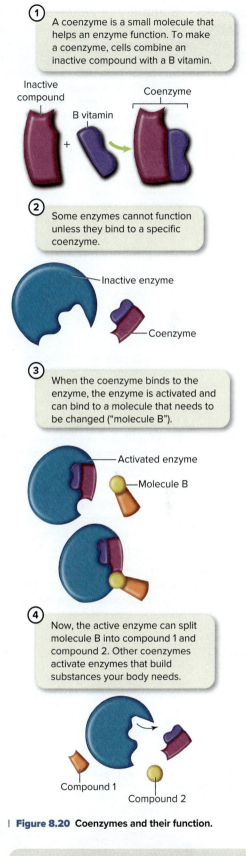

① A coenzyme is a small molecule that helps an enzyme function. To make a coenzyme, cells combine an inactive compound with a B vitamin.

Inactive compound

Coenzyme

B vitamin

② Some enzymes cannot function unless they bind to a specific coenzyme.

Inactive enzyme

Coenzyme

③ When the coenzyme binds to the enzyme, the enzyme is activated and can bind to a molecule that needs to be changed ("molecule B").

Activated enzyme

Molecule B

④ Now, the active enzyme can split molecule B into compound 1 and compound 2. Other coenzymes activate enzymes that build substances your body needs.

Compound 1

Compound 2

Figure 8.20 Coenzymes and their function.

coenzyme small, organic molecule that interacts with enzymes, enabling the enzymes to function

TABLE 8.7   Summary of Water-Soluble Vitamins and Choline

Vitamin	Major Functions in the Body	Adult RDA/AI (adult RDA = bold)	Major Dietary Sources	Major Deficiency Signs and Symptoms	Major Toxicity Signs and Symptoms
Thiamin	Part of coenzyme needed for carbohydrate metabolism and the metabolism of certain amino acids; may help neurotransmitter production	**1.1–1.2 mg**	Pork, wheat germ, enriched breads and cereals, brewer's yeast	Beriberi and Wernicke-Korsakoff syndrome: Weakness, abnormal nervous system functioning	None (Upper limit [UL] not determined)
Riboflavin	Part of coenzymes needed for carbohydrate, amino acid, and lipid metabolism	**1.1–1.3 mg**	Milk, yogurt, and other milk products; enriched breads and cereals; liver	Inflammation of the mouth and tongue, eye disorders	None (UL not determined)
Niacin	Part of coenzymes needed for energy metabolism	**14–16 mg**	Enriched breads and cereals, beef, liver, tuna, salmon, poultry, pork, mushrooms	Pellagra: • Diarrhea • Dermatitis • Dementia • Death	**Adult UL = 35 mg/ day** Flushing of facial skin, itchy skin, nausea and vomiting, liver damage
Pantothenic acid	Part of the coenzyme that is needed for synthesizing fat and releasing energy from macronutrients	5 mg	Beef and chicken liver, sunflower seeds, mushrooms, yogurt, soy milk, fortified cereals	Rarely occurs	Unknown (UL not determined)
Biotin	Needed for synthesizing glucose and fatty acids	30 mcg	Liver, eggs, peanuts, salmon, pork, mushrooms, sunflower seeds	Rarely occurs: Skin rash, hair loss, convulsions, and other neurological disorders; developmental delays in infants	Unknown (UL not determined)
Vitamin B-6	Part of coenzyme needed for amino acid metabolism, involved in neurotransmitter and hemoglobin synthesis	**1.3–1.7 mg**	Meat, fish, and poultry; potatoes, bananas, spinach, sweet red peppers, broccoli	Dermatitis, anemia, depression, confusion, and neurological disorders such as convulsions	**Adult UL = 100 mg/ day** Nerve destruction
Folate	Part of coenzyme needed for DNA synthesis and conversion of cysteine to methionine, preventing homocysteine accumulation	**400 mcg DFE**	Dark green, leafy vegetables, liver, legumes, asparagus, broccoli, orange juice, enriched breads and cereals (folic acid)	Megaloblastic anemia, diarrhea, neural tube defects in embryos	**Adult UL = 1000 mcg/ day** May stimulate cancer cell growth
Vitamin B-12	Part of coenzymes needed for various cellular processes, including folate metabolism; maintenance of myelin sheaths	**2.4 mcg**	Animal foods, fortified cereals, fortified soy milk	Pernicious anemia: Megaloblastic anemia and nerve damage resulting in paralysis and death	None (UL not determined)
Ascorbic acid (vitamin C)	Needed for connective tissue synthesis and maintenance; antioxidant; synthesis of neurotransmitters and certain hormones; immune system functioning	**75–90 mg** (nonsmokers)	Peppers, citrus fruits, papaya, broccoli, cabbage, berries	Scurvy: Poor wound healing, pinpoint hemorrhages, bleeding gums, bruises, depression	**Adult UL = 2000 mg/ day** Diarrhea and GI tract discomfort
Choline	Neurotransmitter and phospholipid synthesis; methionine metabolism	425–550 mg	Widely distributed in foods and human biosynthesis (production)	Liver damage	Fishy body odor and reduced blood pressure

Cornflakes: ©David Toase/Getty Images RF; Mushroom: ©Brand X Pictures/Getty Images RF; Orange: ©Dennis Gray/Cole Group/Getty Images RF; Spinach: ©Florea Marius Catalin/E+/Getty Images RF

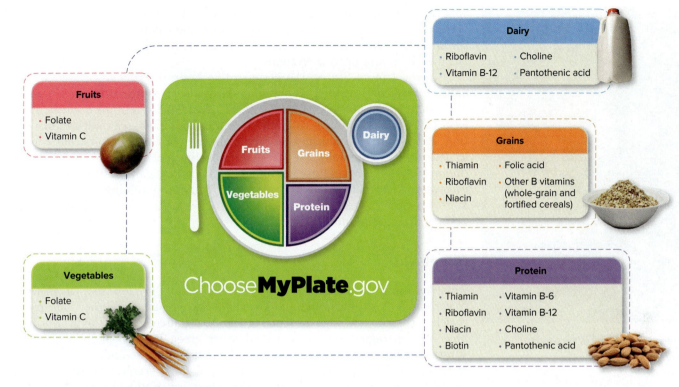

Figure 8.21 MyPlate: Water-soluble vitamins and choline. This illustration highlights MyPlate food groups that generally are good sources of water-soluble vitamins and choline. Source: U.S. Dept. of Agriculture; Mango and Bowl of cereal: ©Stockbyte/Getty Images RF; Carrots: ©Comstock/Getty Images RF; Milk: ©Judith Collins/Alamy RF; Almonds: ©Ingram Publishing/SuperStock RF

Dietary Adequacy

The adult RDA for thiamin is 1.2 mg/day and 1.1 mg/day for men and women, respectively. There are no reports of toxicity from consuming high amounts of thiamin from food or supplements,[15] probably because the excess vitamin is readily excreted in urine. Thus, no UL has been established for thiamin.

TABLE 8.8   Thiamin Content of Selected Foods

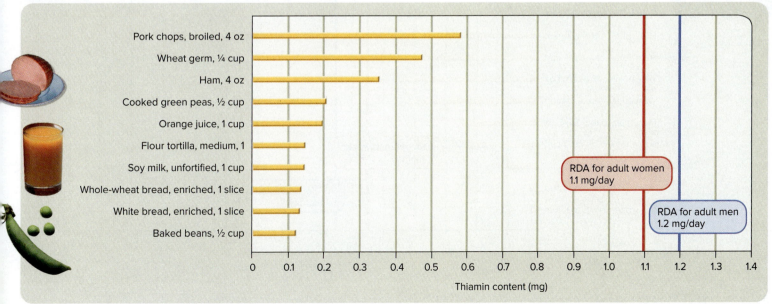

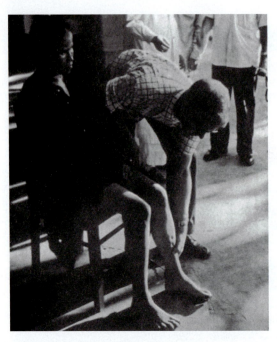

Figure 8.22 **Beriberi.** This woman has a form of beriberi. Source: Centers for Disease Control and Prevention

The thiamin deficiency disease is called **beriberi.** People suffering from beriberi are very weak and have poor muscular coordination (Fig. 8.22). The severe lack of thiamin also negatively affects the functioning of the cardiovascular, digestive, and nervous systems.

In the United States, the degenerative brain disorder associated with thiamin deficiency is called **Wernicke—Korsakoff syndrome** (*vear'—nih—key kor'—sah—koff*). Most cases of Wernicke—Korsakoff syndrome occur in alcoholics because alcohol reduces thiamin absorption and increases the vitamin's excretion. People with alcoholism also tend to have poor eating habits that contribute to deficiencies of thiamin and other vitamins. Signs of Wernicke—Korsakoff syndrome include abnormal eye movements, staggering gait, and distorted thought processes. Treatment involves avoiding alcohol and obtaining thiamin injections. Without prompt treatment, people with Wernicke—Korsakoff syndrome can become disabled permanently or die.

Riboflavin

Riboflavin is a component of two coenzymes that play key roles in metabolism of carbohydrates, lipids, and amino acids. Milk, yogurt, and other milk products; enriched cereals; and liver are among the best sources of riboflavin. Mushrooms, broccoli, asparagus, and spinach and other green leafy vegetables also contain substantial amounts of the vitamin. Table 8.9 lists these and other food sources of riboflavin. Riboflavin's chemical structure is fairly stable, but exposure to light causes the vitamin to break down rapidly. Therefore, riboflavin—rich foods, such as milk and milk products, should not be packaged or stored in clear glass containers.

beriberi thiamin deficiency disease

Wernicke-Korsakoff syndrome degenerative brain disorder resulting from thiamin deficiency that occurs primarily among alcoholics

Dietary Adequacy

The RDA for riboflavin is 1.1 mg/day for women and 1.3 mg/day for men. The average riboflavin intake of adult Americans is about 1.8 mg/day for women and 2.5 mg/day for men.[4] In the United States, riboflavin deficiency rarely occurs because many commonly eaten foods contain riboflavin (see Table 8.9). However,

TABLE 8.9 Riboflavin Content of Selected Foods

Food	Riboflavin content (mg)
Beef liver, cooked, 3 oz	~3.1
All-Bran® cereal, ½ cup	~2.7
Whole-grain Total® cereal, ¾ cup	~1.7
Chicken liver, cooked, 1 oz	~0.85
Wheaties® cereal, ¾ cup	~0.8
Yogurt, plain, low-fat, 8 oz	~0.48
Cottage cheese, 2% fat, 1 cup	~0.45
Chicken, meat only, cooked, ¾ cup	~0.2
Milk, fat-free or 1%, 1 cup	~0.05
Mushrooms, white, raw, 5 medium	~0.05

RDA for adult women 1.1 mg/day

RDA for adult men 1.3 mg/day

Source: Data from U.S. Department of Agriculture, Agricultural Research Service: *USDA national nutrient database for standard reference,* Release 26, 2013.
Cereal ©David Toase/Getty Images RF

TABLE 8.10 Niacin Content of Selected Foods

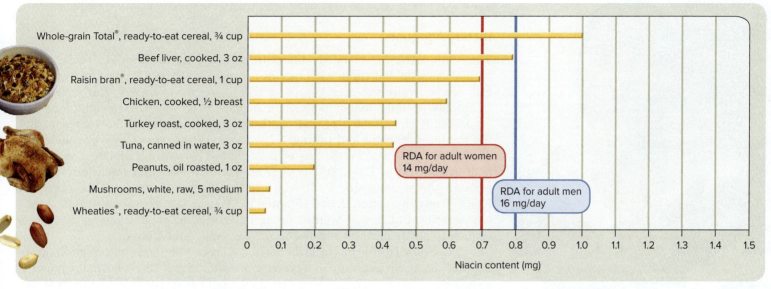

Whole-grain Total®, ready-to-eat cereal, ¾ cup
Beef liver, cooked, 3 oz
Raisin bran®, ready-to-eat cereal, 1 cup
Chicken, cooked, ½ breast
Turkey roast, cooked, 3 oz
Tuna, canned in water, 3 oz
Peanuts, oil roasted, 1 oz
Mushrooms, white, raw, 5 medium
Wheaties®, ready-to-eat cereal, ¾ cup

RDA for adult women 14 mg/day

RDA for adult men 16 mg/day

Niacin content (mg)

Source: Data from U.S. Department of Agriculture, Agricultural Research Service: *USDA national nutrient database for standard reference,* Release 26, 2013.
Bowl of cereal: ©Comstock/Getty Images RF; Roast chicken: ©Getty Images RF; Peanuts: ©C Squared Studios/Getty Images RF

people who do not consume milk, milk products, or enriched breads and cereals may develop mild cases of riboflavin deficiency. A symptom of mild riboflavin deficiency is to become fatigued easily. Riboflavin is not well absorbed by the intestinal tract, so consuming large amounts of the vitamin does not appear to cause side effects.[16] Thus, no UL has been established for riboflavin.

Niacin

The body uses niacin to synthesize two coenzymes that participate in at least 200 reactions, including those involved in the release of energy from macronu—trients. Major food sources of niacin include enriched cereals, beef liver, tuna, salmon, poultry, pork, and mushrooms (Table 8.10). The chemical structure of niacin is very heat stable, so food retains much of its niacin content during usual preparation and cooking methods.

When diets supply plenty of protein—rich foods, the human body can syn—thesize niacin from a precursor, the amino acid tryptophan. It takes about 60 mg of tryptophan to yield about 1 mg of niacin. For example, eggs and milk lack niacin, but they are rich sources of tryptophan that can be converted to the B vitamin.

The niacin content of corn is considerably higher than that of most other vegetables, but the B vitamin is tightly bound to a protein that resists digestion. Thus, people who eat corn as their staple food are prone to develop pellagra. The traditional Mexican diet is corn based, but pellagra was not a widespread disease in Mexico when it was a major health concern in other parts of the world. Why? The Mexican practice of soaking corn kernels in lime water before using them to prepare tortillas helps free the niacin, enhancing its ability to

The traditional Mexican practice of soaking corn kernels in lime water before using them to prepare tortillas helps free the niacin, enhancing its ability to be absorbed. ©Mireille Vautier/Alamy

be absorbed. In the United States, corn products such as hominy and grits are sources of niacin because they have been treated with lime before cooking.

Dietary Adequacy

The adult RDA for niacin is 14 to 16 mg/day. In the United States, people with alcoholism and those with rare disorders that disrupt tryptophan metabolism are generally the only groups at risk of niacin deficiency. Early signs and symptoms of mild niacin deficiency include poor appetite, weight loss, and weakness. If the affected person continues to consume a niacin–deficient diet, the condition worsens and **pellagra** (*peh–lah'–gra* or *peh–lay'–gra*) develops. The classic signs and symptoms of pellagra are dermatitis, diarrhea, dementia, and death—the "4 Ds of pellagra" (Fig. 8.23). In the early twentieth century, pellagra was widespread in the southeastern United States (see the "Did You Know?" box in Section 2.1 of Chapter 2). Today, the disease is rare in Western societies, but it still occurs among impoverished populations in developing countries, particularly in regions of Africa, India, and China.

The adult UL for niacin is 35 mg/day. There have been no reports indicating that the niacin naturally in foods can cause toxicity.[17] Physicians may prescribe megadoses of niacin supplements to treat elevated blood cholesterol levels. However, patients taking very high doses of the vitamin (more than 3 grams) may experience side effects such as gastrointestinal ulcers, loss of vision, and liver damage.[18] The "Vitamins as Medicines" section of this chapter discusses the use of niacin supplements to reduce cholesterol levels.

Vitamin B-6

The body requires vitamin B–6 to make a coenzyme needed for amino acid metabolism, including the conversion of the amino acid tryptophan to niacin and transamination reactions that form nonessential amino acids (see Fig. 7.11). The coenzyme that contains vitamin B–6 also helps convert a toxic amino acid, homocysteine, to cysteine, a nonessential amino acid.

During red blood cell (RBC) production, the coenzyme participates in the synthesis of heme. Heme is the iron–containing portion of **hemoglobin,** the protein in RBCs that transports oxygen. If vitamin B–6 is unavailable for heme synthesis, a type of anemia develops. **Anemia** is a disorder characterized by too few red blood cells and poor oxygen transport in blood. Vitamin B–6 is also involved in the synthesis of *neurotransmitters*, chemicals that nerves produce to transmit messages.

Food Sources of Vitamin B-6

Liver, meat, fish, and poultry are among the best dietary sources of vitamin B–6. Additionally, potatoes, bananas, spinach, sweet red peppers, and broccoli are good sources of vitamin B–6. During the refining process, the vitamin B–6 that is naturally in grains is lost, and the nutrient is not added back to the grain products during enrichment. However, many ready–to–eat and cooked cereals have been fortified with the vitamin. Table 8.11 lists some foods that are major sources of vitamin B–6. During cooking, excessive heat can cause major losses of the vitamin.

Dietary Adequacy

The adult RDAs for vitamin B–6 range from 1.3 to 1.7 mg/day. In the United States, the average adult consumes more than the RDA of the vitamin.[4] Therefore, cases of vitamin B–6 deficiency are rare, but they can result from alcoholism or genetic conditions that affect vitamin B–6 metabolism. Signs and symptoms of vitamin B–6 deficiency include dermatitis, anemia, convulsions, depression, and confusion.

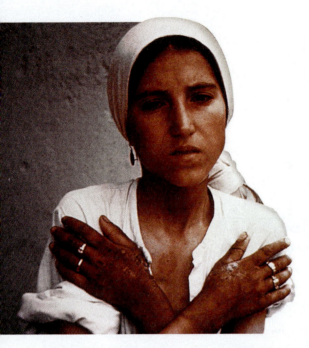

Figure 8.23 Pellagra. This person with pellagra shows one of the classic signs of the niacin deficiency disease: dermatitis, particularly on parts of the body exposed to sun. Source: Centers for Disease Control and Prevention

pellagra niacin deficiency disease

hemoglobin iron-containing protein in red blood cells that transports oxygen

anemia disorder characterized by too few red blood cells and poor oxygen transport in blood

Did *YOU* Know?

In the early 1950s, some babies became unusually irritable and developed convulsions after being fed a commercial infant formula. Scientists determined that the vitamin B-6 in the formula had been destroyed by excessive heating during the manufacturing process. Vitamin B-6 is needed for neurotransmitter synthesis, so the irritability and convulsions may have resulted from a lack of neurotransmitters in the infants' brains. The babies were effectively treated with vitamin B-6.

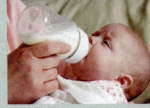

©McGraw-Hill Education. Jill Braaten, photographer

The adult UL for vitamin B−6 is 100 mg/day. Unlike most B vitamins, megadoses of vitamin B−6 are toxic.[19] The "Vitamins as Medicines" section of this chapter provides information about vitamin B−6 toxicity.

Folate

"Folate" is the name for a group of related compounds that includes **folic acid.** Folic acid refers specifically to the synthetic form of the vitamin found in supplements and added to fortify foods. In the body, cells convert all forms of folate to a group of folate−containing coenzymes collectively called **tetrahydrofolic** (*te'−tra−hi−drow−foe−lik*) **acid** or simply **THFA.** THFA accepts a single−carbon group, such as CH_3, from one compound and transfers it to another substance. As a result, THFA participates in many chemical reactions involved in DNA synthesis and amino acid metabolism. As cells prepare to divide, they need THFA to make DNA.

Certain roles of folate and vitamin B−12 are interrelated. THFA can transfer a CH_3 group to vitamin B−12, which, in turn, transfers the CH_3 group to homocysteine, forming the essential amino acid methionine (Fig. 8.24). This

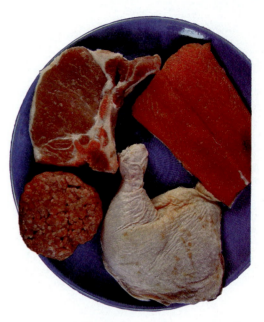

Meat, fish, and poultry are among the best dietary sources of vitamin B-6.
©Wendy Schiff

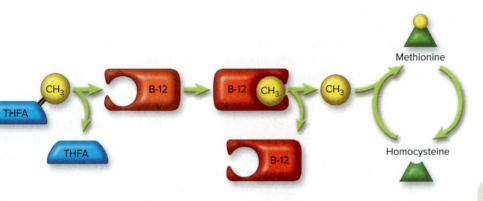

Figure 8.24 Folate and vitamin B-12: Working together. This diagram shows how folate (THFA) works with vitamin B-12 to transfer a methyl group (CH_3).

folic acid form of folate

tetrahydrofolic acid (THFA) folate coenzyme

TABLE 8.11 Vitamin B-6 Content of Selected Foods

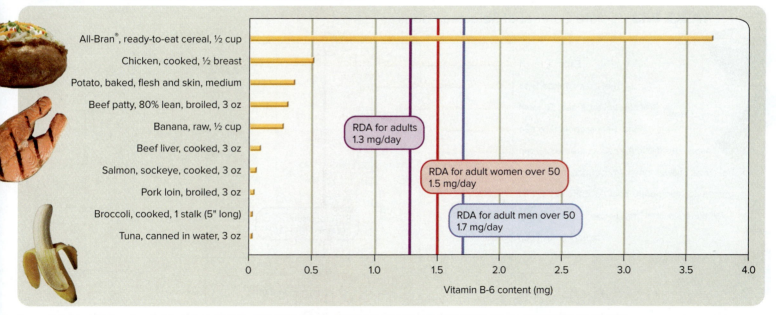

RDA for adults
1.3 mg/day

RDA for adult women over 50
1.5 mg/day

RDA for adult men over 50
1.7 mg/day

All-Bran®, ready-to-eat cereal, ½ cup	
Chicken, cooked, ½ breast	
Potato, baked, flesh and skin, medium	
Beef patty, 80% lean, broiled, 3 oz	
Banana, raw, ½ cup	
Beef liver, cooked, 3 oz	
Salmon, sockeye, cooked, 3 oz	
Pork loin, broiled, 3 oz	
Broccoli, cooked, 1 stalk (5" long)	
Tuna, canned in water, 3 oz	

Vitamin B-6 content (mg)
0   0.5   1.0   1.5   2.0   2.5   3.0   3.5   4.0

Source: Data from U.S. Department of Agriculture, Agricultural Research Service: *USDA national nutrient database for standard reference,* Release 26, 2013.
Baked potato: ©Getty Images RF; Salmon dinner: ©C Squared Studios/Getty Images RF; Banana: ©Stockbyte/Getty Images RF

process recycles methionine. When vitamin B−12 is unavailable, folate cannot be used, and a deficiency of the vitamin occurs, even though dietary intakes of folate are adequate.[20]

Food Sources of Folate

Leafy vegetables, liver, legumes, asparagus, broccoli, and orange juice are good sources of naturally occurring folate. The synthetic folic acid that is used to for−tify or enrich food is better absorbed than naturally occurring forms of folate.

The folate content of foods may be reported as micrograms of *dietary folate equivalents* (*DFEs*). DFE units account for differences in the body's ability to absorb folic acid and natural forms of folate. Table 8.12 lists the folate content of selected foods in micrograms of DFE.

Folate is extremely susceptible to destruction by heat, oxidation, and ultra−violet light. Food processing and preparation can destroy 50 to 90% of the folate in food. By eating fresh fruits and raw or lightly cooked vegetables, you are likely to obtain most of the foods' folate content.

Dietary Adequacy

The adult RDA for folate is 400 mcg (DFE)/day. The diets of most Americans provide adequate amounts of folate.[4] The risk of folate deficiency is highest in alcoholics, women of childbearing age, pregnant women, and people with disor−ders of the intestinal tract that reduce the vitamin's absorption.[21]

Folate deficiency usually results from nutritionally inadequate diets, but excess alcohol consumption and use of certain medications can negatively affect the body's ability to absorb and use folate, resulting in deficiencies of the vita−min. Initially, folate deficiency affects cells that rapidly divide, such as red blood cells. Mature RBCs do not have nuclei, and they live for only about 4 months. Thus, the body must replace old or worn−out RBCs constantly. To keep up with their rapid rate of cell division, the precursor cells that mature into RBCs must actively synthesize DNA. Without folate, RBC precursor cells that reside in bone marrow enlarge, but they cannot divide normally, because they are unable to form new DNA. Bone marrow releases some of the abnormal RBCs into the

TABLE 8.12 Folate Content of Selected Foods

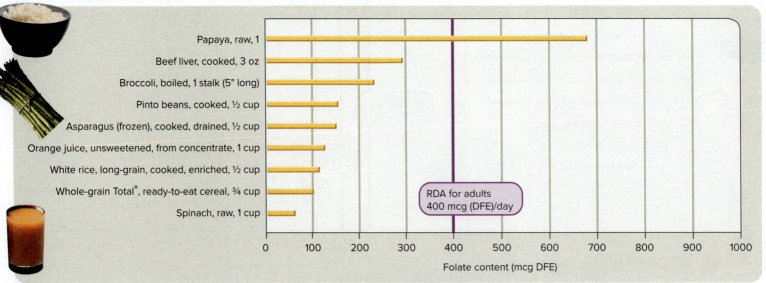

Source: Data from U.S. Department of Agriculture, Agricultural Research Service: *USDA national nutrient database for standard reference,* Release 26, 2013.
Rice: ©Jules Frazier/Getty Images RF; Asparagus: ©Brand X Pictures/Getty Images RF; Juice: ©Stockbyte/Getty Images RF

bloodstream before they mature (Fig. 8.25). This condition, called megaloblastic (*mega* = large; *blast* = immature cell) anemia, is characterized by large, immature RBCs (*megaloblasts*) that still have nuclei and do not carry normal amounts of oxygen.

Because many of folate's metabolic roles are related to those of vitamin B−12, diets that lack either vitamin produce a number of identical deficiency signs and symptoms. For example, being deficient in folate or vitamin B−12 can cause megaloblastic anemia. Therefore, a person with this type of anemia needs further analysis of his or her blood to determine which vitamin is lacking.

Although the folate naturally in foods does not appear to be toxic, the UL for the synthetic form of the vitamin (folic acid) is 1000 mcg/day. The UL was established because taking folic acid supplements can cure not only the anemia that occurs in folate deficiency but also the anemia that is a sign of vitamin B−12 deficiency. Folic acid supplementation, however, does not prevent the serious nervous system damage that accompanies the B−12 deficiency. Furthermore, some medical experts are concerned that taking folic acid supplements and consuming foods that contain the micronutrient may cause excess folic acid to accumulate in blood and produce negative health effects as a result.

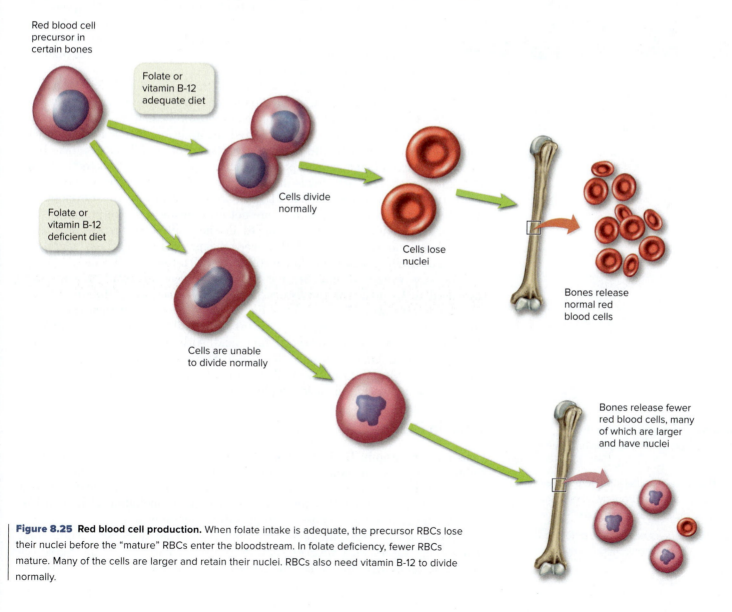

Figure 8.25 Red blood cell production. When folate intake is adequate, the precursor RBCs lose their nuclei before the "mature" RBCs enter the bloodstream. In folate deficiency, fewer RBCs mature. Many of the cells are larger and retain their nuclei. RBCs also need vitamin B-12 to divide normally.

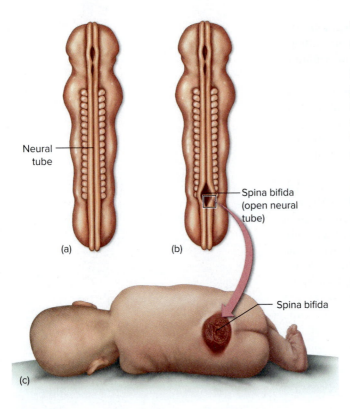

Figure 8.26 Neural tube. (*a*) Normal neural tube in an early embryo. (*b*) Spina bifida (abnormal neural tube) in an early embryo. (*c*) Infant with severe spina bifida.

Thus, more research is needed to determine whether ingesting too much folic acid poses health risks.

Neural Tube Defects   A woman's diet before and during pregnancy provides the raw materials for her developing offspring's needs, as well as her body's needs. Not surprisingly, recommendations for intakes of many nutrients increase during pregnancy. A pregnant woman has an increased requirement for folate because DNA synthesis and cell division take place at a rapid pace during embryonic development.

During the first few weeks after conception, the **neural tube** forms in the human embryo (Fig. 8.26a). This tube eventually develops into the brain and spinal cord. Pregnant women who suffer from folate deficiency have high risk of giving birth to infants with neural tube defects. The two most common neural tube defects are **spina bifida** (*spy'−na bif'−eh−dah*) and **anencephaly** (*an−en−sef'−ah−lee*). Spina bifida occurs when the embryo's spine does not form properly and the bones fail to enclose the spinal cord. As you can see in Figure 8.26c, infants with severe spina bifida have a section of their spinal cord or a sac containing some spinal fluid bulging through an opening in their backs. Often, people with spina bifida are unable to use muscles in the lower part of their bodies, and as a result, they cannot walk independently. Infants born with anencephaly have much of their brain malformed or missing, and they usually die shortly after birth.

In 1992, officials with the U.S. Public Health Service recommended that all women capable of becoming pregnant consume 400 mcg of folic acid daily to prevent neural tube defects. In January 1998, the Food and Drug Administration required the addition of folic acid to enriched flour and cereals. According to medical experts, adequate folic acid intake before and during early pregnancy can prevent many cases of spinal tube defects.[22] For pregnant women, adequate folate status is critical early in pregnancy because the neural tube begins to form about 21 days after conception. This developmental milestone occurs when many women are not even aware they are pregnant.

Each year, about 3000 pregnancies in the United States are affected by anencephaly and spina bifida.[22] However, the prevalence of these neural tube defects has declined since enrichment of grains with folic acid began.

Because women of childbearing age may become pregnant at some point, they need to be aware of the association between the lack of folate and neural tube defects. In addition to including folate−rich foods in their diets, young women can prepare for pregnancy by taking a daily multivitamin supplement that contains 400 mcg of synthetic folic acid. Although folic acid intakes have increased among Americans since the United States began enriching grain products with the vitamin, only 40% of women who are of childbearing age report that they take a daily folic acid supplement.[22]

Vitamin B-12

Cells require vitamin B−12 to make coenzymes that participate in a variety of cellular processes, including the transfer of CH_3 groups in the metabolism of folate (see Fig. 8.24). Vitamin B−12 is also needed to convert folate to coenzyme forms that are needed for metabolic reactions, including DNA synthesis. Vitamin B−12 also participates in homocysteine metabolism.

There is one vital function of vitamin B−12 that does not involve folate: maintaining the *myelin sheaths* that wrap around parts of certain nerve cells, insulating them. Myelin enables the nerves to communicate effectively. Without

neural tube embryonic structure that eventually develops into the brain and spinal cord

spina bifida type of neural tube defect in which the spine does not form properly before birth, and it fails to enclose the spinal cord

anencephaly type of neural tube defect in which the brain does not form properly or is missing

vitamin B−12, segments of myelin sheath gradually undergo destruction that can lead to paralysis. If a person who is vitamin B−12 deficient does not obtain treatment with the vitamin, he or she could die as a result of the deficiency.

Absorbing the vitamin B−12 that is naturally in food requires a com−plex series of steps that are unique for a vitamin (Fig. 8.27). Natural vitamin B−12 is bound to animal protein that prevents its absorption. When the food enters the stomach, the vitamin is released from the protein, primarily by the actions of hydrochloric acid (HCl) in gastric juice. Synthetic vitamin B−12 in dietary supplements or fortified foods is not bound to food protein, so it does not need stomach acid to release the protein.

In the small intestine, vitamin B−12 binds to **intrinsic factor (IF),** a com−pound produced by certain stomach cells. Eventually, the vitamin B−12/intrinsic factor complex reaches the ileum of the small intestine, where the vitamin com−plex is absorbed. Within the absorptive cells, vitamin B−12 is separated from intrinsic factor and attached to transport molecules. The transport molecules enter the bloodstream and travel to the liver via the hepatic portal vein. The liver removes vitamin B−12 from many of the carrier molecules and stores about 50% of the vitamin. A healthy liver has enough vitamin B−12 reserves to last 5 to 10 years.[23] Therefore, a healthy person who decides to follow a diet that com−pletely lacks vitamin B−12 is not likely to experience signs and symptoms of the vitamin's deficiency disorder for as long as 10 years.

> **intrinsic factor (IF)** substance produced in the stomach that facilitates intestinal absorption of vitamin B-12

Food Sources of Vitamin B-12

Plants do not make vitamin B−12; therefore, we rely almost entirely on animal foods to supply the vitamin naturally. Major sources of vitamin B−12 in the typical American diet are meat, milk and milk products, poultry, fish, shellfish, and eggs. Although liver is not a popular food, it is one of the richest sources of vitamin B−12. Many soy products, such as soy milk, and ready−to−eat cereals are fortified with synthetic vitamin B−12. Table 8.13 lists some foods that provide vitamin B−12.

TABLE 8.13   Vitamin B-12 Content of Selected Foods

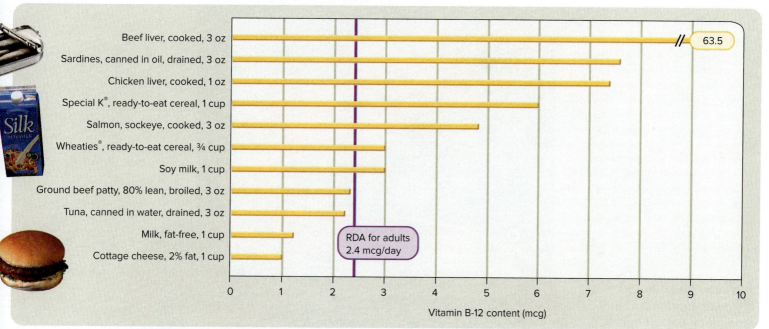

Source: Data from U.S. Department of Agriculture, Agricultural Research Service: *USDA national nutrient database for standard reference,* Release 26, 2013.
Sardines and Burger: ©Brand X Pictures/Getty Images RF; Soy beverage: ©Wendy Schiff

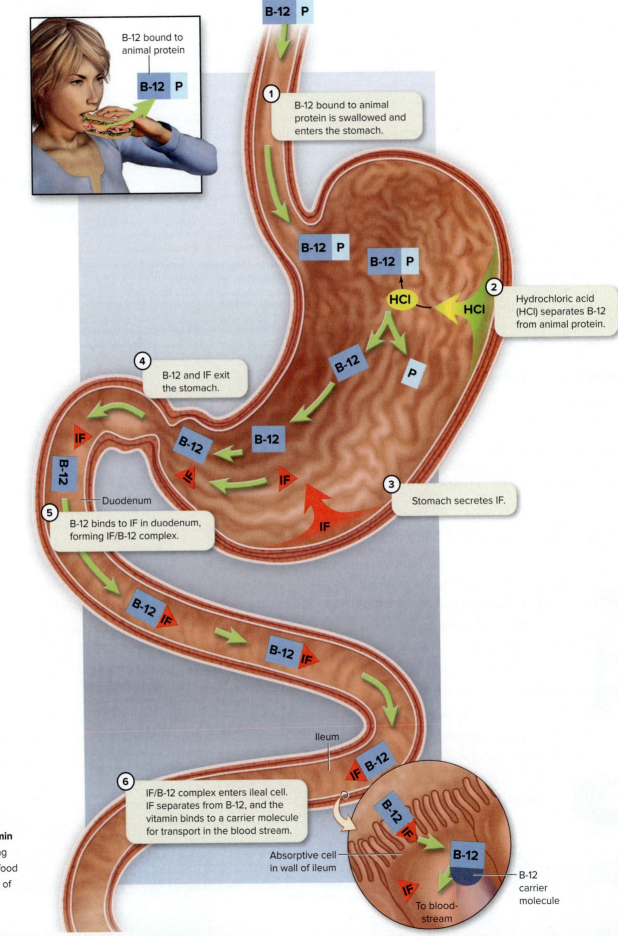

B-12 bound to animal protein

① B-12 bound to animal protein is swallowed and enters the stomach.

② Hydrochloric acid (HCl) separates B-12 from animal protein.

④ B-12 and IF exit the stomach.

③ Stomach secretes IF.

Duodenum

⑤ B-12 binds to IF in duodenum, forming IF/B-12 complex.

Ileum

⑥ IF/B-12 complex enters ileal cell. IF separates from B-12, and the vitamin binds to a carrier molecule for transport in the blood stream.

Absorptive cell in wall of ileum

B-12 carrier molecule

To blood-stream

Figure 8.27 Natural vitamin B-12 absorption. Absorbing natural vitamin B-12 from food requires a complex series of steps.

Dietary Adequacy

The adult RDA for vitamin B−12 is 2.4 mcg/day. Most Americans consume more than the RDA.[4] No UL has been established for vitamin B−12 because no adverse effects have been observed with excess intake from food or dietary supplements.

Vitamin B-12 Deficiency   As many as 15% of Americans have vitamin B−12 deficiency.[24] Vitamin B−12 deficiency is characterized by nerve damage and megaloblastic RBCs. Other common signs and symptoms of the deficiency include muscle weakness, sore mouth, smooth and shiny tongue, memory loss, confusion, difficulty walking and maintaining balance, and numbness and tingling sensations, particularly in the lower extremities. Most cases of vitamin B−12 deficiency result from problems that interfere with intestinal absorption of the vitamin (cobalamin) in foods (*food−cobalamin malabsorption*) and not from inadequate intakes.[20]

As people age, HCl production in their stomachs declines. Thus, many older adults have food−cobalamin malabsorption because they are unable to release vitamin B−12 from animal protein.[20] People with this condition can develop vitamin B−12 deficiency despite consuming diets that contain the vitamin. In addition to advanced age, chronic alcoholism, gastric bypass surgeries for weight reduction, and certain medications, particularly those that reduce stomach acid secretion, can contribute to food−cobalamin malabsorption. People with this form of malabsorption produce intrinsic factor, so they can absorb synthetic forms of the vitamin in dietary supplements that contain B−12.

An estimated 2% of older adults have an autoimmune disorder that causes inflammation and destruction of the cells in the stomach that produce intrinsic factor.[20] (An autoimmune disorder results when a person's immune system attacks his or her own cells.) In these cases, diets may supply adequate amounts of vitamin B−12, but the lack of intrinsic factor prevents most of the micronutrient from being absorbed. Eventually, people who lack intrinsic factor develop a disease called **pernicious** ("deadly") **anemia.** As its name implies, pernicious anemia can lead to vitamin B−12 deficiency and death. Treatment involves bypassing the need for intrinsic factor and intestinal absorption, usually by providing routine vitamin B−12 injections. Furthermore, taking large doses of vitamin B−12 floods the intestinal tract with the vitamin and enables a small amount to be absorbed without the need for intrinsic factor.

In addition to advanced age, family history is a risk factor for pernicious anemia. Therefore, it is a good idea to have your blood tested for signs of vitamin B−12 deficiency as you grow older, especially if you have a close relative with pernicious anemia.

Vegans ("total" vegetarians) avoid eating animal products. Plant foods supply little vitamin B−12, so vegans need to be concerned about their intakes of the nutrient (see the "Vegetarianism" section of Chapter 7). People who eat few or no animal products should consume foods that have been fortified with vitamin B−12, such as fortified soy milk and cereals, or take supplements that supply the vitamin. Vegan women who breastfeed their babies need to be aware that their breast milk may contain inadequate amounts of vitamin B−12. Babies who consume only vitamin B−12–deficient breast milk are likely to develop megaloblastic anemia and serious nervous system problems, including diminished brain growth and spinal cord damage. The signs and symptoms of the deficiency are likely to occur during the first few months of life, particularly when the infants' mothers did not supplement their diets with vitamin B−12 during pregnancy. Providing vitamin B−12 to the deficient babies promptly can prevent permanent damage to the children's nervous systems.

pernicious anemia condition caused by the lack of intrinsic factor and characterized by vitamin B-12 deficiency, nerve damage, and megaloblastic RBCs

Pantothenic Acid

Pantothenic acid is a component of *coenzyme A*, which is critical for energy metabolism and fatty acid production in the body. Pantothenic acid is so wide—spread in foods that a nutritional deficiency is unlikely to occur among healthy people who eat varied diets. Rich sources of pantothenic acid include cereals that have been fortified with the vitamin, beef and chicken liver, sunflower seeds, mushrooms, peas, and soy milk.

Most Americans consume adequate amounts of pantothenic acid, and as a result, deficiencies of the vitamin are rare. When scientists experimentally cause pantothenic deficiency in human subjects, they note signs and symptoms that include headache, fatigue, impaired muscle coordination, and GI tract dis—turbances. People who abuse alcohol may develop pantothenic acid and other B—vitamin deficiencies, particularly if their diets are lacking other nutrients as well. At this time, scientists have not set an UL for the vitamin because there have been no reports of toxicity from taking high doses.

Biotin

Biotin participates in chemical reactions that add carbon dioxide to other com—pounds. By doing so, the vitamin promotes the synthesis of glucose and fatty acids and the breakdown of certain amino acids. Severe deficiencies of biotin rarely occur because intestinal bacteria produce some biotin and the vitamin is in a wide variety of foods. Liver, eggs, peanuts, salmon, pork, mushrooms, and sunflower seeds are good sources of biotin. The typical diet of American adults provides adequate amounts of the micronutrient.

Conditions that reduce intestinal bacteria's biotin production, such as sur—gical removal of a large part of the colon or taking antibiotics for many months, can contribute to a biotin deficiency. Signs and symptoms of biotin deficiency include skin rash, hair loss, convulsions, and some other nervous system disor—ders. Because reports of biotin toxicity are lacking, nutrition scientists have not set an UL for the micronutrient.

Did *YOU* Know?

Avidin is a protein in raw egg whites that binds to biotin, making the vitamin resist digestion. People who consume raw eggs regularly for long periods of time may develop signs of biotin deficiency. Cooking eggs destroys avidin, making biotin available for absorption.

Vitamin C

ascorbic acid vitamin C

Most animals do not need dietary sources of vitamin C (**ascorbic acid**) because they can synthesize all the vitamin they need. Humans and guinea pigs are among the few species that are unable to make vitamin C, and for these animals, the micronutrient is essential.

Vitamin C absorption occurs in the small intestine. As intakes of the vita—min increase, the amount absorbed decreases. The small intestine, for example, absorbs 50% or less of the vitamin when intakes are 1 g or more/day. Addi—tionally, the kidneys increase their excretion of the vitamin in response to high intakes. Therefore, taking megadoses of vitamin C may be wasteful because such high amounts of the vitamin are not well absorbed and excesses are eliminated in urine.

Functions of Vitamin C

Vitamin C does not function as part of a coenzyme as do most of the B vitamins, but the vitamin facilitates certain chemical reactions. Vitamin C also acts as an antioxidant by donating electrons to other compounds. In the body, vitamin C has widespread physiological roles; the following sections describe some of the micronutrient's most well—understood functions.

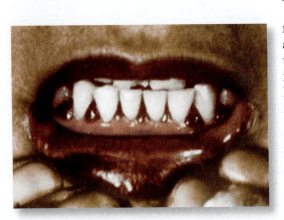

Swollen gums that bleed easily are a sign of scurvy.
Source: Centers for Disease Control and Prevention

Collagen Synthesis   Vitamin C participates in reactions that form and maintain collagen. **Collagen** is a fibrous protein that gives strength to *connective tissue*. Connective tissues, such as bone, cartilage, and tendons, connect and support other structures in the body. During collagen formation, vitamin C helps create numer–ous cross–connections between the amino acids in collagen that greatly strengthen the connective tissue (Fig. 8.28). If vitamin C is unavailable, the body forms weak connective tissue and is unable to maintain existing collagen. Some of the more obvious signs of scurvy, such as swollen gums that bleed easily, teeth that loosen and fall out of their sockets, skin that bruises easily, and poor wound healing, are primarily the result of weak connective tissue.

Antioxidant Activity   Results of some experiments indicate that vitamin C can act as an antioxidant by donating electrons to radicals. Vitamin C also may donate electrons to another antioxidant—vitamin E. Thus, vitamin C recycles vitamin E so it can regain its antioxidant function. Scientists, however, do not know the extent of vitamin C's antioxidant abilities in the human body. Taking excessive amounts of vitamin C may be harmful because in high doses, the vitamin has **prooxidant** effects. A prooxidant promotes radical production.

Other Roles of Vitamin C in the Body   Vitamin C plays a role in the body's immune function, and the vitamin is necessary for the synthesis of bile and certain neurotransmitters. Vitamin C is also involved in the production of vari–ous hormones, including the "stress hormone" cortisol; adolsterone, a hormone involved in blood pressure regulation; and thyroxin, the thyroid hormone that regulates energy metabolism.

Food Sources of Vitamin C

Plant foods are the best dietary sources of vitamin C. Peppers, citrus fruit, papaya, broccoli, and berries contain relatively high amounts of the micronutri–ent (Table 8.14). Potatoes and vitamin C–fortified fruit drinks and cereals also supply vitamin C. Most animal foods are not sources of the micronutrient.

Vitamin C is very unstable in the presence of heat, oxygen, light, alkaline conditions, and the minerals iron and copper. Storing vitamin C–rich foods in cool conditions, such as in the refrigerator, will help preserve the micronutrient. Because vitamin C is easily lost during cooking, eat raw fruits and vegetables whenever possible.

collagen fibrous protein that gives strength to connective tissue

prooxidant substance that promotes free radical production

MY DIVERSE PLATE

MyPlate: Source: U.S. Dept. of Agriculture

Guava

Guava is a tropical fruit that is available in many varieties. Although guavas can be eaten fresh, the fruit is often used to make sauces, jellies, and juices. Guavas are an excellent source of fiber and vitamin C. The white or pink flesh of a guava contains more vitamin C than an orange.

©Wendy Schiff

Figure 8.28 Vitamin C and collagen formation. The action of vitamin C results in the formation of numerous cross-connections between the amino acids in collagen, greatly strengthening the connective tissue.

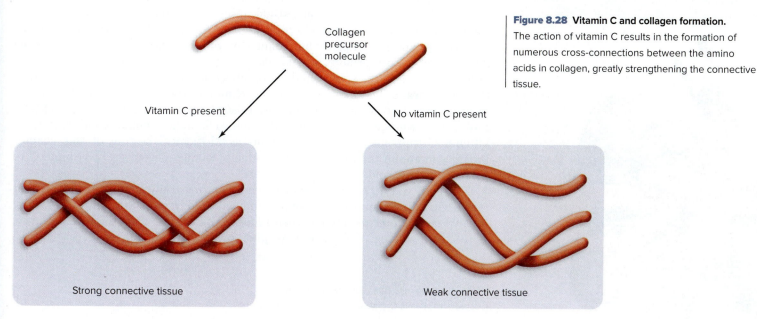

TABLE 8.14   Vitamin C Content of Selected Foods

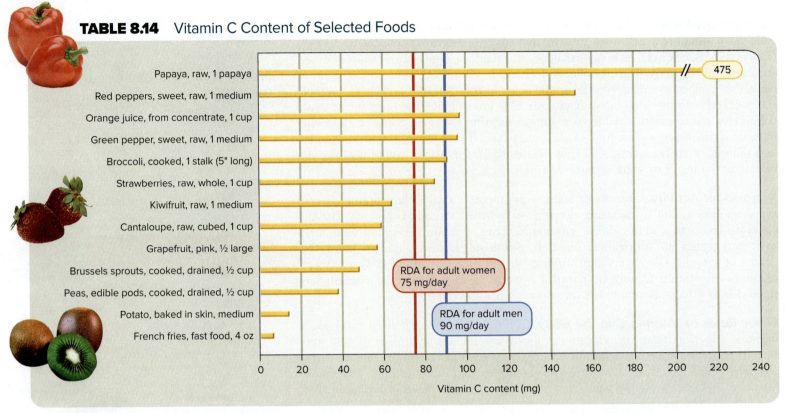

Food	Vitamin C content (mg)
Papaya, raw, 1 papaya	475
Red peppers, sweet, raw, 1 medium	
Orange juice, from concentrate, 1 cup	
Green pepper, sweet, raw, 1 medium	
Broccoli, cooked, 1 stalk (5" long)	
Strawberries, raw, whole, 1 cup	
Kiwifruit, raw, 1 medium	
Cantaloupe, raw, cubed, 1 cup	
Grapefruit, pink, ½ large	
Brussels sprouts, cooked, drained, ½ cup	
Peas, edible pods, cooked, drained, ½ cup	
Potato, baked in skin, medium	
French fries, fast food, 4 oz	

RDA for adult women 75 mg/day

RDA for adult men 90 mg/day

Vitamin C content (mg): 0, 20, 40, 60, 80, 100, 120, 140, 160, 180, 200, 220, 240

Source: Data from U.S. Department of Agriculture, Agricultural Research Service: *USDA national nutrient database for standard reference,* Release 26, 2013.
Peppers: ©Jules Frazier/Getty Images RF; Strawberries: ©Brand X Pictures/Getty Images RF; Kiwifruit: ©Ingram Publishing/Alamy RF

Did *YOU* Know?

People who are exposed to cigarette smoke exhaled by smokers ("passive smokers") need to consume more than the RDA for vitamin C, but no specific amount has been recommended for these persons.[5]

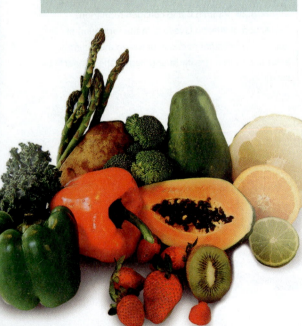

Many kinds of fruits and vegetables are rich sources of vitamin C. ©Wendy Schiff

Dietary Adequacy

The adult RDA for vitamin C is 75 and 90 mg/day for women and men, respectively. Cigarette smokers need to add an extra 35 mg/day to their RDA because exposure to cigarette smoke increases radical formation in their lungs. By including vitamin C–rich fruits and vegetables in their diets, healthy people can obtain adequate amounts of vitamin C.

The adult UL for vitamin C is 2000 mg/day. When people exceed this amount of the vitamin, gastrointestinal upsets, including diarrhea, often occur.[2] Taking megadoses of vitamin C supplements is wasteful because the small intestine reduces absorption of the micronutrient when intakes of the vitamin exceed 200 mg/day.[25] Furthermore, when cells are saturated with vitamin C, the excess vitamin and *oxalate*, a by–product of breaking down vitamin C, circulate in the bloodstream. The kidneys filter and eliminate these unnecessary substances in urine. Excess oxalate excretion may raise the risk of kidney stones.[5] Therefore, people who are susceptible to develop such stones should avoid consuming vitamin C supplements. The "Vitamins as Medicines" section of this chapter provides more information about the value of taking megadoses of vitamin C to prevent or treat colds and other disorders.

Even if you do not regularly eat foods that naturally contain the vitamin or take a vitamin C supplement, you are unlikely to develop a vitamin C deficiency because most people require less than 10 mg of the vitamin daily to prevent scurvy. A 6–ounce serving of fresh orange juice provides about 60 mg of vitamin C, which is well beyond the requirement. Additionally, Americans rarely develop scurvy because vitamin C is added to many processed foods, including fruit and sports drinks, ready—to—eat cereals, and nutrition or power bars. If you would still like to take a vitamin C supplement daily, consider choosing a product that provides up to 200 mg of the vitamin in each tablet.

Choline

The body needs the vitamin—like nutrient choline to produce phospholipids in cell membranes and acetylcholine, a neurotransmitter associated with learning and memory, muscle control, and many other nervous system functions. Addition— ally, the liver uses choline to synthesize a part of a phospholipid (see Chapter 6). Choline is widely distributed in foods. Liver, wheat germ, eggs, beef, and pork are among the richest sources of the nutrient. The source of choline in egg yolk is the phospholipid lecithin (see Chapter 6).

The adult AI for choline is 425 to 550 mg/day. On average, adult Americans consume about 340 mg of choline per person per day.[4] Although the amount of choline that Americans consume is often less than the AI for the micronutrient, the body can make choline from serine, an amino acid. However, the body cannot produce enough choline to meet the amount that is required, especially during some life stages. Vegans may develop choline deficiency because they do not eat animal sources of food.[26] Choline deficiency can cause liver damage.

Concept CHECKPOINT

7. Prepare a table of water-soluble vitamins and choline. For each of these micronutrients, indicate its major function in the body, major food sources, deficiency disorder (if it has a specific name), and major signs and symptoms of the deficiency disorder. If the micronutrient is known to be toxic, also indicate major toxicity signs and symptoms. Check your table against the information provided in Table 8.7.

See Appendix G for responses.

8.4 Vitamins as Medicines

Learning Outcome

1 Evaluate the use of vitamin supplements with respect to their potential health benefits and hazards.

Vitamin supplements are effective for treating people with specific vitamin defi— ciency diseases, metabolic defects that increase vitamin requirements, and a few other medical conditions. However, scientific evidence generally does not support claims that megadoses of vitamins can prevent or treat everything from gray hair to lung cancer.

How did vitamins earn the reputation of being cure—alls? The fact that a very small amount of a vitamin can prevent or cure the vitamin's deficiency dis— ease provides the foundation for beliefs that these micronutrients are useful for preventing or treating serious chronic diseases. Furthermore, many people think that vitamins are helpful and safe in any amount. When ingested in high doses, however, vitamins and related compounds such as carotenoids often have druglike

Food & Nutrition tip

Vitamin C supplements that contain "ester" forms of the vitamin do not provide any advantage over "regular" vitamin C supplements. The ester forms of the supplements are usually more expensive, too.

Did *YOU* Know?

effects in the body. In some cases, these physiological responses are beneficial, but in other instances, vitamin excesses cause unpleasant and even dangerous side effects. Therefore, people should be just as cautious about using mega-doses of vitamins as they need to be when taking medications. This section of Chapter 8 focuses on some current scientific evidence regarding the usefulness and safety of using large doses of vitamins and related compounds as medications.

Niacin as Medicine?

In Chapter 6, we discussed the association between elevated blood levels of LDL cholesterol and increased risk of cardiovascular disease (CVD), the number one killer of Americans. Heart disease and stroke are the major forms of CVD. Physicians may prescribe megadoses of niacin alone or in combination with statins to reduce elevated LDL cholesterol levels.[17] High doses of niacin can be toxic, so people should consult with qualified medical practitioners before using the vitamin as a medicine.

Vitamin B-6 as Medicine?

Popular sources of nutrition information often recommend large doses of vitamin B-6 to treat *premenstrual syndrome (PMS)*, a condition that many women experience a few days before their menstrual period begins. However, studies investigating the value of vitamin B-6 supplementation for relieving PMS provide mixed results.[19] Scientists continue to study the effectiveness of using high doses of vitamin B-6 to treat PMS.

Unlike most other B vitamins, vitamin B-6 is toxic in high doses, caus-ing severe sensory nerve damage when taken in doses that exceed the UL for extended periods. Signs and symptoms of vitamin B-6 toxicity include walk-ing difficulties and numbness of the hands and feet. The nerve damage usually resolves when affected people stop ingesting megadoses of vitamin B-6.

Folic Acid, B-6, and B-12 as Medicine?

Deficiencies of folic acid, vitamin B-6, and vitamin B-12 are associated with elevated blood levels of homocysteine. High homocysteine levels may be a bio-chemical marker (an indicator in the body) or a risk factor for cardiovascu-lar disease. However, results of research do not provide evidence that lowering homocysteine levels by taking these B vitamins reduces the risk of heart disease or stroke.[19]

Some scientists think poor vitamin B-6 status contributes to the cognitive decline that often occurs with aging. Cognitive functions include the ability to remember, understand, and use information. According to results of a few reli-able studies, there is no evidence that short-term use of vitamin B-6, by itself or along with other B vitamins, can prevent or slow cognitive decline among older adults.[19]

Vitamin C as Medicine?

In 1970, Nobel Prize–winning American chemist Dr. Linus Pauling (1901–1994) published *Vitamin C and the Common Cold*. This bestselling book established the popular belief that megadoses of vitamin C could prevent colds. As a result of Pauling's claim, many Americans take megadoses of the micronutrient when they notice the first cold symptoms.

In the years that followed the publication of *Vitamin C and the Common Cold*, Pauling became more convinced of vitamin C's health benefits. He claimed

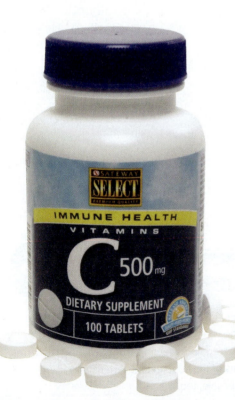

large doses of vitamin C could battle a variety of diseases, including influenza, cancer, and CVD. He even believed the vitamin could slow the aging process. Despite Pauling's impressive credentials in chemistry, many conventional nutrition scientists have approached his ideas about vitamin C's health benefits with caution and skepticism.

Can taking vitamin C protect you against infection by cold viruses? The evidence collected from several scientific studies indicates that routine vitamin C supplementation (200 mg or more of the vitamin daily) does not prevent colds in the general population.[5] However, taking such large doses of the vitamin may reduce the duration of cold symptoms by a day or so. Additionally, vitamin C may reduce the severity of cold symptoms because the micronutrient acts like an antihistamine when taken in very large doses.

Beyond the Common Cold

When LDL cholesterol is oxidized, it is more likely to contribute to atherosclerosis than nonoxidized LDL cholesterol (see Chapter 6). As an antioxidant, vitamin C may reduce the oxidation of LDL cholesterol, lowering the risk of CVD. Studies to determine whether vitamin C can help prevent CVD have not provided consistent evidence that the micronutrient reduces the risk of CVD or dying from the condition.[5] Atherosclerosis takes years and probably decades to result in heart attack, strokes, and other forms of CVD. Thus, more research is needed to determine whether long-term vitamin C supplementation can reduce the risk of this leading killer of Americans.

According to findings of epidemiological studies, people who consume diets containing high amounts of vitamin C–rich fruits and vegetables have lower risk of cancer than people who do not eat much of these foods. Nevertheless, results of studies generally do not support the usefulness of taking vitamin C supplements to prevent cancer.[5] There is some encouraging scientific evidence that intravenous (IV) administration of megadoses of vitamin C may be useful in treating cancer.[5] The "Nutrition Matters" section in this chapter provides more information concerning the role of diet in cancer development and prevention.

It is important to note that complex chronic diseases such as CVD, cognitive decline, and cancer generally do not have simple causes. Inherited factors as well as lifestyle practices other than diet—smoking, obesity, and lack of physical activity—contribute to the development of these health conditions. Therefore, it is unlikely that people will be able to prevent or treat cancer simply by taking vitamin C (or any other supplement).

Vitamin E as Medicine?

Major studies fail to show that high intakes of vitamin E consistently reduce the risk of CVD, cancer, and mild cognitive impairment, a condition characterized by declining thought-processing abilities that can progress to Alzheimer's disease.[13] Furthermore, use of vitamin E supplements has been associated with an increased risk of prostate cancer (men) and hemorrhagic stroke. More clinical research is needed to determine whether combinations of vitamin E and other antioxidant nutrients can prevent or slow the development of chronic diseases, such as CVD, cancer, and Alzheimer's disease.

Did scientists *prove* vitamin E supplements are useless or "bad"? No. Vitamin E has several forms, and it is possible that the alpha-tocopherol form of vitamin E that is typically in supplements does not have any beneficial druglike effects on the body. The dosage of vitamin E and the length of time the supplements are administered during clinical tests may provide other reasons why research findings do not always support epidemiological observations. To detect positive effects on health, scientists may need to test higher doses of the vitamin than have been studied in the past. Additionally, studies that last longer may be necessary; the health benefits of vitamin E supplementation may take several years to become evident.

Vitamin A and Carotenoids as Medicine?

Findings of observational studies suggest an association between eating diets rich in fruits and vegetables and lower risk of certain cancers, heart disease, and *age−related macular degeneration* (see the following section, "Dietary Supplements and AMD"). Such diets provide plenty of beta−carotene and other antioxidant carotenoids. Scientists have conducted numerous large−scale studies to determine whether carotenoid supplements provide health benefits. The following sections summarize research findings regarding the health effects of taking these supplements.

Cancer

Results of clinical studies have not provided support for taking vitamin A or beta−carotene supplements to reduce the risk of cancer.[7] In two major studies, smokers who took beta−carotene supplements were *more* likely to die of lung cancer than smokers who took placebos.[7] Nevertheless, more research is needed to determine whether other carotenoids, such as lycopene and *beta−cryptoxanthin (bay'−ta krip'−toe−zan'−thin)*, protect against various forms of cancer.

Dietary Supplements and AMD

In the United States, age−related macular degeneration (AMD) is one of the leading causes of blindness among older adults.[7] The disease is associated with changes in the *macula*, the region within the eye that provides the most detailed central vision (Fig. 8.29). When the macula is damaged, objects appear to be distorted, as in the grid shown in Figure 8.30 (right side). Major risk factors for AMD are genetics, smoking, and advanced age, but diet also plays a role in the development of the condition.

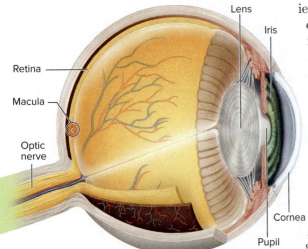

Figure 8.29 **The macula.** The macula is the region within the eye that provides the most detailed central vision.

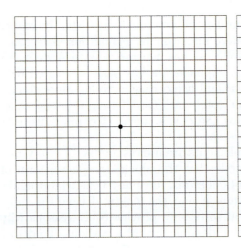
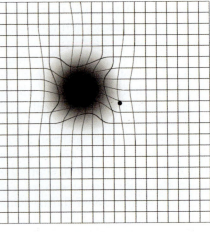

Figure 8.30 Visual effect of macular degeneration. When shown a grid comprised of straight lines, people with normal vision see the grid on the left. However, people with age-related macular degeneration (AMD) would see distorted gridlines, as shown in the right illustration.

The macula contains the carotenoids lutein and zeaxanthin. In the Age–Related Eye Disease Study (AREDS), patients who already had AMD took dietary supplements that contained relatively high amounts of vitamins C and E, beta–carotene, and the minerals copper and zinc.[7] The combination of these substances slowed the progression of vision loss associated with advanced macular degeneration. In a follow–up study, scientists determined that giving beta–carotene supplements to patients with AMD was not helpful. However, the patients who took lutein and zeaxanthin supplements experienced a delay in the progression of AMD. At this point, there is no scientific evidence that taking antioxidant supplements *prevents* healthy people from developing AMD.

Some Final Thoughts

According to a report issued by the U.S. Preventive Services Task Force, there is a lack of credible scientific evidence for or against using dietary supplements, including those with vitamins, to prevent major chronic diseases.[28] However, there is strong evidence to advise against the use of beta–carotene supplements, especially among smokers.[28] Although the health benefits of vitamin supplementation are often uncertain, there is more consistent evidence that a diet high in fruits, vegetables, and legumes has important benefits. It is possible that other constituents besides vitamins may account for the benefits of such diets.

Consuming a wide variety of vitamins, antioxidants, and phytochemicals in their natural states and concentrations (in foods) may be the most effective way to lower your risk of CVD, cancer, and many other serious chronic diseases. Why? These substances probably work together to enhance health, and isolating them from their natural sources or synthesizing and concentrating them into supplements may reduce their usefulness and increase their risks.[30] Therefore, nutrition experts recommend that adults eat a variety of fruits and vegetables each day rather than take antioxidant or phytochemical supplements.

Nutrition experts tend to emphasize the importance of combining a nutritious diet with regular exercise for achieving and maintaining good health. However, an overwhelming amount of scientific evidence links tobacco use to several forms of cancer, heart disease, AMD, and other serious chronic conditions. If you smoke tobacco, quitting may have a greater beneficial impact on your long–term health than improving your diet or increasing your physical activity level while still continuing tobacco use.

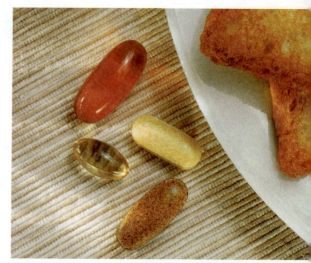
©Comstock/Getty Images RF

Did *YOU* Know?

In 2010, Americans spent over $28 billion on dietary supplements, which included vitamin supplements.[29]

Concept CHECKPOINT

8. Explain why people should be careful about taking megadoses of vitamin supplements.
9. What is a serious side effect that can occur from taking megadoses of niacin?
10. Explain why people should avoid taking high doses of vitamin B-6.
11. A friend of yours takes 1000 mg of vitamin C daily because she thinks the vitamin prevents colds. After reading section 8.4, what would you tell your friend about her vitamin C use?
12. Dorothy is 85 years of age. She has excellent vision, but she takes megadoses of beta-carotene, because she thinks taking the phytochemical helps prevent macular degeneration. Based on the information in section 8.4, what would you tell Dorothy about her beta-carotene use?

See Appendix G for responses.

8.5 Nutrition Matters: Diet and Cancer

Learning Outcomes

1. Define key terms, including *metastasize, carcinogen,* and *malignant tumor.*
2. Identify common cancer sites and causes of cancer deaths for Americans.
3. Identify lifestyle practices associated with increased risk of certain cancers.
4. Identify foods that may increase risk of cancer.
5. Discuss some practical steps that people can take to reduce their risk of cancer.

For many people, no diagnosis evokes more fear than that of *cancer.* Although modern medical technologies have enabled physicians to make great progress in treating many types of cancer successfully, the disease is still the second–leading cause of death in the United States. According to the American Cancer Society, one in four Americans dies as a result of cancer.[31]

In 2017, the three leading sites of new cancer cases (excluding common types of skin cancer) for American men were prostate, lung, and colon and rectal (colorectal) cancers.[31] The three leading sites of new cancer cases in American women were breast, lung, and colorectal cancers. As shown in Figure 8.31, lung cancer is responsible for most cancer deaths. There is good news: A significant number of cancer deaths are preventable.

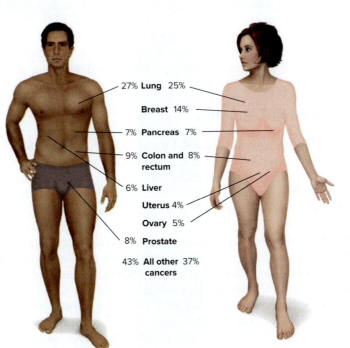

Figure 8.31 Leading cancer sites and deaths. This figure indicates leading sites of cancer deaths and percentages of cancer deaths, according to 2017 estimates. Source: American Cancer Society, *Cancer facts & figures 2017.* www.cancer.org. Accessed: June 4, 2017.

This section focuses on the roles of diet and exercise in the development, progression, and possible prevention of cer–tain cancers. For more information about cancer, including

| Figure 8.32 Cancer development and progression.

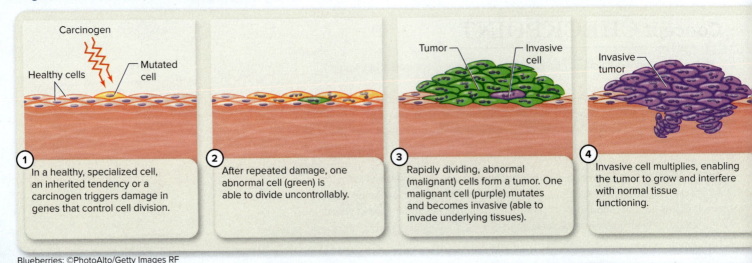

1. In a healthy, specialized cell, an inherited tendency or a carcinogen triggers damage in genes that control cell division.

2. After repeated damage, one abnormal cell (green) is able to divide uncontrollably.

3. Rapidly dividing, abnormal (malignant) cells form a tumor. One malignant cell (purple) mutates and becomes invasive (able to invade underlying tissues).

4. Invasive cell multiplies, enabling the tumor to grow and interfere with normal tissue functioning.

Blueberries: ©PhotoAlto/Getty Images RF

specific forms of cancer, visit the American Cancer Society's website at www.cancer.org or the National Cancer Institute's website at www.cancer.gov.

What Is Cancer?

Cancer is the term for a group of chronic diseases characterized by cells that have undergone damage to certain genes (*mutations*). Genes are portions of DNA that code for the production of specific proteins (see Chapter 7). DNA dictates cellular growth, division, and eventual death. The rate at which healthy cells develop, grow, divide, and die occurs in a controlled fashion. As a normal body cell develops and matures, it acquires specialized functions. Examples include the ability of muscle cells to contract and that of certain stomach cells to secrete hydrochloric acid.

Cancerous (*malignant*) cells are literally "out of control": They divide repeatedly and frequently, and they do not die. If genes that regulate cellular growth, division, and death mutate, abnormal cell development, rapid cell growth, and unchecked cell division can result. When a cell becomes malignant, it does not perform the specialized functions of the cells from which it was derived. A cancerous liver cell, for example, does not remove toxins from the bloodstream or store nutrients properly.

As a result of their rapid growth rate, many types of cancer cells form masses, called **malignant tumors.** Malignant cells often break away from the tumor. These cells can move to and invade other parts of the body. When cancer spreads to other tissues, the disease has **metastasized** (*meh−tass′−tah−sized*).

Some cells multiply excessively and form *benign* (*bih−nine′*) masses or tumors as a result. A benign tumor is not cancerous because the tumor's cells do not destroy nearby tissues or metastasize. Benign tumors are usually harmless. In some cases, however, a benign tumor grows large enough to interfere with the functioning of healthy structures, such as a blood vessel or brain tissue. When this occurs, the tumor needs to be treated to reduce its size or remove it.

A **carcinogen** (*car−sin′−o−jin*) is an environmental factor, such as radiation, tobacco smoke, or a virus, that triggers cancer. Carcinogens can irritate tissues, causing an inflammatory response by the body. Over time, the inflammation may result in cancer development. Some carcinogens damage DNA, causing mutations to genes that control certain cell behaviors. Over time, repeated exposures to various carcinogens take their toll on cells, making malignant cells more likely to develop. In fact, it is not unusual for cancerous cells to develop during a person's lifetime. However, a healthy immune system identifies the malignant cells and destroys them before they multiply uncontrollably. Nutrient deficiencies, the aging process, and environmental insults, such as exposure to radiation and certain chemicals, reduce the effectiveness of the immune system. As a result, cancer cells are able to divide unchecked and eventually metastasize. Figure 8.32 illustrates major steps in the development and behavior of most cancerous cells.

Because of their rapid growth and frequent cell divisions, malignant cells require more nutrients than normal cells. To supply enough nutrients to meet their needs, cancerous tumors stimulate the body to form blood vessels that divert blood away from healthy cells and into the tumor (see Fig. 8.32). Much of the severe body wasting that usually accompanies advanced cases of cancer happens because healthy tissues are unable to obtain adequate supplies of nutrients, and they die.

malignant tumor mass of cancerous cells

metastasized spread to other tissues

carcinogen factor that triggers cancer

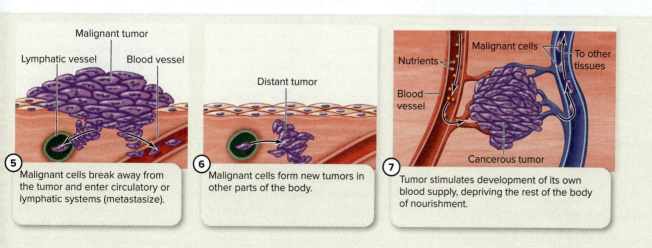

5 Malignant cells break away from the tumor and enter circulatory or lymphatic systems (metastasize).

6 Malignant cells form new tumors in other parts of the body.

7 Tumor stimulates development of its own blood supply, depriving the rest of the body of nourishment.

Regular health checkups and various screening methods can detect cancer in its early stages, when many forms can be effectively treated. Screening methods include using a special scope to view the inside of the lower gastrointestinal tract to detect colorectal cancer (*colonoscopy*). Conventional medical treatments for cancer typically involve surgical removal of cancerous tissue; chemotherapy, medications that are toxic to cancer cells or limit their growth; and radiation that kills cancer cells. Early diagnosis of cancer is very important. Once cancer metastasizes, it is far more difficult to treat.

What Causes Cells to Become Cancerous?

Why do many smokers develop lung cancer and some not develop it? Why do some women have breast cancer and others remain free of the disease? Medical researchers have discovered several risk factors for many forms of the disease, including the following:

- Aging (87% of cancers occur in people over 50 years of age)
- Having a family history of cancer
- Using tobacco
- Being exposed to some forms of radiation
- Being exposed to certain environmental substances, such as irritants
- Having certain viral and bacterial infections
- Having elevated levels of certain hormones
- Consuming alcohol and certain foods
- Being physically inactive and having excess body fat[31,32]

People can lower their risk of cancer by avoiding known carcinogens, especially tobacco smoke. In the United States, approximately one of every three cancer deaths is associated with smoking tobacco.[31] Smoking is responsible for many cases of lung cancer, but mouth, larynx ("voicebox"), esophageal, stomach, pancreatic, kidney, and bladder cancers are also associated with tobacco use. According to the American Cancer Society, over 190,000 Americans were predicted to die in 2017 as a result of smoking cigarettes.[31]

Cancer causation is a complex process. Therefore, it may be impossible to pinpoint a single cause of a patient's cancer. Individuals differ widely in their genetic makeups, lifestyle practices, environmental exposures, and nutritional states. Some forms of the disease are likely to be inherited, but poor diet, alcohol consumption, physical inactivity, and excess body fat are responsible for 20% of the cancers that occur in the United States.[31] The following sections examine relationships between dietary factors and the risk of cancer.

The Role of Diet in Cancer Development

Rates of specific cancers vary widely among different populations. Men and women living in Asian countries, for example, have lower risks of prostate and breast cancer, respectively, than men and women living in Western countries. After Asian men and women migrate to Western countries, their risks of prostate and breast cancer increase and eventually become similar to the risks of their adopted country's native population. Such findings provide epidemiological evidence of associations between cancer and certain lifestyle choices.

According to results of observational and experimental studies, certain substances in foods and beverages promote cancer development. Alcohol, for example, is a carcinogen. People who consume alcoholic drinks daily have higher than average risks of cancers of the mouth, throat, esophagus, larynx, colorectum, liver, and breast.[31] The risk rises as the amount of alcohol consumed increases and when cigarette smoking is combined with drinking. To reduce your risk of cancer, avoid alcoholic beverages or drink in moderation: no more than one standard drink per day for women and no more than two standard drinks per day for men (see the "Nutrition Matters" section of Chapter 6).

Certain molds that can grow on nuts or grains produce a chemical called *aflatoxin* (*ah'–fla–tox'–in*). Consuming foods that are contaminated with these molds increases the risk of liver cancer. Although liver cancer is not common among Americans, populations that consume peanuts and grains that have been stored improperly have high rates of this type of cancer. Chapter 12 discusses toxic molds and ways to protect the food supply from them and other foodborne health threats.

Diets that contain large amounts of processed meats and/or red meat (defined as beef, pork, and lamb) are associated with increased risk of colorectal and prostate cancer.[31] Processed meat ("deli" meat) has sodium nitrate and sodium nitrite added to it during production. Under certain conditions, these chemicals form *nitrosamine* (*ni–tros'–ah–menes*), which are carcinogens. Eating high amounts of smoked or salt–preserved (*pickled*) foods, such as salted fish, may increase the risk of stomach cancer.[33]

The high temperatures used to fry, grill, or broil meat may cause the formation of a group of substances in the food called *heterocyclic* (*het'–eh–ro–si'–klic*) amines. Results of animal studies indicate that these amines are carcinogens. However, it is not known whether heterocyclic amines are human carcinogens.[34] Nevertheless, you may want to consider limiting your intake of grilled meats and avoiding charred parts of charcoal–grilled meats. Also, covering the grate with aluminum foil, poking a few holes in the foil, and placing the meat on top of it will reduce charring of the meat.

Excess Body Fat Diets that provide a surplus of calories result in a person becoming overweight or obese, conditions characterized by excess body fat (see Chapter 10). Obese people have higher risks of cancers of the colon, rectum, breast (in postmenopausal women), uterus, kidney, and esophagus than people who have healthy amounts of body

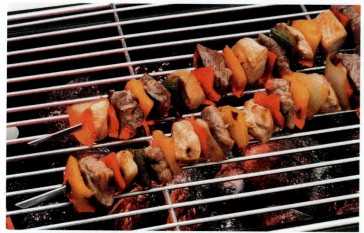
©Ingram Publishing/Alamy RF

TABLE 8.15 Possible Diet-Related Carcinogens

Possibly Carcinogenic	Common Dietary Sources	Possible or Known Action
Aflatoxin	Moldy nuts and grains	Can cause liver cancer
Arsenic	Natural contaminant in drinking water	May increase risk of bladder cancer
Alcohol	Alcoholic beverages	Unclear but may be related to a toxic byproduct of alcohol metabolism
Excess calorie intake	All macronutrients	Excess calorie intake is linked to obesity, which can increase certain hormone levels
Heterocyclic amines	Foods exposed to high temperature, especially grilled meat that has charred areas	Formation of heterocyclic amines that alter DNA of colon cells
Sodium nitrate and nitrite	Cured meats, such as deli meats, hot dogs, and bacon	Formation of nitrosamines

©C. Squared Studios/Getty Images RF

fat.[35] The reasons for the relationship between excess body fat and cancer development are unclear. However, overweight and obese people often have elevated insulin, estrogen, and testosterone levels. Excesses of these and possibly other hormones may stimulate the production of cell factors that promote malignant cell development and growth. In some cases, cancer triggers are easier to identify. For example, overweight and obesity are associated with the increased risk of esophageal cancer. Excess abdominal fat contributes to the reflux of stomach acid into the esophagus by restricting the ability of the stomach to expand during meals. As a result, the gastroesophageal sphincter is unable to keep the stomach's contents from moving into the esophagus. (See Chapter 4 "Nutrition Matters.") Chronic exposure to stomach acid irritates the lining of the esophagus, making cancerous cells more likely to develop in the affected area.

Table 8.15 indicates dietary factors that may be associated with increased risk of various cancers. Currently, there is no scientific evidence that consuming artificial sweeteners, such as aspartame; coffee; fluoridated water; genetically modified foods; or foods preserved by radiation (*irradiated foods*) causes cancer.[36] However, physical activity and some dietary practices may *reduce* the risk of cancer.

Nutrition and Physical Activity Cancer Prevention

Consuming a nutritious diet that contains adequate fluids and a variety of foods, especially plant foods, may prevent or delay the development of certain cancers. Drinking enough water and other nonalcoholic fluids may reduce the risk of bladder cancer because water dilutes carcinogens that may be present in urine.[37] Adequate fluid intake also encourages frequent urination, which reduces the time that carcinogens remain in contact with the walls of the bladder.

High intakes of fiber-rich foods, including fruits and vegetables, may reduce the risk of cancer.[36] Fruits and vegetables are rich sources of fiber and vitamin C, as well as carotenoids and other phytochemicals that may have antioxidant activity in the body. Antioxidants protect DNA from free radical damage, preventing potentially cancer-causing mutations from occurring. Although research is ongoing, results of scientific studies generally do not provide evidence that taking dietary supplements that contain antioxidants reduces the risk of cancer.[36] Some medical experts are concerned that taking antioxidant supplements may *increase* the risk of lung and prostate cancers, especially among smokers and men with family histories of prostate cancer.

Many plant foods naturally contain chemicals that reduce carcinogens' ability to damage DNA. Other phytochemicals inhibit tumor growth by being toxic to cancer cells, interfering with their ability to form supportive blood vessels, or creating conditions that make it difficult for cancer cells to flourish. For example, *cruciferous* (*crew–siff'–er–us*) vegetables, such as broccoli, cabbage, and Brussels sprouts, and *turmeric* (*tur'–mur–ik*), a spice found in curry powder, contain substances that are toxic to cancer cells. Medical researchers do not know whether taking supplements that contain phytochemicals offers the same benefits as consuming the chemicals in their natural forms. Currently, much of the evidence about the cancer-protective benefits of specific plant-based chemicals is from laboratory experiments on animals or cell cultures. Testing the chemicals in clinical settings is necessary to determine whether the results observed in laboratories also occur in people. Thus, more research is needed to support the use of phytochemicals to prevent or treat cancer.

Reducing the Risk Although medical researchers are studying the cancer-fighting potential of various chemicals naturally in food, no major breakthroughs have occurred. Avoiding obesity by establishing healthy eating and physical activity habits, especially early in life, may reduce the risk of cancer. According to results of epidemiological studies, people who exercise regularly have lower risks of certain cancers, including colon and breast cancer. Regular physical activity may reduce the risk by helping to control weight, improving immune system functioning, and enhancing the body's regulation of various hormones. Following the American Cancer Society's recommendations does not guarantee zero risk of cancer. As mentioned earlier in this "Nutrition Matters" section, an individual's cancer risk is ultimately determined by the complex interaction of numerous factors, not just diet and physical activity. However, people may be able to reduce their risk of many types of cancer significantly by improving their dietary choices and increasing their physical activity.

At this point, the best course of action is to take steps to prevent cancer. According to the American Cancer Society, people can change their diets to reduce their risk of cancer by:

- limiting alcohol consumption;
- achieving and maintaining a healthy weight;
- adopting a physically active lifestyle; and
- eating a healthy diet that limits intakes of red and processed meats and emphasizes intakes of plant foods, including fruits, vegetables, and whole grains.[31]

Concept CHECKPOINT

13. Which form of cancer is the leading cause of cancer deaths in the United States?

14. Margaret's breast cancer metastasized to her lungs. Define *metastasize.*

15. List three dietary factors that may contribute to cancer.

16. List three steps people can take to reduce their risk of cancer.

See Appendix G for responses.

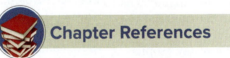

Chapter References

See Appendix H.

Summary

8.1 Vitamins: Basic Concepts

- Vitamins are organic compounds that the body cannot synthesize or make enough of to maintain good health; that naturally occur in commonly eaten foods; that cause deficiency disease when they are missing from diets; and that restore good health when added back to the diet.

- Vitamins play numerous roles in the body, and each vitamin generally has more than one function. In general, vitamins regulate a variety of body processes, including those involved in cell division and development as well as the growth and maintenance of tissues. Vitamins are not a source of energy. Some vitamins have precursors that do not function as vitamins until the body converts them into active forms.

- An oxidation reaction can form a radical. Radicals damage or destroy molecules by removing electrons from them. Cells normally regulate oxidation reactions by using antioxidants such as vitamin E.

- Vitamins A, D, E, and K are fat-soluble vitamins; thiamin, riboflavin, niacin, vitamin B-6, pantothenic acid, folate, biotin, vitamin B-12, and vitamin C are water-soluble vitamins. The body stores extra fat-soluble vitamins. Over time, these vitamins can accumulate and cause toxicity. Water-soluble vitamins are generally not as toxic as fat-soluble vitamins.

- The enrichment program for grains specifies amounts of thiamin, riboflavin, niacin, and folic acid and the mineral iron that manufacturers must add to their refined wheat flour and certain other milled grain products. Fortification involves the addition of one or more vitamins (and/or other nutrients) to a wide array of commonly eaten foods during manufacturing. The vitamins that are added may or may not be in the food naturally.

- Vitamin deficiency disorders generally result from inadequate diets or conditions that increase the body's requirements for vitamins, such as reduced intestinal absorption or higher-than-normal excretion of the micronutrients. Severe vitamin deficiencies are uncommon in the United States. The chances of developing a vitamin deficiency disease increase when the diet consistently lacks the micronutrient and levels of the nutrient in the body become depleted.

- Most commonly eaten foods do not contain toxic levels of vitamins. Vitamin toxicity is most likely to occur in people who take megadoses of vitamin supplements or consume large amounts of vitamin-fortified foods regularly.

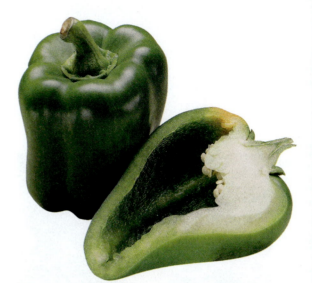

©Stockbyte/Getty Images RF

8.2 Fat-Soluble Vitamins

- Vitamin A is involved in vision, immune function, and cell development. The vitamin A precursor, beta-carotene, functions as an antioxidant. Dietary sources of preformed vitamin A include liver and fish liver oils; provitamin A carotenoids are especially plentiful in dark green and orange fruits and vegetables. Excess vitamin A can be quite toxic and cause birth defects when taken during pregnancy.

- Vitamin D is both a hormone and a vitamin. Exposure to sunlight enables human skin to synthesize a precursor of the vitamin from a cholesterol-like substance. The body can convert this substance to the active form of the vitamin. A few foods, including fatty fish and fortified milk, are dietary sources of the vitamin. Vitamin D helps regulate the level of blood calcium by increasing calcium absorption from the intestine. Infants and children who do not obtain enough vitamin D may develop rickets, and adults with inadequate amounts of the vitamin in their bodies may develop osteomalacia. Older people and breastfed infants often need a supplemental source of the vitamin. Excess intakes of vitamin D can cause the body to deposit calcium in soft tissues.

- Vitamin E functions primarily as an antioxidant. By donating electrons to electron-seeking compounds, vitamin E neutralizes them. Plant oils and products made from these oils are generally rich sources of vitamin E.

8.3 Water-Soluble Vitamins

- Thiamin, riboflavin, and niacin play key roles as part of coenzymes in energy-yielding reactions. These water-soluble vitamins help cells metabolize carbohydrates, fats, and proteins. Enriched grain products are common sources of all three of the vitamins. Beriberi is the severe thiamin deficiency disease; pellagra results from a severe lack of niacin. Excess intakes of niacin can cause toxicity.

- Vitamin B-6 is involved in protein metabolism, especially in synthesizing nonessential amino acids. The vitamin also participates in the synthesis of neurotransmitters and the metabolism of homocysteine. Healthy people can obtain enough vitamin B-6 by eating a varied diet that contains animal foods and rich plant sources of the micronutrient. High doses of vitamin B-6 should be avoided because the vitamin can cause nervous system damage.

- Folate plays important roles in DNA synthesis and homocysteine metabolism. Rich food sources of folate are leafy vegetables, organ meats, and orange juice. Enriched grains have folic acid added to them. Signs of folate deficiency include megaloblastic anemia. Pregnancy increases the body's needs for folate; a deficiency in early pregnancy can result in neural tube defects in offspring. Women of childbearing age can meet the RDA for the vitamin by taking dietary supplements that contain folic acid.

- The body needs vitamin B-12 to metabolize folate and homocysteine, and maintain the insulation surrounding nerves. Although vitamin B-12 does not occur naturally in plant foods, the vitamin is in animal foods and products that have been fortified with the micronutrient. Vitamin B-12 deficiency is more common in older adults. As people age, they produce less stomach acid, which can result in B-12 deficiency even though adequate amounts of the micronutrient are consumed in foods. Loss of intrinsic factor production in the stomach also causes vitamin B-12 deficiency and a condition called pernicious anemia.

- The body uses vitamin C to synthesize and maintain collagen, a major protein in connective tissue. Vitamin C also functions as an antioxidant. Fresh fruits and vegetables, especially citrus fruits, are generally good sources of the micronutrient. Because vitamin C is readily lost in cooking, diets should emphasize fresh or lightly cooked fruits and vegetables. Smoking increases the body's requirement for vitamin C. Scurvy is the vitamin C deficiency disease. Excess vitamin C may cause diarrhea and increase the risk of kidney stones in some people.

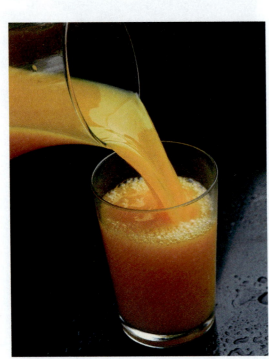

©Pixtal/SuperStock RF

8.4 Vitamins as Medicines

- Although the health benefits of vitamin supplementation remain uncertain, there is consistent epidemiological evidence that a diet high in fruits, vegetables, and legumes may lower the risk of CVD, cancer, and other serious chronic disease. Consuming a wide variety of vitamins, antioxidants, and phytochemicals in their natural states and concentrations (in foods) may be the most effective way to achieve good health. Therefore, people should consume a variety of fruits and vegetables daily rather than take vitamin or antioxidant supplements.

8.5 Nutrition Matters: Diet and Cancer

- Cancer occurs when genes that regulate cellular growth, division, and death mutate, resulting in abnormal cell development, rapid cell growth, and unchecked cell division. Maintaining a healthy body weight, exercising regularly, consuming diets that supply plenty of fruits and vegetables, limiting intakes of red and/or processed meats, and avoiding tobacco smoke and excess alcohol may reduce the risk of cancer.

Recipe for 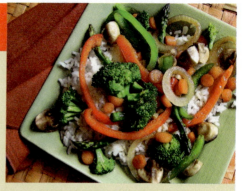 Healthy Living

Stir-Fried Vegetable Medley

"Eat your vegetables!" Does this order bring back some not-so-fond dinnertime memories? If you are like many Americans, cooked vegetables were not high on your list of favorite foods when you were a child. Corn on the cob was fun to eat, but you may have picked at your peas and carrots, and refused to eat broccoli unless it was smothered in a gooey cheese sauce. You probably drew a "line in the sand" when offered Brussels sprouts. Now that you have read Chapter 8, you should appreciate the nutritional contribution that a wide variety of colorful vegetables can make to your diet. Your parents told the truth when they said, "Vegetables are good for you."

©Wendy Schiff

This vegetable medley can be the foundation of a vegetarian meal or a colorful accompaniment to main dishes. You don't need to use all the vegetables in the recipe; feel free to improvise, especially when certain fresh vegetables are in season and plentiful. If you use fresh vegetables, wash them in cool water and drain on paper towels before cutting them into bite-size pieces. If you use frozen vegetables, add them directly to the hot oil, without thawing them first. Be careful because ice from the vegetables can cause hot oil to spatter.

Your goal is to heat the vegetables in a small amount of hot oil only until they are still colorful and crisp—about 4 to 8 minutes. Add the quicker-cooking vegetables (for example, mushrooms) last, so they don't overcook. Use a slotted spoon to drain oil from vegetables and serve immediately.

This recipe (without rice or noodles) makes about four ½-cup servings. Each serving supplies approximately 107 kcal, 3 g protein, 7 g fat, 3 g fiber, 45 mg vitamin C, and 43 mcg folate.

INGREDIENTS:

1 Tbsp low-sodium soy sauce
2 Tbsp water
1 Tbsp brown sugar
⅛ tsp ground black pepper
2 Tbsp vegetable oil
1 large garlic clove, minced
½ cup onions, sliced
1 cup asparagus, cut into 2"-long pieces
½ cup broccoli, small pieces
½ cup carrots, sliced into "coins"
½ medium green pepper, cut in 2" strips, about ¼" wide
½ medium sweet red pepper, cut in 2" strips, about ¼" wide
6 button mushrooms, crosscut into quarters

PREPARATION STEPS:

1. In a small dish, prepare mixture of soy sauce, water, and brown sugar. Set aside.

2. Heat oil in a wok or large deep frying pan over medium-high heat. Add garlic and onions. Stir.

3. When onions and garlic are translucent, add asparagus, broccoli, carrots, peppers, and mushrooms. Stir mixture constantly to coat vegetables with oil.

4. Add soy sauce, water, and brown sugar mixture.

5. Add zucchini. Sprinkle black pepper over vegetables.

6. Do not overcook. If the mixture seems too dry, add another tablespoon of water.

7. Serve immediately over cooked rice or noodles.

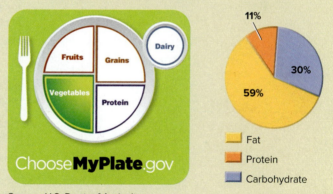

ChooseMyPlate.gov

Source: U.S. Dept. of Agriculture

11%
30%
59%

☐ Fat
☐ Protein
☐ Carbohydrate

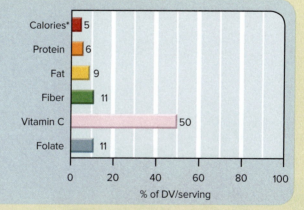

	% of DV/serving
Calories*	5
Protein	6
Fat	9
Fiber	11
Vitamin C	50
Folate	11

*2000 daily total kcal

connect Further analyze this recipe or other recipes through activities located in Connect.

Personal Dietary Analysis

Using the DRIs

1. Refer to your 1- or 3-day food log from the "Personal Dietary Analysis" feature in Chapter 3.

    a. Find the RDA values for vitamins under your life stage/sex group category in the DRI tables (see Appendix I). Write those values under the "My RDA" column in the table of this analysis activity.

    b. Review your personal dietary assessment. Find your 3-day average intakes of vitamins A, E, C, D, folate, B-12, thiamin, riboflavin, and niacin. Write those values under the "My Average Intake" column of the table.

    c. Calculate the percentage of the RDA you consumed for each vitamin by dividing your intake by the RDA amount and multiplying the figure you obtain by 100. For example, if your average intake of vitamin C were 100 mg/day, and your RDA for the vitamin were 75 mg/day, you would divide 100 mg by 75 mg to obtain 1.25. To multiply this figure by 100, simply move the decimal point two places to the right, and replace the decimal point with a percentage sign (125%). Thus, your average daily intake of vitamin C was 125% of the RDA. Place the percentages for each vitamin under the "% of My RDA" column.

    d. Under the ">, <, or =" column, indicate whether your average daily intake was greater than (>), less than (<), or equal to (=) the RDA.

2. Use the information you calculated in the first part of this activity to answer the following questions:

    a. Which of your average vitamin intakes equaled or exceeded the RDA value?

    b. Which of your average vitamin intakes was below the RDA value?

    c. What foods would you eat to increase your intake of the vitamins that were less than the RDA levels? (Review sources of certain vitamins in Chapter 8.)

    d. Turn in your completed table and answers to your instructor.

Personal Dietary Analysis: Vitamins

Vitamin	My RDA	My Average Intake	% of My RDA	>, <, or =
A				
E				
C				
D				
Folate				
B-12				
Thiamin				
Riboflavin				
Niacin				

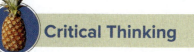

Complete the Personal Dietary Analysis activity located in Connect.

Critical Thinking

1. Choose a vitamin and type the nutrient's name in the search box of an Internet browser. Locate three sites that sell products containing the vitamin. Review the pages of each site, making notes about claims, prices, and the kinds of links provided. Then write a three— to five—page report that describes and compares the information you found at the sites. In your paper, discuss any claims made on behalf of these products that you consider false or misleading. Include the URLs for the sites mentioned in your report.

2. Choose three different websites that sell vitamin sup—plements. Choose three different products and compare prices for the same product at the different websites. Then compare prices of the vitamins from these sites with the prices you would pay at a local supermarket, discount department store, or drugstore. Make sure to compare products with the same chemical composition (single vitamin, for example) and that have the same amount of the vitamin in each dose. Write a one—page report about your findings.

3. While watching an infomercial on TV, you hear a so—called nutrition expert make claims for a substance that he or she claims to be a vitamin. What questions would you ask the expert to ascertain whether the substance truly is a vitamin?

4. One of your friends takes megadoses of vitamin A, C, B−6, and E because she thinks they help her stay healthy. What would you tell her about taking such large doses of these vitamins?

5. According to MyPlate, a person who needs 2000 kcal/day should consume 2 cups of fruit and 2.5 cups of veg—etables daily. Plan a day's meals and snacks that provide these amounts of fruits and vegetables. In your plan, incorporate foods you like to eat. For information concerning how much of a certain form of fruit or type of vegetable equals 1 cup, visit http://www.choosemyplate.gov/MyPlate and click on the "Fruits" and then the "Vegetables" tabs.

Practice Test

Select the best answer.

1. Megadoses of vitamins
   a. are safe to take if the vitamins are water soluble.
   b. prevent certain chronic diseases.
   c. are available naturally from a wide variety of foods.
   d. may be toxic.

2. Vitamins
   a. are metabolized to yield energy.
   b. occur in gram amounts in foods.
   c. are organic molecules.
   d. are macronutrients.

3. People who are unable to absorb fat are likely to develop a _____ deficiency.
   a. vitamin A
   b. folate
   c. vitamin B−12
   d. riboflavin

4. Enriched grain products have specific amounts of _____ added during processing.
   a. vitamin C
   b. vitamin A
   c. vitamin B−12
   d. thiamin

5. The vitamin content of a vegetable can be affected by
   a. soil composition.
   b. the vegetable's maturity when harvested.
   c. sunlight exposure.
   d. All of the above are correct.

6. Which of the following foods is not a rich source of pro−vitamin A?
   a. Beef
   b. Carrots
   c. Squash
   d. Sweet potato

7. Children who lack vitamin D can develop
   a. pellagra.
   b. rickets.
   c. beriberi.
   d. scurvy.

8. During pregnancy, excess _____ intake is known to be teratogenic.
   a. vitamin A
   b. biotin
   c. vitamin K
   d. folate

9. Lack of vitamin _____ causes scurvy.
   a. A
   b. C
   c. D
   d. K

©Brand X Pictures/Getty Images RF

10. Vitamin K can be produced by
   a. skin exposure to ultraviolet radiation.
   b. hydrolysis of seawater.
   c. intestinal bacteria.
   d. conversion of lactic acid into lactate.

11. Diets that lack niacin can lead to
   a. rickets.
   b. beriberi.
   c. pellagra.
   d. pernicious anemia.

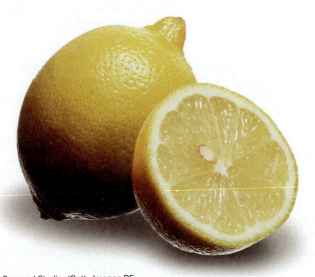

12. To reduce the likelihood of giving birth to babies with neural tube defects, women of childbearing age should obtain adequate

    a. folate.
    b. biotin.
    c. cellulose.
    d. niacin.

13. Major food sources of vitamin B−12 include

    a. enriched grain products.
    b. meat and milk products.
    c. fruit and vegetables.
    d. nuts and seeds.

14. Which of the following statements is false?

    a. Intrinsic factor is needed for vitamin B−12 absorption.
    b. Vitamin B−12 deficiency is common among elderly persons.
    c. Patients with pernicious anemia are treated with high doses of folic acid.
    d. If untreated, pernicious anemia can be deadly.

15. Which of the following foods is a rich source of vitamin C?

    a. Whole milk
    b. Egg white
    c. Hamburger patty
    d. Green pepper

16. Which of the following practices may reduce your risk of cancer?

    a. Eating fruits and vegetables
    b. Eating grilled meats regularly
    c. Smoking no more than 10 cigarettes daily
    d. Consuming two to three standard alcoholic drinks daily

Answers to Quiz Yourself

1. Natural vitamins are better for you because they have more biological activity than synthetic vitamins. **False.** (Section 8.1)

2. Certain vitamins are toxic. **True.** (Section 8.1)

3. Vitamin E is an antioxidant. **True.** (Section 8.2)

4. Vitamins are a source of "quick" energy. **False.** (Section 8.1)

5. According to scientific research, taking large doses of vitamin C daily prevents the common cold. **False.** (Section 8.4)

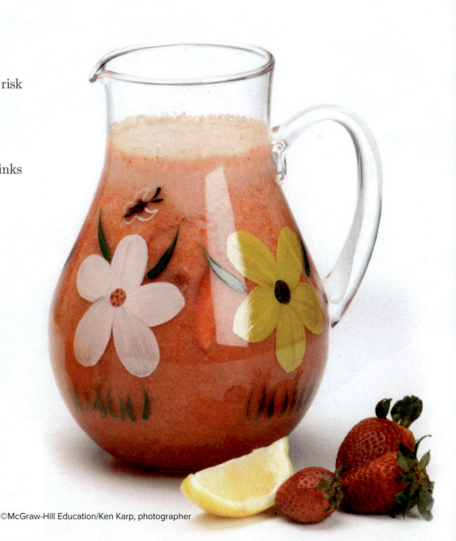

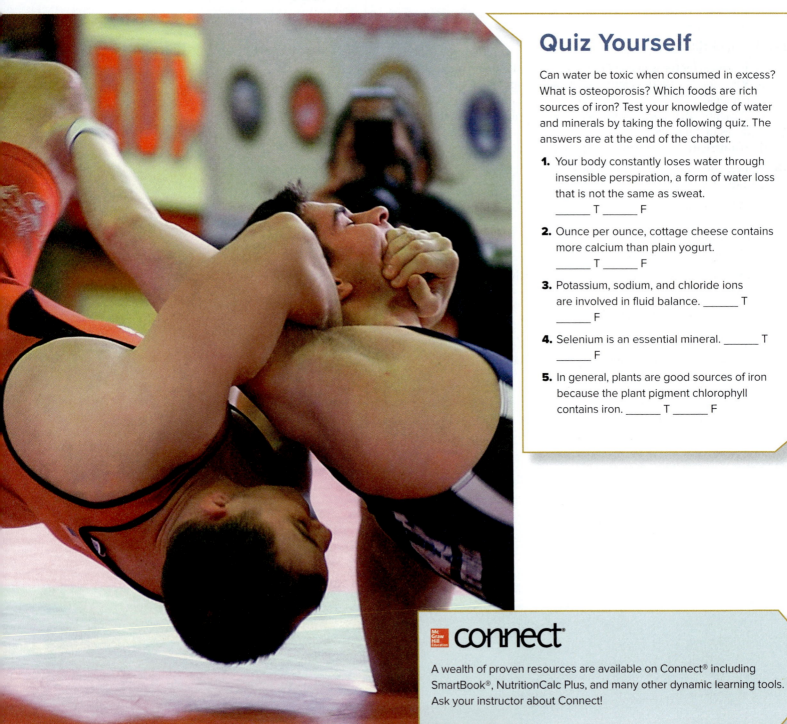

CHAPTER 9

Water and Minerals

Quiz Yourself

Can water be toxic when consumed in excess? What is osteoporosis? Which foods are rich sources of iron? Test your knowledge of water and minerals by taking the following quiz. The answers are at the end of the chapter.

1. Your body constantly loses water through insensible perspiration, a form of water loss that is not the same as sweat.
   _____ T _____ F

2. Ounce per ounce, cottage cheese contains more calcium than plain yogurt.
   _____ T _____ F

3. Potassium, sodium, and chloride ions are involved in fluid balance. _____ T _____ F

4. Selenium is an essential mineral. _____ T _____ F

5. In general, plants are good sources of iron because the plant pigment chlorophyll contains iron. _____ T _____ F

McGraw Hill Education **connect®**

A wealth of proven resources are available on Connect® including SmartBook®, NutritionCalc Plus, and many other dynamic learning tools. Ask your instructor about Connect!

9.1 Introducing Water and Minerals

Learning Outcomes

1 Explain what can happen when dehydration occurs.

2 Classify mineral nutrients as major, trace, or possible essential minerals.

3 Explain the difference between a major mineral and a trace mineral.

In late August 1997, a 19−year−old student wrestler who weighed 233 pounds attended a university in North Carolina. The young man was anxious to lose enough weight to qualify for the 195−pound weight class when the collegiate wrestling season began later that semester. By November 6, the wrestler had lost 23 pounds, but the first tournament was to be held in 2 days and he was still 15 pounds too heavy. To lose ("cut") the extra weight, he engaged in an intense, almost nonstop training session. In a 12−hour period that spanned November 6 and 7, the wrestler restricted his water and food intake severely. Addition−ally, he wore a special suit made from a rubberized material that was *vapor impermeable*, and he even covered it with a cotton warm−up outfit. By wearing this combination of clothing, the young man perspired profusely. Sweating can cause the body to lose a significant amount of "water weight"; however, sweat−ing can also cause **dehydration** (body water depletion), especially when a person restricts his or her fluid intake. Severe dehydration is a life−threatening condition that requires urgent medical care.

At 3 P.M. on November 6, the college wrestler began exercising vigorously in a hot environment. By 11:30 P.M., he had lost 9 pounds. After resting for about 2 hours, the young man resumed his exercise regimen in a desperate effort to lose the remaining 6 pounds. Around 2:45 A.M. on November 7, he had to discon−tinue exercising: he was extremely fatigued and unable to communicate. An hour later, he stopped breathing and his heart ceased beating. Attempts to revive him were unsuccessful. **Hyperthermia** (very high body temperature) is likely to have contributed to his death.[1]

The rapid weight−loss practices that resulted in the death of the young wrestler were prohibited by National Collegiate Athletic Association (NCAA) regulations. However, many wrestlers were determined to lose enough weight prior to a meet so they could gain a competitive edge by wrestling in weight categories that were lower than their preseason weights. Today, NCAA rules prohibit wrestlers from losing weight rapidly by any means, including restrict−ing food and fluid intakes excessively. Failure to follow the NCAA's wrestling guidelines can result in suspension from competition.

We often take water for granted, but this simple molecule is highly essen−tial. You can survive for weeks, even months, if your diet lacks carbohydrates, lipids, proteins, and vitamins. But if you do not have any water, your life will end within a week or two.

Many of water's functions involve certain minerals. About 15 min−eral elements have known functions in the body and are necessary for human health. The body requires these particular micronutrients in milligram or microgram amounts. The essential minerals are classified into two groups: **major minerals** and **trace minerals** (Table 9.1). If we require 100 mg or more of a mineral per day, the mineral is classified as a major mineral; otherwise, the micronutrient is a trace mineral. The body also contains very small amounts of

dehydration body water depletion

hyperthermia very high body temperature

major minerals essential mineral elements required in amounts of 100 mg or more per day

trace minerals essential mineral elements required in amounts that are less than 100 mg per day

©Comstock/Getty Images RF

TABLE 9.1 Minerals with Known or Possible Roles in the Body*

Major Mineral	Trace Mineral	Possible Essential Mineral
Calcium (Ca)	Chromium (Cr)	Arsenic (As)
Chloride (Cl$^-$)	Fluoride (F$^-$)**	Boron (B)
Magnesium (Mg)	Copper (Cu)	Lithium (Li)
Phosphorus (P)	Iodine (I)	Nickel (Ni)
Potassium (K)	Iron (Fe)	Silicon (Si)
Sodium (Na)	Manganese (Mn)	Vanadium (V)
Sulfur (S)	Molybdenum (Mo)	
	Selenium (Se)	
	Zinc (Zn)	

*Chemical symbol is shown in parentheses next to mineral's name.

**Although fluoride is not essential, the mineral plays an important role in strengthening teeth and bones.

other minerals, such as nickel and arsenic. The essential nature of this particular group of minerals has not been fully determined, so we will refer to them as "possible essential minerals" (see Table 9.1).

The mineral nutrients are key components of body structures and play vital roles in metabolism, water balance, muscle movement, and various physiological processes. Mineral deficiencies can cause serious health problems and, in severe cases, death. In this chapter, we will focus on water first and then discuss mineral nutrients, some of which are of major concern for public health officials in the United States and other parts of the world.

Concept CHECKPOINT

1. What is the difference between a major mineral and a trace mineral?
2. List at least five trace minerals.
3. List at least five major minerals.

See Appendix G for responses.

9.2 Water

Learning Outcomes

1. Discuss the functions of water in the body as well as typical sources of intake and loss.
2. Identify foods that have high and low water contents.
3. Discuss how the body maintains its water balance.
4. Explain why dehydration and water intoxication can be life-threatening conditions.

Compared to other nutrients, water is so unusual, it is in a class by itself. Water is a simple compound: A molecule of water is comprised of two hydrogen atoms and one oxygen atom (H_2O). Water does not need to be digested, and it is easily absorbed by the intestinal tract.

Depending on a person's age, sex, and body composition, 50 to 75% of his or her body is water weight. Lean muscle tissue contains more water (about 73%) than fat tissue (about 20%). On average, young adult men have more lean tissue than young women. Approximately 60% of an average young man's body weight is water; the average young adult woman's body has more fat and, therefore, slightly less water than an average young man's body. A person's percentage of body weight that is water declines from birth to old age.

Water is a major solvent; many substances, including glucose, dissolve in water. Water often participates directly in chemical reactions, such as those involved in digesting food. Water's other physiological roles include transporting substances, removing waste products, lubricating tissues, and regulating body temperature and acid−base balance (proper blood pH). Furthermore, water is a major component of blood, saliva, sweat, tears, mucus, and the fluid in joints. Table 9.2 lists roles of water in the body. Although water has numerous functions in the body, this unique nutrient does not provide energy.

Membrane Transport

One reason why water is such a vital nutrient is its role in helping cells obtain materials from their environment and eliminate wastes. To understand some of water's functions in the body, it is necessary to understand how water−soluble substances can become distributed when they are in water. In some instances, substances move by **simple diffusion,** that is, they move from where they are highly concentrated to where they are less concentrated (Fig. 9.1). For example, simple diffusion occurs when a sugar cube is dropped into a cup of hot tea. As the cube dissolves, the concentration of sugar molecules around the cube becomes higher than the concentration of sugar molecules near the surface of the tea. However, the sugar molecules spontaneously diffuse throughout the tea, and eventually, the concentration of sugar molecules and water molecules becomes evenly distributed within the beverage.

TABLE 9.2 Functions of Water in the Body

Water
is a solvent
is a major component of blood, saliva, sweat, tears, mucus, joint fluid
removes wastes
helps transport substances
lubricates tissues
regulates body temperature
helps digest foods
participates in many chemical reactions
helps maintain proper blood pH

Did *YOU* Know?

The layer of fat that is under the skin (*subcutaneous fat*) interferes with the transfer of heat to the skin. This explains why overweight people who are in warm conditions are more uncomfortable and perspire more than slender people.

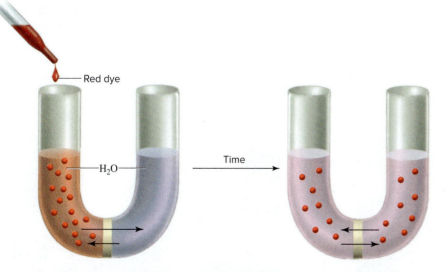

Figure 9.1 Simple diffusion. Simple diffusion can occur when there is a greater concentration of a substance in one region than in another. In this example, the dye is more concentrated on the left side of the container than on the right side. Eventually, the dye molecules diffuse (move) from where they are more concentrated to where they are less concentrated. The diffusion stops when the dye molecules are equally distributed throughout the container.

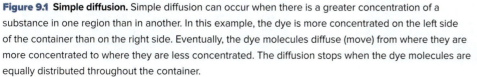

simple diffusion movement of substances from a region of higher to lower concentration

selectively permeable membrane barrier that allows the passage of certain substances and prevents the movement of other substances

osmosis diffusion of a solvent, such as water, through a selectively permeable membrane

intracellular water water that is inside cells

extracellular water water that surrounds cells or is in liquid portion of blood

hydration water status

Simple diffusion also occurs when there is a greater concentration of substances on one side of a *selectively permeable membrane* than on the other. A **selectively permeable membrane** is a barrier that allows the passage of certain substances and prevents the movement of other substances through it. **Osmosis** is the diffusion of a solvent, such as water, through a selectively permeable membrane, such as the plasma membrane of a human cell. The concentration of substances dissolved in the water, such as glucose, influences osmosis. Water moves from a region that has less material dissolved in it (dilute) to a region that has more material dissolved in it (Fig. 9.2). The diffusion stops when the concentrations of the material on either side of the plasma membrane are equal.

To survive, a human cell carefully controls the passage of substances through its plasma membrane. Some materials, such as oxygen and carbon dioxide, easily pass through the cell's plasma membrane by simple diffusion. Large molecules, such as proteins, may be unable to pass through the cell's membrane, unless there are special carrier molecules to help them enter the cell. Chapter 4 discussed other ways cells can obtain substances from their environment.

Body Water Distribution

The body has two major fluid compartments: intracellular water and extracellular water (Fig. 9.3). **Intracellular water** is inside cells. **Extracellular water** surrounds cells (tissue fluid) or is the fluid portion of blood (*plasma*). About two-thirds of the body's water is in the intracellular compartment.

The body maintains the balance of compartmental fluids and proper **hydration,** water status, primarily by controlling concentrations of ions in each compartment. Recall from Chapter 4 that ions are elements or small molecules that have electrical charges. Ions that conduct electricity, such as sodium and potassium ions, are called *electrolytes*. Table 9.3 lists several mineral ions that function in the body.

Maintenance of intracellular water volume depends to a large extent on the intracellular concentration of potassium and phosphate ions. On the other hand, maintenance of extracellular water volume depends primarily on the extracellular concentration of sodium and chloride ions. Changes in the normal

Figure 9.2 Osmosis. Osmosis is the diffusion of a solvent, such as water, through a selectively permeable membrane. Water moves from a compartment that is less concentrated to a compartment that has more material dissolved in it.

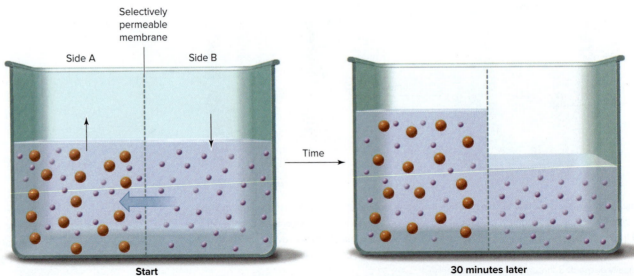

Selectively permeable membrane

Side A   Side B

Time

Start   **30 minutes later**

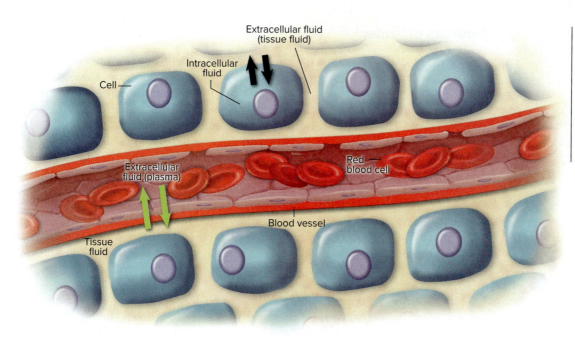

Figure 9.3 Fluid compartments in the body. Intracellular water is inside cells; extracellular water surrounds cells (tissue fluid) or is the fluid in blood (*plasma*). Water is exchanged between plasma and tissue fluid (green arrows) as well as between tissue and intracellular fluids (black arrows).

concentrations of these ions can cause water to shift out of one compartment and move into the other. For example, if extracellular fluid has fewer than normal sodium ions, water moves from the extracellular compartment into cells. When this occurs, the cells swell and can burst (Fig. 9.4a). On the other hand, if extra-cellular fluid has an excess of sodium ions, water moves out of cells. As a result, the cells shrink and die because they lack enough intracellular fluid to function (Fig. 9.4b). Recall from Chapter 7 that edema occurs when an excessive amount of water moves into the space surrounding cells (see Fig. 7.1). To function nor-mally, the body must maintain intracellular and extracellular water volumes within certain limits.

TABLE 9.3 Some Common Ions (Minerals)

Sodium (Na^+)
Calcium (Ca^{2+})
Potassium (K^+)
Magnesium (Mg^{2+})
Chloride (Cl^-)
Phosphate (PO_4^{3-})
Sulfate (SO_4^{2-})

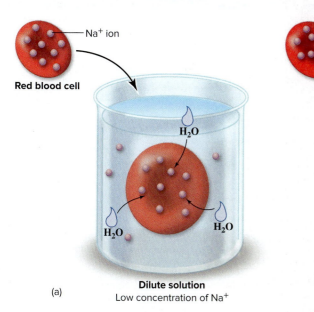
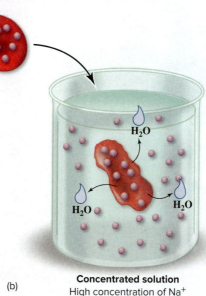

(a) **Dilute solution** Low concentration of Na^+

(b) **Concentrated solution** High concentration of Na^+

Figure 9.4 Maintaining proper hydration. Cells, such as red blood cells, need to maintain their fluid balance. The cell in beaker (*a*) is placed in a solution that contains few sodium ions (Na^+) in relation to the concentration of Na^+ in the cell. As a result, water moves from the solution and into the red blood cell. The cell can swell and burst. The solution in beaker (*b*) has an excess of sodium ions (Na^+) compared to the concentration of Na^+ inside the cell. Water moves out of the red blood cell placed in beaker (*b*). As a result, the cell shrinks and can die.

total water intake water in beverages and foods

metabolic water water formed by cells as a metabolic by-product

Sources of Water

How much water is necessary to drink for good health? Contrary to popular belief, there is no "rule of thumb" recommendation that specifies how many glasses of water to consume each day.[2] Factors such as environmental temperatures, health conditions, physical activities, and dietary choices influence individual water requirements. Thus, total water intakes vary widely. **Total water intake** refers to water ingested by consuming beverages and foods.

The Adequate Intake (AI) for *total* water intake is approximately 11 cups (2.7 L) for young women and approximately 15.5 cups (3.7 L) for young men.[3] These amounts do not need to be consumed in the form of water. Other sources of water include fruit juice, milk, soup, coffee, tea, soft drinks, and flavored bottled water. Most solid foods also contain some water. Fruits and vegetables appear to be solid, but they generally contain 60 to 95% water weight. Table 9.4 lists some commonly consumed foods and their water content by weight. About 80% of our total water intake is from water and other beverages; food supplies the remaining amount of our water intake.[3]

In addition to the water in beverages and foods, a considerable amount of water enters the digestive tract daily through secretions from the mouth, stomach, intestine, pancreas, and gallbladder. The intestinal tract absorbs most of this water, too. Each day, only about 0.4 to 0.8 cup (approximately 100 to 200 ml) of the water that enters the digestive tract is not absorbed. The body eventually eliminates the unabsorbed water in feces.

Cells also form some water as a by–product of metabolism ("metabolic water"). **Metabolic water** also contributes to the body's fluid balance.

The Essential Balancing Act

An average healthy adult consumes and produces approximately 2.6 quarts (2500 ml) of water daily (Fig. 9.5).[4] The body eliminates about 2.6 quarts of water in urine, exhaled air, feces, and perspiration (see Fig. 9.5). Thus, a healthy person's aver–age daily water input equals his or her average daily losses (output).

TABLE 9.4   How Much Water Is in That Food or Beverage?

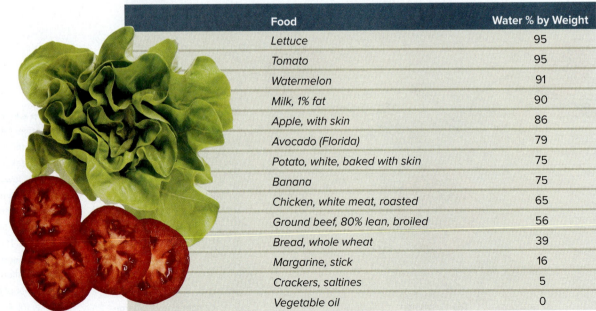

Food	Water % by Weight
Lettuce	95
Tomato	95
Watermelon	91
Milk, 1% fat	90
Apple, with skin	86
Avocado (Florida)	79
Potato, white, baked with skin	75
Banana	75
Chicken, white meat, roasted	65
Ground beef, 80% lean, broiled	56
Bread, whole wheat	39
Margarine, stick	16
Crackers, saltines	5
Vegetable oil	0

Source: Data from U.S. Department of Agriculture, Agricultural Research Service: *USDA national nutrient database for standard reference*, Release 26, 2013. Lettuce: ©Stockbyte/Getty Images RF; Tomatoes: ©Brand X Pictures/Getty Images RF

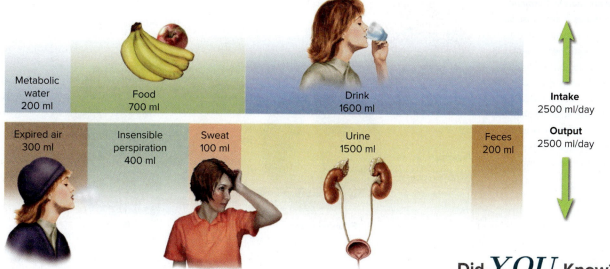

| Metabolic water 200 ml | Food 700 ml | Drink 1600 ml | | Intake 2500 ml/day |
| Expired air 300 ml | Insensible perspiration 400 ml | Sweat 100 ml | Urine 1500 ml | Feces 200 ml | Output 2500 ml/day |

Figure 9.5 Daily water balance. An average healthy adult consumes and produces approximately 2500 ml of water and eliminates about 2500 ml of water daily. Thus, a healthy person's average daily water input equals his or her average daily losses.

Various factors influence a person's fluid input and output. Environmental factors such as temperature, humidity, and altitude can affect body water losses. Physiological conditions, especially fever, vomiting, and diarrhea, as well as life—style practices, such as exercise habits and sodium and alcohol intakes, can also alter the body's fluid balance.

Perspiration is body water that is secreted by sweat glands in skin. When perspiration reaches the skin's surface, it evaporates into the air. This process helps cool the body and maintain its normal temperature. *Insensible perspi—ration* is body water that diffuses through the layers of skin or is exhaled from the lungs instead of being secreted by sweat glands.[4] People are usually unaware that their bodies are constantly losing water in this manner; hence, the term *insensible* perspiration.

Kidneys and Hydration

The kidneys are the major regulator of the body's water content and ion concen—trations. In a healthy person, the kidneys maintain proper hydration by filtering excess ions and water from blood as it flows through the kidney's tissues. Water is the main component of urine. If you drink more watery fluids than your body needs, your kidneys excrete the excess water in urine.

Kidneys also remove drugs and metabolic waste products, such as urea, from the bloodstream. Sometimes, minerals and waste products settle out of urine and collect into crystals. If the crystals enlarge and form a hard mass, the object is called a kidney stone (Fig. 9.6). Kidney stones often contain the mineral calcium.[5] As a kidney stone moves out of the kidney and enters the tube leading to the bladder, it may cause considerable pain and bloody urine until it passes out of the body. Dehydration increases the likelihood of forming kidney stones.

What Is a Diuretic? Caffeine is a **diuretic,** a substance that increases urine production. Coffee, tea, energy drinks, and soft drinks often contain caffeine or caffeine—related compounds. However, the water consumed in caffeinated bever—ages is not completely lost in urine, so drinking these fluids may still contribute to meeting your water needs.[3]

Did *YOU* Know?

Have you ever noticed that your weight increases by a few pounds after you have eaten a lot of salty foods and then consumed beverages? The weight gain is due to a temporary increase in body water volume. If you resume eating foods that supply your usual intake of sodium, your kidneys will eliminate the excess sodium and water in urine within a day. As your body regains its normal fluid balance, your weight also returns to normal.

©Stockbyte/Getty Images RF

diuretic substance that increases urine production

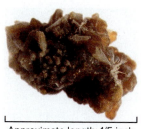

Approximate length: 1/5 inch

Figure 9.6 Kidney stones. Some people form kidney stones. Although small enough to fit on a fingertip, such stones can be quite painful when they move from the kidneys to the bladder and are eliminated in urine.
©Jonathan Kirn/Getty Images

Figure 9.7 Effects of antidiuretic hormone and adolsterone on kidneys. In response to dehydration, the posterior pituitary gland in the brain secretes antidiuretic hormone (ADH), which signals the kidneys to conserve water. Additionally, the adrenal glands secrete the hormone aldosterone. Aldosterone reduces urinary excretion of sodium. When the kidneys retain sodium, they return the mineral to the general circulation. As an result of the actions of these two hormones, body water and sodium are conserved.

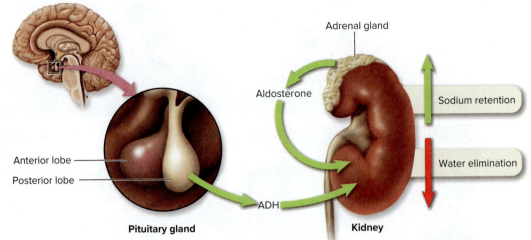

Adrenal gland

Aldosterone

Sodium retention

Water elimination

Anterior lobe
Posterior lobe

ADH

Pituitary gland

Kidney

antidiuretic hormone (ADH) hormone that participates in water conservation

aldosterone hormone that participates in sodium and water conservation

Water Conservation

As mentioned in the opener of this chapter, body water depletion is called dehy—dration. Dehydration can be a life—threatening condition. When you are hot and perspiring heavily, your kidneys try to conserve as much water as possible to avoid dehydration. **Antidiuretic hormone (ADH)** and **aldosterone** (*al—dahs'—te—rown*) are two hormones that participate in the body's efforts to maintain fluid balance. In response to dehydration, the posterior pituitary gland in the brain releases antidiuretic hormone. Antidiuretic hormone stimulates the kidneys to con—serve water. Additionally, the adrenal glands secrete aldosterone. Aldosterone signals kidneys to reduce the elimination of sodium in urine, and as a result, the kidneys return the mineral and water to the general circulation. The diagram in Figure 9.7 summarizes the effects of antidiuretic hormone and aldosterone on the kidneys.

The simplest way to determine if you are consuming enough water is to notice the amount of urine you eliminate. When your fluid intake is adequate, your kidneys will produce enough urine to maintain fluid balance. If you con—sume more fluid than needed, your kidneys will eliminate the excess, and you will produce plenty of urine. On the other hand, if you limit your fluid intake or have high fluid losses such as in sweat, you will produce small amounts of urine.

In addition to urine volume, the color of urine may be a useful indicator of hydration status. Straw—colored (light yellow) urine can indicate adequate hydration, whereas dark—colored urine may be a sign of dehydration. However, the color of urine is not always a reliable guide for judging a person's hydra—tion status.[6] It is important to recognize that having urinary tract infections or ingesting certain medications, foods, and dietary supplements, especially those containing the B—vitamin riboflavin, can alter urine's color.

Alcohol is a diuretic. Normally, antidiuretic hormone signals the kidneys to conserve water (see Figure 9.7). Alcohol, however, inhibits ADH secretion from the pituitary gland in the brain, enabling the kidneys to eliminate more urine than nor—mal. Alcohol consumption actually results in urinary water losses that are greater than the volume of fluid consumed. Therefore, alcohol contributes to dehydration.

Scientists do not know what causes a hangover, the headache, tiredness, thirst, and overall discomfort that occurs a few hours after drinking too much alcohol. Dehydration, the body's immune response, and *congeners* may be responsible for the unpleasant, delayed side effects of excess alcohol consump—tion.[7] Congeners are substances in alcoholic drinks that contribute to the taste and color of the beverages. (Beer and vodka have lower congener contents than red wine and whiskey.) Alcoholic drinks with high congener contents tend to pro—duce more severe hangovers than drinks with lower contents of these substances.

Dehydration

Despite the body's mechanisms to balance its water content, some fluid is constantly being lost, primarily via the skin and lungs. If a person does not consume enough fluids to replace that water, dehydration can occur. Rapid weight loss is a sign of dehydration. Every 16 ounces (about 0.5 L) of water that the body loses represents a pound of body weight. If you lose 1 to 2% of your usual body weight in fluids, you will feel fatigued and thirsty. If you weigh 150 pounds, for example, and your weight drops 3 pounds after exercising in hot conditions, you have lost 2% of your body weight, primarily as water weight.

As the loss of body water approaches 4% of body weight, muscles lose considerable amounts of strength and endurance. By the time body weight is reduced by 7 to 10% as a result of body fluid losses, severe weakness results. At a 20% reduction of body weight, coma and death are likely.

Thirst is the primary regulator of fluid intake.[4] The thirst response alerts you to the need to replenish water that was lost by sweating and other means. The majority of healthy people meet their AI for water by letting thirst be their guide.[3] Thirst stimulates people to drink fluids *before* severe dehydration occurs. However, people who are dehydrated and older than 60 years of age do not sense thirst as accurately as younger adults.[8] Furthermore, older adults may be more susceptible to developing dehydration than younger persons because as kidneys age, they become less able to conserve water when fluid intakes are low. Therefore, it may be necessary to remind older adults to drink more watery fluids, especially when they are physically active or in warm conditions. Nevertheless, healthy elderly persons are generally able to maintain adequate hydration.[8]

People who are sick, especially children with fever, vomiting, diarrhea, and increased perspiration, may need to be given special solutions of water and electrolytes to prevent dehydration. Athletes and other people who work or exercise outdoors, especially in hot conditions, also need to stay properly hydrated to avoid dehydration and heat-related illnesses such as heat exhaustion. Chapter 11 provides information about heat-related illnesses.

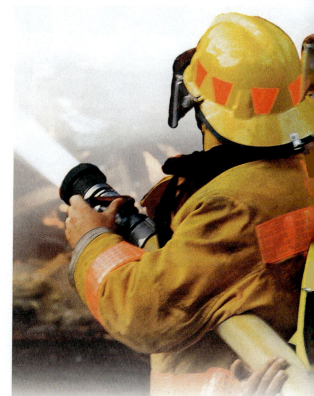

People who work or exercise outdoors, especially in hot conditions, need to stay hydrated to avoid dehydration and heat-related illnesses. ©Comstock/Getty Images RF

Did *YOU* Know?

On October 4, 2016, a powerful hurricane battered the island nation of Haiti. The hurricane devastated the southwestern region of the tiny country and left many Haitians in this area with no access to drinkable water. People can survive for a few days in such conditions before dehydration contributes to their deaths. This photo shows a young Haitian woman receiving bottled water from a U.S. military serviceman during relief efforts.

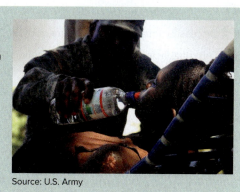

Source: U.S. Army

Can Too Much Water Be Toxic?

There is no Upper Limit (UL) for water. **Water intoxication,** however, can occur when an excessive amount of water is consumed in a short time period or the kidneys have difficulty filtering water from blood. The excess water dilutes the sodium concentration of blood, disrupting water balance. As a result of the imbalance, too much water moves into cells, including brain cells. Signs and symptoms of water intoxication may include drowsiness, nausea and vomiting,

water intoxication condition that occurs when too much water is consumed in a short time period or the kidneys have difficulty filtering water from blood

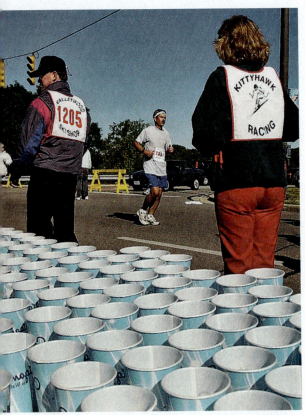

Marathon runners who consume large amounts of plain water in an effort to keep hydrated during competition may be at risk of water intoxication. Source: TSGT Lance Cheung, USAF/DoD Media

confusion, inability to coordinate muscular movements, and weight gain.[9] If the condition is not detected early and treated effectively, coma and death can result.

Healthy people rarely drink enough water to become intoxicated. However, water intoxication can develop in people with disorders that interfere with the kidney's ability to excrete water normally. Marathon runners who consume large amounts of plain water in an effort to keep hydrated during competition may be at risk of water intoxication. Chapter 11 discusses the importance of proper hydration for athletes.

Concept CHECKPOINT

4. List at least five different functions of water in the body.
5. Define *osmosis*.
6. Which ions are found primarily in extracellular water? Which ions are found primarily in intracellular water?
7. Discuss ways the body obtains and loses water.
8. What can happen to cells if the body is unable to regulate its water balance?
9. How do antidiuretic hormone and aldosterone help maintain fluid balance in the body?
10. How much water do healthy young men and women need to consume daily (AI values)?
11. What is a diuretic? Identify two diuretics commonly consumed by Americans.
12. List at least three signs and symptoms of dehydration.
13. List at least three signs and symptoms of water intoxication.

See Appendix G for responses.

9.3 Minerals: Basic Concepts

Learning Outcomes

1. Identify general functions of minerals in the body.
2. Discuss factors that influence the body's ability to absorb and use minerals.
3. Describe factors that can affect retention of minerals during food preparation.

Minerals, such as iron and calcium, are a group of elements in Earth's rocks, soils, and natural water sources. Plants, animals, and other living things cannot synthesize minerals. Plants obtain the minerals they need from soil or fertilizer; animals generally obtain minerals when they consume plants and other animals or substances that contain these elements. About 15 mineral elements have known functions in the body and are necessary for human health.

Several minerals, including lead and mercury, are often found in the human body, but they are environmental contaminants that have no known functions. The body can eliminate most minerals in urine. However, exposure to excessive amounts of minerals can cause toxicity.

Unlike vitamins, minerals are indestructible. Because minerals cannot be destroyed, heating a food or exposing it to most other environmental conditions will not affect the food's mineral content. However, minerals are water soluble, and they can leach out of a food and into cooking water. By using the cooking water to make soups or sauces, you can obtain minerals from the food that would otherwise be discarded.

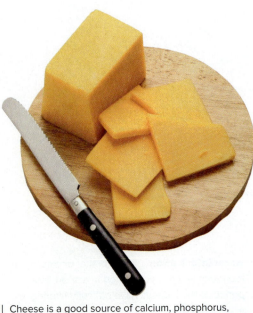

Cheese is a good source of calcium, phosphorus, selenium, zinc, and sodium. ©C Squared Studios/Getty Images RF

Why Are Minerals Necessary?

Essential minerals have diverse roles in the body (Fig. 9.8). Some minerals form inorganic structural components of tissues, such as calcium and phosphorus in bones and teeth. Minerals may also function as inorganic ions, substances that have negative or positive charges (see Chapter 4). For example, calcium ions (Ca^{2+}) participate in blood clotting and sodium ions (Na^+) help maintain fluid balance. Phosphate ions participate in acid–base balance. Some ions, such as magnesium (Mg^{2+}) and copper (Cu^{2+}), are cofactors. A **cofactor** is a metallic ion or small molecule that activates certain chemical reactions. Many minerals are components of various enzymes, hormones, or other organic molecules, such as cobalt in vitamin B–12, iron in hemoglobin, and sulfur in the amino acids methionine and cysteine. Although cells cannot metabolize minerals for energy, certain minerals are involved in chemical reactions that release energy from macronutrients.

In some instances, the digestive tract absorbs more minerals than the body needs, but the excess is excreted, primarily in urine or feces. In other instances, the body stores the extra minerals in the liver, bones, or other tissues. Toxicity signs and symptoms occur when minerals accumulate in the body to such an extent that they interfere with the functioning of cells. Under normal conditions, the human body does not store large quantities of most minerals, and it loses small amounts of these essential elements every day. Therefore, people should choose their diets carefully so their bodies can maintain an adequate supply of minerals.

cofactor metallic ion or small molecule that activates certain chemical reactions

Figure 9.8 Minerals and their functions. Groups of minerals work together to maintain good health.
©Purestock/SuperStock RF

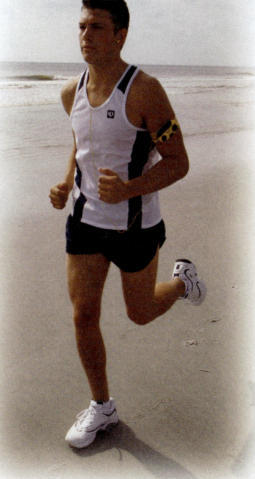

Bone Health

Calcium
Phosphorus
Iron
Zinc
Copper
Manganese
Fluoride
Magnesium

Fluid Balance

Sodium
Potassium
Chloride
Phosphorus
Magnesium

Blood Clotting

Calcium

Transmission of Nerve Impulses

Sodium
Potassium
Chloride
Calcium

Red Blood Cell Formation

Iron
Copper

Muscle Contraction and Relaxation

Sodium
Potassium
Calcium
Magnesium

Cellular Metabolism

Iron
Calcium
Phosphorus
Magnesium
Zinc
Chromium
Iodine
Copper
Manganese

Antioxidant Defense

Selenium
Zinc
Copper
Manganese

Growth and Development

Calcium
Phosphorus
Zinc

Sources of Minerals

Although most foods contain small amounts of minerals, Figure 9.9 indicates food groups from MyPlate that are generally rich sources of various minerals. The digestive tract, however, does not absorb 100% of the minerals in foods or dietary supplements. The body's ability to absorb and use minerals (*bioavailability*) depends on many factors. A major factor is the body's need for the mineral. In general, requirements increase during periods of growth, such as infancy and puberty, and during pregnancy and breastfeeding. During these critical life stages, the bioavailability of minerals also tends to increase to help meet the body's demand.

Compared to plant foods, animal foods tend to be more reliable sources of minerals, such as iron and calcium. Why? Animal products often have higher concentrations of these minerals. Additionally, plant foods can contain substances that reduce the bioavailability of minerals, particularly calcium, zinc, and iron. On the other hand, plants supply more magnesium and manganese than animal foods.

In general, the more processing a plant food undergoes, the lower its natural mineral content. Cereal grains, for example, naturally contain selenium, zinc, copper, and some other minerals, but these micronutrients are lost during refinement. Iron is the only mineral added to grains if they undergo enrichment. To obtain a variety of minerals, include some whole-grain products in your diet each day. By following the recommendations of MyPlate (see Chapter 3) and eating a variety of plant and animal foods, you are likely to obtain adequate amounts of all essential minerals.

Figure 9.9 **MyPlate: Good sources of minerals.**
Each MyPlate food group contributes minerals to the diet. Source: U.S. Dept. of Agriculture

Mango, Kale, and Cereal: ©Stockbyte/Getty Images RF; Milk: ©Ingram Publishing RF; Sardines: ©Caspar Benson/Getty Images RF

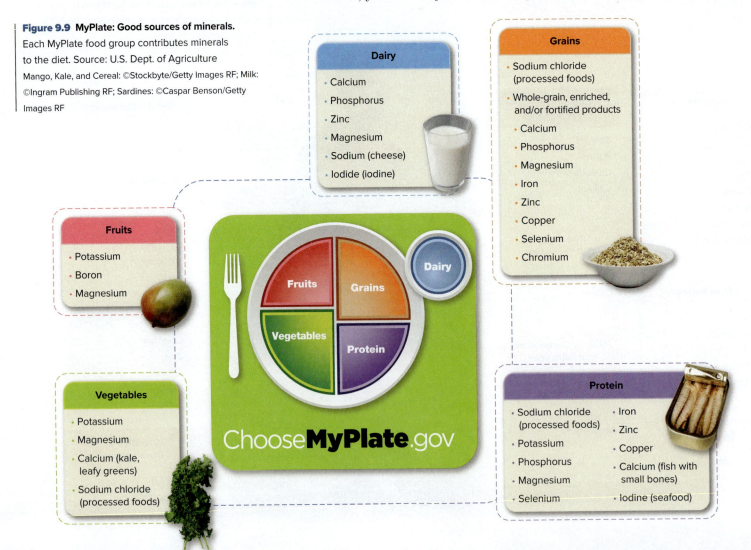

Dairy
- Calcium
- Phosphorus
- Zinc
- Magnesium
- Sodium (cheese)
- Iodide (iodine)

Grains
- Sodium chloride (processed foods)
- Whole-grain, enriched, and/or fortified products
  - Calcium
  - Phosphorus
  - Magnesium
  - Iron
  - Zinc
  - Copper
  - Selenium
  - Chromium

Fruits
- Potassium
- Boron
- Magnesium

Vegetables
- Potassium
- Magnesium
- Calcium (kale, leafy greens)
- Sodium chloride (processed foods)

Protein
- Sodium chloride (processed foods)
- Potassium
- Phosphorus
- Magnesium
- Selenium
- Iron
- Zinc
- Copper
- Calcium (fish with small bones)
- Iodine (seafood)

ChooseMyPlate.gov

Other Sources of Minerals

The tap water in your community may be a source of minerals that you may have overlooked. Fluoride is often added to public water supplies. Although fluoride is not essential for life, the mineral strengthens bones and teeth when consumed in adequate amounts. "Hard" water naturally contains a variety of minerals, including calcium, magnesium, sulfur, iron, and zinc. Water with high mineral content often tastes and smells unpleasant. Many people drink bottled water as a substitute for tap water because they think bottled water tastes better and it is safer. To learn more about bottled water, read the "Nutrition Matters" section at the end of this chapter.

Dietary supplements are another source of minerals. A daily multiple vita-min and mineral supplement is generally safe for healthy people because a dose of this type of supplement does not provide high amounts of minerals. However, people need to be careful when taking dietary supplements that contain indi-vidual minerals, such as iron or selenium. Many minerals have a narrow range of safe intake; therefore, it is easy to consume a toxic amount, especially by taking supplements that contain only a particular mineral (Fig. 9.10). Additionally, an excess of one mineral can interfere with the absorption or metabolism of other minerals. For example, the presence of a large amount of zinc in the intesti-nal tract decreases copper absorption. Single-mineral supplements are usually unnecessary unless they are prescribed to treat a specific medical condition, such as iron deficiency.

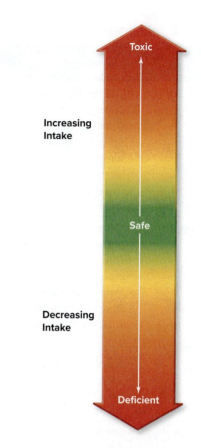

Figure 9.10 Mineral intake. Many minerals have a narrow range of safe intake. As a result, it is relatively easy to consume a toxic amount, especially by taking supplements that only contain a particular mineral.

Concept CHECKPOINT

14. List at least three different functions of minerals in the body, and provide an example of a mineral that performs each function.

15. Explain how foods that are naturally good sources of minerals can become poor sources of those minerals by the time you eat them.

16. Discuss factors that influence mineral absorption in the digestive tract.

17. In the United States, which mineral is added to grain products as part of the grain enrichment program?

See Appendix G for responses.

9.4 Major Minerals

Learning Outcomes

1 List key functions and good food sources of the major mineral nutrients.

2 Discuss deficiency and toxicity disorders associated with the major minerals.

3 Discuss hypertension and osteoporosis, including risk factors.

4 Discuss ways to improve intakes of major minerals without relying on dietary supplements.

This section focuses on the major minerals. Table 9.5 summarizes nutrition-related information about these micronutrients. Unless otherwise noted, RDA/AI values are for adults, excluding pregnant or breastfeeding women. For more information about Dietary Reference Intake values for minerals, see Appendix I.

TABLE 9.5 Summary of Major Minerals

Mineral	Major Functions in the Body	Adult RDA/AI (adult RDA = bold)	Major Dietary Sources	Major Deficiency Signs and Symptoms	Major Toxicity Signs and Symptoms
Calcium (Ca)	• Structural component of bones and teeth • Blood clotting • Transmission of nerve impulses • Muscle contraction • Regulation of metabolism	**1000–1200** mg	Milk and milk products, canned fish, tofu made with calcium sulfate, leafy vegetables, calcium-fortified foods such as orange juice	• Increased risk of osteoporosis • May increase risk of hypertension	UL = 2.0 to 2.5 g/day • Intakes > 2.5 g/day may cause kidney stones and interfere with absorption of other minerals.
Sodium (Na)	• Maintenance of proper fluid balance • Transmission of nerve impulses • Muscle contraction • Transport of certain substances into cells	1500 mg (19–50 years of age)	Luncheon meats; processed and canned foods; pretzels, chips, and other snack foods; condiments; sauces; table salt	• Muscle cramps	UL = 2300 mg/day • Contributes to hypertension in susceptible individuals • Increases urinary calcium losses
Potassium (K)	• Maintenance of proper fluid balance • Transmission of nerve impulses	4700 mg	Fruits, vegetables, milk, meat, legumes, whole grains	• Irregular heartbeat • Muscle cramps	No UL has been determined. • Slowing of heart rate that can result in death
Magnesium (Mg)	• Strengthens bone • Cofactor for certain enzymes • Heart and nerve functioning	Men: **400–420 mg** Women: **310–320 mg**	Wheat bran, green vegetables, nuts, chocolate, legumes	• Muscle weakness and pain • Poor heart function	UL = 350 mg/day (medication-related) • Diarrhea
Phosphorus (P)	• Structural component of bones and teeth • Maintenance of acid-base balance • Component of DNA, phospholipids, and other organic compounds	**700 mg**	Dairy products, processed foods, soft drinks, fish, baked goods, meat	• None reported	UL = 4 g/day • Poor bone mineralization
Chloride (Cl⁻)	• Maintenance of proper fluid balance • Production of stomach acid • Maintenance of acid-base balance	2300 mg (19–50 years of age)	Processed foods, salty snacks, table salt	• Convulsions (observed in infants)	UL = 3600 mg/day • Hypertension (because of the association with sodium in sodium chloride [table salt])
Sulfur (S)	• Component of organic compounds such as certain amino acids and vitamins	None	Protein-rich foods	• None reported	• Unlikely from dietary sources

Calcium (Ca)

Calcium is the most plentiful mineral element in the human body. All cells need calcium, but more than 99% of the body's calcium is in an inorganic compound that forms the structural component of bones and teeth. The remaining calcium is in muscle tissue and extracellular fluid.

Why Is Calcium Necessary?

Although the body needs calcium to form bones and teeth, the mineral is vital to all cells. Calcium is involved in muscle contraction, blood clot formation, nerve impulse transmission, and cell metabolism. Additionally, calcium may play important roles in maintaining healthy blood pressure and functioning of the immune system.

Maintaining Normal Blood Calcium Levels The body has complex hormonal systems to maintain calcium homeostasis. The thyroid and parathyroid glands help regulate blood calcium levels (Fig. 9.11). In response to falling blood calcium levels, the parathyroid glands secrete **parathyroid hormone (PTH),** which signals special bone cells called **osteoclasts** to tear down bone tissue. This process releases calcium from bones so the mineral can enter the bloodstream. PTH also works with vitamin D to increase intestinal calcium absorption and reduce calcium excretion in urine (see Fig. 8.13).

When the level of calcium in blood is too high, the thyroid gland secretes the hormone **calcitonin** (*cal'–sih–toe'–nin*). Calcitonin signals another type of bone cell **(osteoblasts)** to remove excess calcium from blood and build bone tissue. All these physiological responses help maintain your blood calcium level within the normal range.

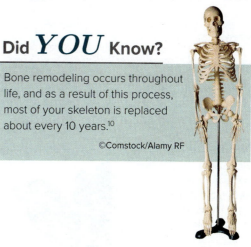

parathyroid hormone (PTH) hormone secreted by parathyroid glands when blood calcium levels are too low

osteoclasts bone cells that tear down bone tissue

calcitonin hormone secreted by the thyroid gland when blood calcium levels are too high

osteoblasts bone cells that add bone to where the tissue is needed

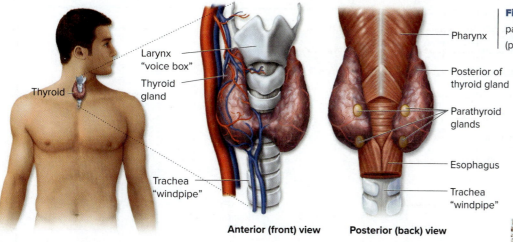

Anterior (front) view   Posterior (back) view

Figure 9.11 Thyroid and parathyroid glands. Four parathyroid glands are imbedded in the back (posterior) of the thyroid.

Bone Development and Maintenance Although your bones do not appear to change shape, they are being remodeled continually in response to the physical stresses placed on them. The remodeling process involves breaking down bone where there is little stress and building bone where there is more stress. For example, if you begin to play tennis regularly and hold the racket in your right hand, osteoblasts in the bones of your right arm build bone tissue where it is needed to help support the muscular activity. As a result, the bones in that arm become denser than the bones in your left arm. Bones that are denser have greater bone mass. As a result, they are stronger and less likely to fracture than less dense bones. Figure 9.12 shows x-rays of bone tissue. By just looking at the photos, can you tell which bone is denser and has greater mass?

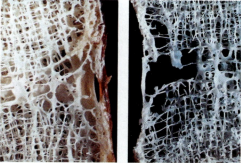

Figure 9.12 Bone tissue. Normal spine tissue is on the left; the spine tissue on the right is from a person with osteoporosis. ©Michael Klein/Photolibrary/Getty Images

MY DIVERSE PLATE

MyPlate: Source: U.S. Dept. of Agriculture

Bok Choy (Pak Choi or Chinese Cabbage)

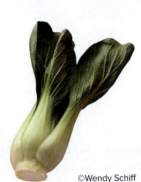

©Wendy Schiff

Bok choy is a cruciferous vegetable that is typically used in Asian cookery. Cruciferous vegetables contain phytochemicals that may have cancer-fighting activity. The leaves and stalks are steamed or sautéed with other vegetables. Bok choy is a good source of minerals, especially iron, calcium, and potassium; the vegetable also contains high amounts of vitamin C.

Sources of Calcium

Table 9.6 includes some foods that are among the richest sources of calcium. Fluid milk, yogurt, and cheese provide most of the calcium in American diets.[5] Moreover, the calcium in milk products is well absorbed and used by the body. Not all products made from milk are rich sources of calcium. Cottage cheese, for example, does not supply as much calcium as the milk from which it is made because the milk loses as much as half of its calcium content when it is processed to make cottage cheese. Although butter, sour cream, and cream cheese are made from whole milk, people generally do not eat enough of these high−fat foods to contribute much calcium to their diets.

Certain foods from plants contain calcium, but the foods also contain *phytic (fi'−tik) acid* or *oxalic (awk−sal'−ik) acid*, naturally occurring substances that interfere with calcium absorption. Phytic acid is a compound in whole grains and in certain seeds and beans. Spinach, collard greens, and sweet potatoes have high amounts of oxalic acid. In fact, rhubarb leaves are toxic because they contain such high amounts of the chemical.

Good plant sources of calcium include broccoli and leafy greens, especially kale, collard, turnip, bok choy, and mustard greens. Nevertheless, the calcium in plant foods is generally not as bioavailable as the calcium in milk and milk products. For example, 1 cup of fat−free milk supplies almost 300 mg of calcium, and about 30% of the calcium in milk is bioavailable.[11] A cup of boiled and drained spinach supplies 116 mg of calcium, but only about 5% of that amount is bioavailable.[11] Figure 9.13 shows approximately how much cooked spinach, broccoli, and kale a person would need to eat to obtain about the same amount of calcium that is in 1 cup of fat−free milk.

TABLE 9.6 Calcium Content of Selected Foods

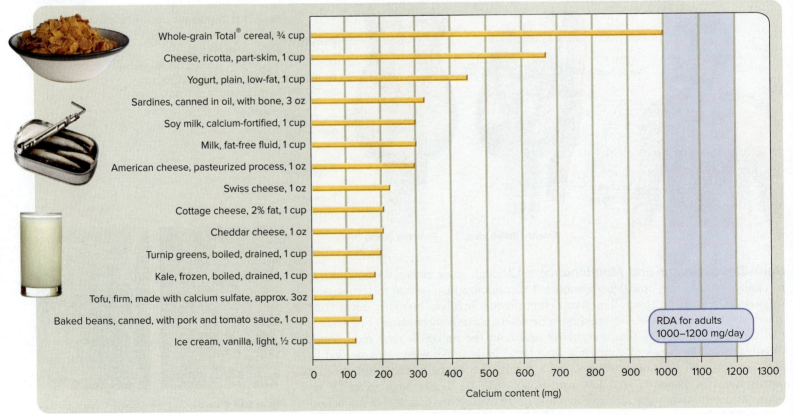

Source: Data from U.S. Department of Agriculture, Agricultural Research Service: *USDA national nutrient database for standard reference,* Release 26, 2013. Bowl of cereal: ©David Toase/Getty Images RF; Sardines: ©Brand X Pictures/Getty Images RF; Milk: ©McGraw-Hill Education/Ken Karp, photographer

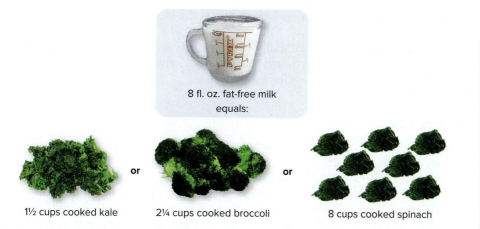

8 fl. oz. fat-free milk equals:

1½ cups cooked kale   or   2¼ cups cooked broccoli   or   8 cups cooked spinach

Figure 9.13 Calcium bioavailability of various foods. To obtain approximately the same amount of calcium that is in 8 fluid ounces of fat-free milk, you would need to consume the amounts of the foods shown.

Measuring glass, Kale, Broccoli, and Spinach: ©Wendy Schiff

Calcium is added to a variety of foods, including fortified orange juice, margarine, soy milk, cereals, and breakfast bars. Another source of calcium is soybean curd (tofu) that is made with calcium sulfate. Figure 9.14 indicates food groups from MyPlate that are good sources of calcium.

Calcium Supplements Many adults find it difficult to consume enough milk products and other calcium–rich foods to achieve adequate intakes of the mineral. Thus, taking calcium supplements or antacids that contain calcium has become a common practice, especially among older adults. If you choose to take a cal–cium supplement, consider products that include vitamin D, because the vitamin

Did *YOU* Know?

Antacids generally contain calcium carbonate, which makes them an inexpensive way of obtaining some calcium. For example, an antacid pill that contains 750 mg of calcium carbonate provides 300 mg of elemental calcium. People, however, should not rely on antacids as a major source of calcium. Long-term ingestion of calcium from antacids may contribute to kidney stones.[5]

A few brands of antacids contain magnesium as well as calcium carbonate. If taken in large doses over a long period, these particular antacids can be toxic.[12] Bone pain is a symptom of toxicity from taking antacids containing calcium carbonate and magnesium. To avoid health problems associated with calcium-containing antacids, consumers should follow dosage recommendations on the labels of the products.

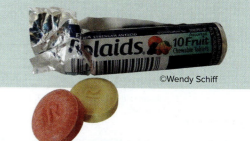

©Wendy Schiff

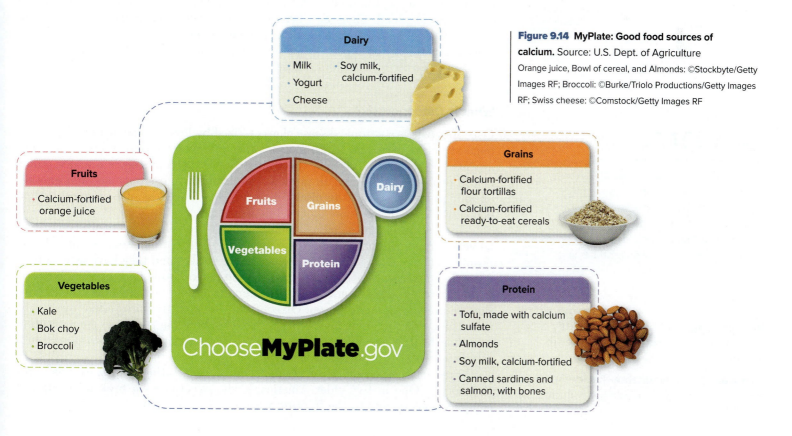

Figure 9.14 MyPlate: Good food sources of calcium. Source: U.S. Dept. of Agriculture

Orange juice, Bowl of cereal, and Almonds: ©Stockbyte/Getty Images RF; Broccoli: ©Burke/Triolo Productions/Getty Images RF; Swiss cheese: ©Comstock/Getty Images RF

Dairy
- Milk
- Yogurt
- Cheese
- Soy milk, calcium-fortified

Fruits
- Calcium-fortified orange juice

Vegetables
- Kale
- Bok choy
- Broccoli

Grains
- Calcium-fortified flour tortillas
- Calcium-fortified ready-to-eat cereals

Protein
- Tofu, made with calcium sulfate
- Almonds
- Soy milk, calcium-fortified
- Canned sardines and salmon, with bones

ChooseMyPlate.gov

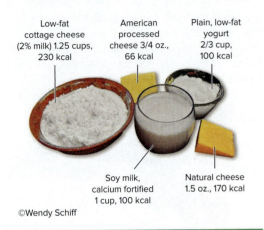
Did *YOU* Know?

Canned fish with edible soft bones, such as sardines and salmon, are good calcium sources. When making salmon patties using canned fish, mash up the bones along with the salmon. The bones are so soft, you won't notice them in the cooked product.

hypercalcemia condition characterized by higher-than-normal concentration of calcium in blood

osteoporosis chronic disease characterized by loss of bone mass and reduced bone structure

enhances calcium absorption. Taking only 500 mg of calcium at a time and ingesting the supplement with meals will also improve the mineral's absorption. Dietary supplements, including calcium supplements, may have a "seal of approval" displayed on the label. As mentioned in Chapter 2, such seals of approval are not a guarantee that products are safe or effective.

Dietary Adequacy

The adult RDA for calcium ranges from 1000 to 1200 mg/day. In the United States, average calcium intakes were 1086 mg/day for men and 852 mg/day for women in 2013–2014.[13] Thus, women tended to consume less than the RDA for calcium. Total vegetarians (vegans) and people who are lactose–intolerant are at risk of calcium deficiency because they often avoid consuming milk and milk products, the most reliable dietary sources of calcium. According to the Dietary Guidelines, calcium is a "nutrient of public health concern" (see Chapter 3).

Healthy adults absorb about 30% of the calcium in foods, but this percentage varies, depending on the type of food.[5] During stages of life when the body needs extra calcium—such as infancy and pregnancy—absorption can be as high as 60%. Vitamin D enhances calcium absorption.

Older people, especially women, do not absorb calcium as well as younger people. Thus, recommendations for calcium intakes are higher for people over 70 years of age than for younger adults. In addition to advanced age, other factors that reduce calcium absorption include vitamin D deficiency and diarrhea.

Calcium Toxicity   The Upper Level (UL) for calcium is 2000 to 2500 mg/day. Normally, the small intestine prevents too much calcium from being absorbed. However, taking too many calcium–containing antacids or supplements, or drinking too much vitamin D–fortified milk can result in excessive calcium absorption and hypercalcemia. **Hypercalcemia** (*hyper* = excess; *calcemia* = calcium in the blood) is a condition characterized by a higher–than–normal concentration of calcium in blood. Signs and symptoms of hypercalcemia include bone pain, muscle weakness, and fatigue, and people with hypercalcemia can develop kidney stones. Treatment for hypercalcemia may include avoiding vitamin D and calcium supplements to reduce calcium absorption.

What Is Osteoporosis?

Osteoporosis is a chronic disease characterized by loss of bone mass and reduced bone structure (see Fig. 9.12). People with osteoporosis have weak bones that are susceptible to fractures. In the United States, osteoporosis is a major public health problem. More than 10 million Americans have osteoporosis, and another 34 million are at risk of the disease because they have loss of bone mass.[5] Most people with osteoporosis are older adult women.

In the United States, half of women and up to one–fourth of men who are over 50 years of age will have an osteoporosis–related fracture at some point.[14] Many people do not realize their bones are becoming weaker and they have osteoporosis until they experience a fracture. People with osteoporosis may break a bone by falling, or they may experience spontaneous fractures in which the fragile bone shatters for no apparent reason. Osteoporosis–related fractures often involve the spine, hip, wrist, or ankle bones. In severe cases, bones in the upper spine fracture and then heal in an abnormally curved position, giving the obvious appearance associated with osteoporosis (Fig. 9.15).

Fractures, especially hip fractures, can be devastating events, especially for the elderly. One in five older Americans who experiences a broken hip dies of complications related to the fracture within 1 year of the injury.[14]

What Causes Osteoporosis? Several factors, including smoking and lack of physical activity, contribute to bone loss and osteoporosis (Table 9.7). Note that some of the factors cannot be modified, but other factors can be changed to prevent or delay the development of the disease.

Around 30 years of age, most healthy young men and women have acquired all of their adult bone mass.[15] Regardless of one's sex, loss of bone tissue begins in mid–adulthood. In men, bone loss is slow and steady beginning around age 30. In women, however, the rate of bone loss increases significantly after *menopause*, that is, after menstrual cycles have ceased. At this time of life, women have the highest risk of osteoporosis. Why? The sex hormones **testosterone** and **estrogen** are needed for normal bone development and maintenance. In women of childbearing age, ovaries are the primary source of estrogen. After menopause, a woman's ovaries no longer produce estrogen, and as a result, her rate of bone loss exceeds the rate of bone replacement. Because estrogen is so important to maintaining strong bones, young adult women should see a physician if they have signs of estrogen deficiency, such as irregular menstrual cycles.

A simple way to monitor bone mass is by tracking height. Losing an inch or more of adult height may be the first sign that a person has experienced fractures of the spine due to osteoporosis.[16] If osteoporosis is suspected, a person can undergo special painless x–ray testing to determine the extent of bone loss. Individuals with a family history of osteoporosis, men who have low testosterone levels, and women who are postmenopausal should ask their physician if testing to determine bone mineral density is necessary. Treatment for osteporosis may include certain medications, calcium and vitamin D supplements, and regular physical activity.

Reducing the Risk of Osteoporosis Efforts to reduce the risk of osteoporosis should begin early in life. Proper diet and regular exercise are especially important from early childhood through late adolescence because the body actively builds bone during these life stages. By following the recommendations of MyPlate, most

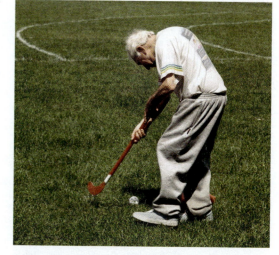

Figure 9.15 Osteoporosis. Severe curvature of the upper spine is a sign of osteoporosis. ©Sally and Richard Greenhill/Alamy

testosterone hormone needed for normal bone development and maintenance

estrogen hormone that plays a role in normal bone development and maintenance

TABLE 9.7 Risk Factors for Osteoporosis

Factors People Cannot Change:
Being a woman
Growing older
Having white or Asian ancestry (confers the highest risk)
Having a family history of osteoporosis
Having a small, thin-boned body frame
Factors People Can Change:
Having low estrogen levels in women, low testosterone levels in men
Having anorexia nervosa
Following long-term diets that contain inadequate amounts of calcium and vitamin D
Being physically inactive
Smoking cigarettes
Consuming excess alcohol

Source: Modified from http://www.niams.nih.gov/Health_Info/Bone/Osteoporosis/overview.asp

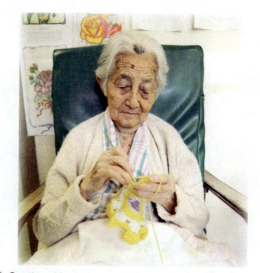

Growing older, being a woman, and having a small, thin-boned body frame are risk factors for osteoporosis that cannot be changed. ©Thinkstock/Getty Images RF

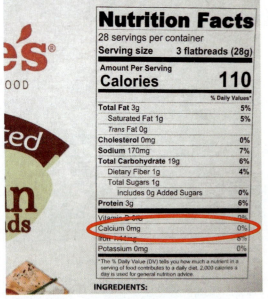

Nutrition Facts

28 servings per container

Serving size   3 flatbreads (28g)

Amount Per Serving	
Calories	**110**

	% Daily Values*
Total Fat 3g	5%
Saturated Fat 1g	5%
Trans Fat 0g	
Cholesterol 0mg	0%
Sodium 170mg	7%
Total Carbohydrate 19g	6%
Dietary Fiber 1g	4%
Total Sugars 1g	
Includes 0g Added Sugars	0%
Protein 3g	6%
Vitamin D 0g	0%
Calcium 0mg	0%
Iron 1.4mg	8%
Potassium 0mg	0%

* The % Daily Value (DV) tells you how much a nutrient in a serving of food contributes to a daily diet. 2,000 calories a day is used for general nutrition advice.

INGREDIENTS:

The Nutrition Facts panel indicates the %DV of calcium in a serving of the food. ©Wendy Schiff

Food & Nutrition tips

The following suggestions can add more calcium to your diet:

- Read the Nutrition Facts panel on food packages and choose foods with high calcium contents whenever possible

- Sprinkle grated low-fat cheeses on top of salads, bean or pasta dishes, and cooked vegetables.

- For a snack, melt a slice of low-fat cheese on half a whole-wheat bagel, whole-wheat crackers, or a slice of rye bread.

- If a recipe calls for water, substitute fat-free milk for water when appropriate. For example, use fat-free milk when making cooked oatmeal or pancake batter.

- Add ¼ cup nonfat milk powder to 1 pound of raw ground meat when preparing hamburgers, meatballs, or meatloaf.

- Make homemade smoothies by blending plain low-fat yogurt with fresh or frozen fruit and fat-reduced ice cream or sherbet (see "Recipe for Healthy Living" at the end of Chapter 4).

people can obtain adequate amounts of calcium from foods. Exposing skin to sunlight can stimulate the body's ability to form vitamin D, but some people will need to take calcium and vitamin D supplements.

Performing weight−bearing activities increases bone mass because contracting muscles keep tension (physical stress) on bones. Table 9.8 lists examples of weight−bearing and non−weight−bearing activities. Regular physical activity that includes weight−bearing muscular movements provides numerous benefits to health, such as improving balance and reducing the likelihood of falling.

Everyone needs to be concerned about his or her risk of osteoporosis and focus on maximizing bone mass while he or she is young. The interactive osteoporosis risk test at the International Osteoporosis Foundation's website (www.iofbonehealth.org/iof−one−minute−osteoporosis−risk−test) can help you determine whether you or someone you know is at risk for the disease.

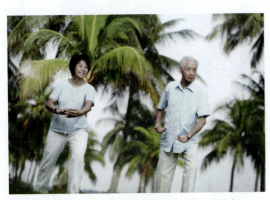

These older adults are performing tai chi, a weight-bearing activity that can improve balance and may reduce the likelihood of falling. ©Floresco Productions/age fotostock RF

TABLE 9.8 Examples of Weight-Bearing and Non-Weight-Bearing Activities

Weight-bearing	Non-weight-bearing
Low-impact aerobics	Lying in bed
Basketball	Swimming
Running or jogging	Water aerobics
Walking or hiking	Cycling
Jumping rope	Traveling in reduced-gravity situations (e.g., space flight)
Dancing	
Stair climbing	
Strength training with weights	
Tennis and other racket sports	

Sodium (Na)

Salt is the primary source of sodium in American diets. The chemical commonly called "table salt" or simply "salt" is actually *sodium chloride*, a compound comprised of two minerals, sodium and chloride. A teaspoon of table salt supplies 2325 mg of sodium. (Unless otherwise noted, we will refer to sodium chloride simply as "salt" or "table salt.") The human digestive tract absorbs almost all of the sodium that is in foods and beverages.

Why Is Sodium Necessary?

As mentioned in the "Water" section of this chapter, sodium plays a major role in maintaining normal fluid balance. The mineral is also necessary for the transmission of impulses by nerves, for transporting small substances such as glucose and amino acids into cells, and for functioning of muscles.

Sources of Sodium

Most uncooked vegetables, raw meats, and grain products are naturally low in sodium. Thus, most of the sodium Americans consume is from foods available from restaurants and the salt that is added to food during processing (including curing, pickling, and canning).[17] As a food additive, salt enhances flavors and can prevent the growth of microorganisms responsible for food spoilage. Other food additives that contain sodium include sodium nitrate, sodium citrate, and *monosodium glutamate (MSG)*, a seasoning that is often added to foods served in Chinese restaurants.

In the United States, the leading sources of dietary sodium include breads and rolls, deli meats, pizza, soups, cheese, salty snacks, and dishes made with meat, such as meatloaf with tomato sauce.[18] Table 9.9 lists some selected foods

TABLE 9.9 Sodium Content of Selected Foods/Food Additives

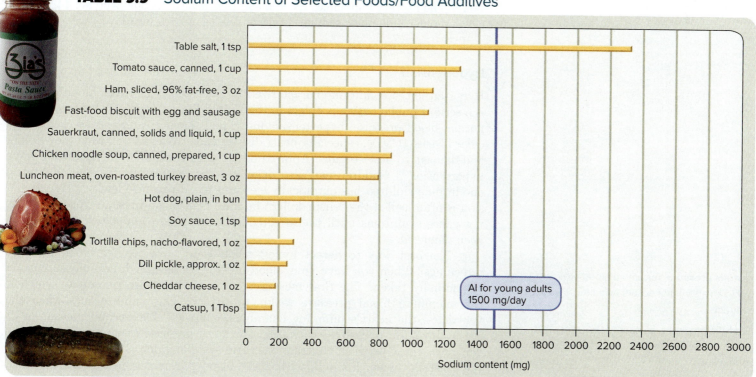

Source: Data from U.S. Department of Agriculture, Agricultural Research Service: *USDA national nutrient database for standard reference,* Release 26, 2013. Pasta sauce: ©Wendy Schiff; Ham and Pickle: ©Brand X Pictures/Getty Images RF

and indicates how much sodium is in a serving of each food. To rate your sodium intake, take the Sodium Intake Assessment that is in this section of the chapter.

Dietary Adequacy

Humans require only about 180 mg of sodium per day, but the AI for adults under 51 years of age is 1500 mg/day. The AI for sodium does not apply for people who perspire heavily, such as marathon runners, or people who work in extremely hot conditions.[3] Sweat contains small amounts of sodium, chloride, and some other minerals. People who perspire extensively can lose large amounts of these minerals in their sweat.

Sodium Deficiency   In the United States, diets generally supply far more sodium than the AI amount, and as a result, an average person is unlikely to become sodium deficient. A healthy body is able to regulate its sodium concentration effectively, but sodium depletion can occur in certain situations. A person who loses more than 2 to 3% of body weight as a result of excessive sweating is at risk of sodium depletion. In most cases, drinking fluids and simply eating some salty foods or adding salt to foods is usually effective for restoring the body's sodium content. However, endurance athletes may need to consume sports drinks during competition to avoid dehydration and sodium depletion. Salt tablets are generally not recommended for sodium replacement. Sodium depletion also can result from diarrhea or vomiting, especially in infants. In these cases, it is necessary to obtain medical care promptly to replace the lost fluids and electrolytes because infants can develop dehydration rapidly.

Sodium Toxicity   The adult UL for sodium is 2300 mg/day. On average, adult Americans consumed almost 3530 mg of sodium per person per day in 2013–2014.[13] High salt (sodium chloride) intakes are associated with increased risk of hypertension.[17] The Dietary Guidelines recommend that healthy people who are 14 years of age and older limit their sodium intake to less than 2300 mg/day.

Hypertension

Hypertension, a condition characterized by persistently elevated blood pressure, is a serious public health problem in the United States. Compared to people with normal blood pressure, hypertensive individuals have greater risk of cardiovascular disease (CVD), especially heart disease and stroke, as well as kidney failure and damage to other organs. Approximately one-third of adult Americans have hypertension.[19] Children can also develop hypertension. In the United States, one in nine children has chronically elevated blood pressure levels.[17] Hypertension is often called the "silent killer" because high blood pressure generally does not cause symptoms until the affected person's organs and blood vessels have been damaged.

The best way to detect hypertension is to have regular blood pressure screenings. When you have your blood pressure determined, two measurements are actually taken. The first measurement is the **systolic pressure,** which is the maximum blood pressure within an artery. This value occurs when the ventricles, the heart's pumping chambers, contract. The second measurement is the **diastolic pressure,** which measures the pressure in an artery when the ventricles relax between contractions. The systolic value is always higher than the diastolic value. For adults, healthy blood pressure readings are less than 120/80 millimeters of mercury (mm Hg). After having your blood pressure

systolic pressure maximum blood pressure within an artery that occurs when the ventricles contract

diastolic pressure pressure in an artery that occurs when the ventricles relax between contractions

Sodium Intake Assessment

For each question, place a check in the column that best describes your sodium intake habits. How often do you . . .	Rarely	Occasionally	Often	Daily
1. Eat cured or processed meats ("deli" meats), such as bacon, sausage, or hot dogs?				
2. Eat canned or frozen vegetables with sauce?				
3. Eat commercially prepared meals, main dishes, or canned or dehydrated soups?				
4. Eat processed cheeses, such as cheese spreads?				
5. Eat salted nuts, popcorn, pretzels, corn chips, or potato chips?				
6. Add salt to cooking water for vegetables, rice, or pasta?				
7. Add salt, seasoning mixes, salad dressings, or condiments—such as soy sauce, steak sauce, pickles, and catsup—to foods during preparation or at the table?				
8. Salt your food before tasting it?				
9. Ignore reading the Nutrition Facts panel for sodium content when buying foods?				
10. Choose menu items that are salty or with sauces when dining out?				

Scoring: The more checks you put in the "often" or "daily" columns, the higher your dietary sodium intake is.

Source: Adapted from USDA, *Home and Garden Bulletin*, No. 232–6, April 1986.

measured, ask the clinician for your systolic and diastolic readings and keep a record of the values.

A person who is under physical or emotional stress can expect his or her blood pressure to rise temporarily. However, persistent systolic blood pressure readings of 120 mm Hg to 139 mm Hg and diastolic readings of 80 mm Hg to 89 mm Hg are signs of **prehypertension.** People with prehypertension are more likely to develop hypertension than people with normal blood pressure. If a person's blood pressure persists at systolic values that are greater than or equal to ($\geq$) 140 mm Hg and diastolic values that are $\geq$ 90 mm Hg, he or she has hypertension. Table 9.10 presents categories for blood pressure levels in adults.

What Causes Hypertension?   Most cases of hypertension do not have simple causes, but advanced age, African–American ancestry, obesity, physical

Did *YOU* Know?

Some homeowners install water-softening machines because "hard water" interferes with the cleansing ability of soap and laundry detergent. Water softeners usually replace calcium and magnesium ions with sodium ions. Therefore, drinking softened water or using the treated water for preparing foods is not recommended because of its high sodium content.

TABLE 9.10   Categories for Blood Pressure Levels in Adults (Ages 18 Years and Older)

Category*	Blood Pressure Level (mm Hg)		
	Systolic		Diastolic
Normal	< 120 and		< 80
Prehypertension	120 to 139	**OR**	80 to 89
Hypertension	$\geq$ 140	**OR**	$\geq$ 90

*When systolic and diastolic blood pressures fall into different categories, the higher category should be used to classify blood pressure level. For example, a person with a blood pressure of 160/80 mm Hg would be classified as having hypertension. In people who are older than 50 years, elevated systolic values are a more significant risk factor for heart disease and stroke than elevated diastolic readings.

Source: Adapted from National Institutes of Health, National Heart, Lung, and Blood Institute, *Description of high blood pressure.* http://www.nhlbi.nih.gov/health/health-topics/topics/hbp Accessed: June 14, 2017.

prehypertension persistent systolic blood pressure readings of 120 mm Hg to 139 mm Hg and diastolic readings of 80 mm Hg to 89 mm Hg

TABLE 9.11 Major Risk Factors for Hypertension

Family history
Advanced age
African-American ancestry
Obesity
Physical inactivity
Consuming excess sodium
Cigarette smoking
Consuming excess alcohol
Type 2 diabetes

inactivity, smoking cigarettes, and excess alcohol and sodium intakes are among the major risk factors for the condition (Table 9.11). Blood pressure usually increases as a person ages, probably in part because plaque builds up in arteries (atherosclerosis) and interferes with the normal functioning of the blood vessels. Healthy arteries are flexible tubes that expand with each heartbeat and recoil in between beats. Atherosclerotic arteries are less flexible and cannot expand as much as healthy arteries. As a result, the heart must work harder to pump blood through the stiff arteries, and blood pressure becomes chronically elevated.

Obesity, a condition characterized by excessive amounts of body fat, is a major risk factor for hypertension. Physical inactivity is another leading risk factor related to hypertension. Obesity and physical inactivity are modifiable risk factors. By exercising and losing some excess fat, obese people who have hypertension may experience reductions in their blood pressure.

Excessive alcohol intake increases the risk of hypertension. To reduce their chances of developing high blood pressure, people should avoid alcohol or limit their consumption to two or fewer drinks/day (men) and only one drink/day (women and older adults). Other important risk factors for hypertension include having diabetes and using tobacco.

As mentioned earlier, a high-sodium diet is associated with increased risk of hypertension.[17] Many medical researchers think some people are genetically "sodium sensitive." A person who is sodium sensitive is more likely to develop hypertension as a result of consuming a high-sodium diet than an individual who lacks this sensitivity.

As mentioned earlier, the Dietary Guidelines recommend consuming less than 2300 mg of sodium daily. One teaspoon of salt contains about 2300 mg of sodium. Members of high-risk populations, particularly people with prehypertension, may need to limit their sodium intake to 1500 mg per day. People who are being treated for hypertension should check with their physician for advice concerning an acceptable sodium intake.

If you want to lower your sodium intake, try gradually reducing your use of salt and consumption of processed foods. By doing so, you will eventually become accustomed to the taste of less salty food. To replace salt as a seasoning,

Nutrition Facts

28 servings per container

Serving size 3 flatbreads (28g)

Amount Per Serving

Calories 110

	% Daily Values*
Total Fat 3g	5%
Saturated Fat 1g	5%
Trans Fat 0g	
Cholesterol 0mg	0%
Sodium 170mg	7%
Total Carbohydrate 19g	6%
Dietary Fiber 1g	4%
Total Sugars 1g	
Includes 0g Added Sugars	0%
Protein 3g	6%
Vitamin D 0mcg	0%
Calcium 0mg	0%
Iron 1.44mg	8%
Potassium 0mg	0%

*The % Daily Value (DV) tells you how much a nutrient in a serving of food contributes to a daily diet. 2,000 calories a day is used for general nutrition advice.

INGREDIENTS:

A serving of these flatbreads provides 7% of the Daily Value for sodium, which is 2300 mg. ©Wendy Schiff

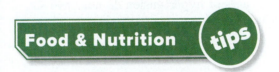

Food & Nutrition tips

To reduce your sodium intake, consider taking these actions:

- Read the Nutrition Facts panels before purchasing packaged foods to determine sodium contents of the items.

- Prepare homemade meals and snacks as much as possible so you have control over your salt intake.

- Do not add salt while preparing foods, even though instructions tell you to "add salt."

- Taste your food *before* salting it. Adjust to eating foods with less salt in them.

- Do not keep a salt shaker on your table.

- When ordering items in restaurants, request that no salt be added to your food while it is being prepared.

try using garlic, citrus juice, and herbs and spices to enhance the taste of foods. Furthermore, avoid buying seasonings with added salt, such as "garlic salt" or "onion salt," and check the ingredient list to purchase seasonings without added salt (garlic *powder* or onion *powder*) instead.

Information about a packaged food's sodium content is a mandatory component of the Nutrition Facts panel. If you take the time to read labels, you can find foods that have little or no salt added to them during processing. For example, an ounce of salted peanuts provides 230 mg of sodium; the same amount of unsalted peanuts has only 2 mg of sodium. The "Food & Nutrition Tip" feature in this section of the chapter provides some suggestions for reducing your salt (sodium) intake.

Even if your blood pressure is normal now, it is important to have regular blood pressure checks as you grow older because the risk of hypertension increases with age. Young adults, however, are not immune to hypertension. Justin Steinbruegge, the college student featured in "Real People, Real Stories" in this section, was 18 when he found out he had hypertension. When was the last time you had your blood pressure measured? What were the systolic and diastolic values?

Treatment for hypertension usually includes taking certain medications, following dietary modifications, and making some other lifestyle changes (Table 9.12). The *Dietary Approaches to Stop Hypertension (DASH)* diet is low in sodium, total fat, and saturated fat, and high in fruits, vegetables, whole grains, and fat−free or low−fat dairy products. Research indicates that people can lower their blood pressure and reduce their risk of CVD by following the DASH diet, losing excess body fat, and increasing their physical activity level.[20] To obtain more information about this diet and some low−sodium recipes, visit the National Heart, Lung, and Blood Institute's website: http://www.nhlbi.nih.gov/health /health−topics/topics/dash.

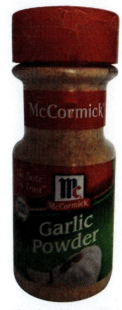

Buy seasonings that do not have added salt.
©Wendy Schiff

TABLE 9.12 Practical Steps to Reduce Your Risk of Hypertension

- Follow the dietary recommendations of MyPlate concerning fruit, vegetable, and low-fat milk intakes. Furthermore, consider using fresh fruit and nuts to replace some empty calories in your daily meals and snacks. (See Chapter 3 for more information about empty calories.)

- Reduce your consumption of salty foods and have your blood pressure checked regularly.

- Attain and maintain a healthy body weight.

- Incorporate more physical activity into your daily schedule. For example, walk more often and use steps instead of elevators or escalators.

- If you drink alcohol, consume alcoholic beverages in moderation—no more than two drinks/day for men and one drink/day for women and older adults.

- Avoid using tobacco products.

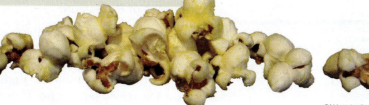

©Wendy Schiff

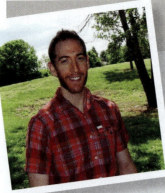
©Wendy Schiff

Justin Steinbruegge

In the spring of his senior year of high school, Justin Steinbruegge was surprised to learn that he had hypertension. "It was a huge shock. I had no signs or symptoms of hypertension. I didn't even know what hypertension was," says Justin. To manage his high blood pressure, he took medication prescribed by his physician, but he had difficulty controlling his sodium intake. "Eating pizzas and salty snacks seemed to keep my blood pressure on a never-ending roller coaster ride," he says.

"When I was 23, I enrolled in a police academy. Four months prior to entering the academy, I started an exercise program. By the time classes began, I thought I was in fantastic shape," says Justin, "but I was training too much, and my diet was horrible—loaded with too many processed foods and not enough fresh fruits, vegetables, and meats. I was ignorant about the importance of proper nutrition to good health."

After finishing at the top of his class at the police academy, Justin focused on improving his health. "I developed a healthy combination of diet and exercise that I continue to follow," he says. "I avoid eating out . . . I eat mainly fresh meats, cheeses, nuts, fruits, and vegetables. I drink only water—no juice, soda, or alcohol. I work out 6 days a week, and I include lifting free weights, rowing, light running, and yoga in my exercise routine. My journey to achieving good health has become a rewarding experience. Now, I don't need to take blood pressure medicine."

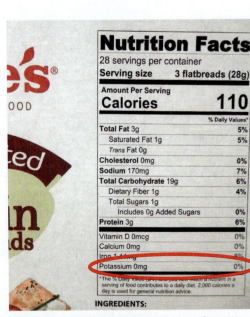
The new Nutrition Facts panel provides information about the food's potassium content. ©Wendy Schiff

Potassium (K)

Potassium is the primary positively charged ion in the intracellular fluid. In fact, most of the body's potassium is in cells. Like sodium, potassium plays a key role in maintaining proper fluid balance. Unlike sodium, potassium is associated with lower, rather than higher, blood pressure values. Potassium is also necessary for transmitting nerve impulses, contracting muscles, and maintaining normal kidney function. Potassium-rich diets, such as the DASH diet, may lower blood pressure.[17] A natural way to counteract high sodium intakes is to consume foods naturally rich in potassium and low in sodium, such as fruits.

Sources of Potassium

Overall, fresh fruits, fruit juice, and vegetables are good dietary sources of potassium. Milk, whole grains, dried beans, and meats are also major contributors of potassium to American diets. Table 9.13 lists foods that are among the richest sources of this mineral. Figure 9.16 indicates food groups that are naturally good sources of potassium. Consumers can read the new Nutrition Facts on food packages to obtain information about products' potassium content. The original Nutrition Facts panel may not include this information.

Dietary Adequacy

The adult AI for potassium is 4700 mg per day. On average, adult Americans consume only about 2660 mg of potassium per day.[13] Because Americans tend to consume less than the AI amount of potassium, the mineral is a "nutrient of public health concern." People can raise their potassium intakes by following the DASH diet.

The body is unable to conserve potassium as well as sodium; therefore, the risk of potassium deficiency is greater than that of sodium deficiency. Individu— als suffering from excessive sweating, vomiting, diarrhea, or kidney diseases that increase potassium excretion are at risk for potassium depletion. Symptoms of the condition generally include loss of appetite, muscle cramps, confusion, and constipation.

Although there is no UL for potassium, taking potassium supplements can upset the GI tract. Moreover, if a person's kidneys are not able to eliminate the excess potassium, the mineral accumulates in the blood and can cause the heart to stop beating. To avoid toxicity, do not take potassium supplements unless you are under a physician's care.

Did *YOU* Know?

Salt substitutes often contain a type of salt called potassium chloride. People who have severe kidney diseases may accumulate toxic levels of potassium in their blood. Therefore, kidney disease patients should consult their physicians before using salt substitutes made with potassium chloride. Fruits and vegetables are recommended sources of potassium instead of potassium chloride.

TABLE 9.13 Potassium Content of Selected Foods

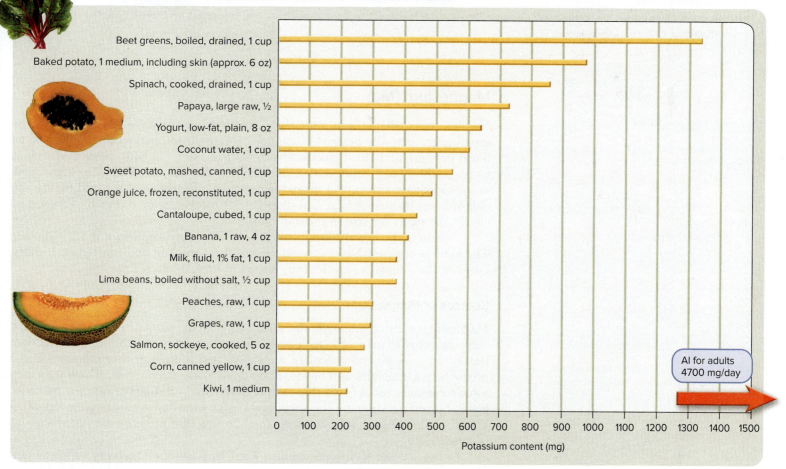

Source: Data from U.S. Department of Agriculture, Agricultural Research Service: *USDA national nutrient database for standard reference,* Release 26, 2013. Beet greens: ©Wendy Schiff; Papaya: ©Brand X Pictures/Getty Images RF; Cantaloupe: ©C Squared Studios/Getty Images RF

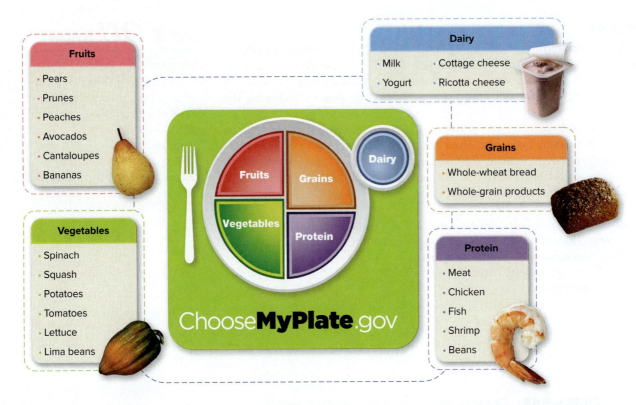

Figure 9.16 MyPlate: Good food sources of potassium. Source: U.S. Dept. of Agriculture

Pear: ©Stockbyte/Getty Images RF; Acorn squash: ©Brand X Pictures/Getty Images RF; Yogurt: ©Ingram Publishing/SuperStock RF; Bread: ©Polka Dot Images/Getty Images RF; Shrimp: ©Comstock/Getty Images RF

Magnesium (Mg)

Magnesium participates in more than 300 chemical reactions in the body.[21] The essential mineral also helps regulate normal muscle and nerve function as well as blood pressure and blood glucose levels. Additionally, the body needs magnesium to maintain strong bones and a healthy immune system. Following diets that supply adequate amounts of magnesium may enhance bone health and reduce the risk of heart disease, stroke, and diabetes.[21] However, more research is needed to clarify the mineral's role in these diseases.

Normally, people absorb about 30 to 40% of the magnesium in their diets.[21] The kidneys regulate blood concentrations of magnesium and can reduce urinary losses of the mineral when the body's level of magnesium is low.

Sources of Magnesium

Magnesium is in chlorophyll, the green pigment in plants. Therefore, it is not surprising that plant foods, such as spinach, green leafy vegetables, whole grains, beans, nuts, seeds, and chocolate are the richest sources of magnesium. Animal products, such as milk and meats, also supply some magnesium. Table 9.14 lists some commonly eaten foods that supply magnesium. Refined grains are generally low in magnesium because the magnesium-rich bran and germ are removed during processing. Figure 9.17 indicates food groups that are naturally good sources of magnesium.

Other sources of magnesium are "hard" tap water and dietary supplements. However, amounts of magnesium in tap water can vary considerably. Moreover, the body does not absorb the form of magnesium (magnesium oxide) in multivitamin/mineral supplements very well. Nevertheless, hard water and magnesium supplements can still contribute to meeting a person's magnesium needs.

Dietary Adequacy

Adult RDAs for magnesium range from 310 to 420 mg/day. Many people in the United States do not consume recommended amounts of magnesium.[13] Despite this, cases of magnesium deficiency rarely occur among healthy members of the population.[21] Nevertheless, alcoholics, people with poorly controlled diabetes, or persons who use certain medications (diuretics) that increase urinary excretion of magnesium have high risk of magnesium deficiency. Older adults are also at risk of magnesium deficiency because their bodies absorb less of the mineral and urinary losses increase with advancing age.

In humans, mild magnesium deficiency can cause tiredness, weakness, loss of appetite, nausea, and vomiting. Signs and symptoms of severe magnesium deficiency often include abnormal heartbeat rhythm, inability to relax muscles, personality changes, and seizures. Chronic magnesium deficiency may increase the risk of osteoporosis because the deficiency lowers the level of calcium in blood.

Magnesium Toxicity Magnesium toxicity rarely occurs from eating too much magnesium-rich food.[21] Toxicity is more likely to occur from ingesting excessive magnesium from laxatives, antacids, or dietary supplements that contain the mineral. Thus, the UL for the micronutrient (350 mg/day) is for magnesium-containing medications and not food sources. A person who consumes too much magnesium often develops diarrhea.

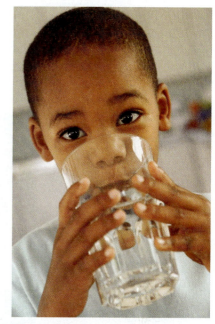

Tap water can be a source of magnesium and other mineral nutrients. ©BananaStock/Getty Images RF

TABLE 9.14 Magnesium Content of Selected Foods

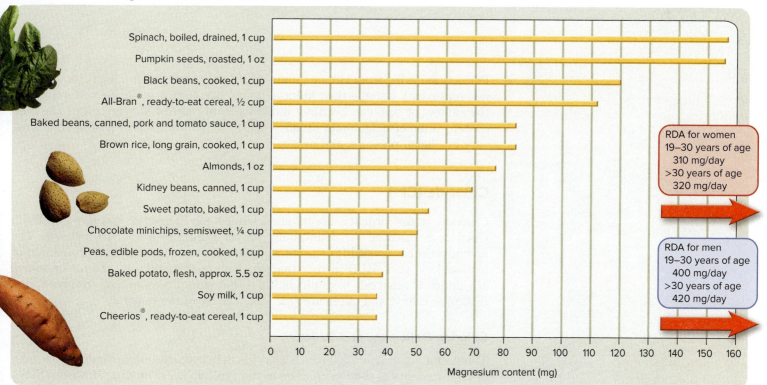

Source: Data from U.S. Department of Agriculture, Agricultural Research Service: *USDA national nutrient database for standard reference*, Release 26, 2013. Spinach: ©Wendy Schiff; Almonds: ©C Squared Studios/Getty Images RF; Sweet potato: ©Stockbyte/Getty Images RF

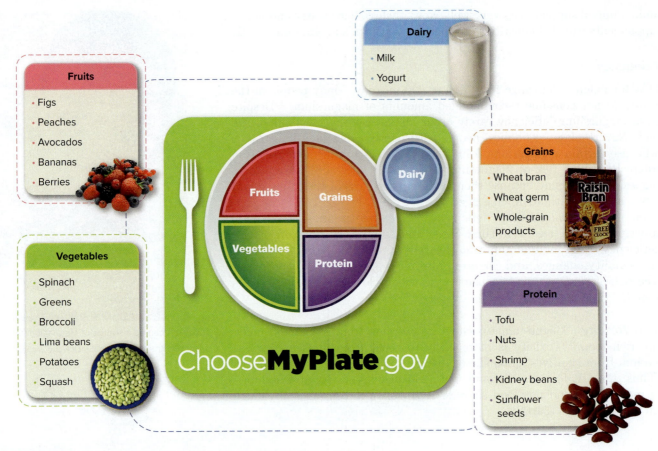

Figure 9.17 MyPlate: Good food sources of magnesium. Source: U.S. Dept. of Agriculture

Berries: ©David Cook/blueshiftstudios/Alamy RF; Lima beans: ©Brand Z Food/Alamy RF; Milk: ©Ingram Publishing RF; Cereal box: ©McGraw-Hill Education/Jill Braaten, photographer; Kidney beans; ©Wendy Schiff

Patients suffering from kidney failure and elderly persons have high risk of mag–nesium toxicity because their kidneys do not excrete the mineral as effectively as the kidneys of younger, healthier individuals. In cases of kidney failure, the high concentration of magnesium in blood causes weakness, nausea, slowed breathing, very low blood pressure, and death.

Chloride (Cl⁻)

Chloride is the primary negatively–charged ion found in extracellular fluid. Chloride is essential for maintaining proper fluid and acid–base balance. The micronutrient is needed for the transmission of nerve impulses and production of hydrochloric acid (HCl) in the stomach. For most Americans, the major source of chloride is table salt (sodium chloride) that is in processed food. Seaweed, rye, tomatoes, celery, and olives are rich food sources of the mineral.

Chloride Deficiency and Toxicity

The AI for chloride is 2300 mg. A chloride deficiency disorder is unlikely because of high amounts of sodium chloride in the typical American diet. However, defi–ciencies may be seen in cases of extreme vomiting, diarrhea, and/or sweating, as well as with diuretic use. Fatigue and loss of appetite are common symptoms of chloride deficiency.

The UL for chloride is 3600 mg/day. Elevated blood chloride levels may result from excessive sodium chloride intake. As in cases of excess sodium ingestion, consuming too much chloride can contribute to hypertension.

Sulfur (S)

Sulfur is a component of several organic compounds, including the amino acids methionine and cysteine, and the vitamins biotin and thiamin. Sulfur is essential for the activity of many enzymes and as part of antioxidant molecules. Protein–rich foods are among the best food sources of sulfur. Some foods and beverages, including many wines, are also sources of sulfur (*sulfites*). In the United States, cases of sulfur deficiency are rare but can occur in people who have severe protein deficiency. Sulfur toxicity is unlikely from dietary sources. Thus, there is no AI, RDA, or UL established for sulfur.

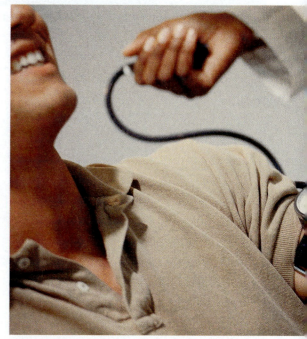
Consuming too much chloride can contribute to hypertension. ©Stockbyte/Getty Images RF

Concept CHECKPOINT

18. What is osteoporosis, and why is it a major public health concern in the United States?
19. Identify at least four major risk factors for osteoporosis. Which risk factors can be modified to reduce the risk of osteoporosis?
20. What is prehypertension? What is hypertension? What are major risk factors for hypertension?
21. What is the DASH diet? Aside from making dietary modifications, what other lifestyle changes can people with hypertension make to lower their blood pressure?
22. Prepare a table for the major minerals that includes information about each mineral's major roles in the body, primary food sources, and signs and symptoms of the mineral's deficiency as well as toxicity disorders. Check your table against the information provided in Table 9.5.

See Appendix G for responses.

9.5 Trace Minerals

Learning Outcomes

1 List key functions and good food sources of trace minerals.

2 Discuss deficiency and toxicity disorders associated with the trace minerals.

Although the body requires trace minerals in very small amounts, obtaining adequate amounts of these important nutrients can be difficult. Iron, for example, is one of Earth's most plentiful metals, but the total amount of iron in the human body is quite small, averaging only about 0.006% of a person's body weight.[4] Table 9.15 summarizes nutrition–related information about iron and other trace minerals. Unless otherwise noted, RDA/AI values are for adults, excluding pregnant or breastfeeding women.

TABLE 9.15   Summary of Trace Minerals

Mineral	Major Functions in the Body	Adult RDA/AI (adult RDA = bold)	Major Dietary Sources	Major Deficiency Signs and Symptoms	Major Toxicity Signs and Symptoms
Iron (Fe)	• Component of hemoglobin and myoglobin that carries oxygen • Energy generation • Immune system function	Women: **18 mg** Men: **8 mg**	Meat and other animal foods, except milk; whole-grain and enriched breads and cereals; fortified cereals	• Fatigue upon exertion • Small, pale red blood cells • Low hemoglobin levels • Poor immune system function • Growth and developmental retardation in infants	UL = 45 mg/day • Intestinal upset • Organ damage • Death
Zinc (Zn)	• Component of numerous enzymes	Women: **8 mg** Men: **11 mg**	Seafood, meat, whole grains	• Skin rash • Diarrhea • Depressed sense of taste and smell • Hair loss • Poor growth and physical development	UL = 40 mg/day • Intestinal upset • Depressed immune system function • Supplement use can reduce copper absorption.
Copper (Cu)	• Promotes iron metabolism • Component of antioxidant enzymes • Component of enzymes involved in connective tissue synthesis	**0.9 mg**	Liver, cocoa, legumes, whole grains, shellfish	• Anemia • Reduced immune system function • Poor growth and development	UL = 10 mg/day • Vomiting • Abnormal nervous system function • Liver damage
Selenium (Se)	• Component of an antioxidant system	**55 mcg**	Meat, eggs, fish, seafood, whole grains	• Muscle pain and weakness • Form of heart disease	UL = 400 mcg/day • Nausea • Vomiting • Hair loss • Weakness • Liver damage
Iodine (I)	• Component of thyroid hormones	**150 mcg**	Iodized salt, saltwater fish, dairy products	• Goiter • Cretinism (intellectual impairment and poor growth in infants of women who were iodine deficient during pregnancy)	UL = 1100 mcg/day • Reduced thyroid gland function
Fluoride (F⁻)	• Increases resistance of tooth enamel to cavity formation • Stimulates bone formation	Women: **3 mg** Men: **4 mg**	Fluoridated water, tea, seaweed	• No true deficiency, but increased risk of tooth decay	UL = 10 mg/day • Stomach upset • Staining of teeth during development • Bone deterioration
Chromium (Cr)	• Enhances insulin action	Women: **20–25 mcg** Men: **30–35 mcg**	Egg yolks, whole grains, pork, nuts, mushrooms	• Blood glucose level remains elevated after meals.	• Unknown but currently under scientific investigation • May interact with certain medications
Manganese (Mn)	• Cofactor for certain enzymes, including some involved in carbohydrate metabolism	Women: **1.8 mg** Men: **2.3 mg**	Nuts, oats, beans, tea	• None in humans	UL = 11 mg/day • Abnormal nervous system function
Molybdenum (Mo)	• Component of certain coenzymes	**45 mcg**	Liver, peas, beans, cereal products, leafy vegetables, low-fat milk	• None in healthy humans	UL = 2000 mcg/day • Rarely occurs from usual dietary sources • Overdoses of dietary supplements containing molybdenum may cause joint pain; side, lower back, or stomach pain; and swelling of feet or lower legs.

Shrimp and Kidney beans: ©Wendy Schiff; Mushrooms: ©C Squared Studios/Getty Images RF; Spinach: ©Royalty-Free/Corbis RF

Iron (Fe)

Do you think of "iron" when you think of "strength"? Associating iron with strength makes sense because muscular strength and endurance are reduced when the body lacks iron. Iron is a component of hemoglobin and *myoglobin* (*my'−o−glow−bin*). **Hemoglobin** is the iron−containing protein in red blood cells that transports oxygen to tissues and some carbon dioxide away from tissues. Hemo−globin is also responsible for the red color of oxygenated blood. **Myoglobin** is the iron−containing protein in muscle cells that controls oxygen uptake from red blood cells. Oxygen is critical for energy metabolism. Cells also contain iron in **cytochromes** (*sigh'−toe−crowms*), a group of proteins that are necessary for certain chemical reactions involved in the release of energy from macronutrients. If the body does not have enough iron to make hemoglobin, myoglobin, and the cytochromes, cells cannot obtain the energy they need to perform work. Thus, fatigue is a major symptom of iron deficiency. Iron also plays roles in immune system function and brain development.

Sources of Iron

Beef, fish, and poultry ("meat") contain more iron than most plant foods. Some of the iron in meat is present as hemoglobin and myoglobin. These forms of iron are collectively referred to as **heme iron.** The remaining iron in meat, as well as all the iron in vegetables, grains, and supplements, is **nonheme iron.**

The intestinal tract absorbs more of the heme iron than nonheme iron in foods.[22] Some plant foods, such as spinach, contain nonheme iron, but oxalic acid in spinach binds to the mineral, reducing its absorption. Other naturally occurring compounds that reduce iron absorption include phytic acid in whole grains, tan−nins in tea, and substances that are chemically related to tannins in coffee.

Meat is the major source of iron in the typical American diet. Other impor−tant sources of iron are fortified cereals and products made from enriched flour, such as breads and rolls. Dairy products are poor sources of iron. Figure 9.18 indicates food groups that are good sources of iron. Table 9.16 lists some foods that are among the richest sources of iron.

hemoglobin iron-containing protein in red blood cells that transports oxygen to tissues and some carbon dioxide away from tissues

myoglobin iron-containing protein in muscle cells that controls oxygen uptake from red blood cells

cytochromes group of proteins involved in the release of energy from macronutrients

heme iron form of iron in hemoglobin and myoglobin

nonheme iron form of iron that is primarily in vegetables, grains, meats, and supplements

Figure 9.18 **MyPlate: Good food sources of iron.** Source: U.S. Dept. of Agriculture

Dried apricots: ©Stockbyte/Getty Images RF; Peas: ©Ingram Publishing/SuperStock RF; Oats: ©McGraw-Hill Education/ Jacques Cornell, photographer; Beef: ©Comstock/Getty Images RF

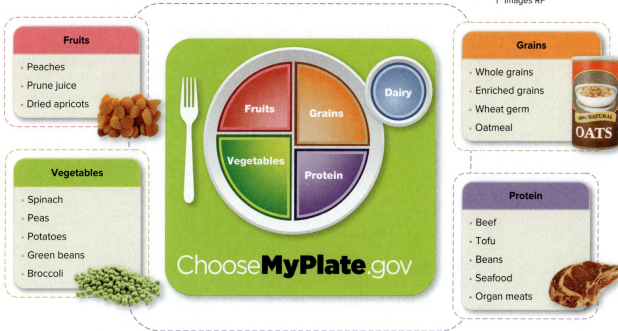

Fruits
- Peaches
- Prune juice
- Dried apricots

Vegetables
- Spinach
- Peas
- Potatoes
- Green beans
- Broccoli

Grains
- Whole grains
- Enriched grains
- Wheat germ
- Oatmeal

Protein
- Beef
- Tofu
- Beans
- Seafood
- Organ meats

ChooseMyPlate.gov

TABLE 9.16 Iron Content of Selected Foods

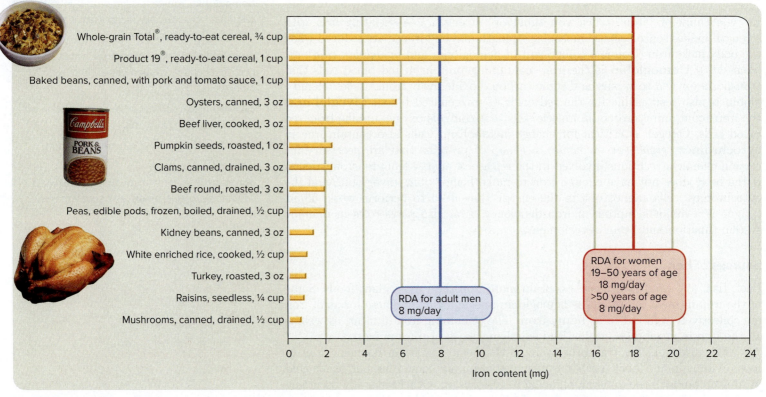

Source: Data from U.S. Department of Agriculture, Agricultural Research Service: *USDA national nutrient database for standard reference,* Release 26, 2013. Cereal: ©Comstock/Getty Images RF; Baked beans: ©Wendy Schiff; Roast poultry: ©Ernie Friedlander/Cole Group/Getty Images RF

Regulating Iron Under normal conditions, the body regulates iron absorption and conservation. The digestive tract absorbs only 5 to 15% of the iron in foods. However, the intestinal tract can absorb more iron when the body's need for the trace mineral increases. Despite iron enrichment, only about 5% of the iron added to grain products is absorbed.[22] The liver, the body's main site for iron storage, incorporates the trace mineral into the protein ferritin (*fer'−ih−tin*) until it is needed.

After red blood cells die, the body breaks them down and conserves most of the iron that was in hemoglobin. By doing so, the body can recycle the trace mineral to make hemoglobin for new red blood cells. Nonetheless, some iron is lost each day via the GI tract, urine, and skin. Any form of bleeding, including menstruation, also contributes to iron losses. Replacing the iron is essential to good health.

Dietary Adequacy

For adult men, the RDA for iron is 8 mg per day; for adult women between 19 and 50 years of age, the RDA for iron is 18 mg/day. The average daily intake for American men is 16.6 mg, whereas the average daily intake for American women is about 12.6 mg/ day.[13] Thus, women between 19 and 50 years of age are more likely than men to have inadequate iron intakes.

iron deficiency condition characterized by low body stores of iron

Iron Deficiency–Related Disorders Low blood iron levels usually result from losing blood, consuming diets that lack iron, or being unable to absorb dietary iron. In cases of **iron deficiency,** the body's iron stores are low but not low enough to result in severe health problems. Nevertheless, iron deficiency can still have widespread negative effects on the body, including interfering with normal growth, behavior, immune system function, cardiac function, and energy metabolism.[23] Furthermore, iron deficiency can lead to iron deficiency anemia.

Anemia occurs when oxygen transport in blood is impaired, generally because there are not enough red blood cells to carry the oxygen or the red blood cells do not contain enough hemoglobin (Fig. 9.19). If oxygen is lacking, cells cannot release considerable amounts of energy from macronutrients, so symptoms of iron deficiency anemia include lack of energy and difficulty concentrating on mental activities. Furthermore, the heart of a person suffering from anemia has to work harder to circulate oxygen–poor blood throughout the body. Over time, anemia can cause rapid or irregular heartbeat, chest pain, an enlarged heart, and even heart failure. Table 9.17 lists common signs and symptoms of iron deficiency anemia.

There are many different kinds of anemia, but iron deficiency anemia is the most common form. According to the World Health Organization, over 30% of the world's population suffers from anemia, and many cases of the condition are due to iron deficiency.[24] In the United States, iron deficiency is the most common nutritional deficiency. An estimated 16 million American children and adolescents have iron deficiency anemia.[25]

Substantial blood loss is a common cause of iron deficiency anemia. Such losses of blood often result from serious intestinal diseases, severe physical injuries, and excessive menstrual bleeding. Diseases that reduce red blood cell formation or increase red blood cell destruction also cause anemia. It is important to note that some types of anemia are the result of genetic defects and not dietary deficiencies. Blood testing can determine which kind of anemia a person has developed, so the condition can be treated properly.

Women of childbearing age generally lose some iron during menstruation. Women with heavy menstrual blood losses are especially prone to iron deficiency anemia. Although pregnant women do not have to contend with menstrual blood losses, they still need to be concerned about their iron intake. According to the Dietary Guidelines, iron is a "nutrient of public health concern" for women who are pregnant or able to become pregnant. The "Food & Nutrition Tips" feature in this section suggests practical ways to increase dietary sources of iron.

Iron deficiency anemia is especially harmful for pregnant women as well as children. During pregnancy, a woman's need for iron increases as her blood supply expands and new tissues are added to both her body and that of her fetus.

TABLE 9.17 Signs and Symptoms of Iron Deficiency Anemia

Pale skin
Fatigue and weakness
Irritability
Difficulty concentrating and thinking
Brittle nails
Headache

Source: U.S. Library of Medicine (Medline), National Institutes of Health, MedlinePlus: *Iron deficiency anemia.* 2016. www.nlm.nih.gov /medlineplus/ency/article/000584.htm Access date: June 14, 2017.

Did *YOU* Know?

Donating 1 pint (approximately 0.5 L) of blood represents a loss of 200 to 250 mg of iron. Even when a person consumes adequate amounts of iron, his or her body generally needs several weeks to replace the iron that was in the donated blood. According to the American Red Cross, healthy people can give whole blood every 56 days.[26] Iron deficiency can result from donating blood too often.[27]

©liquidllibrary/Getty Images RF

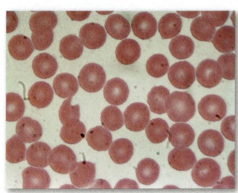
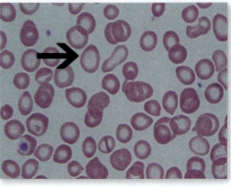

(a)　　　(b)

Figure 9.19 **Iron-deficient red blood cells.** (*a*) Normal red blood cells. (*b*) Iron-deficient red blood cells. Arrow points to one of the deficient cells.
Normal RBCs: ©Dr. R. King/Science Source; Iron deficient RBCs: ©McGraw-Hill Education

Did *YOU* Know?

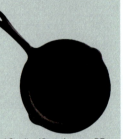

Cooking utensils may be a source of dietary iron. When acidic foods, such as tomato sauce, are cooked in cast-iron cookware, some iron migrates from the cookware and enters the food. Replacing the heavy iron cookware with lighter stainless steel and aluminum pots and pans can reduce the amount of iron in diets.

©C Squared Studios/Getty Images RF

Pregnant women who suffer from iron deficiency anemia have higher risk of dying during pregnancy than healthy pregnant women. Anemic pregnant women are also more likely to give birth to premature or low–birth–weight infants. Premature babies are born before the 37th week of pregnancy; normally, preg–nancies last about 40 weeks from the date of the mother's last menstrual period. A low–birth–weight baby weighs less than 5½ pounds at birth. Compared to healthy newborns, premature or low–birth–weight infants are more likely to die during their first year of life. Iron supplementation can prevent pregnant women from developing iron deficiency and iron deficiency anemia before they give birth.

Because of their rapid growth rates, infants and toddlers have higher needs for iron than older children. Furthermore, iron appears to be necessary for nor–mal nervous system functioning, including brain development. Iron–deficient infants can experience delays in the development of normal motor and mental functions.

Consuming too much milk may play a role in the development of iron deficiency in children. Milk is a poor source of iron. Thus, children who drink excessive amounts of milk may not have the appetite to eat foods that are more reliable iron sources. The calcium that is in milk may interfere with iron absorption when the beverage is consumed with foods that contain the min–eral.[27] To reduce the risk of iron deficiency, children should be encouraged to eat more iron–rich foods, such as meat, products made from soybeans, and iron–fortified cereals.

Total vegetarians have a higher risk of iron deficiency–related disorders than people who eat meat because meat provides heme iron. Combining a small amount of meat with plant foods improves the bioavailability of the plant's nonheme iron. Vegetarians, however, may reject recipes that include any meat, especially red meats. Some plant foods contain high amounts of oxalic acid and phytic acid, substances that can depress iron absorption. On the other hand, vegetarian diets usually are rich in vitamin C, a factor that increases nonheme iron absorption. Thus, vegetarians should consume vitamin C–rich foods along with plant foods, especially those that contain appreciable amounts of iron, such as spinach, lentils, and soybeans. Eating iron–fortified ready–to–eat cereals

Nutrition Facts

28 servings per container

Serving size	3 flatbreads (28g)

Amount Per Serving

Calories	110

	% Daily Values*
Total Fat 3g	5%
Saturated Fat 1g	5%
Trans Fat 0g	
Cholesterol 0mg	0%
Sodium 170mg	7%
Total Carbohydrate 19g	6%
Dietary Fiber 1g	4%
Total Sugars 1g	
Includes 0g Added Sugars	0%
Protein 3g	6%
Vitamin D 0mcg	0%
Calcium 0mg	0%
Iron 1.44mg	8%
Potassium 0mg	0%

*The % Daily Value (DV) tells you how much a nutrient in a serving of food contributes to a daily diet. 2,000 calories a day is used for general nutrition advice.

INGREDIENTS:

The Nutrition Facts panel indicates the %DV of iron in a serving of the food. ©Wendy Schiff

Food & Nutrition tips

The following suggestions can add more iron to your diet:

- Read the Nutrition Facts panel for information about a packaged food's iron content; choose foods with high iron contents whenever possible.
- Eat lean meat, poultry, or fish with plant sources of iron.
- Combine soybeans with tomatoes or tomato sauce.
- Add orange segments or chopped tomatoes to spinach salads or cooked spinach.
- Add chopped onions and green peppers to peas or beans.
- Serve sweet potatoes with fresh orange segments or dried apricots.
- Add raspberries, strawberries, raisins, or dried apricots to cereal.
- Drink orange juice when eating peanut butter or soy nut butter sandwiches.
- Consume watermelon, dried plums, dried apricots, or raisins for snacks.

can also be helpful for vegetarians, even though the form of iron used to fortify cereals is not as well absorbed as heme iron. Finally, vegetarians can take a multivitamin/mineral supplement that contains iron and vitamin C to ensure their iron and other mineral intakes are adequate.

Treatment for iron deficiency anemia generally includes iron supplements and the addition of iron—rich foods to the diet. It is also important to find and treat factors that may be causing the deficiency, such as intestinal bleeding.

Iron Toxicity The UL for iron is 45 mg/day. Although not having enough iron in the body interferes with normal growth, development, and functioning, ingesting too much iron poses the risk of toxicity. Between 1983 and 2000, 43 American children died as a result of accidentally taking too many iron—containing dietary supplements.[27] Early signs of acute iron poisoning include vomiting and diarrhea that may progress to coma and death.

In 1997, the U.S. Food and Drug Administration (FDA) required a warning statement on the packaging of iron supplements to reduce the number of iron poisoning cases among young children. The agency also required unit—dose packaging of oral iron supplements that contained 30 mg of iron or more per dose. The individually wrapped supplements were designed to make it difficult for young children to ingest large quantities of the supplements at a time. After these rules were instituted, only one child died from iron poisoning between 1998 and 2002.[27] In 2003, however, a federal court ruled that the FDA did not have the legal authority to require special unit—dose packaging of iron supplements. The agency, however, could continue to require warning statements on supplement labels.

Iron Overload: Hereditary Hemochromatosis *Iron overload* is a condition characterized by excess iron in the body. Iron overload occurs when toxic amounts of iron supplements are ingested, but the condition also results from certain genetic diseases. **Hereditary hemochromatosis** (*he'—mo—crow'—ma—toe—sis*) is the most common type of iron overload disease.[28] People who have hereditary hemochromatosis (HH) absorb too much iron. The body has no way to eliminate the excess iron, so the mineral accumulates in tissues and can cause joint pain, abnormal bronze skin color, diabetes, and damage to the liver, heart, adrenal glands, and pancreas.

HH most often affects people who have northern European ancestors. In the United States, about 5 of every 1000 non—Hispanic white Americans are susceptible to developing the disease.[28] Men are more likely to be diagnosed with HH than women. Additionally, men tend to develop health problems from the excess iron at a younger age than women with the condition.

Common signs and symptoms of HH include joint pain, fatigue, weight loss, abdominal pain, loss of sex drive, and abnormal skin color (gray or bronze). Even though people with HH begin accumulating iron early in life, they often do not report any signs and symptoms of the disease until they are over 40 years of age. Testing is available to determine the presence of the genes that are responsible for the disease.

Many people who have HH experience vague symptoms or no symptoms at all. If the disease is not detected early and treated effectively, the organ damage resulting from the condition can be deadly. Treatment usually includes visiting a clinic periodically to have blood removed. This process stimulates the tissues that produce red blood cells to use storage iron for hemoglobin production. People with HH should avoid taking dietary supplements that contain iron as well as vitamin C supplements (vitamin C enhances iron absorption).

MY DIVERSE PLATE

MyPlate: Source: U.S. Dept. of Agriculture

Although the kiwano (*Cucumis metuliferusis*) is native to southern Africa, this odd-looking relative of the cucumber is grown in California. The green pulpy seeds can be scooped out of the rind and eaten as a snack or added to salads. Kiwano is a good source of protein (almost 4 g), iron (2.3 mg), and vitamin C (11 mg). The pulp, however, has a slimy texture and not much flavor. In Africa, kiwano is generally considered to be an edible weed that is not eaten unless other foods are unavailable.

Kiwano, whole and kiwano, cut ©Wendy Schiff

hereditary hemochromatosis most common type of iron overload disease

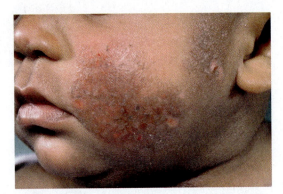

Figure 9.20 **Sign of zinc deficiency in a baby.** Zinc is necessary for healthy skin and normal physical growth. This child has a type of dermatitis that is a sign of zinc deficiency.

©Medical-on-Line/Alamy

Zinc (Zn)

In 1958, physician Ananda Prasad was working in Iran when he examined a 21-year-old man with dwarfism, intellectual disability, iron deficiency anemia, and underdeveloped sexual organs.[29] Prasad noted that the young man ate unleavened ("flat") bread almost exclusively. After examining other patients in Iran and Egypt with similar health problems and dietary practices, Prasad hypothesized that diet was responsible for the condition. Eventually, medical researchers determined that Prasad's patients had severe zinc deficiencies. After these patients were given zinc supplements, they began to grow and develop normally. Prasad later determined that girls also experienced stunted growth and delays in sexual maturation as a result of zinc deficiency.[30]

In the regions where the men who were zinc deficient lived, the typical diet was comprised primarily of unleavened whole-wheat bread and little animal protein. Unleavened whole-wheat bread is naturally high in phytic acid and fiber, substances that decrease zinc bioavailability. In places where people use yeast to leaven (raise) bread dough, severe zinc deficiency is less likely to occur. Yeast reduces the binding effects of phytic acid and fiber, making zinc more bioavailable. Consuming zinc-rich sources of animal protein, such as meat and milk, also reduces the likelihood of zinc deficiency.

Other factors that influence the bioavailability of zinc include the body's need for the mineral and the presence of large amounts of certain other metals. During times when a healthy body needs zinc, the small intestine absorbs more. However, the presence of excess copper or iron in the small intestine interferes with zinc absorption. Thus, iron supplements should be taken between meals instead of with them.

Why Is Zinc Necessary?

Zinc is a component of about a hundred enzymes.[31] Zinc is necessary for wound healing, the sense of taste and smell, DNA synthesis, healthy skin, and proper functioning of the immune system (Fig. 9.20). Zinc is also essential for growth and development during pregnancy, childhood, and adolescence.

Sources of Zinc

Zinc is widespread in foods (Table 9.18). Red meat and poultry products supply most of the zinc in the typical American diet. Figure 9.21 indicates MyPlate food groups that have foods that are good sources of zinc.

Dietary Adequacy

Adult RDAs for zinc range from 8 mg to 11 mg/day. In the United States, the average adult consumes adequate amounts of zinc.[13] Thus, zinc deficiency is not a widespread problem in the United States. However, alcoholics have high risk of zinc deficiency because alcohol reduces zinc absorption and increases excretion of the mineral in urine. Making matters worse, many people who suffer from alcoholism do not consume nutritious diets. Vegetarians need more zinc than people who eat meat because the GI tract does not absorb zinc from plant foods as well as from animal foods.[31] Older adults are at risk of zinc deficiency because they often consume foods that do not provide adequate amounts of the trace mineral.

Although breast milk contains zinc, the milk does not supply enough of the trace mineral for infants who are older than 6 months of age. To increase the likelihood that their diets contain enough zinc, breastfed babies who are between 6 and 12 months of age need to consume foods that contain the trace mineral, such as zinc-fortified infant cereal.

In children and adolescents, zinc deficiency can cause growth retardation and delayed sexual maturation. Adult men who are zinc deficient may experience sexual dysfunction, particularly the inability to attain an erection. Other signs of zinc deficiency include loss of appetite, diarrhea, hair loss, dermatitis, poor wound healing, impaired sense of taste, and mental slowness.[31]

TABLE 9.18 Zinc Content of Selected Foods

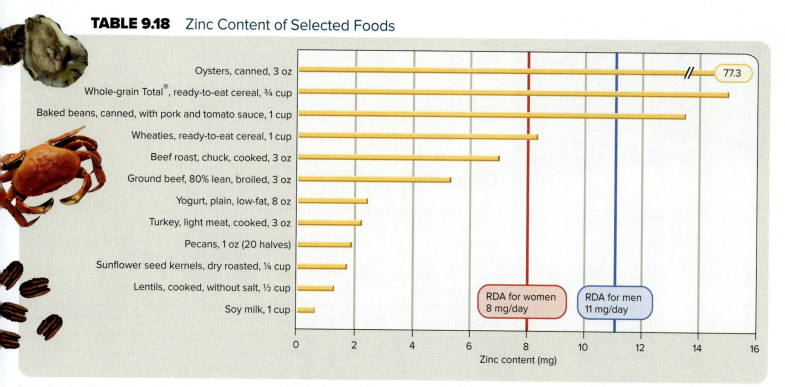

Source: Data from U.S. Department of Agriculture, Agricultural Research Service: *USDA national nutrient database for standard reference, Release 26*, 2013. Oysters: ©Wendy Schiff; Crab, Pecans: ©C Squared Studios/Getty Images RF

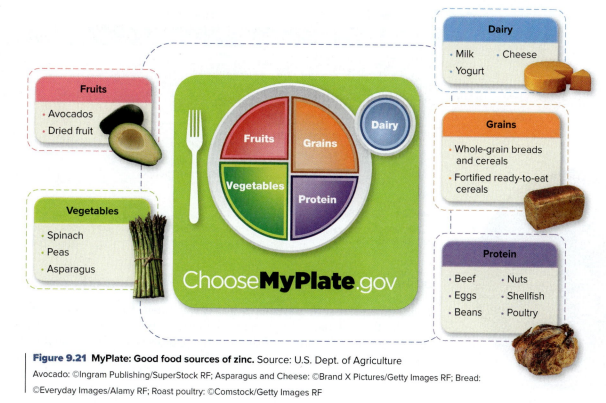

Figure 9.21 MyPlate: Good food sources of zinc. Source: U.S. Dept. of Agriculture

Avocado: ©Ingram Publishing/SuperStock RF; Asparagus and Cheese: ©Brand X Pictures/Getty Images RF; Bread: ©Everyday Images/Alamy RF; Roast poultry: ©Comstock/Getty Images RF

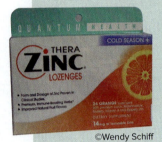
Zinc Toxicity The UL for zinc is 40 mg/day. Zinc intakes that exceed the UL can reduce beneficial HDL cholesterol levels in blood. Ingesting more than 150 mg of zinc per day can also result in diarrhea, cramps, nausea, vomiting, and depressed immune system function.[31] Additionally, megadoses of zinc may interfere with copper absorption. Therefore, people should avoid high intakes of zinc, unless they are under a physician's supervision.

In 2009, the FDA warned the public about using two *intranasal* ("within the nose") forms of a nonprescription, zinc–containing product. The agency had received several reports that the alternative medical treatment for the common cold may result in loss of sense of smell.[31] In response to FDA actions, the manufacturer voluntarily removed the product from the marketplace. Results of studies do not provide consistent evidence that zinc helps reduce the severity or duration of colds, but more research is needed to clarify whether cold products that contain zinc may be beneficial.

Copper (Cu)

The body uses copper to make several enzymes that act as antioxidants. The mineral is also involved in iron metabolism, immune function, and collagen production. A wide variety of foods contain copper, but the foods listed in Table 9.19 are among the richest sources of the micronutrient.

The adult RDA for copper is 0.9 mg/day, and Americans typically consume more than this amount.[13] Consuming high amounts of iron or zinc can interfere with the intestinal tract's ability to absorb copper, so taking these supplements may cause copper deficiency. People with chronic digestive system diseases may also develop copper deficiency because their bodies' ability to absorb the mineral is depressed. A deficiency of copper can lead to anemia, impaired functioning of the immune and nervous systems, abnormal skin pigmentation, and poor growth (children). Copper toxicity rarely occurs.

TABLE 9.19 Copper Content of Selected Foods

Food	mg
Beef liver, 3 oz, cooked	12.40
Crab meat, ½ cup, canned	1.10
Cashews, 1 oz, dry roasted	0.63
Mushrooms, ½ cup, white, cooked, drained	0.40
Soybeans, ½ cup, mature, boiled, drained	0.35
Chocolate, ¼ cup, semisweet	0.30
Baked beans, ½ cup, canned, with pork and tomato sauce	0.27
Sunflower seeds, 1 oz, dry roasted	0.26

RDA adults = 0.9 mg/day

Source: Data from U.S. Department of Agriculture, Agricultural Research Service: *USDA national nutrient database for standard reference*, Release 26, 2013.

Iodine (I)

During World War I, physicians noted that men drafted into the U.S. military from the Great Lakes region were far more likely to have goiter (*goy'–ter*) than men from some other areas of the country. Goiter is an enlargement of the thyroid gland that is not the result of cancer (Fig. 9.22). Goiters often occur among populations living in areas that have iodine–depleted soil. In general, these regions are inland and far from an ocean. If people in these communities limit their diets to locally produced foods, they might not have enough iodine in their diets.

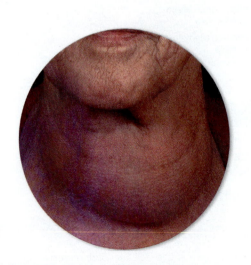

| **Figure 9.22 Goiter.** ©Biophoto Associates/Science Source

Iodine (I₂) is poisonous, but most ingested iodine loses an electron to become the iodide ion (I⁻) in the digestive tract.[22] Iodide is the form of iodine that the body uses. Most of the iodide in an adult's body is located in the thyroid gland. Under normal conditions, the kidneys filter and eliminate excess iodide from blood.

From 1917 to 1922, researchers in Ohio conducted an experiment on a group of girls in which one group of the children received doses of iodine, whereas the other group (the control group) did not receive the trace mineral. The results of the study indicated iodine was nearly 100% effective in preventing goiter in the healthy children. Moreover, the majority of the girls who already had goiters when they received the iodine experienced a reduction in the size of their thyroid glands by the end of the study. In 1924, iodine was added to table salt in the United States, and as a result, cases of goiter caused by iodine deficiency rarely occur in this country. Today, use of iodized salt is the major method of preventing iodine deficiencies in developed nations, but inadequate iodine intake and goiters are still common in central Asia and central Africa.

Why Is Iodine Necessary?

People require iodine for normal thyroid function and for the production of two thyroid hormones, collectively referred to as **thyroid hormone.** Thyroid hormone controls the rate of cell metabolism, that is, the rate at which cells obtain energy. The thyroid gland traps iodide from the bloodstream and accumulates the element for thyroid hormone synthesis. If a person's iodine intake is too low, the pituitary gland in the brain releases a hormone that causes the thyroid gland to enlarge. As a result, the larger thyroid gland tries to remove as much iodide as possible from the bloodstream. It is important to note that an enlarged thyroid gland can also be a sign of some diseases and conditions that are not related to iodine intake.

Sources of Iodine

Major sources of iodine include saltwater fish; seafood; seaweed; some plants, especially the leaves of plants grown near oceans; and iodized salt. A half teaspoon of iodine–fortified salt supplies the adult RDA for iodine. Iodine fortification of salt is voluntary in the United States, so not all salt has the trace mineral added to it. Other dietary sources of iodine include food additives that contain the mineral, such as certain dough conditioners and food dyes. Table 9.20 lists some foods that are good sources of iodine.

Dietary Adequacy

The adult RDA for iodine is 150 mcg/day. Most Americans have adequate iodine intakes.[32] As many Americans, particularly older adults, try to reduce their risk of hypertension by using less salt, iodine intakes may decline to marginal or inadequate levels.

Iodine Deficiency In cases of iodine deficiency, the thyroid gland produces insufficient amounts of thyroid hormone and goiter develops. As a result of the lack of thyroid hormone, iodine–deficient people generally have low metabolic rates and elevated blood cholesterol levels. Other signs and symptoms of iodine deficiency include fatigue, difficulty concentrating on mental tasks, weight gain, intolerance of cold temperatures, constipation, and dry skin.

Throughout the world, millions of people are at risk of iodine deficiency. Pregnant women who are iodine deficient have high risk of stillbirths (giving birth to a dead infant) or low–birth–weight babies. During fetal life, thyroid hormone is crucial for normal brain development. Thus, infants of iodine–deficient women are likely to be born with a condition called **cretinism** (*kre'–tin–ih–zim*). Babies with cretinism have permanent brain damage, reduced intellectual functioning,

Did YOU Know?

Sea salt forms when the water in naturally occurring salt-water evaporates, leaving mineral deposits, including sodium chloride. Table salt is made by processing natural forms of sodium chloride to remove other minerals. In the United States, manufacturers often add iodine to table salt to make "iodized salt." The sea salt that is usually sold in supermarkets is not a good source of iodine because it has not been fortified with the mineral. It is wise to avoid excess sodium from all sources, including sea salt.

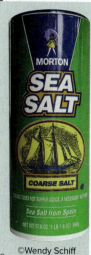
©Wendy Schiff

Did YOU Know?

Raw vegetables, particularly turnips, cabbage, brussels sprouts, cauliflower, and broccoli, contain **goitrogens**. These compounds inhibit iodine metabolism by the thyroid gland and, as a result, reduce thyroid hormone production. Unless people eat large amounts of raw vegetables that contain goitrogens or they are iodine deficient, they do not need to be concerned about eating these foods.[32] Furthermore, cooking vegetables destroys goitrogens.

thyroid hormone hormone that regulates the body's metabolic rate

goitrogens compounds that inhibit iodine metabolism by the thyroid gland

cretinism condition affecting infants of women who were iodine deficient during pregnancy

TABLE 9.20 Iodine Content of Selected Foods

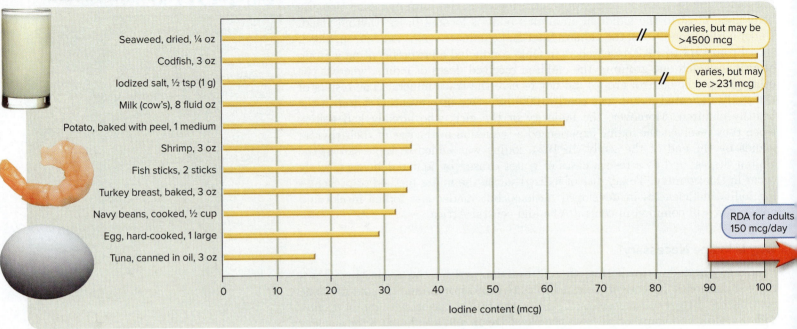

Source: Data from Higdon, J, "Iodine," *Micronutrient Information Center,* Linus Pauling Institute, Oregon State University. 2015. http://lpi.oregonstate.edu/infocenter/minerals/iodine/ Accessed: June 14, 2017. Milk: ©McGraw-Hill Education/Ken Karp, photographer; Shrimp: ©Ingram Publishing/Alamy RF; Egg: ©Siede Preis/Getty Images RF

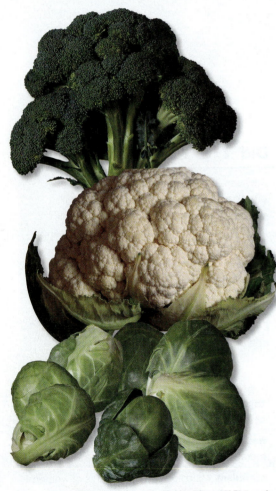

Broccoli, Cauliflower, and Brussels sprouts: ©Brand X Pictures/Getty Images RF

and growth retardation. Worldwide, iodine deficiency is the most common cause of preventable intellectual disability.[32] Pregnant women can reduce the risk of giving birth to infants with cretinism by consuming adequate amounts of iodine throughout pregnancy.

Iodine deficiency is a serious threat to health in places where soils are iodine deficient and commonly eaten foods are not fortified with the trace mineral, such as regions of Latin America, India, Southeast Asia, and Africa. Currently, international health organizations are engaging in efforts to eliminate iodine deficiency, primarily by promoting the use of iodized salt or iodine-fortified vegetable oils.

Iodine Toxicity The UL for iodine is 1.1 mg/day. Over time, consuming very high amounts of iodine can cause thyroid gland enlargement and reduced production of thyroid hormone. These side effects are the same as those that occur when diets are deficient in iodine. Excess iodine is also associated with an increased risk of a form of thyroid cancer.[32]

Nuclear power plant accidents, such as the one that occurred after a major earthquake struck Japan in 2011, may release radioactive iodine (iodine-131) into the environment. When people are exposed to radioactive iodine, the element can enter their bodies and be picked up by their thyroid glands. Exposure to a high amount of the radiation increases the risk of thyroid cancer, especially in children.[32] People who have iodine deficiency are more likely to accumulate the radioactive iodine in their thyroid glands than people who are not iodine deficient. To reduce the risk of thyroid cancer, people who are exposed to radioactive iodine can take supplements that contain 16 to 130 mg of potassium iodide, depending on their age, until the risk of extreme radiation exposure ends.[32] The thyroid gland picks up the potassium iodide, which helps block the thyroid gland's uptake of the radioactive form of the element.

Fluoride (F⁻)

Although fluoride is not an essential nutrient, the mineral strengthens bones and teeth when ingested in small amounts. In the some parts of the United States, well water contains high amounts of the trace mineral. To ensure that people living in other sections of the country obtain healthful amounts of fluoride, the mineral is often added to public water supplies, toothpastes, and dental rinses. Tea naturally contains fluoride.

Long–term consumption of too much fluoride can cause *fluorosis*. In cases of skeletal fluorosis, excess fluoride builds up in bones, causing joint stiffness and bone pain. Skeletal fluorosis rarely occurs in the United States. Dental fluorosis often affects young children who drink well water that contains high amounts of fluoride, but it also can occur in children who routinely swallow toothpaste and dental rinses. Children with severe fluorosis develop permanently stained teeth that do not resist decay as do healthy teeth (Fig. 9.23). Parents should teach their children to place a pea–sized amount of toothpaste on their brush, rinse with water, and spit out the excess fluid.

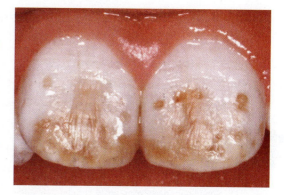

Figure 9.23 **Dental fluorosis.** Source: Centers for Disease Control and Prevention

Selenium (Se)

Selenium is widespread in Earth's crust, but soils can vary widely in their content of the essential trace mineral. Areas of the western United States, including parts of Colorado and South Dakota, have unusually high concentrations of selenium in soil. Certain types of plants that grow in these places accumulate toxic levels of the mineral. Livestock that graze on the selenium–rich plants often ingest poisonous amounts of the trace mineral. In horses and cattle, selenium toxicity can cause hair and weight loss, malformed hooves that can separate from the animals' feet, muscle weakness and loss of muscular function (paralysis), and death.

Why Is Selenium Necessary?

In the body, selenium functions as a component of several proteins referred to as selenoproteins (*sell'–in–oh–pro'–teens*). Many selenoproteins are antioxidants. Other selenoproteins are necessary for the normal functioning of the immune system and thyroid gland.

Sources of Selenium

Although the selenium content of foods varies, nuts, whole–grain products, seafood, and meats are generally rich sources of the trace mineral (Table 9.21). Because Brazil nuts can have very high selenium contents, people should not eat these nuts regularly.

Dietary Adequacy

Most Americans' diets meet the RDA for selenium. In the United States, selenium deficiency is uncommon, but the condition may occur in people who have serious digestive tract conditions that interfere with the mineral's absorption. Selenium deficiency reduces thyroid gland activity and can lead to goiter. The deficiency also depresses immune system function and may contribute to the development of heart disease and cancer. In parts of China where the soil lacks selenium and the population consumes locally produced foods, diets typically contain inadequate amounts of selenium. Certain types of cancer and a form of heart disease are common in these areas of China. There is not enough scientific evidence, however, to support the use of selenium supplements to prevent or treat cancer or CVD.[33]

Brazil nuts have high selenium contents. ©Wendy Schiff

TABLE 9.21 Selenium Content of Selected Foods

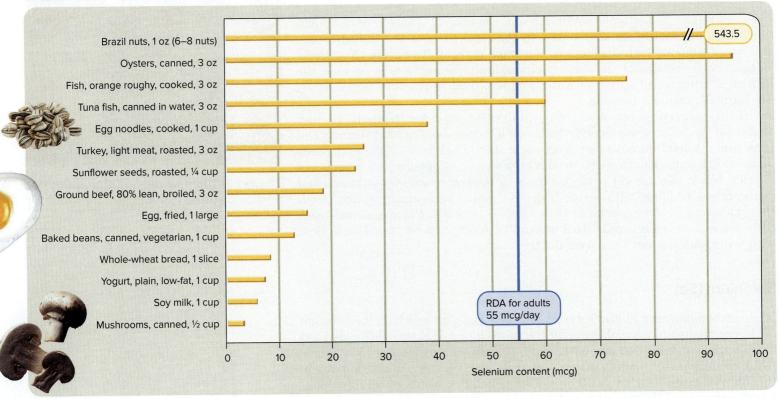

Food	Selenium content (mcg)
Brazil nuts, 1 oz (6–8 nuts)	543.5
Oysters, canned, 3 oz	~95
Fish, orange roughy, cooked, 3 oz	~75
Tuna fish, canned in water, 3 oz	~60
Egg noodles, cooked, 1 cup	~38
Turkey, light meat, roasted, 3 oz	~26
Sunflower seeds, roasted, ¼ cup	~24
Ground beef, 80% lean, broiled, 3 oz	~18
Egg, fried, 1 large	~15
Baked beans, canned, vegetarian, 1 cup	~12
Whole-wheat bread, 1 slice	~8
Yogurt, plain, low-fat, 1 cup	~7
Soy milk, 1 cup	~6
Mushrooms, canned, ½ cup	~3

RDA for adults 55 mcg/day

Source: Data from U.S. Department of Agriculture, Agricultural Research Service: *USDA national nutrient database for standard reference*, Release 26, 2013. Sunflower seeds: ©McGraw-Hill Education/ Jacques Cornell, photographer; Fried egg: ©Brand X Pictures/Getty Images RF; Mushrooms: ©C Squared Studios/Getty Images RF

Selenium Toxicity The UL for selenium is 400 mcg/day. In the United States, selenium toxicity (selenosis) (*sell′−in−o′−sis*) is rare. Chronic selenosis, however, can occur from drinking well water that naturally contains too much selenium. Selenium toxicity can develop by taking megadoses of dietary supplements. In humans, signs and symptoms of chronic selenosis include brittle fingernails, loss of hair and nails, garlicky body odor, nausea, vomiting, and fatigue.

Chromium (Cr)

The importance of chromium as an essential trace mineral in human diets has been recognized only for about the past 40 years. The results of scientific stud−ies suggest that chromium plays an important role in maintaining proper car−bohydrate and lipid metabolism. The concentration of chromium in the body is generally low, because the digestive tract absorbs only about 0.4 to 2.5% of the chromium in foods; the remainder is excreted in the feces.[34] Vitamin C and the B−vitamin niacin enhance the intestinal tract's ability to absorb chromium.

Why Is Chromium Necessary?

Most cells require the hormone insulin to obtain glucose from the bloodstream. Chromium may enhance insulin's action on cell membranes and, in a way, help to "hold the door open" for glucose's entry into the cells. Can people who have diabetes experience better blood glucose regulation by taking chromium supple−ments? A review of scientific research indicated mixed results when people took chromium supplements to improve their blood glucose levels. In some of the studies, chromium supplements were helpful for people with diabetes, but the results of other studies indicated no such benefits.

Whole grains are good sources of chromium.
©Nancy R. Cohen/Getty Images RF

Sources of Chromium

Although chromium is widely distributed in foods, most foods contain less than 2 mcg of the mineral per serving.[34] Information regarding the chromium content of various foods is difficult to find because most reliable food composition tables do not include this trace mineral. In general, meat, whole–grain products, yeast, fruits, and vegetables are good sources of chromium. Like selenium, the amount of chromium in plant foods reflects the chromium content of soils where crops are grown.

Dietary Adequacy

The adult AIs for chromium are 25 mcg/day for young women and 35 mcg/day for young men. Well–balanced diets typically contain these amounts of chromium. On average, American adults consume diets that meet or exceed their AIs for chromium.[34]

Chromium Deficiency Signs of chromium deficiency are impaired glucose tolerance and elevated blood cholesterol and triglyceride levels. The mechanism by which chromium influences cholesterol metabolism is not known but may involve enzymes that control the body's cholesterol production. Cases of chromium deficiency have been reported in people maintained on special–formula diets that did not contain chromium, as well as in severely malnourished children.

Chromium Toxicity The form of chromium that is naturally in foods has not been shown to produce toxicity, so no UL has been set for the trace mineral. The long–term safety of taking various chromium supplements is unknown.[34] Therefore, taking supplemental chromium may be risky.

Manganese (Mn)

Manganese is an important component and activator of many enzymes in the body. These manganese–dependent enzymes play a role in wound healing, metabolism, bone and cartilage formation, and antioxidant function.[35] Some experts suspect that the trace mineral may play a role in preventing osteoporosis, diabetes, and epilepsy. Food sources of manganese include leafy vegetables, whole grains, nuts, and tea. Small amounts of manganese are in natural sources of water.

Manganese deficiency rarely occurs in humans. Results of animal studies indicate that manganese deficiency interferes with reproduction, impairs growth, alters carbohydrate and lipid metabolism, and causes skeletal abnormalities.[35] Although a small amount of manganese is essential, too much is highly toxic. Overconsumption of manganese, which can occur from drinking water that is contaminated with the mineral, causes a nervous system disorder that is similar to Parkinson's disease. Cases of manganese toxicity from food consumption have not been reported.[35]

Molybdenum (Mo)

Molybdenum is a cofactor that is needed for the functioning of four enzymes:

- Aldehyde oxidase
- Mitochondrial amidoxime
- Sulfite oxidase
- Xanthine oxidase

Legumes, grains, and nuts are excellent sources of molybdenum. There have been no reports of molybdenum deficiency in healthy persons, and excesses of the trace mineral generally have low toxicity.[36]

Concept CHECKPOINT

23. What are the signs and symptoms of iron deficiency anemia? Which members of the population are most at risk of iron deficiency?

24. Identify at least three signs or symptoms of hemochromatosis. How is the condition treated?

25. What is a goiter? What is cretinism? How can cretinism be prevented?

26. Prepare a table for trace minerals that includes information about each trace mineral's major role or roles in the body, food sources, and signs and symptoms of the mineral's deficiency as well as toxicity disorders. Check your table against the information provided in Table 9.15.

See Appendix G for responses.

Did YOU Know?

Arsenic is naturally in water, soil, and air. Plants, especially rice, take up arsenic from the environment and store the metal. Inorganic arsenic is quite toxic, and rice is a leading source of inorganic arsenic in diets.[37] The FDA tests foods, including rice, for arsenic. In 2016, the agency proposed a limit for the amount of inorganic arsenic that is allowed in infant cereals that contain rice.

9.6 Minerals with Possible Physiological Roles

Learning Outcome

1 Discuss the six minerals, including arsenic, that may have roles in the body.

A few minerals, including nickel, arsenic, and silicon, are found in small amounts in the body, but their roles in the body are unclear (Table 9.22). At present, this group of minerals is not classified as essential nutrients. Although there are reports of severe illness and deaths resulting from environmental exposure to high amounts of these minerals, foods generally do not contain toxic amounts of them. Rice, however, can contain high levels of arsenic.

TABLE 9.22 Summary of Six Possible Essential Minerals

Mineral	Possible Functions	Suggested Daily Human Intakes	Dietary Sources
Arsenic (As)	Methionine metabolism, growth, and reproduction (animal studies)	No UL has been established; however, inorganic arsenic is highly toxic. Long-term exposure to arsenic may contribute to heart disease and certain cancers.	Fish, rice, fruits, vegetables
Boron (B)	Steroid hormone metabolism	1–13 mg (UL: 20 mg/day)	Fruit, leafy vegetables, peanuts, beans, wine
Lithium (Li)	Reproduction; maintenance of appropriate mood	1000 mcg (No UL has been established)	Water supply, grains, vegetables
Nickel (Ni)	Amino acid and fatty acid metabolism	25–35 mcg (UL: 1 mg/day)	Chocolate, nuts, beans, whole grains
Silicon (Si)	Connective tissue, including bone formation	25–30 mg (Insufficient data to determine UL)	Root vegetables, whole grains
Vanadium (V)	Glucose metabolism; tooth and bone mineralization	10 mcg (UL: 1.8 mg/day)	Shellfish, mushrooms, black pepper, parsley, dill

Sources: Data from Food and Nutrition Board, Institute of Medicine: *Dietary Reference Intakes for Vitamin A, Vitamin K, Arsenic, Boron, Chromium, Copper, Iodine, Iron, Manganese, Molybdenum, Nickel, Silicon, Vanadium, and Zinc* and *Standing Committee on the Scientific Evaluation of Dietary Reference Intakes*, National Academy Press, 2006; Schrauzer GN: Lithium: Occurrence, dietary intakes, nutritional essentiality. *Journal of the American College of Nutrition* 21(1):14, 2002.

Concept CHECKPOINT

27. Identify at least four minerals that are classified as possible essential minerals.

28. Prepare a table for arsenic, boron, lithium, nickel, silicon, and vanadium that includes information about each mineral's possible function and major food sources. Check your table against the information provided in Table 9.22.

See Appendix G for responses.

9.7 Nutrition Matters: Bottled Water Versus Tap Water

Learning Outcomes

1 Explain the roles of the FDA and EPA in regulating water safety in the United States.

2 Discuss the pros and cons of drinking bottled water.

3 Discuss the significance of the Safe Drinking Water Act.

4 Explain health risks associated with BPA.

Today, preparing for a class often involves bringing into the classroom a notebook, something to write with, and a bottle of cold water. Even many college instructors keep a bottle of water nearby as they lecture. Not long ago, most Americans got their water from a faucet ("tap water"). Now, millions of Americans are turning away from the tap and choosing to drink bottled water instead. If you prefer drinking bottled water over tap water, you are part of a growing trend. According to the International Bottled Water Association,

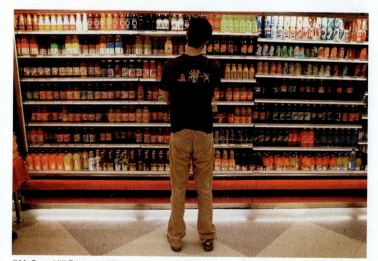

©McGraw-Hill Education/Gary He, photographer

Blueberries: ©PhotoAlto/Getty Images RF

each American consumed, on average, about 36.5 gallons of bottled water in 2015.[38]

Why do so many Americans drink bottled water when tap water is much less costly? Among adults, taste, convenience, and health concerns were major reasons they chose bottled water over other beverages. For most Americans, however, bottled water is usually unnecessary and expensive, as it is often very similar to tap water. Consumers need to be aware that the water in some bottled water products actually comes from a municipal water supply. However, when public water supplies are disrupted by hurricanes, tornadoes, or earthquakes, drinking bottled water may be a consumer's only option. What is bottled water? Is it safe to drink?

The Environmental Protection Agency (EPA) regulates the sanitation of public water supplies in the United States. Another federal agency, the FDA, regulates bottled water products that are marketed for interstate commerce. Neither agency "certifies" bottled water.[39]

The FDA requires bottled water producers to:

- process, bottle, hold and transport bottled water under sanitary conditions;
- protect water sources from bacteria, chemicals, and other contaminants;
- use quality control processes to ensure the bacteriological and chemical safety of the water; and
- sample and test both the source of water and the final product for contaminants.[40]

Bottled water is sealed in containers and has no added ingredients other than a substance that prevents the growth of microbes, such as bacteria. Bottled water may have fluoride added, but amounts must meet FDA guidelines. If bottled water manufacturers add flavorings or other ingredients to their products, the name of the product must indicate the added ingredients; "Bottled Water with Cherry Flavor," for example. These drinks are often called "flavored water beverages." Flavored waters may simply contain additives that make the beverage taste good, but a growing number of flavored waters also have added nutrients other than sugars, such as sodium, potassium, and amino acids. The beverage's label must identify the additives in the list of ingredients.

Safety standards for bottled water are similar to those established by the EPA for tap water. According to FDA guidelines, bottled water manufacturers are responsible for producing safe products. Production procedures for bottled water must follow manufacturing regulations established and enforced by the FDA. Additionally, the FDA inspects water bottling facilities regularly.

Because of FDA regulations and oversight, consumers can be assured that their supply of bottled water is safe. Additionally, most Americans can trust the safety of their tap water because the vast majority of municipal water systems in the United States are regulated by the *Safe*

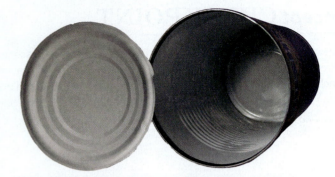

Figure 9.24 **BPA and epoxy resins.** The epoxy resin that is used to coat the inside of cans contains BPA.
©Wendy Schiff

Drinking Water Act (SDWA). As a result of this law, most tap water undergoes a thorough purification process and is constantly tested for safety. If such testing indicates the water supply may pose a threat to public health, consumers are warned through media, and a "boil order"—requirement to boil water for 10 minutes to kill harmful microorganisms—may be issued.

Although bottled water is safe to drink, the plastic used to contain it may have toxic effects on health. *Bisphenol (biss'–feen–ol) A*, which is also called *BPA*, is a chemical used to make polycarbonate plastics and epoxy resins. Polycarbonate plastics are in many consumer products that come in contact with foods and beverages, including some water bottles and older baby bottles. The epoxy resin that contains BPA is used to coat the inside of certain food cans. The coating prevents the can's metal from coming in contact with and being damaged by the food (Fig. 9.24). However, BPA can leach from polycarbonate plastic containers or epoxy resin–coated cans and enter the food or beverage stored within them.

Scientists are studying BPA to determine the extent to which the chemical can affect human health. Concern over the safety of BPA has encouraged some manufacturers to discontinue using the chemical in their products. Plastic containers that are marked with recycle codes 1, 2, 4, 5, and 6 most likely do not contain BPA. Some plastics that are marked with recycle codes 3 or 7 may be made with BPA (Fig. 9.25).[41] To reduce exposure to BPA, consider taking these actions:

- Avoid heating foods in polycarbonate plastic containers.
- Avoid plastic containers that have the symbol shown in Figure 9.25.
- Do not wash polycarbonate containers in the dishwasher or with harsh detergents.
- Reduce intake of foods in cans lined with epoxy resins.
- Cook or store foods and beverages in glass, porcelain, or stainless steel containers.

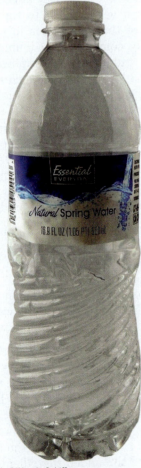

©Wendy Schiff

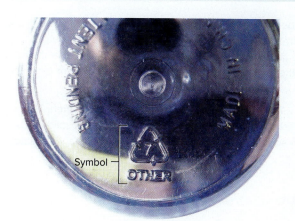

Figure 9.25 Where's the BPA? This symbol indicates that the plastic used to make this water bottle may contain BPA.
©Wendy Schiff

Concept CHECKPOINT

29. What is the significance of the Safe Drinking Water Act?
30. List three ways to reduce your exposure to BPA.

See Appendix G for responses.

Chapter References

See Appendix H.

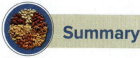

Summary

9.1 Introducing Water and Minerals

• Dehydration can be deadly. A mineral nutrient can be classified as a major, trace, or possible essential mineral.

9.2 Water

• Water is a simple compound that does not undergo digestion. In the body, water is a major solvent that often participates directly in chemical reactions. Water's other physiological roles include transporting substances, removing waste products, lubricating tissues, and regulating body temperature and acid-base balance. Water does not provide energy for the body.

• The body maintains a balance between intracellular and extracellular fluids primarily by controlling concentrations of ions in each fluid compartment. If the normal concentrations of these ions change too much, water shifts out of a compartment, and cells shrink or swell as a result.

• Total water intake includes water from beverages and foods. Most of the water that enters the digestive tract is absorbed. Metabolic water is another source of water for the body.

Groceries: ©Brand X Pictures/Getty Images RF; Apple: ©lynx/iconotec.com/Glow Images RF

Stacked books: ©Stockbyte/Getty Images RF; Nuts: ©C Squared Studios/Getty Images RF

- The body loses water in urine, perspiration, exhaled air, feces, and insensible perspiration. A healthy person's average daily total water input equals his or her average output. Environmental factors, physiological conditions, and lifestyle practices can alter the body's fluid balance. The kidneys are the major regulator of the body's water content and mineral ion concentrations.

- The AI for total water intake is 2.7 L for young women and 3.7 L for young men. These amounts do not need to be consumed in the form of fluids, because most solid foods and metabolic water contribute some water to the body. Thirst is the primary regulator of fluid intake.

9.3 Minerals: Basic Concepts

- Some minerals function as inorganic ions, cofactors, or structural components of tissues; other minerals are components of various enzymes, hormones, or other organic molecules. Cells cannot metabolize minerals for energy. The body, however, needs certain minerals to catalyze specific chemical reactions that release energy from macronutrients. Excessive amounts of minerals in the body can disrupt normal cell functioning, causing toxicity. Most foods contain small amounts of minerals. When the body's needs for minerals increase, the bioavailability of minerals generally increases to meet the demand.

9.4 Major Minerals

- Calcium is a major structural component of bones and teeth, and the mineral is necessary for blood clotting, muscle contraction, nerve transmission, and cell metabolism. Calcium absorption depends on vitamin D. Milk and milk products are rich calcium sources. Although people, especially women, are at risk of developing osteoporosis as they age, various lifestyle modifications may help reduce this risk.

- Sodium, the major positively charged ion found outside cells, is vital for maintaining fluid balance and transmitting nerve impulses. The typical American diet provides high amounts of sodium, primarily from processed and canned foods. Diets high in sodium are associated with increased risk of hypertension.

- Hypertensive individuals have greater risk of CVD, kidney failure, and damage to other organs than people with normal blood pressures. Advanced age, African-American ancestry, obesity, physical inactivity, cigarette smoking, and excess alcohol and sodium intakes are major risk factors for hypertension. Treatment for hypertension usually includes following dietary modifications and making some other lifestyle changes.

- Potassium, the major positively charged ion found inside cells, has functions that are similar to those of sodium. Potassium-rich diets may lower blood pressure. Plant foods, meat, and milk are good sources of potassium.

- Magnesium is a cofactor for numerous chemical reactions and is needed for nerve and heart function. Plant foods are good sources of magnesium.

9.5 Trace Minerals

- Iron is a critical component of hemoglobin, myoglobin, and cytochromes. Hemoglobin in red blood cells transports oxygen from the lungs to the tissues. Iron deficiency can result in iron deficiency anemia. Iron absorption depends on the body's need for the mineral and the form of iron in food. Heme iron is better absorbed than nonheme iron.

- Women of childbearing age have higher needs for iron than men because of menstrual blood loss. Throughout the world, iron deficiency–related disorders are common. People who have hereditary hemochromatosis develop iron toxicity, because they absorb too much iron.

- Zinc functions as a cofactor that activates many enzymes. Zinc is involved in growth and development, antioxidant activity, immune function, and taste. Zinc deficiency can result in growth failure and decreased immune function. Iodine is needed to make thyroid hormone. When the diet lacks iodine, the thyroid gland enlarges, forming a goiter. Cretinism can occur in infants born to women who were iodine deficient during pregnancy. Iodine deficiency is rare in the United States because table salt is often fortified with iodine.

- Selenium functions as a component of selenoproteins, many of which are antioxidants. Other selenoproteins are involved in the normal functioning of the immune system and thyroid gland. Meat, fish, nuts, whole grains, and seeds are good sources of selenium. Chromium enhances the action of insulin. Chromium is found in meats and whole grains. More research is needed to determine the effects of taking chromium supplements.

9.6 Minerals with Possible Physiological Roles

- A few minerals, including nickel and silicon, are found in very small amounts in the body, but their roles in the body are unclear. At present, these particular minerals are not classified as essential nutrients. Inorganic arsenic, however, is very toxic.

9.7 Nutrition Matters: Bottled Water Versus Tap Water

- In the United States, bottled water is usually unnecessary and expensive, and it is often derived from a municipal water supply. The Environmental Protection Agency regulates the sanitation of public water supplies in the United States. The Food and Drug Administration regulates bottled water products that are marketed for interstate commerce. The Safe Drinking Water Act helps ensure the safety of tap water. Although more research is needed to clarify the role of BPA in health, it is wise to avoid products that contain the chemical.

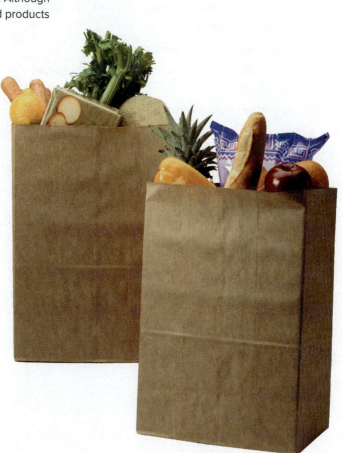

©David Buffington/Getty Images RF

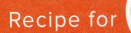

Recipe for Healthy Living

Egg Salad

Egg salad is an easy-to-make meal or snack. This recipe makes about three ⅓-cup servings. Each serving supplies approximately 144 kcal, 8.5 g protein, 11 g fat, 252 mg cholesterol, 0.84 mg iron, and 190 mg sodium.

©Jonelle Weaver/Getty Images RF

INGREDIENTS:

2 Tbsp peeled, finely chopped yellow onion
4 hard-cooked large eggs*
2 Tbsp reduced-fat mayonnaise
1 tsp pickle relish
dash of black pepper

*To hard-cook eggs:

1. Place the eggs in a small saucepan and cover the eggs completely with about 2 inches of water.

2. Heat water and eggs to a boil, then cover the saucepan with its lid, and remove it from the heat.

3. Allow the eggs to remain in the hot water for approximately 20 to 25 minutes (large eggs).

4. Remove eggs from the saucepan and cool by immersing in cold water.

PREPARATION STEPS:

1. Place chopped onion in small mixing bowl.

2. Peel hard-cooked eggs and discard peels. Chop eggs on a cutting board.

3. Add chopped eggs to onions.

4. Add reduced-fat mayonnaise and pickle relish to the egg and onion mixture. Blend together. Mixture should be moist.

5. Serve as a spread on whole-wheat crackers or on rye bread.

6. Egg salad is perishable, so cover any leftover salad and store in the refrigerator for no longer than a day.

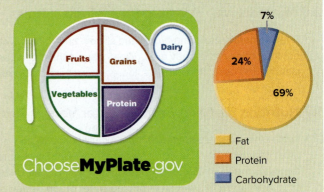

ChooseMyPlate.gov

Source: U.S. Dept. of Agriculture

- Fat 69%
- Protein 24%
- Carbohydrate 7%

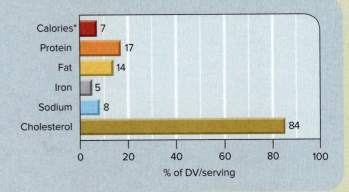

*2000 daily total kcal

- Calories* 7
- Protein 17
- Fat 14
- Iron 5
- Sodium 8
- Cholesterol 84

% of DV/serving

Further analyze this recipe or other recipes through activities located in Connect.

Personal Dietary Analysis

Using the DRIs

1. Refer to your 3-day food log from the "Personal Dietary Analysis" feature in Chapter 3.

   a. Find the RDA/AI values for minerals under your life stage/sex group category in the DRI tables (see Appendix I). Write those values under the "My RDA/AI" column in the table that accompanies this analysis activity.

   b. Review your personal dietary assessment. Find your 3-day average intakes of iron, calcium, zinc, sodium, potassium, and magnesium. Write those values under the "My Average Intake" column of the table.

   c. Calculate the percentage of the RDA/AI you consumed for each mineral by dividing your intake by the RDA/AI amount and multiplying the figure you obtain by 100. For example, if your average intake of iron was 9 mg/day, and your RDA for the mineral is 18 mg/day, you would divide 18 mg by 9 mg to obtain .50. To multiply this figure by 100, simply move the decimal point two places to the right, and replace the decimal point with a percentage sign (50%). Thus, your average daily intake of iron was 50% of the RDA. Place the percentages for each mineral under the "% of My RDA/AI" column.

   d. Under the ">, <, or =" column, indicate whether your average daily intake was greater than (>), less than (<), or equal to (=) the RDA/AI.

2. Use the information you calculated in the first part of this activity to answer the following questions:

   a. Which of your average mineral intakes equaled or exceeded the RDA/AI?

   b. Which of your average mineral intakes was below the RDA/AI?

   c. What foods would you eat to increase your intake of the minerals that were less than the RDA/AI levels? (Review sources of the minerals in this chapter.)

   d. Turn in your completed table and answers to your instructor.

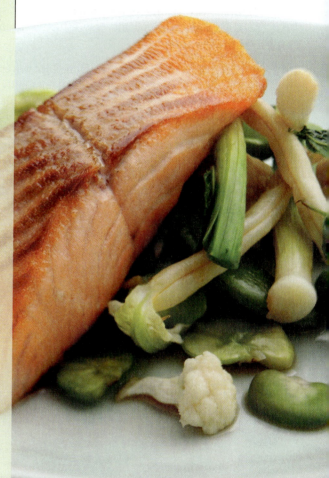

©Ingram Publishing/SuperStock RF

Personal Dietary Analysis: Minerals

Mineral	My RDA/AI	My Average Intake	% of My RDA/AI	>, <, or =
Iron				
Calcium				
Zinc				
Sodium				
Potassium				
Magnesium				

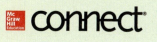 Complete the Personal Dietary Analysis activity located in Connect.

Raspberry: ©Stockbyte/Getty Images RF

Critical Thinking

1. Before the advent of refrigeration, salting meat was a common way of preventing microbes from spoiling the food. Explain why salting was effective as a means of food preservation.

2. A friend of yours refuses to drink tap water because she thinks it is contaminated. She drinks only bottled water or well water. If she asked you to explain why you drink tap water, what would you tell her?

3. A group of food manufacturers is considering fortifying some of their products with iron, chromium, boron, and iodine. Explain why you think they should or should not fortify the foods with each of these minerals.

4. Ben is a total vegetarian (vegan). What advice would you give to him concerning his need for calcium, iron, potassium, magnesium, and zinc?

5. Consider your family history and lifestyle to determine whether you are at risk of osteoporosis. If you are at risk, what steps can you take at this point in your life to reduce your chances of developing this disease?

6. Consider your family history and lifestyle to determine whether you are at risk of hypertension. If you are at risk, what steps can you take at this point in your life to reduce your chances of developing this disease?

7. In a blog, a person claiming to be a doctor recommends taking megadoses of zinc, iron, and selenium supplements to enhance muscular strength and endurance. Discuss why you would or would not follow this person's advice.

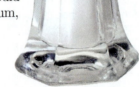

©Brand X Pictures/Getty Images RF

Practice Test

Select the best answer.

1. Which of the following statements is false?

   a. Lean tissue contains more water than fat tissue.
   b. Water is a major solvent.
   c. Generally, young women have more body water than young men.
   d. Water does not provide energy.

2. If the extracellular fluid has an excess of sodium ions,

   a. sodium ions move into cells.
   b. intracellular fluid moves to the outside of cells.
   c. phosphate and calcium ions are eliminated in feces.
   d. blood levels of arsenic and oxalate increase.

3. Which of the following foods has the lowest percentage of water?

   a. Tomatoes
   b. Oranges
   c. Whole-grain bread
   d. Vegetable oil

4. In the United States, table salt is often fortified with

   a. iron.
   b. selenium.
   c. potassium.
   d. iodine.

5. Which of the following foods is not a good source of calcium?

   a. Butter
   b. American cheese
   c. Canned sardines
   d. Kale

6. Henry is concerned about his risk of osteoporosis. Which of the following characteristics is a modifiable risk factor for this chronic condition?

   a. Family history
   b. Racial/ethnic background
   c. Physical activity level
   d. Age

Pineapple, radish: ©Stockbyte/Getty Images RF

7. The primary source of sodium in the typical American diet is

   a. bottled water.
   b. unprocessed food.
   c. fruit.
   d. salt.

8. Which of the following populations has the highest risk of hypertension?

   a. People with African–American ancestry
   b. Young, physically active Asian men
   c. Hispanic women who do not drink alcohol
   d. Young adults who consume high amounts of fruit

9. Sources of heme iron include

   a. fortified grain products.
   b. beef.
   c. spinach.
   d. cast–iron cookware.

10. Worldwide, the most common nutrient deficiency disorder is _____ deficiency.

    a. iodine
    b. cobalt
    c. iron
    d. calcium

11. Which of the following statements is false?

    a. Iodine is necessary for normal thyroid function.
    b. In the United States, milk is usually fortified with iodine.
    c. Having too much or too little iodine in the diet can cause the thyroid gland to enlarge.
    d. Saltwater fish and other seafood are sources of iodine.

12. Which of the following statements is true?

    a. Safety standards for bottled water are similar to those for tap water.
    b. Most brands of water bottled in the United States contain unsafe amounts of arsenic and lead.
    c. The EPA inspects and certifies water bottling facilities at least three times a year.
    d. The majority of Americans should drink bottled water because water from municipal systems is unsafe.

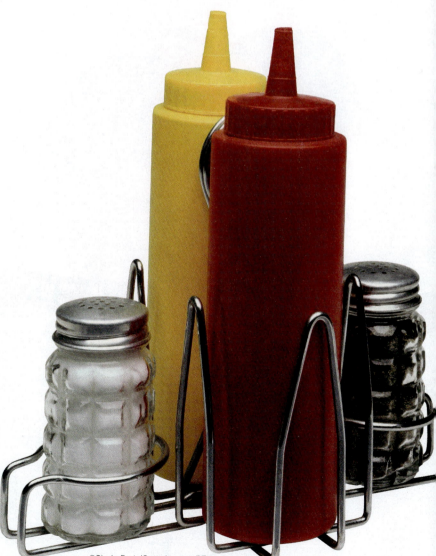

©Siede Preis/Getty Images RF

Answers to Quiz Yourself

1. Your body constantly loses water through insensible perspiration, a form of water loss that is not the same as sweat. **True.** (Section 9.2)

2. Ounce per ounce, cottage cheese contains more calcium than plain yogurt. **False.** (Section 9.4)

3. Potassium, sodium, and chloride ions are involved in fluid balance. **True.** (Section 9.2)

4. Selenium is an essential mineral. **True.** (Section 9.5)

5. In general, plants are good sources of iron because the plant pigment chlorophyll contains iron. **False.** (Section 9.4)

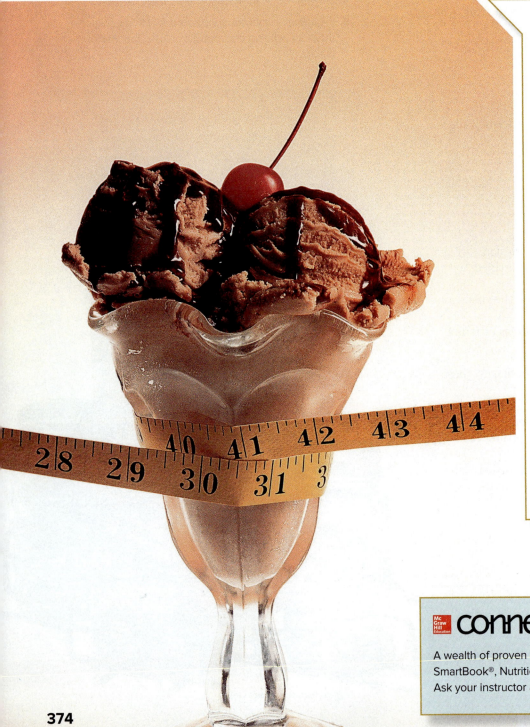

CHAPTER 10

Energy Balance and Weight Control

Quiz Yourself

What is the difference between overweight and obesity? Why do most people gain body fat as they age? How can you tell whether a person is following a fad diet or a diet that is likely to be safe and effective? Are there any medications or dietary supplements that help people lose weight? Test your knowledge of energy balance and weight management concepts by taking the following quiz. The answers are at the end of the chapter.

1. You can determine whether you have an unhealthy amount of body fat simply by measuring your waistline. _____ T _____ F

2. The safest way to lose a lot of weight and keep it off is to follow a low-carbohydrate, high-fat diet, such as the Atkins diet. _____ T _____ F

3. As people age, their muscle cells turn into fat cells. _____ T _____ F

4. When a person consumes more protein than needed, the excess can be converted to fat and stored in fat cells. _____ T _____ F

5. Cellulite is a unique type of fat that can be eliminated by taking certain dietary supplements. _____ T _____ F

connect

A wealth of proven resources are available on Connect® including SmartBook®, NutritionCalc Plus, and many other dynamic learning tools. Ask your instructor about Connect!

©Comstock Images RF

10.1 The Obesity Epidemic

Learning Outcomes

1 Explain the difference between overweight and obesity.

2 Discuss how the prevalence of obesity in the United States changed between 1988–1994 and 2013–2014.

In the United States, overweight and obesity are widespread nutritional problems that have reached epidemic proportions (Fig. 10.1). According to the National Heart, Lung, and Blood Institute, **overweight** refers to having extra body weight that is contributed by bone, muscle, body fat, and/or body water.[1] A professional basketball player, for example, may be "overweight" because of his muscular body build—not because he has excess body fat. **Obesity** is a condition characterized by excessive and unhealthy amounts of body fat. Unless noted otherwise, we will use the term *overweight* to describe people who have too much body fat but are not obese.

It is important to recognize that some body fat is essential for good health. However, people who are overweight or obese ("overfat") have a greater risk for serious chronic health conditions and diseases than people who have healthy body weights.

overweight having extra weight from bone, muscle, body fat, and/or body water

obesity condition characterized by excessive and unhealthy amounts of body fat

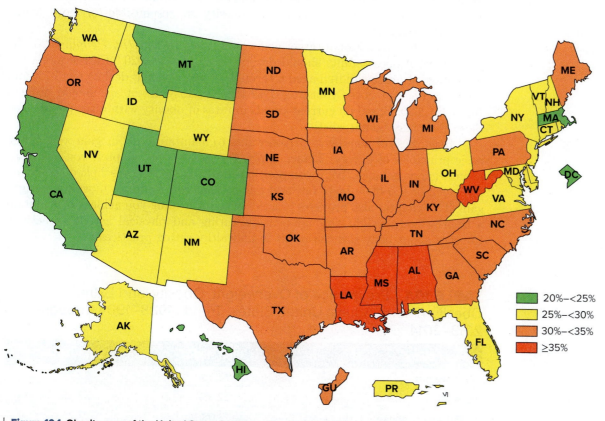

20%–<25%
25%–<30%
30%–<35%
≥35%

Figure 10.1 **Obesity map of the United States (states and territories), 2015.**

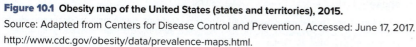
Source: Adapted from Centers for Disease Control and Prevention. Accessed: June 17, 2017.
http://www.cdc.gov/obesity/data/prevalence-maps.html.

Prevalence of Overweight and Obesity

body mass index (BMI) numerical value of relationship between body weight and risk of certain chronic health problems associated with excess body fat

To determine whether a person's weight is healthy, overweight, or obese, medi–cal experts generally use the **body mass index (BMI).** BMI is a numerical value based on the relationship between body weight and risk of chronic health problems associated with excess body fat. According to data collected from a national survey, more than 70% of American adults over the age of 20 were either overweight or obese in 2013–2014.[2] About one–third of these Americans were overweight and more than one–third of them were obese. As shown in Table 10.1, the percent of obese adults increased by almost 66% between 1988–1994 and 2013–2014. People who are classified as being obese can be further categorized into a subgroup of individuals who are "extremely obese." In 2013–2014, over 7% of adult Americans were classified as being extremely obese. This percentage more than doubled since 1988–1994.

Compared to non–Hispanic white adults, overweight and obesity are more common among non–Hispanic black and Hispanic–American adults, particularly among non–Hispanic black women.[2] Behavioral, educational, and environmental factors contribute to racial/ethnic differences in obesity rates.[3]

The prevalence of obesity among American children and adolescents has also risen sharply over the past 25 years. In 2011–2014, approximately 17% of children aged 2 through 19 were obese.[4] Public health experts are very concerned about the high prevalence of obesity among children, because these youngsters are more likely to mature into obese adults than are children who are not obese. See Chapter 13 for a discussion of childhood obesity.

Overweight and obesity rates are also rising rapidly throughout the world ("globesity"). In 2014, the World Health Organization (WHO) estimated that worldwide, 1.3 *billion* adults were overweight and 600 million adults were obese.[5] Throughout the world, overweight and obesity are responsible for more deaths than underweight.[5]

According to national target goals established in *Healthy People* 2020, the percentage of obese adults should decline to 30.5% by 2020.[6] Furthermore, the percentage of obese children aged 6 through 11 years should decline to 15.7% and the percentage of obese youth aged 12 through 19 years of age should drop to 16.1% by 2020. Based on current trends in rates of obesity within the population, these goals may be unrealistic.

Regardless of whether a person wants to maintain, lose, or gain weight, the basic principles of energy balance apply. By reading this chapter, you will learn about energy balance, body composition, health consequences linked to having too much or too little body fat, and factors that contribute to unwanted weight gain. This chapter also provides practical tips for helping you achieve or maintain a healthy body weight through sensible eating and physical activity practices. Concern about body size can result in unhealthy eating practices.

TABLE 10.1 Prevalence of Overweight, Obesity, and Extreme Obesity Among Adults: United States, Trends 1988–1994 through 2013–2014

Weight Status	1988–1994	2013–2014
Overweight	33.1%	32.7%
Obese	22.9%	37.9%
Extremely obese	3.0%	7.7%

Source of data: Fryar CD and others: *Prevalence of overweight, obesity, and extreme obesity among adults aged 20 and over: United States, 1960–1962 through 2013–2014.* July 18, 2016. Accessed: June 17, 2017. http://www.cdc.gov/nchs/data/hestat/obesity_adult_13_14/obesity_adult_13_14.htm

Concept CHECKPOINT

1. Calvin is overweight, but he has a healthy percentage of body fat. Explain why this situation can occur.
2. What percentage of adult Americans were obese in 2013–2014?

See Appendix G for responses.

10.2 Body Composition

Learning Outcomes

1. List the components of the two major body compartments.
2. Discuss the difference between subcutaneous fat and visceral fat.
3. Describe the various ways body fat is measured and the pros and cons of each method.
4. Explain why it is important to have healthy amounts of body fat.

The body is composed of two major compartments: **fat—free mass** (lean tissues) and **total body fat**. (Some scientists who study body composition divide the body into four compartments: body water, bone mineral, fat—free mass, and total body fat.) Fat—free mass is comprised of body water, mineral—rich tissues such as bones and teeth, and protein—rich tissues, including muscles and organs. Total body fat includes "essential fat" and *adipose tissue*. Essential fat is in cell membranes, certain bones, and nervous tissue. Essential fat is vital for survival. Adipose tissue contains white adipose cells (fat cells) that are specialized for storing energy in the form of triglycerides (see Fig. 6.13). Overweight and obese people have excessive amounts of fat stored in their adipose tissue. Furthermore, obese people often store triglycerides in other tissues, particularly the liver and muscles. Such fat deposits are harmful because they interfere with normal cell function and contribute to inflammation.

fat-free mass body compartment that is comprised of body water, mineral-rich tissues, and protein-rich tissues

total body fat essential fat and adipose tissue

Adipose Tissue

When food is plentiful, adipose cells remove excess fat from the bloodstream for storage. As the amount of fat stored in adipose cells increases, the size of each cell expands, and the body gains weight. The body develops more fat cells when over—eating occurs in adulthood, especially in cases of extreme obesity.[8] Once fat cells form, scientists think the cells remain until they die or are surgically removed.

When the body needs energy, adipose cells release fat for other cells to use as fuel. As each adipose cell loses some fat, it becomes smaller. If adipose cells continue to release fat, the body eventually loses weight as a result. In addition to storing and releasing fat, adipose cells secrete hormones and other substances, some of which have roles in regulating food intake, glucose metabolism, and immune responses.

Did YOU Know?

In addition to white fat cells, the body has deposits of beige fat and brown fat cells.[7] As a result of brown fat and beige fat cell activity, the body wastes energy as heat (thermogenesis). Thus, such cells can help regulate body temperature when a person is exposed to chilly conditions.

Subcutaneous Fat and Visceral Fat

Subcutaneous (*sub* = under; *cutaneous* [*qu—tay′—nee—us*] = skin) tissue holds skin in place over underlying tissues such as muscles. Subcutaneous tissue also contains adipose cells. When subcutaneous tissue has more adipose cells than other kinds of cells, it is referred to as *subcutaneous fat*. Subcutaneous fat helps

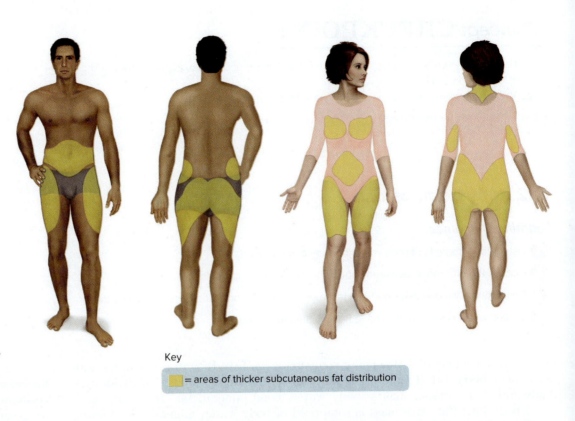

Figure 10.2 **Uneven subcutaneous fat distribution.** Subcutaneous fat is unevenly distributed.

Key

= areas of thicker subcutaneous fat distribution

Did *YOU* Know?

Cellulite, lumpy-appearing skin on thighs and buttocks of most women, is not a unique type of fat or the result of a disease. Scientists have no clear understanding of why cellulite occurs, but it may simply be subcutaneous fat that is loosely held in place by irregular bands of connective tissue. At this point, there is no treatment that effectively smooths the skin's dimpled appearance.[9]

insulate the body against cold temperatures and protects muscles and bones from bumps and bruises. Subcutaneous fat is unevenly distributed. This layer of fat is thicker in certain regions of men's and women's bodies, especially in the abdominal area, thighs, and buttocks (Fig. 10.2).

In addition to subcutaneous fat, the body has *visceral (viss'–eh–rol)* fat. Visceral fat also contains adipose cells, but this type of body fat is in the *omentum*, a structure that is under the abdominal muscles and hangs over the intestines (Fig. 10.3). Although there are some racial differences, women generally have more subcutaneous fat than men, whereas men tend to have more visceral fat than women.[10] Excessive amounts of visceral fat and/or subcutaneous abdominal fat result in what is commonly called a "beer belly" or the "middle–age spread."

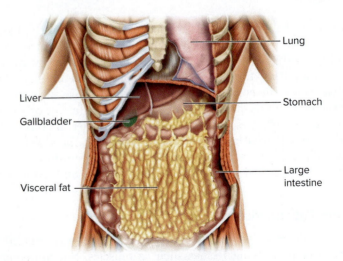

Lung

Liver

Gallbladder

Stomach

Visceral fat

Large intestine

Figure 10.3 **What is visceral fat?** Visceral fat is in the omentum that is under abdominal muscles and hangs over the intestines.

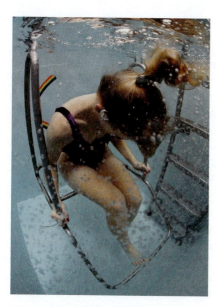

Figure 10.4 Underwater weighing.
©David Madison, Photographer's Choice/Getty Images

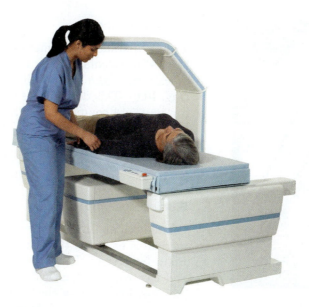

Figure 10.5 Dual-energy x-ray absorptiometry (DXA).
Source: Photo Courtesy of Hologic, Inc.

Visceral fat makes substances that cause inflammation in the body. These inflammatory factors may increase risks of type 2 diabetes and cardiovascular disease (CVD). Section 10.5 discusses an easy way to determine whether you have too much visceral fat.

Measuring Body Fat

When you weigh yourself on a scale, you cannot determine whether your weight is healthy. Why? It is healthier to have more fat–free tissue than fat tissue, but the scale does not distinguish between these two major components of your body. Information concerning your body's composition, especially its *percentage* of fat, can help you predict your risk of obesity–related diseases.

There is no direct way to measure a living person's percentage of body fat. The following sections describe some indirect methods of assessing body composition, including their advantages and disadvantages.

Underwater Weighing

Underwater weighing involves comparing a person's weight "on land" to his or her weight when completely submerged in a tank of water (Fig. 10.4). Lean tissue is denser than water; fat tissue is not as dense as water. Thus, a person who has more body fat will weigh less when under water than a person who has more lean tissue. The underwater weighing method can be an accurate way of assessing body composition. However, the method is not a convenient, easy, inexpensive, or practical way to estimate body fat because it requires special testing facilities.

Dual-Energy X-Ray Absorptiometry

Dual–energy x–ray absorptiometry (DXA) involves the use of multiple low–energy x–rays to scan the entire body. The method provides a detailed "picture" of internal structures, including fat deposits (Fig. 10.5). During the scanning process, the equipment emits a dose of radiation that is lower than that used for a chest x–ray. Although DXA is a highly accurate way to estimate body fat content, the equipment is very expensive and not widely available outside of clinical settings.

underwater weighing technique of estimating body composition that involves comparing weight on land to weight when completely submerged in a tank of water

dual-energy x-ray absorptiometry (DXA) technique of estimating body composition that involves scanning the body with multiple low-energy x-rays

air displacement method of estimating body composition by determining body volume

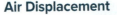

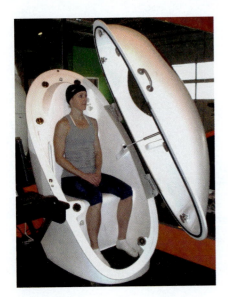

Figure 10.6 BOD POD.
©Mary Dean Coleman-Kelly

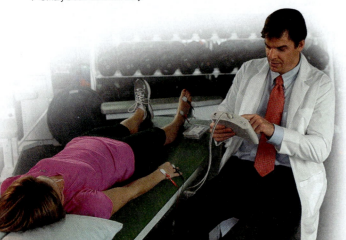

Figure 10.7 Bioelectrical impedance.
Source: RJL Systems

Air Displacement

The **air displacement** method assesses the volume of a person's body, which can be used to calculate his or her body composition. After being weighed on a very precise scale, the subject sits in the chamber of a device called the BOD POD (Fig. 10.6). This device measures the volume of air in the chamber with the person in it and compares the value with the volume of air that was in the chamber when it was unoccupied. The person's volume is the volume of air that was displaced after the subject entered the chamber. Air displacement measurements provide highly accurate estimates of body fat content, but the measuring device is expensive and not practical for most consumers to use.

Bioelectrical Impedance

Bioelectrical impedance is a quick way to estimate body fat content. This method is based on the principle that water and electrolytes conduct electricity. Body fat resists the flow of electricity, because fat tissue contains less water and electrolytes than lean tissue. The bioelectrical impedance device sends a painless, low-energy electrical current via wires connected to electrodes placed on the subject's skin (Fig. 10.7). Within a few minutes, the device converts information about the body's electrical resistance into an estimate of total body fat. The method can be accurate, as long as the subject's hydration status is normal. Dehydration results in an overestimation of total body fat. Consumers can purchase a bioelectrical impedance device that resembles a bathroom scale, but scientific data about the machine's accuracy is lacking.

Skinfold Thickness

A common technique for estimating total body fat involves taking **skinfold thickness measurements** at multiple body sites, such as over the triceps muscle of the arm (Fig. 10.8). The width of a skinfold indicates the depth of the subcutaneous fat at that site. To perform

bioelectrical impedance technique of estimating body composition in which a device measures the conduction of a weak electrical current through the body

skinfold thickness measurements technique of estimating body composition in which calipers are used to measure the width of skinfolds at multiple body sites

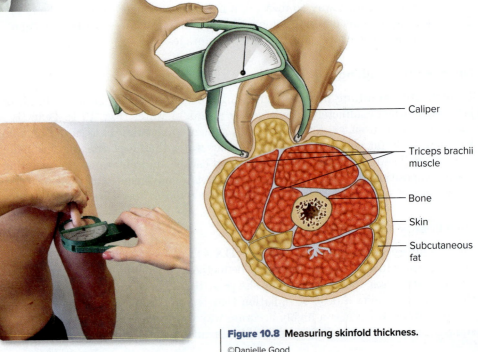

Caliper

Triceps brachii muscle

Bone

Skin

Subcutaneous fat

Figure 10.8 Measuring skinfold thickness.
©Danielle Good

the measurements, a trained person pinches a section of the subject's skin, gently pulls it away from underlying muscle tissue, and uses special calipers to measure the thickness of the fat. After taking the measurements, the values are incorporated into a mathematical formula that provides an estimate of the subject's amount of body fat.

Skinfold thickness measurements are relatively easy and inexpensive to perform, but the method's accuracy largely depends on the skill of the person performing the measurements. Also, the technique may underestimate total body fat when used on overfat subjects. However, by combining data collected from skinfold, waist and hip circumference, and body frame (skeletal joint) measurements, researchers can obtain more reliable estimates of an individual's total body fat.

How Much Body Fat Is Too Much?

Some body fat is essential for good health, but too much adipose tissue, especially visceral fat, can interfere with the body's ability to function normally. Percentages of body fat can be used to develop weight classifications for adults. According to one such classification system, a man is overweight when his body is 22 to 25% fat; a woman is overweight when her body is 32 to 37% fat (Table 10.2).[11] It is important to note that the average healthy young woman has more body fat than the average healthy young man because she needs the extra fat for hormonal and reproductive purposes.

Adults tend to gain adipose tissue as they age, but for elderly persons, some additional fat does not necessarily contribute to serious health problems. The extra fat may provide some health benefits, such as providing an energy reserve for a very ill person who cannot eat. Furthermore, the extra padding of fat may protect a person from being injured by falling.

TABLE 10.2 Adult Body Weight Classification by Percentage of Body Fat

Classification	Body Fat (%) Men	Body Fat (%) Women
Healthy	13 to 21%	23 to 31%
Overweight	22 to 25%	32 to 37%
Obese	26 to 31%	38 to 42%
Extremely obese	32% or more	43% or more

Source: Adapted from: Food and Nutrition Board, National Institute of Health: *Dietary Reference Intakes for energy, carbohydrate, fiber, fat, fatty acids, cholesterol, protein, and amino acids (macronutrients).* Table 5.5, page 126. Washington, DC: National Academies Press, 2005.

Concept CHECKPOINT

3. Which tissues comprise total body fat and which comprise fat-free mass?
4. Why is it necessary to have some body fat?
5. List three roles for subcutaneous fat and visceral fat.
6. Describe three different methods of measuring body fat, including drawbacks of each method.
7. A young man's body is 23% fat. According to information in Table 10.2, is he overweight, obese, or healthy?

See Appendix G for responses.

energy capacity to perform work

10.3 Energy for Living

Learning Outcomes

1. Define *basal metabolism*.
2. Use the "rule of thumb" method to estimate a person's daily basal metabolic energy needs.
3. Discuss the three major ways the body uses energy.
4. Describe factors that influence the basal metabolic rate.

Regardless of what you are doing—eating, watching television, studying, exercising, even sleeping—your body needs a constant supply of energy to function. **Energy** is defined as the capacity to perform work. There are several forms of energy, but heat, mechanical, chemical, and even electrical energy occur in living things. The total amount of energy is *constant*; that is, the amount remains the same, because energy cannot be created or destroyed. Nevertheless, the various forms of energy can be stored, released, moved, or transformed from one kind to another. The following sections discuss how human cells obtain and use energy.

Energy Intake

Just as a car engine uses a mixture of gasoline, ethanol, and oxygen to run properly, your body uses a mixture of *biological fuels* and oxygen to do its work.

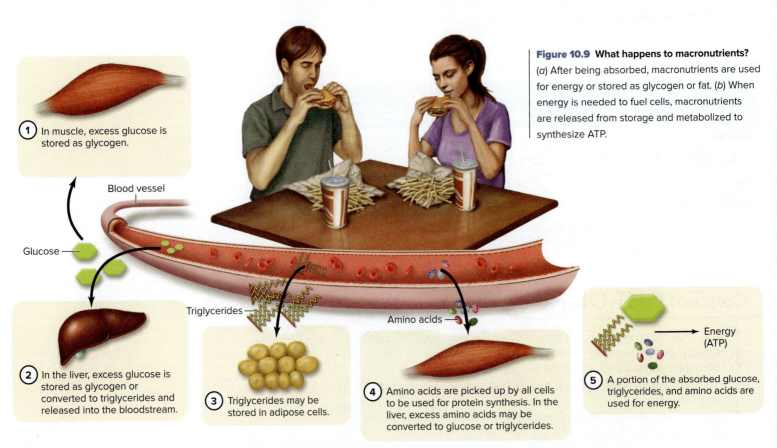

Figure 10.9 What happens to macronutrients? (*a*) After being absorbed, macronutrients are used for energy or stored as glycogen or fat. (*b*) When energy is needed to fuel cells, macronutrients are released from storage and metabolized to synthesize ATP.

1. In muscle, excess glucose is stored as glycogen.

Blood vessel

Glucose

2. In the liver, excess glucose is stored as glycogen or converted to triglycerides and released into the bloodstream.

Triglycerides

3. Triglycerides may be stored in adipose cells.

Amino acids

4. Amino acids are picked up by all cells to be used for protein synthesis. In the liver, excess amino acids may be converted to glucose or triglycerides.

Energy (ATP)

5. A portion of the absorbed glucose, triglycerides, and amino acids are used for energy.

(a)

For humans, biological fuels are foods and beverages that contain macronutrients (**energy intake**). For some individuals, nonnutrient alcohol (ethanol) also provides energy. Under normal conditions, our cells metabolize primarily glucose and fatty acids, but small amounts of amino acids are also used for energy.

Cells release the energy stored in biological fuels by breaking bonds within the compounds' molecules. The energy that is released can be captured and stored in special compounds, such as **adenosine triphosphate (ATP),** until it is needed. Cells obtain only about 40% of the energy that was in macronutrients by forming ATP. Cells release the remaining energy as heat. Figure 10.9 summarizes events that result in macronutrient storage or breakdown for energy. The diagram in Appendix C summarizes the complex chemical pathways that most cells use to generate ATP from the metabolism of glucose, fat, and amino acids.

Energy Output

Energy output (*energy expenditure*) refers to the energy (calories) cells use to carry out their activities. For example, muscle cells need energy to contract, liver cells use energy to convert toxic compounds to safer substances, and intestinal cells need energy to absorb certain nutrients. The following sections discuss the major ways the body uses food energy.

Basal and Resting Metabolism

Metabolism refers to all chemical changes, or reactions, that constantly occur in living cells. Anabolic reactions require energy to occur; catabolic reactions release energy.

energy intake calories from foods and beverages that contain macronutrients and alcohol

adenosine triphosphate (ATP) molecule that stores energy

energy output calories cells use to carry out their activities

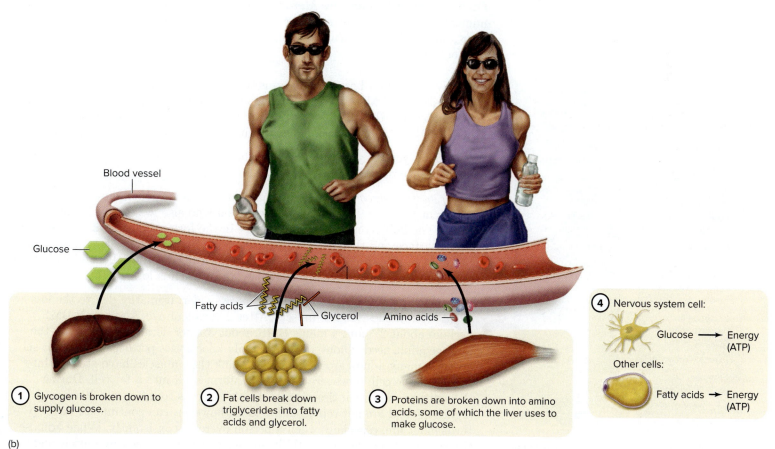

Blood vessel

Glucose

Fatty acids

Glycerol

Amino acids

1. Glycogen is broken down to supply glucose.

2. Fat cells break down triglycerides into fatty acids and glycerol.

3. Proteins are broken down into amino acids, some of which the liver uses to make glucose.

4. Nervous system cell:

Glucose → Energy (ATP)

Other cells:

Fatty acids → Energy (ATP)

(b)

basal metabolism minimal number of kilocalories the body uses to support vital activities after fasting and resting for 12 hours

resting metabolic rate (RMR) body's rate of energy use a few hours after resting and eating

Basal metabolism is the minimal number of calories the body uses for vital physiological activities after fasting and resting for 12 hours. Basal metabolic processes include breathing, circulating blood, and maintaining constant liver, brain, and kidney functions. Basal metabolism does not encompass energy needed for skeletal muscle movements (physical activity), digestion of food, and absorption and processing of nutrients. Generally, basal metabolism accounts for most of the body's total energy use.[12]

The **resting metabolic rate (RMR)** refers to the body's rate of energy use a few hours after resting and eating. A person's RMR is slightly higher than his or her BMR (basal metabolism rate). Although there is a difference between the BMR and the RMR, researchers often use the terms interchangeably in their publications.

Thyroid hormone, secreted by the thyroid gland, regulates metabolism (see Fig. 9.11). A person who has an overactive thyroid gland produces too much thyroid hormone. As a result, this person has a higher-than-normal metabolic rate. Signs and symptoms of excess thyroid hormone production (*hyperthyroidism*) include feeling warm, sweaty, nervous, and restless; having rapid heart rate and chronic diarrhea; fatigue; and losing weight despite having an increased appetite. You might think that hyperthyroidism is the key to treating unwanted weight gain, but the condition can have serious side effects, such as elevated blood pressure and heart failure. A person who suffers from *hypothyroidism* does not produce enough thyroid hormone, and as a result, he or she has a lower-than-normal metabolic rate. This individual typically complains of feeling cold, lacking energy and interest in usual activities, being constipated, and gaining weight easily. Treatment for a hypoactive thyroid gland generally includes medication that contains a form of thyroid hormone.

Factors That Influence the Metabolic Rate In addition to thyroid hormone, numerous factors can increase or decrease basal metabolic rates (Fig. 10.10). Thus, metabolic rates vary among individuals. Factors that influence basal metabolism include:

- *Body composition* Lean body mass is the major factor that influences the metabolic rate.[11] Muscle tissue, a component of lean body mass, is more metabolically active than fat tissue. In general, a person who has more muscle mass will have a higher metabolic rate than someone with less muscle tissue.

- *Sex* Males generally have higher metabolic rates than women because they tend to have more lean body mass.

- *Body surface area* A tall, slender person who weighs 150 pounds has a higher metabolic rate than a shorter person who also weighs 150 pounds. Why? The body constantly loses energy in the form of heat that moves to the skin's surface and then into the environment. Because the taller person's body has more surface area than the shorter person's body, the taller individual has to generate more heat energy to replace that which is lost.

- *Age* Basal metabolism declines as one grows older, primarily due to the loss of fat-free tissues such as muscle. After 20 years of age, a woman's BMR declines about 2% and a man's BMR about 3% per decade.[13] Therefore, the average adult needs about 150 fewer daily kilocalories per decade as he or she ages. As many adults grow older, they think their muscles have "turned into" fat. A muscle cell, however, cannot transform itself into a fat cell. During the aging process, lean tissue mass shrinks, as cells from muscle, bone, and organs die and are not replaced. Fat cells, however, can continue to develop throughout life, especially when a person overeats consistently. When adipose tissue expands in size, it can fill in spaces formerly occupied by muscle and

Factors That Increase BMR

- Increased muscle mass
- Body temperature (Fever increases metabolism.)
- Excess thyroid hormone
- Periods of growth (e.g., pregnancy)
- Greater body surface area (tall height)
- Lactation (milk production for breastfeeding)
- Exercise recovery
- Stimulant drugs (e.g., caffeine)
- Emotional stress

Factors That Decrease BMR

- Decreased muscle mass
- Starvation or very-low-calorie diets
- Low thyroid hormone
- Aging
- Lower body surface area (short height)

| **Figure 10.10** Factors that influence the metabolic rate.

organ tissues. Regular exercise helps build and preserve lean body mass, and to some extent, people can maintain a higher metabolic rate by being physically active as they grow older.

- *Calorie intake* Calorie intake also affects the metabolic rate. The body conserves energy use when calorie intakes are very low or lacking altogether. To enhance the rate of weight loss, an overfat person should reduce caloric intake while maintaining a normal metabolic rate. Because very–low–calorie diets reduce the metabolic rate, such diets are not generally recommended for weight loss.

As listed in Figure 10.10, the following factors increase the metabolic rate:

- *Fever*
- *Stimulant drugs* (caffeine, for example)
- *Pregnancy*
- *Milk production in a female who has given birth*
- *Recovery after exercise* (*metabolic aftereffects of exercise*)
- *Emotional stress*

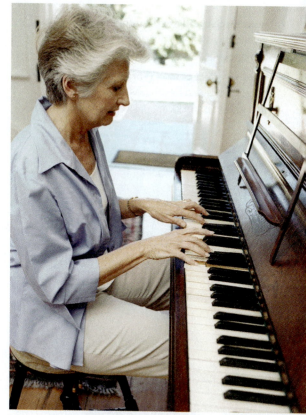

As people grow older, their calorie needs decline.
©BananaStock/Alamy RF

Calculating Metabolic Energy Needs   The basal metabolic rate is fairly constant from day to day.[14] Thus, a young adult can estimate his or her daily metabolic rate by following a "rule of thumb" formula:

$$\text{Formula for men} = 1.0 \text{ kcal/kg/hr}$$

$$\text{Formula for women} = 0.9 \text{ kcal/kg/hr}$$

To estimate the number of calories you need for your basal metabolism, first convert your weight in pounds to kilograms by dividing your weight by 2.2. (A kilogram is approximately 2.2 pounds.)

_____ lb ÷ 2.2 lb = _____ kg

Then, depending on your sex, use one of the following formulas:

_____ kg × 0.9 (women) = _____ kcal/hr

_____ kg × 1.0 (men) = _____ kcal/hr

Finally, use this hourly basal metabolic rate to estimate your basal metabolic rate for an entire day by multiplying the hourly value by 24.

_____ kcal/hr × 24 hr = _____ kcal/day

These calculations only provide a rough estimate of your daily metabolic rate. To estimate your Estimated Energy Requirement (EER) for a 24–hour period, you need to add kilocalories used for physical and other activities to your BMR figure.

Physical Activity

Physical activity, voluntary skeletal muscle movement, increases energy expenditure above basal energy needs. The number of kilocalories expended for a particular physical activity depends largely on the type of activity, how long it is performed (duration), the degree of effort (intensity) used while performing the activity, and the weight of the person. A heavy person expends more kilocalories when performing the same activity, for the same duration, and at the same intensity than a lighter person. Why? The muscles of the heavier person must work harder to move the larger body.

nonexercise activity thermogenesis (NEAT) involuntary skeletal muscular activities such as fidgeting

thermic effect of food (TEF) energy used to digest foods and beverages as well as absorb and further process the macronutrients

To estimate your energy needs for physical activity, visit https://www.supertracker.usda.gov/ and click on "Physical Activity Tracker." Table 10.3 lists various physical activities and the approximate number of kilocalories an individual who weighs 150 pounds expends while performing each activity for a minute. For example, a 150−pound person who walks for 30 minutes (3.5 mph) burns approximately 180 kcal during the walk (30 × 6).

The number of calories you need for physical activity can vary widely, depending on how active you are each day. Because you can control the type, intensity, and duration of your physical activities, you can manipulate your energy output to increase, decrease, or maintain your weight.

Nonexercise Activity Thermogenesis Nonexercise activity thermogenesis (*thermo* = heat; *genesis* = production) or **NEAT** refers to *involuntary* skeletal muscle activity, that is, physical activity that a person does not consciously control. NEAT activities include shivering, fidgeting, maintaining muscle tone, and maintaining body posture when not lying down. Some people may expend as much as 700 kcal daily as NEAT.[15] It is possible that some individuals resist weight gain from overeating because they have higher−than−average energy expenditures for NEAT. Nevertheless, the contribution of NEAT to overall calorie needs is fairly small for most people.

Thermic Effect of Food

The body needs a relatively small amount of energy to digest foods and beverages as well as to absorb and further process the macronutrients. The energy used for these tasks, generally 5 to 10% of total caloric intake, is referred to as the **thermic effect of food (TEF)**. For example, if your energy intake was 3000 kcal/day, TEF would account for 150 to 300 kcal.

©Jules Frazier/Getty Images RF

TABLE 10.3 Approximate Energy Expenditures of Selected Physical Activities (150-pound person)

Physical Activity	Approximate kcal/min.
Sitting and texting	2
Canoeing (4 mph)	4
Dancing (ballroom)	4
Weight training	5
Bowling	6
Walking (3.5 mph)	6
Bicycling (10–12 mph)	10
Walking (4.5 mph)	10
Hiking (with pack, 3 mph)	12
Tennis (singles, recreational)	12
Touch football (vigorous)	12
Swimming (vigorous breaststroke)	15
Running/jogging, steady pace (6 mph)	15
Bicycling (15 mph)	15
Martial arts	15

Source: https://supertracker.usda.gov/physicalactivitytracker.aspx Accessed: June 17, 2017

Putting It All Together

To estimate your daily energy expenditure, you could add the kilocalories you burned for basal metabolism, physical activity, and TEF in a day. However, another method is to use one of the formulas published by the Food and Nutrition Board of the Institute of Medicine, which is in the Personal Dietary Analysis activity at the end of this chapter.[11]

energy equilibrium calorie intake equals calorie output

Did *YOU* Know?

Results of scientific studies suggest that watching television is associated with obesity among children and adults.[16,17] Television watching is a sedentary activity that may include viewing food advertisements and eating foods that are high in empty calories. Health experts recommend that people limit their nonwork-related screen time (including activities involving computers and video games) to no more than 2 hours/day.[18]

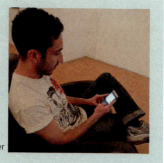

©McGraw-Hill Education/David Moyer, photographer

Concept CHECKPOINT

8. Using the "rule of thumb" formula, estimate the daily basal metabolic energy needs of a woman who weighs 185 pounds.
9. List the three major ways the body uses energy, and identify the one that is most easily altered.
10. For most people, which form of energy expenditure uses the most energy on a daily basis?
11. Discuss at least five factors that influence basal metabolic rate.

See Appendix G for responses.

10.4 Energy Balance

Learning Outcomes

1 Explain the concept of energy balance.
2 Compare states of positive and negative energy balance.

Understanding the concept of *energy balance* is critical to understanding why most people gain, lose, or maintain weight. Your body is in a state of **energy equilibrium** and "balanced" when your calorie intake from food and beverages equals your calorie output for basal metabolism, physical activity, and TEF (Fig. 10.11). By maintaining a balanced energy state, your weight will remain relatively stable over time.

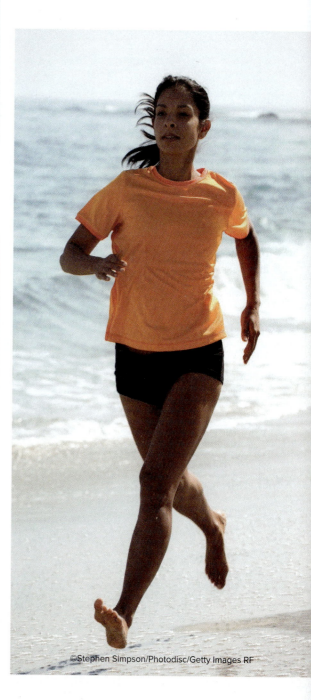

©Stephen Simpson/Photodisc/Getty Images RF

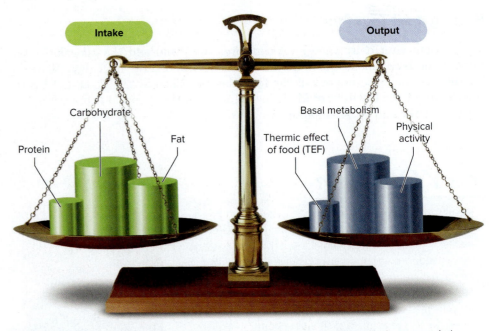

Figure 10.11 Energy balance. Your energy state is in equilibrium and "balanced" when your calorie intake from food and beverages equals your calorie output for basal metabolism, physical activity, and TEF.

negative energy balance calorie intake is less than calorie output

positive energy balance calorie intake is greater than calorie output

If your calorie intake is lower than your calorie output, you are in **negative energy balance.** In this state, your body needs more calories to carry out its activities than your diet is supplying. Therefore, your body metabolizes stored fat for energy. Weight loss results from being in a negative energy state. Over time, you will notice your clothes have become baggy as your adipose tissue shrinks.

If your calorie intake from macronutrients (and alcohol) is greater than your calorie output, you are in a state of **positive energy balance.** In this state, your body stores excess dietary fat in adipose cells. Additionally, the body converts surplus dietary carbohydrate, protein, and alcohol to fat and stores that fat in adipose cells. Weight gain results from being in a positive energy state, and eventually, you will notice that your clothes seem to have shrunk.

Positive energy balance is necessary for pregnant women because extra calories are needed to add new tissues that support the pregnancy. Positive energy balance also occurs during periods of growth, such as during fetal development, infancy, childhood, and adolescence. Over time, however, even a small positive energy balance can cause anyone's weight to increase, regardless of his or her age. Maintenance of energy balance—matching calorie intake to calorie output over the long term—is critical for controlling body weight (Fig. 10.12).

Did *YOU* Know?

Have you heard of the "freshman 15," the popular belief that college students gain 15 pounds during their freshman year? Results of scientific studies confirm that freshmen are likely to gain weight, but the increase is much less than 15 pounds—7.5 pounds on average.[19] Factors that contribute to the weight gain include feeling "stressed out," eating too much unhealthy food, drinking too much alcohol, and being less physically active than before entering college.

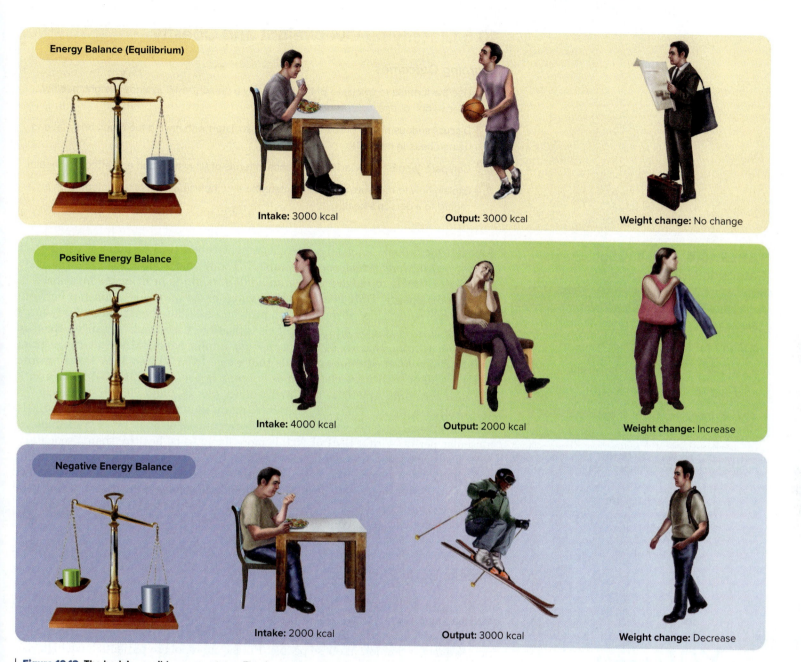

Figure 10.12 The body's possible energy states. This figure presents three possible energy states.

Concept CHECKPOINT

12. What happens to a person's body weight when he or she is in a state of positive energy balance?

13. When is it desirable for a person to be in a positive energy balance state?

14. When is a person in a negative energy balance state?

See Appendix G for responses.

10.5 Classifying Overweight and Obesity

Learning Outcomes

1 Use the formula to calculate BMI, and classify a person's BMI as underweight, healthy, overweight, obese, or extremely obese.

2 Discuss serious health problems that are associated with having too much body fat and being obese in particular.

3 Compare "apple" to "pear" body shapes in terms of fat distribution and effects on health.

4 Explain how to measure waist circumference and the usefulness of this information in regard to a person's health.

TABLE 10.4 Adult Weight Status Categories (BMI)

BMI	Weight Status
Below 18.5	Underweight
18.5 to 24.9	Healthy
25.0 to 29.9	Overweight
30.0 to 39.9	Obese
40 and above	Extremely obese

Source: National Heart, Lung, and Blood Institute: "The practical guide: Identification, evaluation, and treatment of overweight and obesity in adults," *NIH Publication* 00-4084, 2000. Accessed July 22, 2017. www.nhlbi.nih.gov/guidelines/obesity/prctgd_c.pdf

At one time, people referred to height/weight tables to determine whether their body weights were "ideal" or "desirable." Today, medical experts use the body mass index (BMI) to judge whether an adult's weight is healthy. As mentioned in the chapter opener, BMI is a numerical value based on the relationship between body weight and risk of chronic health problems associated with excess body fat.[11]

Table 10.4 presents adult weight classifications based on BMI ranges. Healthy BMIs range from 18.5 to 24.9. *Overweight* adults have BMIs that range from 25.0 to 29.9; *obese* adults have BMIs that range from 30.0 to 39.9. People whose BMIs are 40 or higher are classified as *extremely obese*. In 2011–2014, the average BMI for adult American men and women was 28.7 and 29.2, respectively.[20]

Muscle is denser than fat; therefore, many muscular people may have BMIs in the overweight range, yet have healthy percentages of body fat. For example, a muscular person with a BMI of 25.0 is more likely to be healthy than a sedentary (physically inactive) person who also has a BMI of 25.0. The BMI may underestimate body fat in people who have lost muscle tissue as a result of aging or illness. Therefore, BMIs should not be applied to highly muscular individuals, people who are elderly, or chronically ill persons. However, sedentary people with BMIs of 30 or higher generally have excess body fat.

Excess Body Fat: Effects on Health

People with BMIs greater than 25 have increased risks of type 2 diabetes, hypertension, and CVD. Many types of cancer, including cancers of the gallbladder, pancreas, cervix, uterus, breast (postmenopausal women), colon, rectum, and kidney, are more common in obese people. Furthermore, obese patients have high risk of experiencing serious complications during and after surgery. Such patients often require more anesthesia, and their incisions are more likely to become infected than surgical patients whose weights are within the healthy range. Extremely obese people are far more likely to develop the serious chronic diseases associated with excess body fat and to die prematurely than people who have BMIs that range from 18.5 to 24.9.[21]

Overweight and obese people are more likely to develop osteoarthritis, a painful chronic condition that affects joints and interferes with the person's ability to move. Obese people typically have difficulty carrying out routine daily activities, especially those that require walking, carrying, kneeling, and stooping. Additionally, obese people are more likely to suffer from chronic heartburn as well as *sleep apnea*, a condition that causes breathing to stop periodically during sleep.

Obese men and women are more likely to have fertility problems than people with healthy BMIs. *Polycystic ovary disease* often affects obese women and can reduce the women's chances of becoming pregnant. During pregnancy, obese women have high risk of *gestational diabetes* and a form of hypertension that

Did *YOU* Know?

You can use the following formula to calculate your BMI:

$$\frac{\text{weight (lb)}}{[\text{height (in)}]^2} \times 703$$

For example, a person who weighs 140 pounds and is 5-feet, 3-inches (63 inches) tall has a BMI of approximately 24.8. This person's BMI is almost at the upper limit of the healthy range.

Calculation: $[140 \div (63)^2] \times 703$

$(140 \div 3969) \times 703 =$

$0.03527 \times 703 = 24.8$

can be deadly (see Chapter 5). Additionally, obese pregnant women are at greater risk for stillbirths or giving birth to babies with birth defects than are pregnant women who have lower BMIs.

A person's mental health and self—esteem can be negatively affected by his or her "weight problem." Many Americans admire slim and muscular body builds over overfat body shapes. Thus, overfat people often suffer from poor self—images because they think their bodies are unattractive. The general public often views obesity as a condition that results from lack of willpower and the inability to "push oneself away from the table." Thus, many overfat people also deal with the negative attitude (stigma) that many people have toward them. People who are not overfat often characterize obese persons as lazy, stupid, and sloppy.[22] The stigma of obesity can result in discriminatory practices that limit an obese person's chances for career opportunities and access to adequate health care. It is not surprising that depression tends to accompany obesity. Table 10.5 lists these and other major health problems associated with excessive body fat.

Body Fat Distribution: Effects on Health

The results of medical research suggest that the distribution of excess body fat has a closer association with obesity—related diseases than does the percentage of total body fat. Women tend to store extra subcutaneous fat below the waist, primarily in the buttocks and thighs (Fig. 10.13a). Having this particular pattern of fat distribution (a "pear shape") adds stress to hip and knee joints that must carry the extra weight, but the pattern is not associated with increased risk of more serious chronic such as type 2 diabetes.

Men tend to store extra visceral fat in the abdominal or central region of their bodies.[23] **Central—body obesity** is characterized by a large amount of visceral fat ("spare tire") that spreads beyond buttocks and thighs. A person with central—body obesity is sometimes described as having an "apple" body shape (see Fig. 10.13b). Men or women with central—body obesity have higher risks of serious chronic diseases, especially cardiovascular disease and type 2 diabetes ("diabesity"), than people who have waists that do not extend beyond their hips.

A quick and easy method to determine your risk of obesity—related disorders is to measure your *waist circumference*, which is an indicator of central—body obesity. Figure 10.14 shows a recommended placement of the tape measure. Note

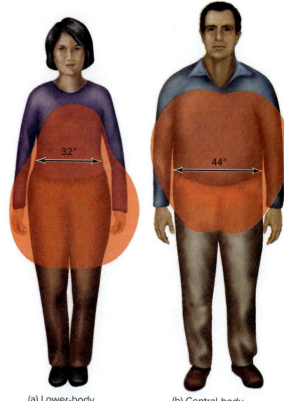

(a) Lower-body fat distribution (pear shape)

(b) Central-body fat distribution (apple shape)

Figure 10.13 Body fat distribution: Typical differences. Women tend to store extra subcutaneous fat below the waist (*a*). Men tend to store extra visceral fat in the central region of their bodies (*b*).

TABLE 10.5 Health Problems Associated with Excess Body Fat

Overweight and obesity increase the risk of:	
Cardiovascular disease (CVD)	Chronic low back pain
Hypertension	Loss of mobility
Type 2 diabetes	Fatty liver disease (not alcohol related)
Metabolic syndrome	Erectile dysfunction in men (impotence)
Polycystic ovary syndrome	Low-grade inflammation
Infertility	Gastroesophageal reflux disorder (GERD)
Elevated blood lipid levels	Psychological depression
Gallstones	Certain cancers
Sleep apnea	Skin ulcers
Osteoarthritis	

Sources: Jackson Y and others: "Summary of the 2000 Surgeon General's listening session: Toward a national action plan on overweight and obesity," *Obesity Research* 10(12):1299, 2002; Virji A, Murr MM, "Caring for patients after bariatric surgery," *American Family Physician,* 73(8):1403, 2006.

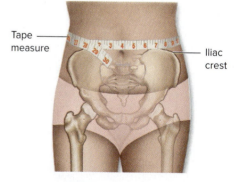

Tape measure

Iliac crest

Figure 10.14 Measuring waist circumference. A quick and easy method to determine a person's risk of obesity-related disorders is to measure the individual's waist circumference.

central-body obesity condition characterized by excessive visceral fat

the positioning of the tape at the top of the hip bones and not necessarily at the narrowest point. It is also important to use a measuring tape that does not stretch and to hold the tape around the waist, parallel to the floor. Central–body obesity is defined by a waist circumference of greater than 40 inches in men and greater than 35 inches in women.[24]

Concept CHECKPOINT

15. A young woman's BMI is 31.2. According to this information, is this woman likely to be healthy, overweight, obese, or extremely obese?

16. List at least six different serious health problems that are associated with having too much body fat and being obese in particular.

17. What is the "stigma" of obesity?

18. Which of the two major types of body fat distribution is more likely to pose serious health risks? Which chronic diseases are more likely to develop in people who have this pattern of excess fat deposition?

19. What is a quick and easy way to determine whether a person's body fat distribution is likely to result in serious health problems, such as type 2 diabetes?

See Appendix G for responses.

10.6 What Causes Overweight and Obesity?

Learning Outcomes

1 Identify factors that can influence the development of excess body fat.

2 Discuss factors that influence hunger and satiety.

3 Discuss the roles of hormones and peptides in regulating hunger.

4 Explain what is meant by having "thrifty genes."

5 Discuss how the set-point theory can explain why people often regain the weight they lose.

Although an excess intake of calories in relation to calorie output causes weight gain, there is no simple *cause* of obesity. To lose weight, a person needs to create a negative energy state by eating fewer calories, expending more calories than the amount consumed, or taking both actions. For many people, however, it is not easy to alter calorie input and output. Numerous factors, including physiological, environmental, behavioral, and psychological forces, influence a person's calorie intake and expenditure.

Physiological Factors

From a physiological standpoint, eating behavior is complex and largely involves interactions among the nervous, endocrine, and digestive systems as well as fat tissue. *Hunger* and *satiety* are key sensations that regulate eating behavior. **Hunger** is an uncomfortable feeling that drives a person to consume food. Thus, hunger is the need to eat. **Satiety** is the sense that enough food or beverages have been consumed to satisfy hunger.

Physical sensations influence eating behavior. As time between meals increases, the stomach signals "it's time to eat" by contracting, causing hunger pangs. As the contractions become stronger, the person usually eats or drinks something to relieve the discomfort. The size of the stomach influences satiety.

hunger uncomfortable feeling that drives a person to consume food

satiety sense that enough food or beverages have been consumed to satisfy hunger

During meals, the stomach stretches as it fills. The sensation that the stomach has reached its capacity can make a person stop eating. Nevertheless, many overfat persons do not recognize the sensation of stomach fullness, and as a result, they may eat even when they should not be hungry.

An area of the *hypothalamus*, a structure in the brain, controls hunger and satiety. Scientists think this region functions as a "hunger/satiety center." The stomach, intestines, and fat tissue produce certain proteins, such as hormones and *peptide YY*, that stimulate nerve cells involved in the regulation of hunger and satiety. **Ghrelin** (*grel′−in*), a hormone secreted mainly by the stomach, stimulates eating behavior. Some scientists think that reducing ghrelin production or activity is the key to helping people lose or maintain their weight. The small and large intestines release peptide YY, a protein that signals the stomach to reduce ghrelin secretion. The small intestine also releases *cholecystokinin* (*CCK*), the hormone that stimulates the gallbladder to contract and the pancreas to release digestive enzymes (see Chapter 6). Additionally, CCK stimulates the brain and other nervous tissue, suppressing appetite as a result.

Fat cells secrete **leptin,** a hormone that reduces hunger and inhibits fat storage in the body. A person's blood leptin level is directly proportional to his or her amount of body fat.[25] The brain obtains information about the status of body fat stores by monitoring the level of leptin in blood. When researchers administer leptin to genetically engineered mice that cannot synthesize the hormone, the rodents lose weight. Studies involving humans, however, generally find that obese people produce high amounts of leptin, but their bodies resist the hormone's hunger−suppressing action.[25] Figure 10.15 illustrates the complex effects of ghrelin, leptin, CCK, and peptide YY on hunger and satiety.

ghrelin hormone that stimulates eating behavior

leptin hormone that reduces hunger and inhibits fat storage in the body

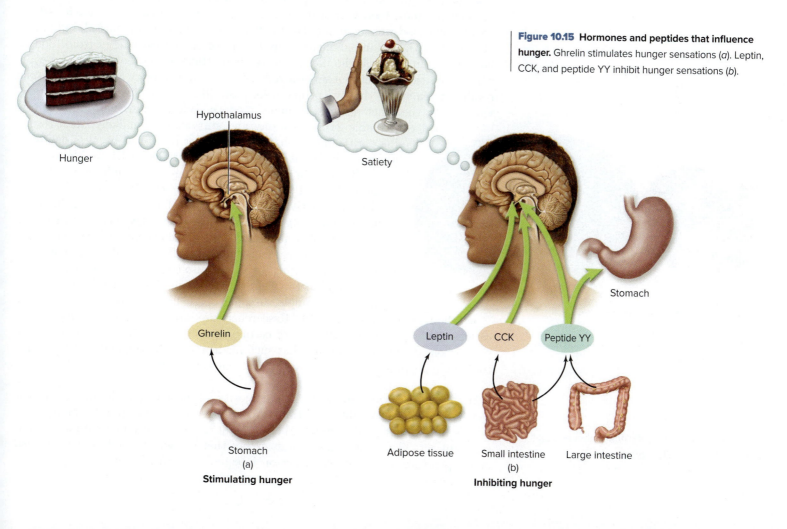

Figure 10.15 Hormones and peptides that influence hunger. Ghrelin stimulates hunger sensations (*a*). Leptin, CCK, and peptide YY inhibit hunger sensations (*b*).

Hunger

Hypothalamus

Satiety

Ghrelin

Stomach

Stomach
(a)
Stimulating hunger

Leptin

CCK

Peptide YY

Adipose tissue

Small intestine

Large intestine
(b)
Inhibiting hunger

Did *YOU* Know?

Prader-Willi syndrome is a rare genetic condition that results from the lack of genes in a particular section of a chromosome. People with this condition have skeletal deformities, delayed motor development, decreased intellectual functioning, food cravings, and insatiable appetites. If their access to food is not restricted, children with Prader-Willi syndrome eat constantly and become obese. There is no cure for Prader-Willi syndrome.

Food Composition Factors

Dietary factors, particularly amounts of fat and certain carbohydrates in diets, can influence body fat production and appetite. Fatty foods are more energy dense than foods that contain more carbohydrate, protein, and water than fat. Thus, high—fat diets are associated with excess calorie intakes and rising obesity rates. However, fatty foods often contain a lot of added sugars. Some medical researchers think the consumption of the simple sugars fructose is associated with the current obesity epidemic. High fructose intakes stimulate fat synthesis in the liver, which contributes to the development of nonalcoholic fatty liver disease.[26] For a more extensive review of the role that carbohydrates may play in weight gain, see the "Are Carbohydrates Fattening?" section of Chapter 5. Chapter 5 also includes information about nonalcoholic fatty liver disease.

Genetic Factors

Genetics play a major role in the development of obesity. Most physical characteristics are inherited, including metabolic rate, hormone production, body frame size, and pattern of fat distribution. All of these characteristics affect body weight.

Some rats and mice are genetically predisposed to become obese because they have inherited genes for "thrifty metabolisms." Rodents with thrifty metabolisms have bodies that are more efficient at storing excess energy as fat than rodents who do not have such metabolisms. It is possible that humans who gain weight easily have genes that code for thrifty metabolisms as well. In ancient times, food was often scarce, and people had to eat as much as they could when food was available. During times when food was plentiful, individuals who had thrifty metabolisms stored more of the excess energy from food as body fat than persons who did not have such efficient metabolisms. The people who lacked thrifty metabolisms wasted the excess food energy as body heat. As a result, the energy—"thrifty" people were more likely to survive periods of starvation than the other persons. In many modern societies, however, high—calorie food is available 24 hours a day and starvation is unlikely. As a result, having thrifty metabolisms is no longer beneficial because depositing excess body fat often results in serious health problems.

If you gain weight easily, you may have inherited a thrifty metabolism. To prevent becoming overfat, you need to be physically active and make careful food choices. On the other hand, you probably do not have a thrifty metabolism if you can eat a lot of food and have difficulty gaining weight.

Medical researchers have identified several genes that contribute to human fatness. Genes also control hormones that regulate growth and metabolism, as well as ghrelin and leptin production. Certain mice, for example, become obese because they lack genes for synthesizing leptin (Fig. 10.16). Researchers are interested in developing medications that regulate the influence of certain genes over metabolism and hormone production. If research indicates that such medications are safe and effective, they could help people manage their weight over the long term.

Figure 10.16 **Genetic obesity in mice.** Certain genetically engineered mice (the mouse on the right) become obese because they lack genes for synthesizing leptin.

What's the Set-Point Theory? The majority of people who intentionally lose weight regain the weight over time. According to the **set—point theory,** the body's fat content (and therefore, body weight) is genetically predetermined. The set point acts like a home thermostat, except that it regulates body weight instead of temperature. For example, a person infected with an intestinal virus tends to

set-point theory scientific notion that body fat content is genetically predetermined

lose weight because he or she has no interest in eating for a few days. During and after recovery, the person generally regains the lost weight. This observation provides support for the set—point theory. Results of studies involving mice support the set—point theory.[27]

When calorie intakes are reduced, blood thyroid hormone levels decline, depressing the normal basal metabolic rate. Additionally, the caloric cost of performing weight—bearing activities decreases when a person loses weight. As a result, an activity that required 100 kcal before weight loss may burn only 80 kcal after weight loss. Furthermore, weight loss appears to make the body become more efficient at storing calories from macronutrients as fat. When a person gains weight and stays at that weight for a while, his or her body tends to establish a new and higher set point. According to the theory, all these changes protect the body from losing weight and explain why weight loss is so difficult to achieve and maintain.

Opponents of the set—point theory argue that weight does not remain constant throughout adulthood: The average person gains weight slowly, at least until old age. Thus, body weight may result more from lifestyle practices and environmental influences than predetermined biological controls such as a set point.

appetite desire to eat appealing food

Environmental Influences

Consider your eating behavior during a typical holiday meal that includes a variety of attractive, tasty foods. After eating the meal, your hunger should be satisfied, but as soon as pie or cake is placed on the table, do you "find some room" in your stomach for some dessert? If you often eat when you are not hungry or when you see a favorite food, then you are probably aware of the effect your environment can have on your appetite. **Appetite** is the desire to eat appealing food.

Food advertising is an aspect of the environment that has a power—ful influence on your food choices. To entice you to buy their products, food manufacturers usually appeal to your senses, emphasizing the appearance and taste of food, in particular. Recently, a television ad for a fast—food chain promoted a hamburger that has three beef patties, three slices of cheese, and six bacon slices topped with mayonnaise. According to information at the fast—food company's website, this burger provides 800 kcal. The site, how—ever, does not tell you that 800 kcal is more than one—third of a day's calorie needs for an average person! How do you respond when you see food adver—tisements on television? Do the ads make you hungry or eager to try a new food product?

Our environment also affects whether we choose to be sedentary or physi—cally active. In our homes, we rely on a variety of "energy—saving" devices such as dishwashing machines, TV remote controls, and garage door openers to work for us. Outside our homes, we use cars, elevators, escalators, and other motor—ized devices, instead of our feet, to move us from place to place. With the help of machines, our lives are considerably easier; however, we are consuming more calories than in the past.

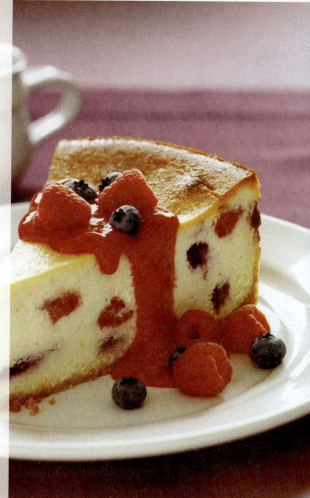

How does the presence of such appealing food affect your appetite? ©Edward ONeil Photography Inc./ iStockphoto/Getty Images RF

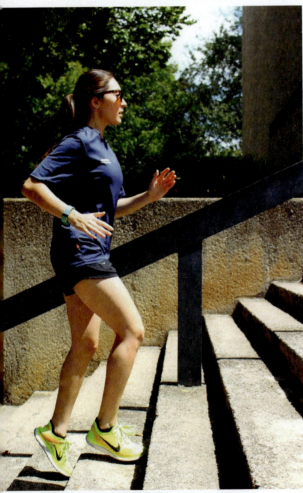

©Elise Westmoreland

In 2013–2014, the average energy intake in one day of American men and women who were 20 to 29 years of age was 2704 kcal and 1993 kcal, respectively.[28] Overall, Americans are consuming more food energy than they consumed in the early 1970s (see Table 1.4). The increase in energy intake may help explain why the prevalence of overweight and obesity has increased among Americans over the past 45 years. According to the principles of energy balance, excess energy intake in relation to energy output results in weight gain.

By becoming more physically active, people can increase their energy output. Many Americans, however, have "desk jobs" that require little muscular movement. When we have some leisure time, we often spend it performing tasks that involve sitting—watching television, playing computer games, or chatting with people on the Internet. Only about 50% of American adults meet recommendations for leisure-time physical activity.[29] According to experts with the Centers for Disease Control and Prevention, healthy adults should perform at least 150 minutes of moderate-intensity physical activity (brisk walking, for example) per week. Adults who include exercise in their weight-loss plan may need to engage in at least 60 minutes of moderate-intensity activity each day to achieve long-term maintenance of lower body weight. ChooseMyPlate.gov has information about physical activity, including examples of activities that are moderate or vigorous.

If you live on or near a university or college campus, your environment probably provides ample opportunities for engaging in exercise and sports, such as tennis courts, swimming pools, and weight-training rooms. It is relatively easy to be physically active while you are in college, *if you choose to be*. After you graduate, consider what you will do to maintain a healthy level of physical activity each day, especially if you have a sedentary job. How likely are you to use the staircase in a building when you see the elevator? Will you keep a pair of comfortable shoes at work so you can walk for at least 20 minutes during lunch?

Genes and Environment: Interactions

It is difficult to determine the extent to which an obese person's genetic makeup or environment contributes to his or her excess body weight. Children are more likely to become overweight or obese if their biological parents were overfat prior to becoming pregnant.[30] This finding appears to support the hypothesis that obesity is an inherited trait. Nevertheless, genes do not control everything about our health, including our weight. Environmental and other factors can modify the expression of genes. For example, children whose mothers are obese may have inherited genes that increase risk for obesity. However, these children may avoid becoming obese if they adopt a physically active lifestyle and do not overeat. On the other hand, these children may become obese if their parents have poor eating habits and sedentary lifestyles and the youngsters follow their parents' practices.

Other Factors That Influence Weight

Psychological factors such as mood and self–esteem influence eating behaviors and body weight. Many people eat not because they are hungry but because they are bored, anxious, angry, or depressed. Obesity may increase the likelihood of depression, especially in American non–Hispanic white women.[32] Researchers, however, cannot easily determine whether being obese causes depression or being depressed causes obesity.

Among some segments of American society, the ideal female figure is slim but curvy, and the ideal male physique is trim and muscular. As a result, societal pressures inspire many young women to idealize underweight. Con–sider the body shapes of many fashion models, professional ballerinas, and successful young actresses. These young women have so little subcutane–ous fat that some of their bones protrude under their skin. In their relentless efforts to pursue such unrealistic body shapes, many young women adopt unhealthy and potentially life–threatening eating practices. The "Nutri–tion Matters" section of this chapter focuses on eating disorders, including *anorexia nervosa.*

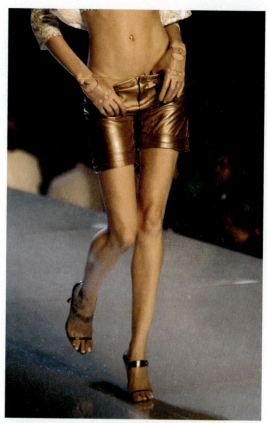

Societal pressures inspire many young women to idealize underweight people, especially thin female models and celebrities. ©Lars A. Niki RF

Concept CHECKPOINT

20. What is hunger? What is satiety?
21. Discuss the roles of leptin and ghrelin in regulating hunger.
22. Under what conditions would having "thrifty genes" benefit a person?
23. What is the set-point theory?
24. What is the difference between hunger and appetite?
25. Describe how the environment influences a person's food intake and physical activity level.
26. Provide at least three examples of ways that physiological, psychological, and environmental factors can influence eating behavior.

See Appendix G for responses.

10.7 Weight Loss and Its Maintenance

Learning Outcomes

1 Identify four key elements that are important for weight loss and maintenance.

2 Describe features of reliable weight-loss plans or programs.

3 Discuss practical steps that overfat people can take to reduce their body fat.

4 Explain what members of the National Weight Control Registry do to maintain their reduced body weights.

Before you embark on an effort to lose (or gain) weight, an important first step is determining whether it is even necessary to change your weight. The need for changing your weight should be based on your overall health and family history of weight–related diseases. If you are dissatisfied with your body weight and shape, consider the following questions. Are you physically healthy at your pres–ent weight? If your BMI is within the healthy range, why do you think you need to lose or gain weight?

Using a BMI calculator (http://www.nhlbi.nih.gov/health/educational /lose_wt/BMI/bmicalc.htm) or consulting a BMI table such as the one in Figure 10.17 that indicates the range of healthy weights for a particular height (BMIs of 18.5 up to 24.9) can be helpful. According to this chart, an adult who is 5−feet, 5−inches tall has a healthy weight range of about 111 to 149 pounds.

To determine your BMI range using the table in Figure 10.17, locate your height in the left−most column with your left index finger, then locate your weight along the bottom line of the graph with your right index finger. Read across the row with your left finger and up from the bottom with your right finger, until your fingers meet. Note the color of the BMI range where the two fingers meet and compare it to the color key in the upper left−hand corner of the figure. According to this graph, is your BMI in the healthy range?

The next step, if necessary, is setting a reasonable and realistic goal weight. It is important to note that an overweight or obese person does not have to shed a lot of weight to reduce risk factors associated with CVD, stroke, and type 2 diabetes. Just losing 5 to 10% of excess weight can increase beneficial high−density lipoprotein levels (HDL cholesterol), reduce elevated blood pressure and triglyceride levels, and improve glucose tolerance.[24]

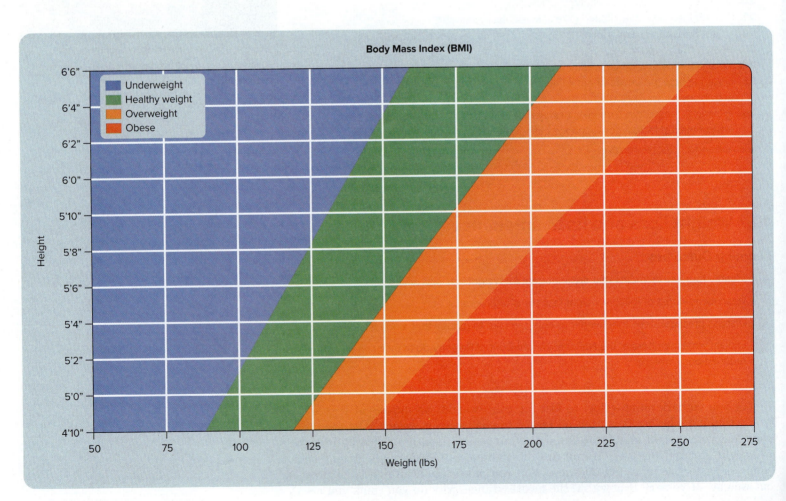

| **Figure 10.17 Adult BMI chart.** Are you at a healthy weight?

Features of Medically Sound Weight-Loss Plans

Table 10.6 presents some important features of reliable weight–loss plans. To lose excess pounds safely, the diet plan needs to be individualized as well as nutrition–ally adequate.[33] Such plans should be safe and effective, as well as flexible enough to meet the person's nutritional, psychological, and social needs. A medically sound weight–loss diet should emphasize a wide variety of low–calorie, readily available nutritious foods and be adaptable to the person's food likes and dislikes. Furthermore, reliable weight–loss plans should provide suggestions for altering environments that foster overeating and sedentary behaviors. Before beginning any weight–loss diet, overfat people should obtain their physician's approval, especially if they have serious health conditions, such as type 2 diabetes.

Key Factors

Despite claims made in advertisements and infomercials, there are no quick cures for overweight and obesity. Key factors for successful weight loss and long–term weight maintenance include motivation, calorie reduction, regular physical activity, and behavior modification.

Motivation

The motivation to lose weight and keep it off requires an overfat person to rec–ognize that there is a need to change his or her behavior and become committed to making those changes permanent. For some people, this recognition occurs when they are diagnosed with a health disorder that is associated with excess body fat. Nevertheless, many overfat people choose not to lose weight. The com–mitment to lose weight and enjoy better health must become far more important than the desire to overeat.

Weight–loss "triggers" often serve as motivators. For some people, seeing themselves in an unflattering photograph, being advised by their physicians to lose weight, or being unable to enjoy activities because being obese restricts their movement triggers the decision to lose weight.

Calorie Intake Reduction

Reasonable calorie intakes for adults who want to lose weight range from 1200 to 1500 kcal/day for women and 1500 to 1800 kcal/day for men.[24] At these calorie intake levels, careful food choices are necessary to obtain nutritionally adequate diets. Certain diets severely limit food intake and provide fewer than 800 kcal/day. Such *very–low–calorie diets* are not recommended without close medical supervision.[24] People who follow very–low–calorie diets may lose a lot of weight rapidly, but they tend to regain the weight quickly after they "go off" the diet and return to their former eating habits.

The healthy way to lower intake of total calories is to reduce consumption of added sugars, solid fats, and alcohol. People can also achieve negative energy states by reducing total calorie intake *and* increasing physical activity.[34]

No particular food has a "metabolic advantage" by promoting greater calorie burning by the body. A dieter's goal should be reducing total calorie intake while obtaining all essential nutrients.

Preparing nutritionally adequate but calorie–reduced meals and snacks can be easier when dietary experts have already done the calculations for con–sumers. For example, MyPlate provides patterns of food choices for 12 different calorie levels (1000 to 3200 kcal/day) that incorporate all food groups (www.choosemyplate.gov/MyPlate–Daily–Checklist). Chapter 3 provides more

TABLE 10.6 Some Key Features of Safe and Reliable Weight-Loss Plans

A safe and reliable weight-loss plan:
• Is safe and effective.
• Meets nutritional, psychological, and social needs.
• Incorporates a variety of common foods from all food groups.
• Fosters slow but steady weight loss.
• Does not require costly devices or diet books.
• Accommodates family and restaurant meals, parties and special occasions, ethnic foods, and food likes.
• Does not make the person feel deprived.
• Emphasizes readily available nutritious foods.
• Promotes changing habits that lead to overeating.
• Encourages regular physical activity.
• Provides suggestions for obtaining social support.
• Can be followed for a lifetime.

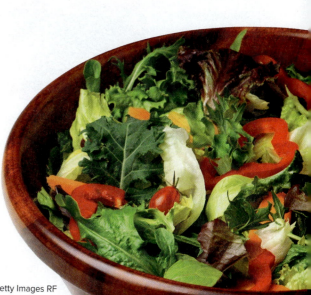

information about MyPlate. For more general information about weight control, obesity, and nutrition, visit the Weight–control Information Network (WIN) at https://www.niddk.nih.gov/. Other reliable sites for weight control information include the Academy of Nutrition and Dietetics at: www.eatright.org.

Eventually, a person who intentionally loses weight by reducing calorie intake and increasing physical activity reaches a weight *plateau*. When this occurs, the individual is in energy balance. To continue losing weight, the person must reduce his or her calorie intake or increase physical activity beyond the present levels. For someone who is consuming only 1000 to 1200 kcal/day, cutting calories even further can lower the metabolic rate, hindering weight loss.

A pound of body fat contains about 3500 kcal. This fact is often used to estimate how changes in caloric intake relate to weight changes: You should lose or gain approximately one pound of weight in a year for every 10 kcal/day reduction or increase of your caloric intake (10 kcal/day × 365 days = 3650 kcal). However, estimating the number of pounds that can be lost or gained in a period of time is not a simple calculation. Factors such as a person's age, weight, height, sex, and physical activity level contribute to his or her rate of weight change over time. According to a new formula, cutting your caloric intake by 10 kcal/day would enable you to lose only about half a pound in one year, and it would take over 3 years for you to lose a pound of weight, after which no further weight would be lost.[35] This formula helps explain why many people who reduce their usual calorie intakes do not lose as much weight as they expect over time and eventually their weight plateaus. To estimate your caloric intake to achieve weight change by using this formula, visit https://www.supertracker.usda.gov/bwp/index.html.

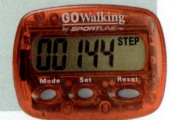
Regular Physical Activity

It is difficult to burn much energy without being physically active. By increas—ing their physical activity level and burning more calories, people do not have to limit their food intake as excessively as they would by relying on calorie reduc—tion alone to lose weight. You do not need to jog for 10 miles to reap the benefits of engaging in regular physical activity. Moderate—intensity activities, such as brisk walking, are recommended for people who want to lose or manage their weight. Chapter 11 discusses the healthful benefits of a physically active lifestyle.

Behavior Modification

Controlling calorie intake and increasing physical activity are easier to accom—plish if overfat persons analyze their faulty behaviors, identify eating *cues* and "problem" habits, and develop ways to change the behaviors. Eating cues are usually environmental factors that stimulate eating behavior, such as seeing an ad for a fast—food restaurant or smelling freshly baked brownies when walk—ing past a bakery. Identifying such cues can enable people to recognize effects of the signals and avoid inappropriate ones, whenever possible. By analyzing their food—related behaviors and habits, overfat individuals can often determine in which circumstances they tend to overeat.

Cues can also help overfat people lose weight. If, for example, you are trying to lose weight, posting an unflattering photograph of yourself on the refrigera—tor or pantry door can serve as a reminder to stay on course with your behavior modification plan.

Although the process may seem slow, people are more likely to change ingrained habits by focusing on changing one behavior at a time. For example, many people snack on energy—dense foods and drinks while watching television. To change this habit, a person could decide to eat only at the kitchen table and avoid all food and beverage consumption while sitting in front of a TV.

For individuals who want to lose (or gain) weight, keeping records of food intake and physical activities can be helpful for estimating daily calorie input and output. However, overfat persons often underestimate their calorie intake[36] and overestimate their energy output.[37] Therefore, people need to record information about food choices and physical activity habits accurately.

Tips for Modifying Food- and Exercise-Related Behaviors   The following suggestions may help a person lose excess weight as well as maintain a lower, healthier body weight.

- **Planning Menus**

  1. Plan meals and snacks to cover three or more days, then use the plan to prepare grocery lists.
  2. When menu planning, include sources of protein, unsaturated fat, and complex carbohydrates in meals and snacks.
  3. Avoid labeling certain foods as "off limits." Depriving yourself of such items can result in bingeing on the "forbidden" food. Learning to analyze why you have difficulty controlling your intake of these foods and developing strategies to learn how to reduce your intake of them can be very helpful.

- **Grocery Shopping**

  1. To reduce the likelihood of making impulsive food choices, shop for food *after* eating.
  2. Shop from a grocery list. If a food is not on your list, ask yourself if you really need to buy it and if it will hinder or help your weight-loss efforts.
  3. Read food labels to compare calorie and fat contents per serving.

- **Food Preparation**

  1. Reduce the use of solid fat in cooking; bake, broil, or roast meats instead of frying them.
  2. Add less solid fat to foods such as cooked vegetables before serving or eating them.
  3. If you sample foods while preparing them, consider the amounts you ate and at mealtimes reduce your portion sizes accordingly.
  4. Prepare only enough food to provide one limited-size portion for yourself. Using measuring cups and a small scale for weighing food can be helpful.
  5. Take your usual-size portion and return one-third to one-half of it to the serving dish or container.
  6. Remove serving dishes from the table. Keeping foods or their containers in sight can encourage overeating.

- **Eating Behavior**

  1. Keep nutrient-dense, low-calorie snack foods, such as fresh fruits and vegetables, on hand.
  2. Eat meals and snacks at scheduled times; do not skip meals, especially breakfast.
  3. Eat all food in a "dining" area; avoid eating while engaged in other activities, such as reading a book, texting, or watching television.
  4. Leave some food on your plate.
  5. Become a "defensive eater." Practice ways to refuse food graciously or request smaller portions. Be aware of people, especially relatives and friends, who *sabotage* your weight-loss efforts. Examples of such sabotage include a person who repeatedly offers calorie-dense foods to you, even though you have turned down the food and this person knows you are trying to lose weight.

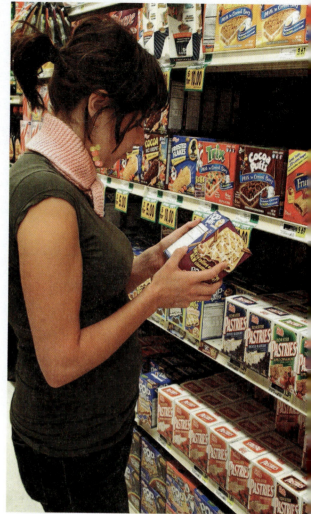

Read Nutrition Facts panels to compare calorie and saturated fat contents of packaged foods. ©McGraw-Hill Education/Andrew Resek, photographer

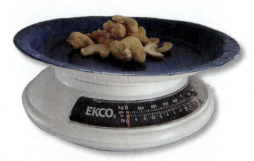

Using a small scale for weighing food can be helpful for limiting portion sizes. ©Wendy Schiff

- When you are hungry, drink some water or fat-free milk or eat a banana, an apple, a few whole dates, or a handful of raisins.

- Skipping meals can contribute to fatigue. Eating a nutritionally balanced breakfast and small between-meal snacks can provide the carbohydrates needed to maintain blood glucose levels.

- Include foods that supply some protein, healthy fat, and fiber in each meal to provide a sense of fullness and satiety.

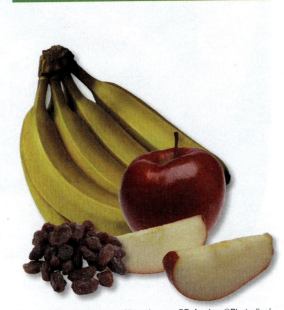

Bananas: ©Brand X Pictures/Getty Images RF; Apples: ©Photodisc/Getty Images RF; Raisins: ©McGraw-Hill Education/Jacques Cornell, photographer

- **Holidays and Parties**

  1. Beforehand, think about what you will eat and drink while attending the event. Practice polite ways to decline food.
  2. Consider limiting your food intake before the special occasion to avoid consuming too many calories for the day.
  3. Eat a low-calorie snack about an hour before the occasion.
  4. Drink fewer alcoholic beverages. Replace alcoholic beverages with ice water or diet soft drinks.

- **Restaurants**

  1. Avoid fried menu items or those made with butter, gravy, or cream sauce.
  2. Choose pasta with red sauce instead of white sauce.
  3. Request salad dressing "on the side" so you can control the amount.
  4. Think "small." Order an entrée and share it with another person.
  5. Do not be a member of the "clean plate club." Ask your server for a carryout container when he or she brings your order to the table. Then divide the food in half, and place one-half in the container. Be sure to refrigerate the leftovers within 2 hours after the meal, and eat them for a meal the following day.
  6. If you choose a dessert item, share it with others.
  7. Avoid eating regularly at fast-food outlets.
  8. When at fast-food outlets, make substitutions, such as a salad instead of a fried fish sandwich, a regular hamburger instead of a specialty burger, or a roasted chicken sandwich instead of a breaded and fried chicken sandwich. Order a diet soft drink or water instead of a regular soft drink. If possible, order a baked potato instead of fries.

- **Physical Activity**

  1. Choose physical activities that you enjoy and can do without the need for expensive equipment.
  2. Increase the time you spend walking each day. Keep walking shoes where you can see them.
  3. Reduce the amount of time you spend sitting. For example, do more household chores yourself.
  4. Take stairs instead of elevators or escalators whenever possible.
  5. Park your car farther from your destination and walk, if you feel it is safe to do so.
  6. Perform calisthenics or lift handheld weights while watching television.
  7. Adopt moderate-intensity activities for your leisure time. For example, join a co-ed volleyball club or take a ballroom dancing class.

- **Self-Monitoring**

  1. Keep a special notebook to use as a food and exercise diary where you can see it—near the kitchen table, refrigerator, or pantry, for example.
  2. In the diary, note the time and place of eating as well as the type and amount of food eaten. Also record who was present and your mood when you ate meals and snacks.
  3. Use the diary to identify your food-related problem areas, such as eating when bored or depressed.
  4. In the exercise section of the diary, record the form of moderate-intensity exercise you performed and the number of minutes you spent engaging in that activity each day. Try to achieve at least 150 minutes of moderate-intensity activities each week.
  5. Measure your waistline weekly and keep a record of the measurements.

6. Weigh yourself at least once a week, preferably at the same time and without clothing. However, do not rely only on your weight as an indication of your progress. Regular exercise often increases muscle mass that can result in weight gain or failure to lose weight. However, adding muscle mass is healthier than maintaining too much body fat.

- **Rewards for New Behaviors**

  1. Plan nonfood motivators or rewards for specific behaviors. For example, "I'll buy a pair of jeans that are one size smaller than what I currently wear and hang them where I can see them," or "I'll buy those earbuds I've wanted when I lose 5 pounds."
  2. Encourage family and friends to provide praise and encouragement for your efforts to manage your weight. Let family, friends, and associates know that you are trying to lose weight and you would appreciate their help and support. Thank them when you receive their praise and support.

- **Changing Negative Thought Patterns**

  1. Do not get discouraged by occasional setbacks; relapses can be expected when changing behaviors. For example, instead of thinking, "I can't lose weight. I'm a failure," say to yourself, "OK, so I lost control and had too much to eat at the wedding. That's to be expected. I just need to get back on track. I'll pull in the reins on my eating for the next day and exercise more."
  2. Think positively about progress. "I didn't lose any weight this week, but I didn't gain any either. I must be losing fat and getting trimmer; those slacks fit better than they did 2 months ago."
  3. Counter negative thoughts with positive statements. "Next time, I'll eat two cookies instead of four. This afternoon, I'll just have to walk a little longer and harder to burn off those extra calories."

Community-Based Weight-Loss Programs

Many communities offer a variety of weight–loss programs. Registered dietitian nutritionists (RDNs) often conduct weight–loss classes at hospitals or universities. If a physician prescribes dietary counseling by an RDN, the patient's health insurance may cover the cost of such treatment.

Some commercial weight–loss programs, such as *Weight Watchers*, have diet plans that have been developed by RDNs. Members who have lost weight while following the plan often conduct local meetings. Before joining any weight–loss program, consumers should obtain answers to the following questions:

- How much does the program cost? Do I pay when I attend meetings? Do I need to sign a contract? If so, for what length of time?

- Do I have to buy special foods or dietary supplements?

- Is nutrition counseling provided? Do the persons providing nutrition counseling and information have degrees in nutrition and dietetics from accredited colleges or universities? How much contact will I have with a counselor?

- Was the diet plan developed by RDNs? Does the plan emphasize the importance of making lifestyle changes, including ways to increase physical activity?

- Does the program's advertising include questionable weight–loss claims and deceptive testimonials?

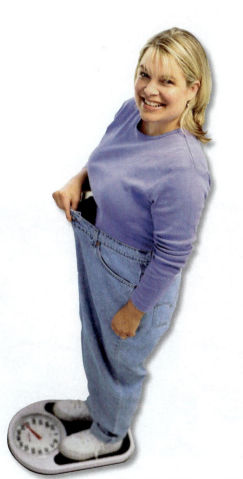

©Ryan McVay/Getty Images RF

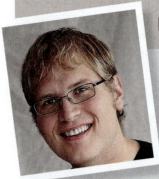

REAL PEOPLE   REAL STORIES

Jan Haapala

Early in 2005, 24-year-old Jan Haapala did not feel well. He slept poorly at night, and during the day, extreme fatigue seemed to be his constant companion. Frequent indigestion added to his general discomfort. Concerned about her husband's health, Jan's wife, Valerie, urged him to see a doctor and have a physical exam. That trip to the doctor's office would prove to be a major turning point in Jan's life.

©Valerie Haapala

During the physical exam, Jan was shocked to learn he had hypertension. The physician prescribed medication to reduce his dangerously elevated blood pressure.

At the time of his doctor's appointment, Jan weighed 335 pounds and his BMI was over 45, which is in the "extremely obese" range. If Jan could not reduce his blood pressure and maintain it at a healthy level, he was very likely to die prematurely. Taking medication can reduce elevated blood pressure and keep it under control, but losing excess fat often cures hypertension, making the medication unnecessary.

Jan was aware that his lifestyle contributed to his extreme obesity. He typically ate two doughnuts and a 20-ounce serving of a sugar-sweetened soft drink for breakfast. Lunches and dinners were "big" meals, often comprised of fast foods, especially double cheeseburgers and large portions of French fries and soft drinks. Candy bars were among his favorite snacks. "I knew those foods were unhealthy, but that didn't change what I ate once I sat down to eat." In addition to his poor food choices, Jan was physically inactive.

After returning home from the doctor's office, Jan made up his mind to improve his health. He recalls, "I didn't want to take medicine to stay alive." Determined to lose weight, Jan heeded his wife's suggestion to join Weight Watchers, one of the oldest and most reliable commercial group weight-loss programs in the country.

Although some people can lose weight on their own, others benefit from participating in group weight-loss programs that offer sensible and safe nutritional guidance, including tips for controlling the size of food portions and increasing physical activity. Group membership also provides emotional support from other members, a factor that is often critical for weight-loss success and maintenance.

By joining Weight Watchers, Jan acquired the information he needed to change his lifestyle to a healthier one. He also developed the motivation to follow a personalized diet and exercise plan that was very different from his past eating and physical activity patterns. In addition to choosing less fatty and sugary foods, he started a walking regimen that eventually became a running regimen. The pounds seemed to melt away from his body, and not long after he began to lose weight, he was able to discontinue taking the medication for hypertension.

When Jan joined the weight-loss program, his waistline measured 46 inches and he wore shirts with a 21-inch neck size. By the time he reached his goal weight of 210 pounds, his waistline was a trim 35 inches and his neck size measured only 15 ½ inches. Although it took 3 years, Jan had lost 125 pounds! The gradual but steady weight loss was an indication that he was making the kinds of behavioral and lifestyle changes that would be permanent.

Today, Jan is "feeling great" and running races from 5Ks to half-marathons. He has even completed his first marathon. His advice to overfat people who are worried about what strangers will think while they exercise: "Don't be embarrassed about doing something in public that's good for you. People won't judge you negatively for trying to become healthier." Clearly, Jan is a role model and inspiration for anyone who is overweight or obese and wants to get his or her weight under control.

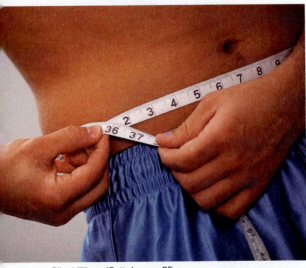

©liquidlibrary/Getty Images RF

Successful Losers: How Do They Manage Their Weight?

The National Weight Control Registry tracks a group of over 10,000 adult Americans, mostly women, who have lost at least 30 pounds and maintained the weight loss for at least 1 year.[38] Information about members' nutrition— and exercise—related practices provides some insights into lifestyle practices that foster losing excess weight and maintaining the lower weight. The majority of registry members:[38]

- eat low—calorie, low—fat diets.
- eat breakfast every day.
- weigh themselves at least once a week.
- exercise, on average, for 60 minutes each day.
- limit television watching to less than 10 hours per week.

Concept CHECKPOINT

27. What are four key elements that are important for weight loss and maintenance?
28. List at least six features of reliable weight-loss plans or programs.
29. What questions would it be wise for consumers to have answered before they join a weight-loss group or plan?
30. List at least three steps that members of the National Weight Control Registry often take to maintain their reduced body weights.

See Appendix G for responses.

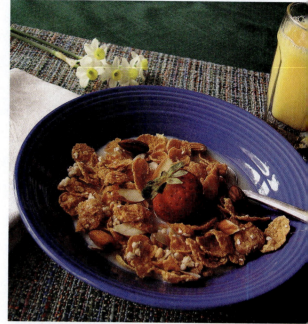

Individuals who lose excess weight and maintain the weight loss tend to eat regular meals, including breakfast. ©Wendy Schiff

10.8 Medical Treatments for Obesity

Learning Outcomes

1. Discuss medications and surgeries that are options for treating obesity.
2. Explain the pros and cons of bariatric surgical procedures.

Obese patients are often unsatisfied with the amount of weight they lose while following fad as well as conventional diets. The frustration of repeated dieting leads some obese persons to turn to physicians for prescription medication and surgical procedures for managing their weight.

Weight-Loss Medication

As of 2015, the U.S. Food and Drug Administration (FDA) has approved a few weight—loss medications that can be prescribed for long—term use, including Contrave®, Saxenda® Belviq®, Qsymia®, and Xenical® (orlistat). Some of these medications suppress or regulate appetite, but orlistat reduces fat digestion by about 30%. The undigested fat is eliminated in the feces and can cause an oily, unpleasant discharge. The fat carries fat—soluble vitamins along with it, and these micronutrients are eliminated in feces as well. Therefore, patients using orlistat often need to take a multiple vitamin supplement. Women who are pregnant or may become pregnant should consult their physicians before using these medications. Although prescription medication can aid weight—loss efforts, their use does not replace the need to reduce calorie intake and increase physical activity.

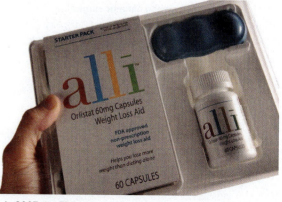

In 2007, the FDA approved sales of the nonprescription form of orlistat (Alli®) as a weight-loss aid for adults.
©McGraw-Hill Education/Jill Braaten, photographer

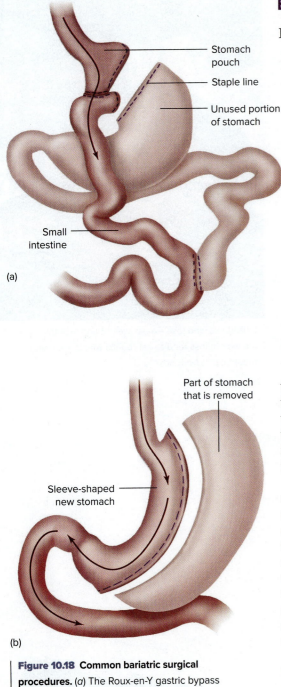

Stomach pouch

Staple line

Unused portion of stomach

Small intestine

(a)

Part of stomach that is removed

Sleeve-shaped new stomach

(b)

Figure 10.18 Common bariatric surgical procedures. (a) The Roux-en-Y gastric bypass procedure. (b) The sleeve gastrectomy procedure.

bariatric medicine medical specialty that focuses on the treatment of obesity

Bariatric Surgical Procedures

Bariatric ($bar-ee-a'-tric$) **medicine** is the medical specialty that focuses on the treatment of obesity. Bariatric surgery can an effective method of treating people who are extremely obese (have BMIs greater than or equal to 40) or have BMIs of greater than or equal to 35 and serious health problems because of their obesity.[24] Such surgical procedures drastically reduce the size of an obese person's stomach, markedly limiting his or her food intake. Patients who have bariatric surgery may lose significant amounts of their excess weight. Most patients, however, regain some weight within 10 years after the surgery.[39] Aside from helping obese people lose considerable amounts of weight and maintain the loss, bariatric surgery can produce dramatic health benefits. Patients often achieve normal blood pressure, glucose levels, and triglyceride levels after surgery. Furthermore, overall death rates are lower for extremely obese people who lose weight after undergoing bariatric surgery. Such surgeries are relatively safe: Fewer than 1% of patients die as a result of a bariatric surgical procedure.[39]

In the United States, two common surgical approaches to treating obesity are the *Roux-en-Y* ($ru-en-wi'$) *gastric bypass* and *gastric banding procedures*. Both of these operations can be performed *laparoscopically*, that is, by using several small incisions that allow surgeons to insert instruments and a video camera into the abdomen. Laparoscopic bariatric surgical procedures reduce recovery time and the risk of infections.

During the Roux-en-Y gastric bypass operation, the surgeon staples across the upper part of the stomach to create a small pouch. This procedure reduces the obese patient's stomach capacity to about 1.5 oz, which is approximately the volume of one egg. (Normally, the stomach's capacity is about 32 oz.) Additionally, the surgeon cuts the small intestine and attaches the lower end of it to the newly formed stomach pouch (Fig. 10.18a). The "bypassed" section of the intestine does not receive food, so digestion and absorption are reduced as a result of the surgery.

Sleeve gastrectomy is another form of bariatric surgery that reduces the stomach's size. During this procedure, the surgeon staples the stomach to form a banana-shaped pouch that holds about 2 to 5 ounces of food. The surgery does not involve bypassing a section of the small intestine, so nutrient absorption is not reduced (Fig. 10.18b). People who have undergone sleeve gastrectomy can eat only small portions of solid foods, which contributes to rapid weight loss. These patients also lose weight because they are not as hungry as they were before having the surgery. Why? The portion of the stomach that secretes ghrelin is removed during surgery, and as a result, hunger sensations are reduced. Sleeve gastrectomy surgery is irreversible because the unused portion of the stomach is removed.

Complications often associated with gastric bypass surgery include intestinal blockage and bleeding, leaks along the staple site, blood clot formation, and wound infections. After surgery, gastric bypass patients can develop micronutrient deficiencies and some bone loss. However, patients can reduce their risk of nutrient deficiencies by taking vitamin and mineral supplements.

By performing the *adjustable gastric banding* procedure, the bariatric surgeon creates the small stomach pouch with an adjustable band instead of fixed surgical staples (Fig. 10.19). By adjusting the tightness of the band, the surgeon determines the size of the stomach. Laparoscopic gastric banding procedure is easier to perform and safer than the other types of bariatric surgery.[39] The procedure is also reversible. However, obese people who undergo the procedure lose weight more slowly and they lose less weight than those who undergo gastric bypass or sleeve gastrectomy procedures.

Bariatric surgeries result in weight loss partly because the stomach pouch fills quickly with food and patients experience satiety sooner than prior to surgery.

Moreover, overeating causes discomfort or vomiting. Thus, people who undergo such surgical procedures must make major lifestyle changes, such as learning to plan and consume frequent, small meals. Engaging in regular exercise and avoiding "soft calories" (energy–dense, high–calorie foods such as milk shakes and ice cream) are also important for maximizing weight loss and maintaining the lower body weight over time.

Other Surgical Approaches

Recently, the FDA approved two unique weight loss devices for certain obese adults. The Maestro Rechargeable System is a rechargeable electrical pulse generator that is surgically implanted under the skin in the patient's abdomen, along with its electrodes and wire leads. The device delivers intermittent electrical pulses to the major nerve that sends messages from the brain to the stomach. This particular nerve is involved in regulating stomach emptying after meals. The nerve also signals the brain to sense that the stomach is empty or full. The patient is able to recharge the pulse generator with a special external charger. According to results of a clinical study, the device helped adult obese patients lose weight, but ongoing research will provide more information about the pulse generator's long–term safety and effectivenss.[40]

In 2016, the FDA approved the AspireAssist device for use in obese persons who have BMIs of 35 to 55 and have been unable to lose or maintain weight using nonsurgical methods, such as reduced–calorie diets.[41] The device is surgically implanted into the stomach and has a tube leading from the stomach to an opening port that is on the patient's abdominal skin. After a meal, the person is able to open the port and drain a portion of his or her stomach's contents into the toilet. As a result, about 30% of the calories that were consumed do not enter the small intestine, and some weight loss occurs.[41] As is often the case, more research is needed to support the use of this device for weight loss among obese people.

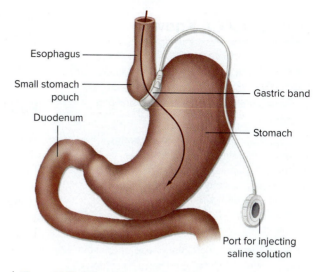

Esophagus

Small stomach pouch

Duodenum

Gastric band

Stomach

Port for injecting saline solution

Figure 10.19 Adjustable gastric banding.

Concept CHECKPOINT

31. Explain how certain prescribed medications can aid weight-loss efforts.

32. Describe common types of bariatric surgery in the United States. Why is bariatric surgery effective? Compared to gastric stapling procedures, what is a major advantage of gastric banding?

See Appendix G for responses.

10.9 Unreliable Weight-Loss Methods

Learning Outcome

1 Identify characteristics of weight-reduction methods that are likely to be unsafe and unreliable.

There are numerous products and services available for adults who want to lose weight. Some overweight or obese people join commercial weight–loss programs that have good track records for encouraging successful weight loss and maintenance. Other overfat persons obtain individual dietary counseling from an RDN to help them lose weight. By recognizing that it took months and probably years to gain

Did *YOU* Know?

According to surveys, 50 to 70% of obese American adults are trying to lose excess body fat.[42] To lose weight, the obese people reported the following actions as being most helpful:

- participation in weight-loss programs,
- eating more fruits and vegetables,
- replacing unhealthy snacks with healthy ones,
- reducing carbohydrate intake,
- limiting portion sizes,
- performing different kinds of exercise, and
- monitoring body weight.

It is interesting to note that obese people did not identify fad diets, liquid diets, "diet foods," or over-the-counter weight-loss products as useful weight-loss tools.

fad trendy practice that has widespread appeal for a period, then becomes no longer fashionable

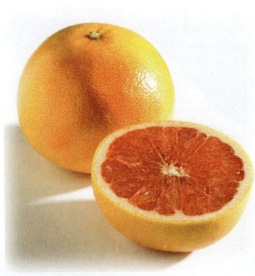

©Purestock/SuperStock RF

the excess fat, individuals may be more likely to accept advice and diets that result in slow but steady weight loss. However, many overweight and obese people seek quick fixes to lose weight, such as *fad* diets and dietary supplements promoted to "burn" or "melt" fat fast.

Fad Diets

A **fad** is a trendy practice that has widespread appeal among a population. After a period, however, people lose interest in the practice, and it becomes no longer fashionable. People often lose weight while following fad diets; however, they usually regain much of the weight that was lost while on the diet when they resume their prior eating and other lifestyle habits. Too often, people think of a weight—loss diet as a temporary change in their eating habits. Achieving a healthy body weight and maintaining that weight requires making lifestyle changes that a person adopts for the rest of his or her life.

Fad diets often rely on *gimmicks*. A gimmick is a novel feature that makes the diet seem to be unique and more likely to work than other diets. Some fad diets use the gimmick of emphasizing one food or food group while excluding almost all others. The cabbage soup and grapefruit diets are examples of fad diets that promote eating single foods. Overfat people may lose some weight while following eating plans that restrict food variety, but the weight loss occurs because the diet is low in calories, not because cabbage, grapefruit, or other "special food" contains compounds that cause rapid weight loss. Following such diets for a few days often results in boredom and monot—ony. Eventually, people who are trying to lose weight abandon such restrictive menu plans because they just cannot face another cup of cabbage soup or bowl of grapefruit. Weight regain occurs when the people return to their former eating habits—the habits that contributed to their original over—weight or obese conditions.

Fad diets will come and go. However, if you examine any diet plan carefully, you can determine whether it is probably a fad. A typical fad diet:

- offers a quick fix; that is, the diet promotes rapid weight loss without calorie restriction and increased physical activity.

- is nutritionally imbalanced. The diet limits food selections from a few food groups and may dictate specific rituals, such as eating only fruit for breakfast or eating only certain food combinations.

- requires buying a book or various gimmicks, such as expensive dietary supplements, weight—loss patches, or cellulite—reducing creams.

- uses outlandish and unscientific claims to support its usefulness. For example, *The Beverly Hills Diet* book promoted the notion that people become fat because food "gets stuck" in their bodies, rots, and produces toxins. Another author of a fad diet book claimed people can lose weight by following diet plans based on their blood types. These notions and recommendations are not supported by scientific evidence.

- relies on testimonials from famous people or connects the diet to trendy places such as Beverly Hills, California, and South Beach, Florida.

- does not emphasize the need to change eating habits and physical activity patterns.

Low-Carbohydrate Approaches

Fad weight—loss diets that limit carbohydrate intakes are high in protein and fat. A weight—reduction diet is low carbohydrate if it eliminates or severely restricts the intake of carbohydrate—rich foods such as breads, cereals, fruits, vegetables, and sweets. The lack of variety often leads to boredom with the selection of foods, and as a result, people lose weight because they tend to eat less.

Low—carbohydrate diets usually produce rapid weight loss initially, primarily because the body loses water. Why? The body produces less glycogen when carbohydrate intake is low and uses much of its stored glycogen to supply glucose for energy. Tissues maintain about 3 grams of water with each gram of glycogen, so a reduction in body glycogen content results in the need for less water to store with it. The kidneys eliminate the excess water in urine. Furthermore, a very—low—carbohydrate intake causes the liver to produce glucose, mostly from certain amino acids supplied by the body's tissue proteins. Protein tissue also contains a lot of water. When protein—rich tissues are dismantled and their amino acids used for energy, the water that was stored with the proteins also ends up in urine.

Not all forms of carbohydrate are unhealthy. Foods that are rich sources of dietary fiber, such as whole grains, beans, and whole fruits and vegetables, are considered to be sources of "high—quality carbs." The human digestive tract digests such foods more slowly than foods that have more refined carbohydrates, which may promote satiety. Eating a low—carbohydrate diet may produce rapid weight loss, but choosing foods that are low in refined carbohydrates and rich sources of less refined carbohydrates may help individuals achieve and maintain a healthy body weight.

An analysis of nearly 50 studies indicated that over the long term, people lose similar amounts of weight regardless of whether they follow a low—carbohydrate or a low—fat diet.[43] Low—carbohydrate diets, however, can result in more favorable high—density lipoprotein ("good cholesterol") and serum triglyceride levels.[44] Recall from Chapter 6 that increased high—density lipoprotein levels and decreased serum triglyceride levels are associated with lower risk of cardiovascular disease.

Very-Low-Fat Approaches

Very—low—fat diets are actually very—high—carbohydrate diets. These diets supply approximately 5 to 10% of calories from fat and generally result in rapid weight loss when followed consistently. The most notable are the Pritikin Diet and Dr. Dean Ornish's "Eat More, Weigh Less" diet plans. Very—low—fat diets are not harmful for healthy adults, but they are difficult to follow for the long term. Fat contributes to the flavor and texture of foods. Extremely low—fat diets are not tasty, and they eliminate many foods that are usually high on peoples' favorite foods lists, such as ice cream and meat. Although grains, fruits, and vegetables are nutrient—dense foods, eating them repeatedly and without fat can cause "diet boredom."

Dietary Supplements for Weight Loss

Many overweight and obese people are attracted to dietary supplements for weight loss because they believe promoters' claims that their products are "magic bullets" for shedding unwanted weight quickly and effortlessly. Although several different types of weight—loss supplements are available, these products generally have not been scientifically tested in humans for safety and effectiveness.

In 2004, the FDA banned the sale of most dietary supplements that contained the natural stimulant ephedra ($eh-feh'-dra$) or ephedra—related compounds, after the agency received reports of serious side effects and even deaths resulting from use of these products. The death in 2003 of Steve Bechler, Baltimore Orioles baseball player, was linked to ephedra (Fig. 10.20). Table 10.7 presents science—based findings about some popular weight—loss supplements, including their potential usefulness and safety concerns. At this point, medical experts do not recommend any dietary supplement for weight loss.[45]

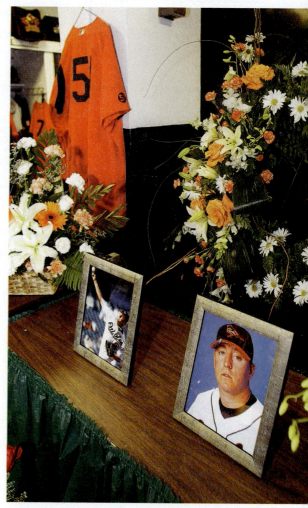

Figure 10.20 Toxic herbal supplement. In 2003, Baltimore Orioles pitcher Steve Bechler's death was linked to ephedra. Bechler had taken a large dose of an ephedra-containing supplement a few hours before he died.

©AP Photo/Roberto Borea

TABLE 10.7 Summary of Selected Weight-Loss Supplements

Supplement	Usefulness	Side Effects/Safety Concerns (Usual Doses)
Bitter orange	May increase metabolic rate and suppress appetite Mixed results concerning weight loss	Some negative effects reported, including chest pain, and increased blood pressure and heart rate
Chitosan	Little effect on weight loss	May cause gastrointestinal discomfort including nausea, constipation, and intestinal gas
Chromium	May enhance weight loss to a small extent	Headache, diarrhea, dizziness
Conjugated linoleic acid	Has minimal effect on reducing body weight	Appears to be safe, but can cause gastrointestinal upset
Ephedrine (ma huang, ephedra, ephedra sinica, sida cordifolia, pinellia, and ephedrine with caffeine)	Ephedrine-containing products promote short-term weight loss but also increase risk of serious side effects. Ephedra-containing dietary supplements are banned in the United States.	May cause rapid heart rate, elevated blood pressure, dizziness, sweating, headache, and sleep disturbances. Linked to heart attacks, strokes, and deaths
Garcinia cambogia (hydroxycitric acid, HCA)	Overall evidence does not suggest usefulness.	May cause headache, nausea, and gastrointestinal discomfort
Glucomannan	Little or no effect on body weight	Tablet forms can block esophagus. Diarrhea, intestinal gas, and abdominal discomfort
Green tea and green tea extracts	May enhance weight loss to a small extent	Contains caffeine Concentrated extracts linked to severe liver damage
Guar gum	Not effective	May cause diarrhea and intestinal gas
Hoodia	Not effective	Can increase blood pressure and heart rate
Pyruvate	Possible but minimal effect on body weight	None reported, but long-term safety is unknown
Raspberry ketone	Lack of scientific support for effectiveness	Unknown
Spirulina (blue-green algae)	Not effective	Unknown
Yohimbe	Not effective	Serious negative health effects including hypertension and rapid heart rate

Source: National Institutes of Health, Office of Dietary Supplements: *Dietary supplements for weight loss.* Updated 2015. Accessed: June 17, 2017. https://ods.od.nih.gov/factsheets/WeightLoss-HealthProfessional/

Analyzing Advertising Hype for Weight-Loss Supplements

Maybe you have heard or read remarkable claims for weight–loss products such as "Lose weight while you sleep," "Lose 30 pounds in just 30 days," and "Eat anything you want and still lose weight." In general, advertising claims that a product promises quick and easy weight loss are too good to be true.

A Federal Trade Commission (FTC) study identified several features, includ–ing typical claims, for popular weight–loss products and services. The agency's report also provided reasons why you should be skeptical of such features when they are used in magazine ads, in television infomercials, or on Internet websites. According to the FTC, you should be wary of claims that the product or service:

- *causes rapid and extreme weight loss.* Ads commonly use outrageous claims such as "Lose up to 18 pounds in one week!" to attract consumers. The use of the modifier "up to" means that the person using the product could lose considerably less than 18 pounds a week.

- *requires no need to change dietary patterns or physical activity.* Principles of energy balance do not support claims such as "Lose weight without dieting or strenuous exercise" and "Eat as much as you want—the more you eat, the more you'll lose." Regular exercise and moderate energy intake are necessary for weight loss and long−term maintenance.

- *results in permanent weight loss.* Claims such as "Discover the secret to permanent weight loss" and "Lose weight and keep it off" often appear in ads. These claims target consumers who have lost weight but gained it back and are wary of weight−loss products. Long−term weight loss is difficult to achieve without calorie reduction and regular exercise, and claims that permanent weight loss can result simply from using a product are questionable.[45]

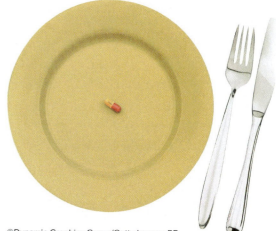

©Dynamic Graphics Group/Getty Images RF

- *is scientifically proven or doctor endorsed.* Some ads claim their product or service has been "clinically tested," "scientifically proven," or "physician recommended." Scientific testing of the product or service supposedly occurred at "respected" or "leading" medical centers or universities. However, most ads do not provide information about testing sites or journals where the results were published. Such information is critical for assessing the reliability of claims. Endorsements by "doctors" or medical professionals can be misleading. A doctor could be someone with a bogus doctorate degree (PhD) or a PhD in a nonscientific field. Moreover, consumers need to be aware that the "professionals" pictured or featured in the ads may be models or fictional characters.

- *includes a money−back guarantee.* Consumers should recognize that a product does not necessarily work just because it is guaranteed. The FTC frequently sues companies that fail to return money to dissatisfied consumers, as their ads guaranteed.

- *is safe or natural.* Ads may include safety−related claims, such as "proven 100% safe" or "safe, immediate weight loss." Additionally, the term *natural* often accompanies safety claims, implying that "natural" weight−loss products are safer than prescribed weight−loss treatments. Despite such assurances, weight−loss supplement manufacturers usually have little scientific evidence to support safety claims, particularly concerning long−term use of their products. Furthermore, "natural" does not indicate safety. Mushrooms are natural, but many species of the fungi are highly toxic and even deadly.

- *is supported by satisfied customers.* Ads for weight−loss products or services typically feature testimonials from satisfied users. The assumption is that if the product worked for the person providing the testimonial, it should work for anyone. According to the FTC, testimonials generally provide little reliable information about what consumers can expect from using the product.

- *displays before−and−after photos.* Many ads use photos of "satisfied" customers to support claims that their weight−loss products are effective. In the typical "before" photo, the subject has poor posture, no smile, unkempt hair, and unfashionable, unflattering clothing. In the "after" photo, the person stands with his or her shoulders held back and abdomen tucked in. Additionally, the subject is usually smiling and appears more attractive than in the "before" photo. If you read carefully, you may find disclaimers in small print, such as "results not typical," at the bottom of the "after" photo.

Did *YOU* Know?

The U.S. Federal Trade Commission can prosecute promoters making fraudulent claims about the effectiveness of their weight-loss products. Enforma Natural Products, Inc., had to pay $10 million in fines after the company used false claims in ads for its "Fat Trapper" and "Exercise in A Bottle" products.

Concept CHECKPOINT

33. What is a "fad" diet? List at least four typical features of fad diets.
34. Why do fad diets and dietary supplements promoted for weight loss appeal to overfat people?
35. Identify at least four popular dietary supplements that are promoted for weight loss, and indicate whether each supplement is safe and effective.
36. Discuss at least three features or claims that are commonly used in ads for weight-loss products or services.

See Appendix G for responses.

10.10 Gaining Weight

Learning Outcomes

1 Explain why some people are underweight.

2 Discuss ways to gain weight safely and sensibly.

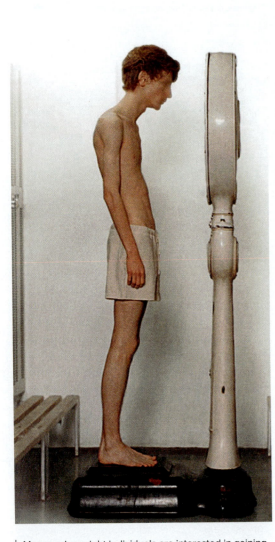

Many underweight individuals are interested in gaining weight, especially muscle mass. ©fStop/Getty Images RF

In 2013–2014 about 2% of Americans who were 20 to 39 years of age were under-weight.[46] An **underweight** individual has a BMI that is less than 18.5. Factors that contribute to underweight include genetics, lifestyle practices, serious chronic diseases, and psychological disturbances.

It is often difficult to pinpoint a cause of underweight; multiple factors contribute to having a lower–than–average body weight. Individuals who inherit higher resting metabolic rates, tall body frames, or both may find it difficult to gain weight. Excessive physical activity can result in low body weight. Compared to sedentary adults, the bodies of rapidly growing, physically active children and adolescents have higher energy needs. If these children do not consume enough energy, they can lose weight. Chronic diseases such as cancer, tuberculosis, AIDS, and *inflammatory bowel disease* often result in severe weight loss that is difficult to treat. Some people who suffer from depression fail to eat enough food to support their energy needs, and they lose weight as a result.

If a person's BMI was within the healthy range before excessive weight loss occurred, an evaluation by a physician may be necessary to determine the cause or causes of the loss, especially when the underweight person has not tried to shed pounds. A thorough medical examination can rule out possible reasons for unintentional weight loss, such as hormonal imbalances, depression, cancer, and infectious or digestive tract diseases.

Many underweight individuals want to gain weight, especially muscle mass. For an underweight person, gaining weight can be just as challenging as losing weight is for an overfat person. To gain weight, underweight adults can gradually increase their consumption of calorie–dense foods, especially those high in healthy fats. Fatty fish, such as salmon; olives; avocados; seeds; low-fat cheeses; nuts and nut butters; bananas; and granola made with dried fruit, seeds, and nuts are high–calorie nutritious food choices with low saturated–fat content. Additionally, underweight people can replace beverages such as soft drinks with more nutritious calorie sources, such as 100% fruit juices, smoothies, and milk shakes made with peanut butter and fat–reduced ice cream. Following a regular meal and snack schedule also aids in weight gain and maintenance.

Sometimes people who are underweight are too busy to eat, and as a result, their caloric intakes are too low to support weight gain. If physical activity habits

underweight describes person with a BMI of less than 18.5

contribute to their inability to increase their weight, underweight people can find ways to be less active. If their weight remains low, underweight persons can add muscle mass through a *resistance−training* (weight−lifting) program, but they must increase their calorie intake to support the additional exercise. Otherwise, gaining muscle tissue is not likely to occur.

In many instances, healthy underweight people may have to accept their body builds. Furthermore, they can realize the health benefits of being lean and the sheer enjoyment of being able to eat a variety of foods without gaining weight. For the typical slim person, the passage of time is usually all that is necessary for weight gain to occur, as the aging process is often accompanied by increasing body fat.

Concept CHECKPOINT

37. List at least three health conditions that are often associated with being underweight.

38. Discuss at least three measures an underweight person can take to gain lean mass safely.

See Appendix G for responses.

10.11 Nutrition Matters: Eating Disorders and Disordered Eating

Learning Outcomes

1 Explain the difference between having an eating disorder and practicing disordered eating.

2 List the major types of eating disorders and their signs.

3 Identify risk factors for eating disorders, disordered eating practices, and the female athlete triad.

4 Describe the health consequences of eating disorders and professional forms of treatment for these conditions.

Many American adolescents and young adults are dissatisfied with their body shape and weight. Among some segments of society, the ideal female figure is slim but curvy, and the ideal male physique is lean and muscular. The media con−stantly bombard consumers with images of the "ideal" body. Television shows and movies often portray thin women or muscular men as happy and successful. As a result, societal pressures inspire many young people to idealize underweight. In their efforts to pursue such unrealistic slender body shapes, young people may adopt unhealthy and potentially life−threatening eating practices. This "Nutrition Matters" focuses on eating disorders and disordered eating behaviors.

Eating disorders are psychological disturbances that lead to abnormal physiological changes and dangerous health complications. An eating disorder is not the same as disordered eating. **Disordered eating** is chaotic and abnormal food−related practices, such as skipping meals, limiting food choices, following fad diets, and bingeing on food. Disordered eating behaviors are temporary, and they often occur when a person is under a lot of stress or wants to lose weight quickly. When a person adopts disordered eating behaviors as a lifestyle, the practices can become harmful and lead to serious eating disorders.

Major Types of Eating Disorders

According to guidelines published in the fifth edition of the American Psychiatric Association's (APA's) *Diagnostic and*

eating disorders psychological disturbances that lead to certain physiological changes and serious health complications

disordered eating chaotic and abnormal food-related practices

TABLE 10.8 Risk Factors for Eating Disorders

Being female
Being an adolescent (AN and BN)
Having a history of frequent dieting
Having a first-degree relative with an eating disorder
Placing a high degree of importance on having an "ideal" body shape
Being dissatisfied with one's body shape
Having a poor self-image and low self-esteem
Having a perfectionist personality
Being from a dysfunctional family
Being teased or bullied about one's weight
Being in an occupation or sport that emphasizes a lean body build

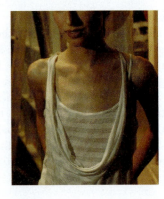

Figure 10.21 Risky occupation. People in occupations that encourage thinness, such as ballet, have an increased risk of developing an eating disorder.
©Lars A. Niki RF

Statistical Manual of Mental Disorders (DSM−5), physicians can diagnose three main types of eating disorders:[47]

- Anorexia nervosa (AN);
- Bulimia nervosa (BN); and
- Binge−eating disorder (BED).

Eating Disorders: Risk Factors There are several known risk factors for eating disorders. These factors include being female, having a poor self−image, having low self−esteem and a perfectionist personality, being in a dysfunctional family environment, and being teased about weight. Table 10.8 lists these and several other risk factors.[48,49]

A person's age is a major factor in predicting his or her risk of a particular eating disorder. Binge−eating disorder is more likely to occur in adults, while AN and BN tend to begin during adolescence.[50] Results of studies of adolescent girls conducted over a long period of time indicated that 13% developed an eating disorder.[51] Factors that contribute to an adolescent's vulnerability to develop AN or BN generally include:

- increases in body weight and size, as well as changes in body shape that normally occur as a teenager develops into an adult;
- greater dependence on peers for their emotional support and social approval; and
- greater freedom from parental control over food choices and eating practices.

Causes of Eating Disorders

The causes of eating disorders are complex and include genetic, biological, social, psychological, and environmental factors. The following sections discuss several of these factors.

Genetic and Biological Factors People who have a first−degree relative (a sister or mother, for example) with AN are 10 times more likely to have an eating disorder than people

who do not have any relatives with AN.[52] Specific genes that modify the brain's ability to regulate moods may have a role in development of eating disorders.[53] More research, however, is needed to clarify how genes affect eating behavior.

Psychological and Personality Factors Mood and anxiety disorders, as well as substance abuse, often accompany eating disorders. It is not clear whether eating disorders cause psychological problems or are the result of emotional disturbances. Furthermore, people with eating disorders typically have a distorted view of their body weight or shape, and they often place a great deal of importance on "ideal" body weight, shape, or specific body parts. Having a poor self−image and being dissatisfied with one's body shape are risk factors for developing an eating disorder.

Other Factors National origin, income level, occupation, and lifestyle choices contribute to the development of eating disorders in people who are vulnerable to developing them. Eating disorders are more prevalent in industrialized, high−income countries such as the United States, Australia, Canada, Japan, and many European nations.[54] Individuals who participate in activities or occupations that encourage thinness such as ballet, acting, and fashion modeling have an increased risk for developing an eating disorder, especially AN and BN (Fig. 10.21). Athletes, especially those participating in endurance running, swimming, and gymnastics, are also at risk.[50] Additionally, athletes who have to "make weight," such as wrestlers and jockeys, have a higher likelihood of developing eating disorders than athletes in sports that do not require low body weight for participation.

Adolescents who are at risk of an eating disorder, such as AN, may develop the condition in response to a stressful life event (a "trigger"). Moving away from home to attend college is an example of a trigger. Additionally, the manner in which a family interacts and functions can increase the risk of developing an eating disorder, especially among adolescents. Teenagers with eating disorders tend to think their parents are more controlling and less affectionate than the parents of healthy youths.[55] In general, individuals with eating disorders describe having a poor emotional connection to their family.

Parents can influence whether their children develop an eating disorder because they play a role in establishing healthy attitudes about body weight and shape, as well as healthy eating practices. Adolescents may model unhealthy behaviors of their parents, especially when the teens' mothers are overly focused on their own weight.[56] Furthermore, parents who tease their children about their body weight may foster the development of disordered eating behaviors.[56,57] On a positive note, parents and other caregivers can play an important role in preventing eating disorders among their children by modeling healthy eating behaviors and expressing a positive attitude toward their own bodies.

The following sections provide more specific information about anorexia nervosa, bulimia nervosa, and binge–eating disorder. We also discuss other conditions that are characterized by unhealthy eating and exercise patterns, and we describe measures to prevent and treat these conditions.

Anorexia Nervosa

It is not unusual for *anorexia*, loss of appetite, to occur when a person is ill. The anorexia generally resolves as the individual recovers. **Anorexia nervosa (AN)** is a severe psychological disturbance characterized by self–imposed starvation that results in malnutrition and very low body weight (*emaciation*). A BMI of 18.5 is the lowest limit of what is generally considered a normal or healthy body weight for adults.[58]

According to estimates, about 0.5% of American females have AN.[59] Although males also develop AN, females comprise three times more cases than males.[50]

Signs and Symptoms People with AN have distorted body images and severely restrict their food intake, which leads to rapid weight loss and maintenance of an unhealthy low body weight. Even when they are emaciated, the patients deny they are too thin, and they are overly concerned or fearful about becoming fat. The fear of weight gain or becoming fat compels people with AN to act in ways that hinder weight gain. These behaviors can include frequent food restriction (dieting), fasting, or exercising excessively.

Some forms of AN involve bingeing and purging behaviors. **Purging** includes activities that limit calorie intake (self–induced vomiting after eating, for example) or increase calorie output by performing more physical activity than is necessary for optimal health. Although AN does not typically involve purging behaviors, when fasting or food restriction becomes difficult to maintain, someone with AN may try to compensate for eating by self–induced vomiting, misuse of laxatives or diuretics, or excessive exercise.[59]

Because people with AN are so thin, they lack adequate amounts of subcutaneous fat to insulate their bodies and have trouble maintaining their body heat as a result. Therefore, individuals with the disorder often wear layers of clothing to keep warm and hide their emaciated appearance. People with AN also have lanugo (*la–new'–go*), which is dense, fine white hair that grows on the face and other parts of the body. Lanugo may help retain body heat. Table 10.9 lists lanugo and some other common signs of AN.

TABLE 10.9 Common Health Consequences of Anorexia Nervosa[60]

Severe constipation
Slow heart rate
Hypotension (low blood pressure)
Loss of normal menstrual cycles (women)
Low bone mineral density
Lanugo (delicate, dense, white hair on the skin)
Low thyroid hormone and decreased metabolic rate
Muscle wasting and weakness

AN has the highest mortality rate of any psychological disorder.[59] As many as 6% of people with AN eventually die as a result of the disorder.[59] Primary causes of death include suicide, heart failure, and alcoholism.[61]

Bulimia Nervosa

Bulimia nervosa (BN) is a severe psychological condition characterized by repeated episodes of binge eating followed by purging, such as self–induced vomiting, to prevent weight gain. **Binge eating** involves consuming an amount of food that is much larger than what a normal person would eat in a brief period of time, such as 2 hours. People with BN feel they have no control over their eating behavior during binge episodes. After a binge, people with BN attempt to prevent weight gain with inappropriate purging methods, such as self–induced vomiting, abuse of laxatives and/or diuretics, fasting, or excessive exercise. As with AN, a major underlying personal characteristic of BN is having a distorted body image.

BN usually begins in adolescence or young adulthood. An estimated 2 to 3% of American females bulimia nervosa.[59] Females are more likely to have BN than males.

Signs and Symptoms Unlike people who have anorexia nervosa, individuals with bulimia nervosa are often difficult to identify by their appearance because they tend to have BMIs in the normal or overweight range (18.5 to less than 30). However, people with BN are often ashamed of their food–related behaviors and attempt to conceal their binge–purge practices from others.

> **anorexia nervosa (AN)** severe psychological disturbance characterized by self-imposed starvation
>
> **purging** activities that limit calorie intake or increase calorie output
>
> **bulimia nervosa (BN)** severe psychological condition characterized by repeated episodes of binge eating followed by unhealthy behaviors to prevent weight gain
>
> **binge eating** consuming a much larger amount of food than is normally eaten in a brief period

People with BN frequently induce vomiting by thrust-ing fingers deep into their mouths and, as a result, scrape their knuckles. Thus, characteristic signs of bulimia nervosa are bite marks and scars on the knuckles. Dentists often identify people who practice bulimic behaviors because the acid in vomit erodes the enamel on the surfaces of teeth, especially the backs of teeth. Eroded teeth develop many dental caries (cavities) and may become chipped and ragged in appearance.

Persons with bulimia nervosa often have low self-esteem and feel guilty or depressed after a binge. Bingeing usually involves eating "forbidden" foods such as cakes, cookies, ice cream, and other high-fat, high-carbohydrate foods dur-ing binges. In cases of BN, different triggers may bring on a binge, including stressful situations, extensive dieting, and negative feelings about body weight, body shape, or food.

The bingeing activities can help the person with BN feel better in the short term; but guilt, emotional distress, and depression persist in the long term and worsen the disorder. The compelling need to binge and purge eventually becomes a preoccupation for people with BN, and as a result, they become less involved in social activities and more isolated.

Some people show behavioral characteristics of both anorexia nervosa and bulimia nervosa because the illnesses can overlap. About half of the women diagnosed as having anorexia nervosa eventually develop signs or symptoms of bulimia.

Health Risks Self-induced vomiting and diuretic abuse can cause fluid and electrolyte imbalances that can be life threatening. Frequent vomiting also causes tears, ruptures, or bleeding of the esophagus and stomach. Someone who abuses laxatives may become dependent on their use in order to stimulate bowel movements. As many as 4% of people with BN die as a result of the disorder.[54] Nearly one in four of these deaths is due to suicide.

Several psychological disorders are associated with BN. Compared to people who do not have an eating disorder, people with BN are more likely to have low self-esteem and bipolar, depressive, and personality disorders. Some people with BN also abuse alcohol or other drugs.

Binge-Eating Disorder

Binge-eating disorder (BED) is an eating disorder that features recurrent episodes of overeating that are not fol-lowed by purging behaviors.[47] As mentioned earlier, binge eating involves consuming a much larger amount of food than most people would eat under similar circumstances in a brief period of time, such as within 2 hours.

In the United States, BED affects more people than the other eating disorders.[60] According to one report, 3.5% of adult American women and 2% of adult American men have been diagnosed with binge-eating disorder.[54]

People with BED can be normal weight, overweight, and obese. Table 10.10 lists typical signs and symptoms of binge-eating disorder.

TABLE 10.10 Common Signs and Symptoms of Binge-Eating Disorder[60]

A person with BED:
• Is extremely distressed over the binge-eating behavior.
• Eats large amounts of food when not hungry.
• Eats more rapidly than normal and eats until uncomfortably full.
• Eats alone because of feeling embarrassed by how much is consumed.
• Feels depressed, guilty, or disgusted with him- or herself after the binge.
• Frequently restricts food intake to lose weight.

People with BED often have other psychological ill-nesses, such as bipolar, depressive, anxiety, and substance use disorders. Furthermore, stressful events and feelings of loneliness, anxiety, depression, anger, isolation, and frus-tration can trigger a food binge. During binges, a person with BED typically isolates him- or herself and consumes large quantities of calorie-dense foods, such as ice cream, cookies, sweets, and potato chips. While bingeing, the per-son may feel better, but after the episode of overeating, the individual usually feels depressed, ashamed, guilty, and disgusted with his or her abnormal eating behavior.

As with the other eating disorders, BED usually begins during adolescence and young adulthood. However, people with BED are usually older than people who have AN or BN.[50]

Other Disordered Eating Behaviors

The *DSM-5* also describes "other specified" feeding and eating disorders, which include less severe versions of the three main eating disorders, as well as a condition called *night eating syndrome*. Physicians use the specific criteria reported in the *DSM-5* to diagnose someone with one of the eating disorders. Some disordered eating behaviors, such as "diabulimia," are publicized in the media, but these unusual food-related practices are not recognized as eating disorders by the APA. The following sections describe night eating syndrome and some popularized unhealthy eating practices.

Night Eating Syndrome People with **night eating syndrome (NES)** experience episodic food binges that are not followed

binge-eating disorder (BED) eating disorder featuring recurrent episodes of binge eating that are not followed by purging behaviors

night eating syndrome (NES) episodic food binges that are not followed by purging; binges take place after the evening meal or when the person wakens from sleep during the night

by purging. These binges take place after the evening meal or when the person wakens from sleep during the night. People with NES are aware of their actions and can recall their overnight eating practices the next day. Approximately 1 to 2% of the general population may have NES.[62,63]

Diabulimia Insulin treatment often causes weight gain in people who are recently diagnosed with type 1 diabetes. Accepting the weight can be difficult for a person who has a poor body image. However, some people with the chronic disease discover they can manipulate their body weight by skipping insulin injections or using less insulin than prescribed. This abusive practice, which affects an estimated 11 to 42% of young women with type 1 diabetes, is often referred to as **"diabulimia."**[64] The signs and symptoms of diabulimia include those that are associated with poorly controlled type 1 diabetes (see Table 5.9). Complications of long-term diabulimia are very serious and can include blindness, kidney failure, hypertension, heart attack, permanent heart damage, stroke, and nerve damage.[65]

Muscle Dysmorphia

Muscle dysmorphia is an unhealthy preoccupation with the body being too small or not muscular enough. This condition occurs almost exclusively in men, and it is common among body builders. More than 50% of men with muscle dysmorphia have used anabolic steroids to help gain weight and increase muscle size.[66] People with muscle dysmorphia exercise obsessively and may lift weights for hours every day. They can become so obsessed with exercise that they continue to train despite injury and they allow exercise to take priority over work, school, and friends. Individuals who have muscle dysmorphia are more likely to be dissatisfied with their lives, abuse drugs, and commit suicide when compared to people who do not have the condition.[67]

Female Athlete Triad

Women and girls participating in competitive sports or sports and activities that benefit from a low body weight, such as gymnastics, dance, and distance running, are at risk of developing one or more components of the **female athlete triad** (Fig. 10.22). This condition is characterized by three interrelated components:

- **Low energy availability** (negative energy balance);
- Menstrual disturbances that often include loss of menstrual cycles; and
- Reduced bone mineral density that may lead to osteoporosis.

As many as 16% of female athletes have all three components of the triad.[68]

Female athletes may restrict their calorie intake to improve athletic performance, lose weight, or maintain a

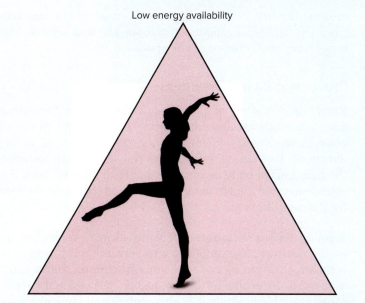

Low energy availability

Menstrual disturbances

Reduced bone mineral density

Figure 10.22 Female athlete triad. Women and girls participating in competitive sports or sports and activities that benefit from a low body weight are at risk of developing one or more components of the female athlete triad.
©Digital Vision/Getty Images RF

lean physique. Other female athletes may lack the appetite, nutrition knowledge, or time to consume enough energy to meet their high needs and maintain a healthy BMI, especially during periods of intense physical training.

Females of childbearing age need adequate amounts of energy to maintain normal menstrual cycles. Low energy availability is associated with a deficiency of the "female hormone" estrogen.[69] The lack of estrogen causes menstrual disturbances, such as longer-than-normal intervals between menstrual periods and absence of menstrual periods. Estrogen is needed to build and maintain bone mineral mass. Female athletes who have low energy availability and no menstrual periods can have low bone mineral density and an increased risk for bone fractures.

When the lack of estrogen occurs during adolescence, a critical time for bone growth, the female athlete's bone

diabulimia popular term used to describe people with type I diabetes who skip insulin injections or use less insulin than prescribed to control their body weight

muscle dysmorphia unhealthy preoccupation with the body being too small or not muscular enough

female athlete triad condition that is characterized by low energy availability, menstrual problems, and reduced bone mineral density in female athletes

low energy availability state of negative energy balance

mineral density may not improve even after she recovers from the triad.[70] Premature osteoporosis is a serious and long—term consequence of the triad.

Preventing Eating Disorders

Early identification of people with risk factors for eating disorders, such as disordered eating patterns and distorted body images, can help prevent the development of eating disorders. Prevention efforts generally focus on fostering the individual's body acceptance, improving his or her self—confidence, and encouraging the person to challenge the idea that being thin is ideal.

Treating Eating Disorders If someone you know has an eating disorder, it is important to encourage the person to seek help as soon as possible to avoid serious health consequences. In academic environments, professional help is often available at student health centers and student guidance or counseling facilities on campus.

It may be difficult to talk with someone who you suspect has an eating disorder. When approaching the individual to discuss your concerns, you can follow these recommendations:[71]

- Meet with the person privately and without distractions.
- Share your feelings and concerns in a caring and supportive manner.
- Describe occasions when you observed behaviors that were signs of an eating disorder.
- Avoid using harsh, judgmental language and instead explain how you feel. For example, instead of stating "You've lost too much weight: You look like you're starving!" say "I feel very worried about how much weight you've lost."
- Do not suggest simple solutions, such as: "If you'd just have meals with the family again, you'd eat and feel better."
- Suggest that he or she discuss your concerns with an expert who treats eating disorders, such as a psychotherapist or RDN. Offer to help find such an expert, make an appointment, or accompany him or her on the first visit.
- Avoid conflict. If the person denies that he or she has an eating disorder, repeat your concerns and indicate that you will be available if the person decides to get help in the future.

- End the conversation by expressing your desire to be supportive. For example, remind the person that you want him or her to be happy and healthy.

A multidisciplinary group of experts in nutrition, mental health, and medicine is necessary for optimal treatment of eating disorders.[50] Treatment should include psychotherapy while also addressing critical nutritional needs and other medical conditions. RDNs play a critical role in assessing and treating eating disorders, including providing nutritional counseling. RDNs can help stabilize healthy eating patterns and improve patients' nutrient status by providing appropriate medical nutrition therapy. Furthermore, experts in nutrition can play an important role in helping patients avoid relapse once recovery is underway.

Treatment for eating disorders can occur in several settings. Inpatient hospitalization or residential care in a facility that specializes in the treatment of the disorders may be required when the patient's medical complications become life threatening. However, eating disorder treatment most often occurs in outpatient care settings. Outpatient care may involve individual, group, or family counseling. Treatment of eating disorders may also include prescription medications. Participation in eating disorder support groups may help prevent relapse.

Cognitive behavioral therapy (CBT) is a major treatment approach for BN and BED.[50] CBT is a general term used to describe psychological therapy approaches that address unhealthy emotions and behaviors. The therapy teaches people healthy coping strategies to use when under stress instead of fasting, bingeing, purging, or excessive exercise.

> **cognitive behavioral therapy (CBT)** psychological therapy approaches that address unhealthy emotions and behaviors

Concept CHECKPOINT

39. Keira usually skips breakfast. Explain whether her behavior is a sign of an eating disorder.

40. List the major types of eating disorders and their signs.

41. List at least four risk factors for eating disorders.

42. What are three serious health consequences of anorexia nervosa?

See Appendix G for responses.

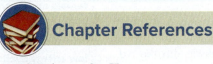

Chapter References

See Appendix H.

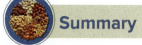

Summary

10.1 The Obesity Epidemic

- The prevalence of overweight and obesity has reached epidemic proportions in the United States and throughout the world. Over 70% of American adults were either overweight or obese in 2013–2014; about 38% of the adults were obese. The prevalence of obesity among Americans has risen sharply over the past 25 years.

10.2 Body Composition

- The body is composed of two major compartments: total body fat and fat-free mass. Overfat people have excessive adipose tissue. Percentage of body fat is associated with risks of obesity-related diseases. Medical researchers use several methods to estimate body composition.

10.3 Energy for Living

- Biological fuels are foods and beverages that contain macronutrients and the nonnutrient alcohol. Under normal conditions, human cells metabolize primarily glucose and fatty acids, but small amounts of amino acids are also used for energy. Cells release the energy stored in biological fuels by breaking bonds within the molecules. Cells obtain only about 40% of the energy that was in macronutrients by forming ATP. Cells release the remaining energy as heat.

- Basal or resting metabolism, physical activity, and TEF account for total energy use by the body. Metabolism accounts for the largest share of an average person's daily energy needs. Various factors including thyroid hormone, body composition, gender, and age influence the metabolic rate. Physical activity is energy use by skeletal muscle movement. NEAT is energy use for involuntary skeletal muscle activities, such as shivering. TEF is the increase in energy needs that occurs during digestion, absorption, and processing of nutrients in food.

10.4 Energy Balance

- Energy balance is a state in which a person's calorie intake from food and beverages equals his or her calorie output for metabolism, physical activity, and TEF. Negative energy balance occurs when calorie output is greater than calorie intake, resulting in weight loss. Positive energy balance occurs when calorie intake is greater than calorie output, resulting in weight gain.

10.5 Classifying Overweight and Obesity

- In addition to percentage of body fat, medical experts use BMI to determine whether one's weight is healthy. BMIs of 18.5 to 24.9 are healthy; BMIs of 25.0 to 29.9 are in the overweight range. Persons with BMIs of 30.0 or more are obese.

- People with BMIs greater than 25 have increased risks of CVD, hypertension, type 2 diabetes, and certain cancers. Compared to people with healthy BMIs, obese people are more likely to die prematurely from all causes. Body fat distribution is associated with obesity-related diseases. Excessive central-body fat (apple shape) is associated with increased risks of CVD, type 2 diabetes, and hypertension. Waist circumferences that exceed 40 inches (men) or 35 inches (women) are linked to obesity-related diseases.

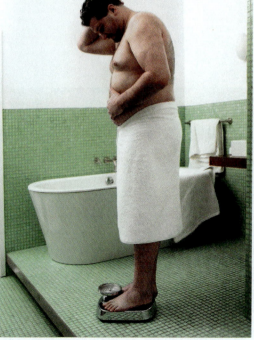

©Digital Vision/Getty Images RF

Nuts: ©C Squared Studios/Getty Images RF

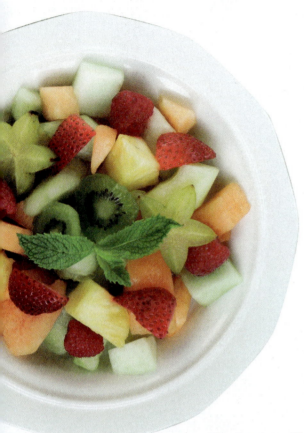

10.6 What Causes Overweight and Obesity?

- There is no simple cause for obesity. From a physiological standpoint, eating behavior is complex and largely involves interactions among the nervous, endocrine, and digestive systems, as well as fat tissue. Dietary and inherited factors also influence body weight. Additionally, overfat people may have inherited genes for "thrifty metabolisms." According to the set-point theory, the body's fat content is genetically predetermined. The set point may protect the body from losing weight and explain why weight loss is so difficult to achieve and maintain.

- Environmental factors can have a powerful influence on food choices and appetite. The environment also influences people's patterns of physical activity.

10.7 Weight Loss and Its Maintenance

- A reliable weight-loss plan is safe and effective, and the plan should meet the person's nutritional, psychological, and social needs. Successful weight loss and long-term weight maintenance involves motivation, calorie reduction, regular physical activity, and behavior modification.

- A pound of body fat contains about 3500 kcal. If energy output exceeds calorie intake, a person can expect to lose weight. A healthy way to lower total calorie intake is to reduce consumption of added sugars, added fats, and alcohol. A goal of a person who wants to lose weight should be reducing total calorie intake while obtaining all essential nutrients.

10.8 Medical Treatments for Obesity

- At present, the FDA has approved a few medications for weight loss. Orlistat can improve weight loss to a small degree, when it is combined with a plan that includes calorie restriction and regular exercise. Bariatric surgeries reduce the stomach volume of people with extreme obesity.

10.9 Unreliable Weight-Loss Methods

- People can lose weight while following fad diets, but they usually regain much of the weight that was lost when they resume their prior eating and other lifestyle habits. Achieving a healthy body weight and maintaining that weight requires making lifestyle changes that a person adopts for the rest of his or her life. No dietary supplement is recommended for weight loss.

10.10 Gaining Weight

- Underweight can be caused by various factors, such as genetics, excessive physical activity, and certain diseases. To gain weight, an underweight person generally needs to increase portion sizes, eat more calorie-dense foods, and reduce physical activity, if excessive.

10.11 Nutrition Matters: Eating Disorders and Disordered Eating

- Disordered eating, involving temporary chaotic and abnormal food-related practices, often occurs when a person is under a lot of stress or wants to lose weight. When a person adopts disordered eating behaviors as a lifestyle, the practices can become harmful and difficult-to-treat eating disorders. Eating disorders are psychological disturbances that lead to behavioral changes and serious health complications. Anorexia nervosa, bulimia nervosa, and binge-eating disorder are the major types of eating disorders. Treatment of eating disorders is complex, involving more than just dietary counseling.

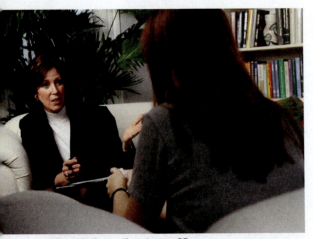

Recipe for Healthy Living

Did You Make That Dip?!

When it's time to entertain your friends, you can make a fiesta dip that will disappear quickly and provide plenty of compliments, too. Fresh cilantro and dried cumin give recipes a distinctive "Mexican" flavor. Bean dip recipes often include canned refried beans and cheeses that are high in fat. This lower-fat version uses canned red beans and reduced-fat cheese. You can save time by using canned fat-free "refried" beans (yes, there is such a product). You can also substitute commercially prepared salsa for the homemade version, but you may find that making salsa with fresh ingredients is worth the extra effort. If you like a hotter salsa, use jalapeño peppers instead of mild green chili peppers. When preparing hot peppers, be careful to avoid touching your eyes or the inside of your nose until after you have thoroughly washed your hands with soap and water. The peppers contain *capsaicin*, the highly irritating chemical used in pepper spray that causes intense burning when in contact with mucous membranes.

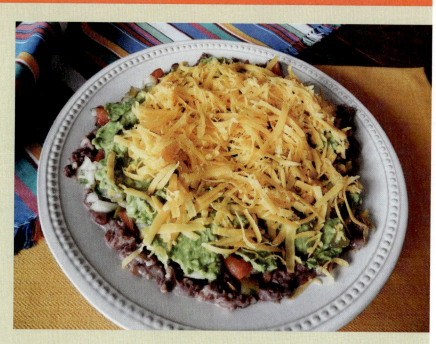

©Wendy Schiff

This recipe makes approximately eight ¼-cup servings. Each serving (without tortilla) supplies approximately 157 kcal, 10 g protein, 5 g fat, 110 mcg folate, 439 mg potassium, 1.6 mg iron, and 5 g fiber.

SALSA LAYER INGREDIENTS:

1 large, fresh ripe tomato
¼ medium onion
1 clove garlic finely minced
1 4-oz can of mild green chilies (peeled and diced)
3 Tbsp fresh cilantro leaves

GUACAMOLE LAYER INGREDIENTS:

1 ripe, black-skinned avocado (slightly soft)
juice of ½ lime
¼ tsp dried cumin (a spice)
⅛ tsp ground black pepper

OTHER LAYERS:

1 14-oz to 16-oz can red beans (no added salt)
1 cup shredded fat-reduced cheddar cheese
⅓ cup fat-free plain yogurt (optional)

PREPARATION STEPS:

1. Set aside an 8" dinner plate.

2. Wash cilantro in cool water and shake off excess water. Wash tomato, avocado, and lime in cool water. Set cilantro and fruits aside on paper towels.

3. Use a sharp knife to *mince* (finely chop) onion, garlic, and cilantro on a cutting board. Place in a small bowl.

4. Add chilies to the onion, garlic, and cilantro mixture. Stir gently until well mixed.

5. *Dice* (cut into small pieces) tomato and add to minced ingredients. You've made *salsa*.

6. To make guacamole, cut the avocado in half lengthwise and remove the round seed. Using a large spoon, scoop out the soft green flesh, and place it in a small bowl. Discard the skin. Dice the avocado into small pieces and sprinkle with lime juice. Mash avocado and lime mixture. Add cumin and black pepper to avocado mixture, stir, and set aside.

7. Drain juice from beans and rinse them with cool water. Mash beans with the back of a large spoon; bean mixture will be lumpy.

8. Spread mashed beans evenly on the plate, leaving about ¾" from the edge of the plate free of beans.

9. Cover beans with individual layers of salsa and guacamole, and top with shredded cheese. If desired, place yogurt in the center as a low-fat substitute for sour cream and top with the cheese.

10. Loosely cover layered dip with clear plastic wrap and refrigerate.

11. To serve, spoon dip on pieces of soft whole-wheat tortillas.

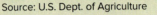

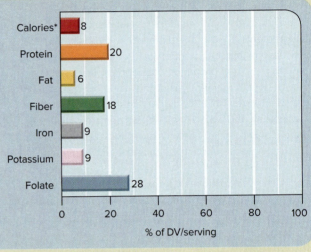

Source: U.S. Dept. of Agriculture

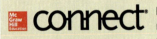 Further analyze this recipe or other recipes through activities located in Connect.

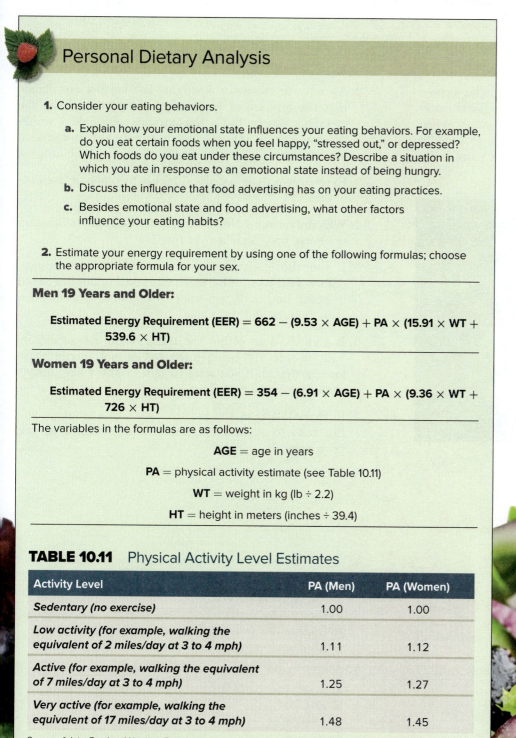

Personal Dietary Analysis

1. Consider your eating behaviors.

    a. Explain how your emotional state influences your eating behaviors. For example, do you eat certain foods when you feel happy, "stressed out," or depressed? Which foods do you eat under these circumstances? Describe a situation in which you ate in response to an emotional state instead of being hungry.

    b. Discuss the influence that food advertising has on your eating practices.

    c. Besides emotional state and food advertising, what other factors influence your eating habits?

2. Estimate your energy requirement by using one of the following formulas; choose the appropriate formula for your sex.

Men 19 Years and Older:

Estimated Energy Requirement (EER) = 662 − (9.53 × AGE) + PA × (15.91 × WT + 539.6 × HT)

Women 19 Years and Older:

Estimated Energy Requirement (EER) = 354 − (6.91 × AGE) + PA × (9.36 × WT + 726 × HT)

The variables in the formulas are as follows:

AGE = age in years

PA = physical activity estimate (see Table 10.11)

WT = weight in kg (lb ÷ 2.2)

HT = height in meters (inches ÷ 39.4)

©iStockphoto/Getty Images RF

TABLE 10.11 Physical Activity Level Estimates

Activity Level	PA (Men)	PA (Women)
Sedentary (no exercise)	1.00	1.00
Low activity (for example, walking the equivalent of 2 miles/day at 3 to 4 mph)	1.11	1.12
Active (for example, walking the equivalent of 7 miles/day at 3 to 4 mph)	1.25	1.27
Very active (for example, walking the equivalent of 17 miles/day at 3 to 4 mph)	1.48	1.45

Source of data: Food and Nutrition Board, National Institute of Medicine: *Dietary Reference Intakes for energy, carbohydrate, fiber, fat, fatty acids, cholesterol, protein, and amino acids (macronutrients)*. Washington, DC: National Academies Press, 2005

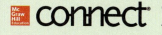 Complete the Personal Dietary Analysis activity located in Connect.

Raspberry: ©Stockbyte/Getty Images RF

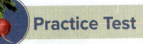

Critical Thinking

1. Kim and Kevin weigh the same and have similar swimming skills. While in a swimming pool, Kim floats easily when she extends her arms and legs in the water. When Kevin extends his arms and legs and tries to float in the pool, he sinks. Why is Kim able to float more easily than Kevin?

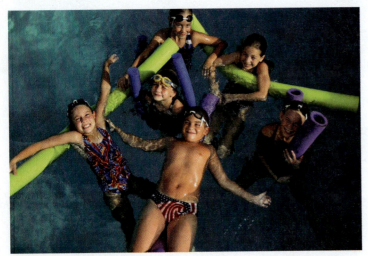

©Scott T. Baxter/Getty Images RF

2. An advertisement for a weight–loss supplement claims that the mixture of herbs in the product increases the metabolic rate by 150%. Explain why you would or would not recommend this product to someone who wants to lose weight.

3. Explain why it is usually difficult to pinpoint a *cause* of obesity.

4. Why are most people who lose weight unable to maintain the lower body weight over time?

5. If your BMI is within the overweight or obese range, discuss your reasons for being interested or not interested in losing weight. If you want to lose weight, what life–style changes will you make?

6. If your BMI is within the underweight range, discuss your reasons for being interested or not interested in gaining weight. If you want to gain weight, what lifestyle changes will you make?

7. If your BMI is in the healthy range, discuss steps you can take to maintain a healthy body weight as you grow older.

Practice Test

Select the best answer.

1. Body mass index (BMI) is
   a. a standard used to calculate a person's body fat percentage.
   b. based on a relationship between weight and risk of chronic disease.
   c. gradually being replaced by more reliable height/weight tables.
   d. a chart used to predict one's caloric intake.

2. _____ cells are specialized to store fat.
   a. Carcinoma
   b. Megaloblastic
   c. Neural
   d. Adipose

3. _____ fat deposits are in the omentum, which is under the abdominal muscles.
   a. Subcutaneous
   b. Visceral
   c. Cellulite
   d. Bulimic

4. _____ relies on the principle that lean tissue is denser than water.
   a. Bioelectrical impedance
   b. Direct calorimetry
   c. Underwater weighing
   d. Air displacement

5. A healthy body fat percentage for women is
   a. 3–10%.
   b. 23–31%.
   c. 32–37%.
   d. 40–50%.

6. _____ raises a person's metabolic rate.
   a. High–fructose corn syrup
   b. Orlistat
   c. Gastrin
   d. Thyroid hormone

7. Basal metabolism includes energy needs for
   a. breathing and circulating blood.
   b. performing physical activity.
   c. digesting food.
   d. absorbing nutrients.

8. Which of the following statements is true?
   a. Women generally have higher metabolic rates than men.
   b. Thyroid hormone levels influence BMR.
   c. A person who has more muscle mass will have a lower BMR than someone with less muscle tissue.
   d. When a person has a fever, his or her BMR drops below normal.

9. Negative energy balance occurs when
   a. the body needs more calories than the diet supplies.
   b. fat storage in the body increases.
   c. energy intake is higher than energy output.
   d. the thermic effect of food equals NEAT.

10. _____ is a hormone that reduces hunger and inhibits fat storage in the body.
    a. Coumadin
    b. Leptin
    c. Ghrelin
    d. Dexadrin

11. Members of the National Weight Control Registry tend to
    a. skip breakfast regularly.
    b. follow low–carbohydrate/high–protein diets.
    c. exercise two to three times per week.
    d. eat meals regularly, including breakfast.

12. Joseph's BMI is 23. When he is under a lot of stress, he eats a large amount of cake, cookies, and ice cream. Soon after eating these foods, he goes to a bathroom and makes himself vomit. Based on this information, Joseph probably has
    a. diarexia psychosis.
    b. anorexia nervosa.
    c. cystic fibrosis.
    d. bulimia nervosa.

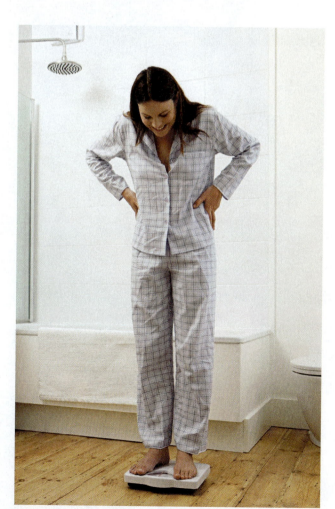

©Image Source, all rights reserved RF

CHAPTER 11

Nutrition for Physically Active Lifestyles

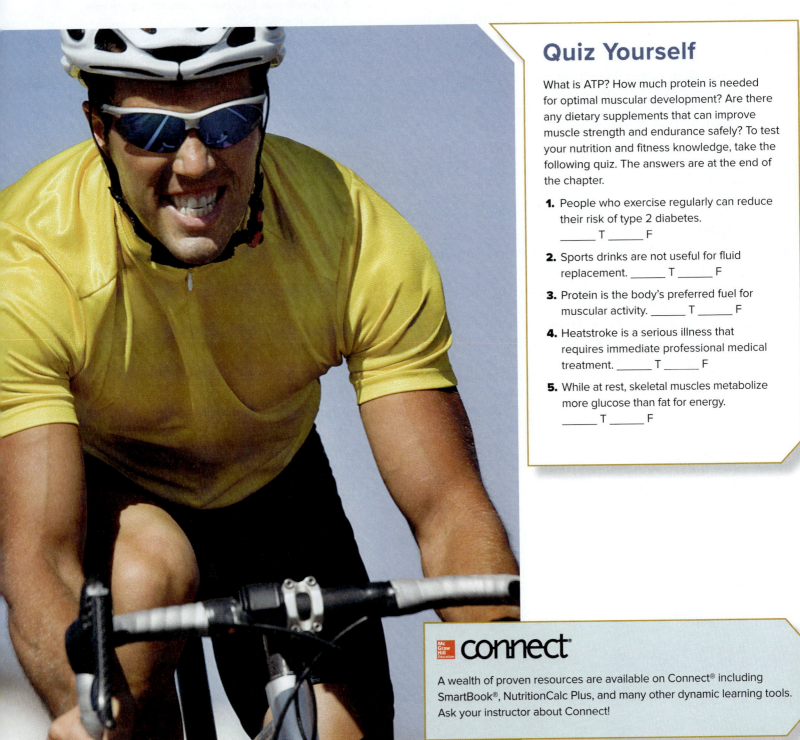

Quiz Yourself

What is ATP? How much protein is needed for optimal muscular development? Are there any dietary supplements that can improve muscle strength and endurance safely? To test your nutrition and fitness knowledge, take the following quiz. The answers are at the end of the chapter.

1. People who exercise regularly can reduce their risk of type 2 diabetes.
   _____ T _____ F

2. Sports drinks are not useful for fluid replacement. _____ T _____ F

3. Protein is the body's preferred fuel for muscular activity. _____ T _____ F

4. Heatstroke is a serious illness that requires immediate professional medical treatment. _____ T _____ F

5. While at rest, skeletal muscles metabolize more glucose than fat for energy.
   _____ T _____ F

connect®

A wealth of proven resources are available on Connect® including SmartBook®, NutritionCalc Plus, and many other dynamic learning tools. Ask your instructor about Connect!

11.1 Introduction to Nutrition for Fitness and Sport

Learning Outcomes

1 Explain the difference between physical activity and exercise.

2 Define *physical fitness*.

3 Discuss recommendations concerning the duration and intensity of physical activity to achieve good health.

Bicycling for weeks through quaint villages and over steep mountains in France; swimming for miles in the chilly English Channel while being buffeted by waves; lifting metal disks that weigh more than the weight lifter—the extent to which some people push their bodies is truly amazing. Superior athletes seem to thrive on performing grueling physical feats that require extraordinary stamina, strength, and energy. Millions of Americans admire competitive athletes for their physical accomplishments and enjoy watching them perform. Many Americans, however, lead *sedentary* lives; that is, their daily activities do not require much muscular exertion. In 2016, almost 50% of Americans who were 18 years of age or older did not obtain recommended amounts of moderate or vigorous physical activity.[1] Even when Americans have the time, many chose not to be physically active.

The human body is designed for **physical activity,** movement that results from skeletal muscle contraction. Most of the physical activities you perform each day are *unstructured*, for example, shopping for groceries or doing house—hold tasks. **Exercise** refers to physical activities that are usually planned and structured for a particular purpose, such as having fun or increasing muscle mass. Both forms of physical activity can benefit your health.

Physical fitness may be defined as the ability to perform moderate— to vigorous—intensity activities for a reasonable amount of time, without becoming excessively fatigued. A *physically fit* person has the strength, endurance, flexibil—ity, and balance to meet the physical demands of daily living, exercise, and sports. Proper nutrition is essential for optimal physical fitness and sports performance.

Regardless of whether you aspire to be a world—class athlete or simply want to be healthier, regular exercise should be a part of your daily routine. Physically inactive people do not have to perform high—intensity structured workouts daily to improve their health. According to recommendations of the U.S. Department of Health and Human Services, healthy adults under 65 years of age should perform:

- moderate—intensity physical activity for 150 minutes a week,

or

- vigorous—intensity (high—intensity) physical activity for 75 minutes a week,

and

- eight to 10 strengthening exercises (eight to 12 repetitions of each exercise) that focus on major muscle groups at least twice a week.[2]

By reading this chapter, you will learn about the benefits of a physically active lifestyle, different cellular energy systems, and dietary practices that are appropriate for athletes and other physically active people. This chapter also provides practical tips for planning an exercise routine that you can follow for a lifetime.

physical activity movement resulting from contraction of skeletal muscles

exercise physical activities that are usually planned and structured for a purpose

physical fitness ability to perform moderate-to vigorous-intensity activities for a reasonable amount of time, without becoming excessively fatigued

Concept CHECKPOINT

1. What is the difference between exercise and physical activity?
2. What is the difference between a physically fit person and someone who is not physically fit?
3. To obtain some health benefits, what is the minimum amount of time an adult should spend engaging in exercise each week?

See Appendix G for responses.

11.2 Benefits of Regular Exercise

Learning Outcomes

1 Describe the health benefits of performing exercise on a regular basis.

2 Describe the physical activity pyramid, and explain how it can be used as a guide for developing a personal exercise plan.

3 Calculate a person's target heart rate range.

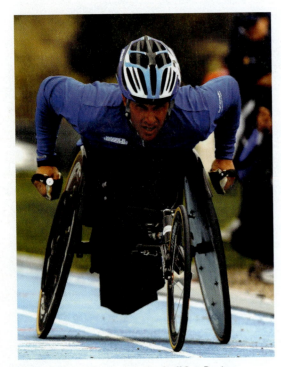

Source: U.S. Air Force photo by Staff Sgt. Desiree N. Palacios

People who exercise regularly can help reduce their risks of serious chronic conditions, including cardiovascular disease, type 2 diabetes, hypertension, obesity, osteoporosis, and certain cancers.[3] Maintaining a physically active lifestyle is one of the most important steps that people can take to improve their health. In 2008, the U.S. Department of Health and Human Services issued the *2008 Physical Activity Guidelines for Americans* (http://www.health.gov/paguidelines/). These guidelines provide evidence−based physical activity recommendations to help Americans reduce the risk of chronic diseases that contribute to millions of premature deaths each year.[4] The *2015–2020 Dietary Guidelines for Americans* support the *2008 Physical Activity Guidelines for Americans*.

Determining the Intensity of Physical Activity

As Figure 11.1 illustrates, you can gain physical as well as psychological benefits by performing moderate−intensity physical activity regularly. Furthermore, you may achieve even greater health benefits by increasing the duration, frequency, and intensity of your exercise routine.

Intensity refers to the level of exertion (physical effort) used to perform an activity. Duration and type of physical activity, as well as body weight, influence the intensity of skeletal muscle movement. Thus, activities such as walking and bicycling can be classified as either moderate−or vigorous−intensity physical activity, depending on the rate at which the activities are performed as well as the weight of the person performing them. Visit http://www.cdc.gov /physicalactivity/basics/measuring/index.html for examples of physical activities that are generally classified as moderate or vigorous intensity.

There are a few ways to determine the intensity of exercise. One way is to judge your level of exertion based on physical signs, such as breathing rate and sweat production. While exercising at the moderate−intensity level, you should be aware of your muscular effort, but you should also be able to chat with an exercise partner comfortably.

A popular method of estimating the intensity of exercise is to use a percentage of your *age−related maximum heart rate*. To calculate your age−related maximum heart rate, subtract your age from 220, the age−related maximum heart rate. (Some experts suggest using a slightly lower age−related maximum heart rate for women.)

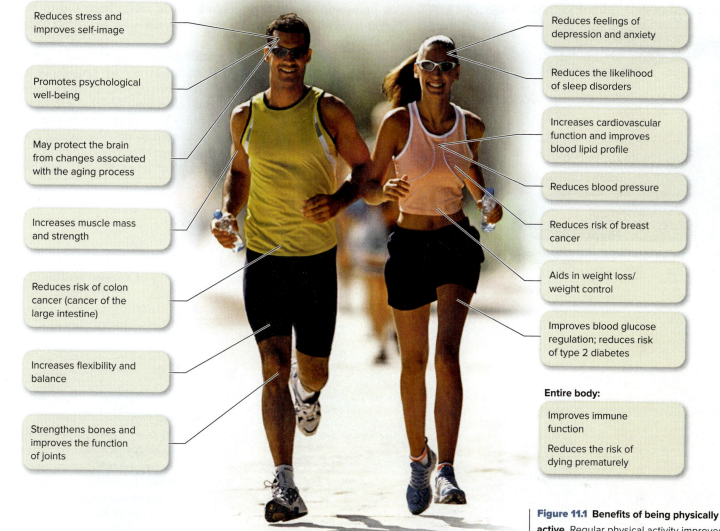

Reduces stress and improves self-image

Promotes psychological well-being

May protect the brain from changes associated with the aging process

Increases muscle mass and strength

Reduces risk of colon cancer (cancer of the large intestine)

Increases flexibility and balance

Strengthens bones and improves the function of joints

Reduces feelings of depression and anxiety

Reduces the likelihood of sleep disorders

Increases cardiovascular function and improves blood lipid profile

Reduces blood pressure

Reduces risk of breast cancer

Aids in weight loss/ weight control

Improves blood glucose regulation; reduces risk of type 2 diabetes

Entire body:

Improves immune function

Reduces the risk of dying prematurely

Figure 11.1 Benefits of being physically active. Regular physical activity improves health in several ways. Couple running: ©Image Source/Getty Images RF

Your **target heart rate zone** is the range of heart rate that reflects the intensity of your exertion during physical activity. For moderate-intensity physical activity, your target heart rate zone should be 50 to 70% of your age-related maximum heart rate.[5] To determine your moderate-intensity "zone," take your age-related maximum heart rate and multiply this figure by 0.50 and 0.70. For example, the age-related maximum heart rate of a 20-year-old person is 200 beats per minute (220 minus 20). Multiply 200 beats per minute (bpm) by 0.50 to calculate the 50% value and multiply 200 bpm by 0.70 to obtain the 70% level. This person's target heart rate zone for moderate-intensity activities is 100 to 140 bpm.

Moderate-intensity physical activities expend 3.5 to 7.0 kcal/min.[6] To "burn" (*oxidize* or *metabolize*) more energy and give your heart a more vigorous workout, you can engage in physical activities that expend more than 7 kcal/min. Such physical activities usually require considerable muscular effort and result in significant increases in breathing rate and perspiration. Examples of vigorous physical activities include jogging, running, aerobic dancing, swimming laps, and bicycling uphill.

To exercise vigorously, your target heart rate should be 70 to 85% of your age-related maximum heart rate.[5] To calculate this range, follow the same formula that you used to determine the range for moderate-intensity activity, except that you need to change "0.50 and 0.70" to "0.70 and 0.85." A 20-year-old person, for example, would have an estimated maximum age-related heart rate of

target heart rate zone heart rate range that reflects intensity of physical exertion

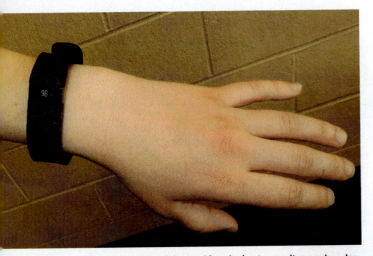

Figure 11.2 Using an activity tracking device to monitor one's pulse.
©Wendy Schiff

200 bpm, and the 70 to 85% levels would range from 140 to 170 bpm. If you have any serious health problems, ask your physician to help you determine your target zone.

You can measure your heart rate (pulse) easily by finding the *radial artery* in your wrist. Locate the radial artery by gently placing your index and middle fingers on the underside of your wrist by the thumb. Count your pulse for 10 seconds, and then multiply that number by 6 to determine your heart rate for 1 minute. Your heart rate begins to decline as soon as you stop exercising, so you need to practice taking your pulse while still working out. By wearing an activity tracking device on your wrist, however, you can easily check your heart rate without having to stop, find your radial artery, and count your pulse (Fig. 11.2).

Physical Activity Pyramid

The physical activity pyramid shown in Figure 11.3 provides practical suggestions for increasing the intensity of various routine activities.

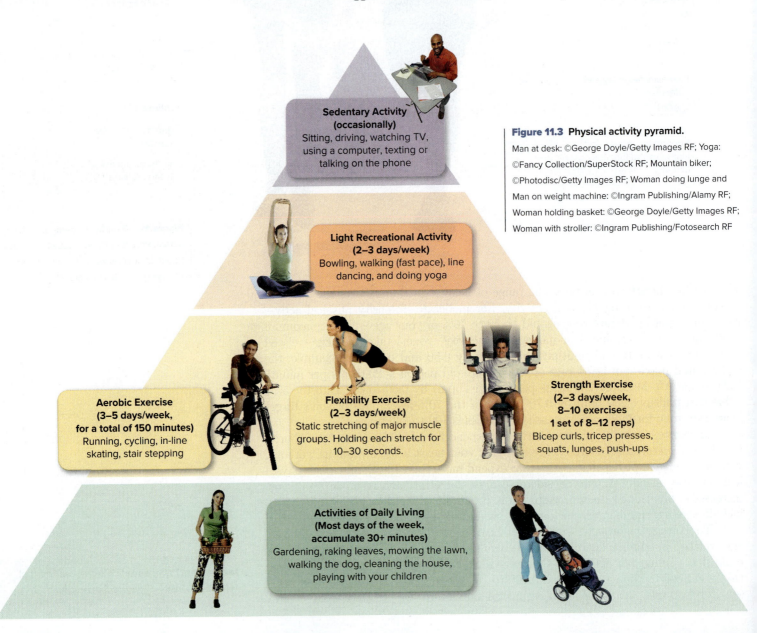

Figure 11.3 Physical activity pyramid.

Man at desk: ©George Doyle/Getty Images RF; Yoga: ©Fancy Collection/SuperStock RF; Mountain biker; ©Photodisc/Getty Images RF; Woman doing lunge and Man on weight machine: ©Ingram Publishing/Alamy RF; Woman holding basket: ©George Doyle/Getty Images RF; Woman with stroller: ©Ingram Publishing/Fotosearch RF

Sedentary Activity (occasionally)
Sitting, driving, watching TV, using a computer, texting or talking on the phone

Light Recreational Activity (2–3 days/week)
Bowling, walking (fast pace), line dancing, and doing yoga

Aerobic Exercise (3–5 days/week, for a total of 150 minutes)
Running, cycling, in-line skating, stair stepping

Flexibility Exercise (2–3 days/week)
Static stretching of major muscle groups. Holding each stretch for 10–30 seconds.

Strength Exercise (2–3 days/week, 8–10 exercises 1 set of 8–12 reps)
Bicep curls, tricep presses, squats, lunges, push-ups

Activities of Daily Living (Most days of the week, accumulate 30+ minutes)
Gardening, raking leaves, mowing the lawn, walking the dog, cleaning the house, playing with your children

For example, you will exert more physical effort and expend more energy if you use stairs instead of elevators or jog instead of walk the dog.

Low—intensity, unstructured physical activities that involve usual daily living activities, such as routine household chores, form the foundation of the physical activity pyramid. The next level of the activity pyramid recommends adding *aerobic* exercise to foundation activities at least three times a week. **Aerobic exercise** involves sustained, rhythmic contractions of large muscle groups in the legs and arms. Such activities raise your heart rate, giving your heart a more effective workout. Running, jogging, rapid walking, and swimming are aerobic activities. Additionally, the second level of the pyramid recommends performing resistance and stretching exercises at least two times a week to increase muscle mass, strength, and flexibility. Resistance exercises, such as weight lifting, can also increase bone mass. The third level of the pyramid encourages regularly performing recreational activities that are physical, such as yoga and line dancing. The top of the pyramid depicts activities that expend little energy, such as watching television or using a personal computer. The pyramid recommends spending little time being sedentary. The "Nutrition Matters" section in this chapter provides information concerning how to design a more formal physical fitness plan.

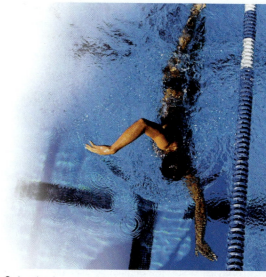

Swimming is an aerobic exercise. ©Ryan McVay/Getty Images RF

Concept CHECKPOINT

4. List at least five health benefits of performing moderate-intensity exercise regularly.
5. What are at least two benefits of performing resistance exercise regularly?
6. Calculate the target heart rate range for a 24-year-old person performing moderate-intensity physical activity.

See Appendix G for responses.

aerobic exercise physical activities that involve sustained, rhythmic contractions of large muscle groups

11.3 Energy for Muscular Work

Learning Outcomes

1. Explain how cells make and use ATP.
2. Discuss how each energy system supplies ATP for muscles and under what conditions a particular energy system functions.
3. Explain how a person can improve his or her aerobic capacity.
4. Discuss the body's use of macronutrients as energy sources.

To move, muscles must contract, and to contract, muscles must have a source of energy. Under normal conditions, most cells, including muscle cells, metabolize a mixture of biological fuels, especially glucose and fatty acids. Muscle cells also metabolize a small amount of amino acids from proteins to obtain energy.

Energy Metabolism

Cells obtain energy by means of a complex series of chemical reactions that progressively break down (*catabolize*) macronutrients and alcohol to release the energy that is stored within them. Cells lose much of this energy as heat, but they capture some of the energy in *high—energy compounds* such as adenosine triphosphate (ATP). ATP forms when an *inorganic phosphate* group (P*i*) bonds

Figure 11.4 ATP. Cells capture and store energy by forming ATP from ADP and inorganic phosphate (P_i).

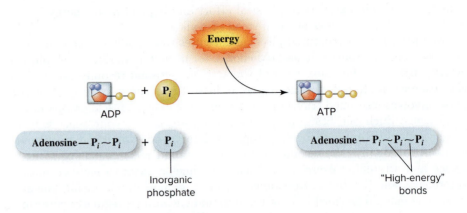

adenosine diphosphate (ADP) high-energy compound; by-product of ATP use

anaerobic conditions that lack free oxygen

aerobic conditions that require free oxygen

glycolysis first stage of glucose oxidation

pyruvate compound that results from anaerobic breakdown of glucose

mitochondria cellular structures that release energy from macronutrients; singular, mitochondrion

Figure 11.5 Obtaining energy.
(a) During glycolysis, the first stage of glucose oxidation, cells degrade glucose into pyruvate under anaerobic conditions.
(b) If oxygen is available, pyruvate undergoes further degradation in mitochondria, forming CO_2, H_2O, and ATP, at certain points.

with **adenosine diphosphate (ADP)** and traps energy in the process (Fig. 11.4). Note in Figure 11.4 that ADP has two inorganic phosphate groups and ATP has three inorganic phosphate groups.

Glucose is the most useful biological fuel because the simple sugar can be catabolized when free oxygen (O_2) is unavailable **(anaerobic)** or available **(aerobic).** Catabolic processes involve *oxidation*, the removal of electrons from compounds to create new compounds. During **glycolysis** (*glyco* = carbohydrate [particularly sugar]; *lysis* = breakdown), the first stage of glucose oxidation, glucose is degraded to form **pyruvate** under anaerobic conditions (Fig. 11.5a). Glycolysis produces a small amount of ATP.

If oxygen is available, pyruvate undergoes further oxidation in a stepwise series of chemical pathways called *aerobic respiration*. Pyruvate moves from the fluid within cells (cytoplasm) into **mitochondria** (Fig. 11.5b). Mitochondria are

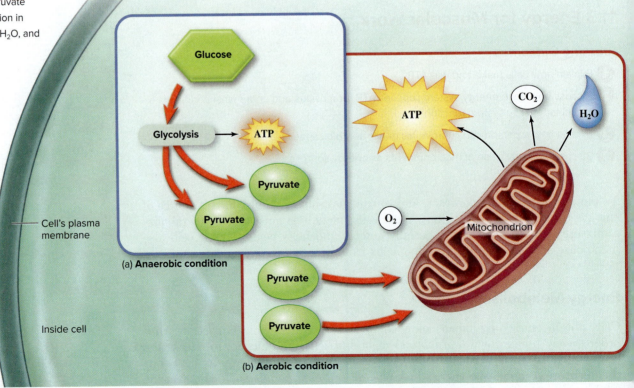

(a) **Anaerobic condition**

(b) **Aerobic condition**

often referred to as "powerhouses" because much of the energy stored in glucose or other biological fuels is released within these cellular structures. In mitochon—dria, pyruvate undergoes complete degradation, and as a result, cells generate more ATP than during glycolysis. Oxygen is a key player in this phase of the process because the element bonds to hydrogen atoms that were released from pyruvate, forming water (H_2O) (see Fig. 11.5b). When cells completely oxidize glucose to release energy, the end products are ATP, carbon dioxide (CO_2) and H_2O. Most of the CO_2 is exhaled, and the H_2O produced metabolically can help maintain proper body water volume. Besides glucose, triglycerides (fat), amino acids, and alcohol are also sources of ATP. Figure 11.6 summarizes the pathways that dietary protein, carbohydrate, and fat follow during energy metabolism. For more detailed illustrations of the metabolic pathways that biological fuels undergo, see Appendix C.

Did *YOU* Know?

Human cells can convert certain amino acids into glucose, but the cells are unable to make glucose from fatty acids.

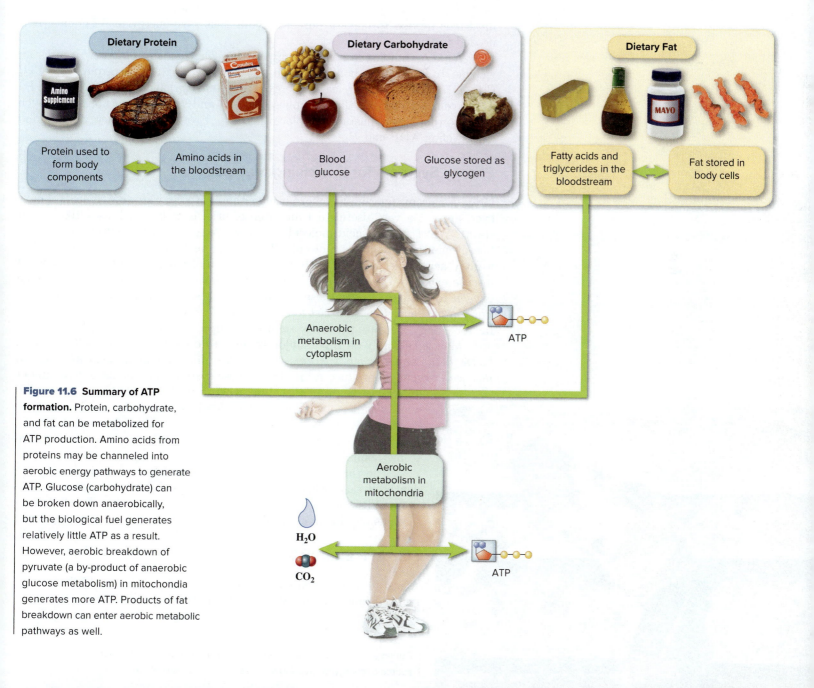

Figure 11.6 Summary of ATP formation. Protein, carbohydrate, and fat can be metabolized for ATP production. Amino acids from proteins may be channeled into aerobic energy pathways to generate ATP. Glucose (carbohydrate) can be broken down anaerobically, but the biological fuel generates relatively little ATP as a result. However, aerobic breakdown of pyruvate (a by-product of anaerobic glucose metabolism) in mitochondia generates more ATP. Products of fat breakdown can enter aerobic metabolic pathways as well.

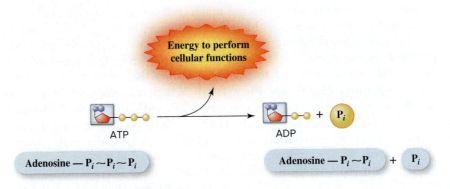

Figure 11.7 Energy from ATP. When a cell needs energy to drive a chemical reaction, it uses an enzyme to break the bond between the last two phosphate groups of ATP, releasing energy and reforming ADP and P_i.

How Do Cells Use ATP?

ATP is the primary source of direct energy for all cells. ATP is often referred to as "energy currency," because it functions like money. Just as you save money until it is needed to make a purchase, your cells save energy in ATP until it is needed to power cellular work.

When a cell needs some energy to drive a chemical reaction, it uses an enzyme to break the bond between the last two phosphate groups of ATP (Fig. 11.7). This process releases energy ($ATP-energy$) and reforms ADP and P_i. Thus, cells can recycle their supplies of ADP and P_i. Cells do not store much ATP, so they must constantly replace their supply of the high−energy compound by recycling ADP and P_i.

Energy Systems for Exercising Muscles

Gram for gram, fat supplies more energy than carbohydrate. Fatty acids, how−ever, are not a very useful fuel for intense, brief exercise, such as a 100−meter sprint. Why? A fatty acid molecule has fewer oxygen atoms in relation to car−bon atoms than a glucose molecule. Thus, cells need more oxygen to metabolize a fatty acid molecule than to burn a glucose molecule. During a brief bout of intense exercise, the heart and lungs do not have enough time to deliver much oxygen to muscles. Under these conditions, glucose is a major source of energy. For physical activities that last longer and are less intense, muscles can use more fat for energy, because the lungs are able to supply them with enough oxygen.

Muscle cells rely on three major systems to obtain energy: the $PCr-ATP$, *lactic acid*, and *oxygen systems*. The PCr−ATP and lactic acid systems do not need oxygen to produce ATP. Thus, these systems metabolize glucose under anaerobic conditions, such as when a person holds his or her breath while sprinting or lifting a heavy load. As the duration of the activ−ity increases, muscle cells need to form considerably more ATP. To meet this demand, muscle cells depend heavily on the oxygen system to metabolize glucose and fat.

The three energy−releasing systems do not function indepen−dently of each other during intense physical exertion; each contrib−utes ATP−energy to power intense muscular activity. The following sections provide more information about these major energy systems.

PCr-ATP Energy System

A resting muscle cell contains only a small amount of ATP that can be used immediately. Muscle cells have another type of high−energy

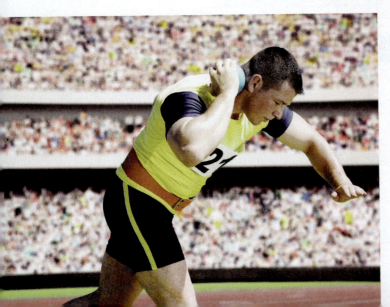

During a brief bout of intense anaerobic exercise, glucose is a major source of energy for working muscles. ©Robert Daly/age fotostock RF

Figure 11.8 PCr. Muscle cells break down PCr into creatine and inorganic phosphate, releasing energy to form ATP from ADP and P$_i$ (a). When the intense activity stops and there is no need to maintain high levels of ATP, an inorganic phosphate group bonds with creatine to recycle PCr (b).

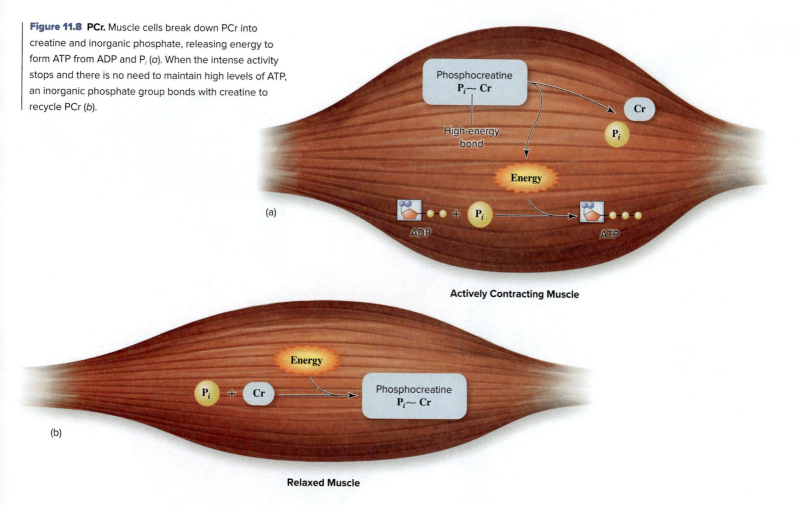

(a)

Actively Contracting Muscle

(b)

Relaxed Muscle

compound—**phosphocreatine (PCr)**—that enables the cells to produce more ATP quickly under anaerobic conditions. To make the ATP, cells break down PCr into *creatine* and P_i, releasing energy to form ATP from ADP and P$_i$ (Fig. 11.8a). Cells do not use PCr directly to power their activities; the compound provides the energy to resupply ATP.

By breaking down PCr to form ATP, muscle cells can obtain enough energy to function during intense events lasting only about 10 seconds.[7] However, the PCr–ATP system can be activated instantly, replenishing ATP fast enough to meet the energy demands of the swiftest and most powerful muscle movements, such as jumping, lifting, throwing, and sprinting. When the intense activity stops and there is no need to maintain high levels of ATP, an inorganic phosphate group bonds with creatine to recycle PCr (see Fig. 11.8b). Muscle cells, however, do not make or store much PCr.

Lactic Acid Energy System

When physical activity lasts longer than about 10 seconds, the PCr–ATP energy system cannot keep up with the demand for energy, and muscle cells must metabolize glucose to generate more ATP. The immediate source of glucose for working muscles is glycogen that is stored in muscles. The liver also helps supply glucose for muscles by degrading glycogen and releasing glucose molecules into the bloodstream.

In anaerobic conditions, muscle cells metabolize glucose to pyruvate and then convert pyruvate to **lactic acid** (Fig. 11.9.1). The degradation of glucose to lactic

phosphocreatine (PCr) high-energy compound used to reform ATP under anaerobic conditions

lactic acid compound formed from pyruvate during anaerobic metabolism

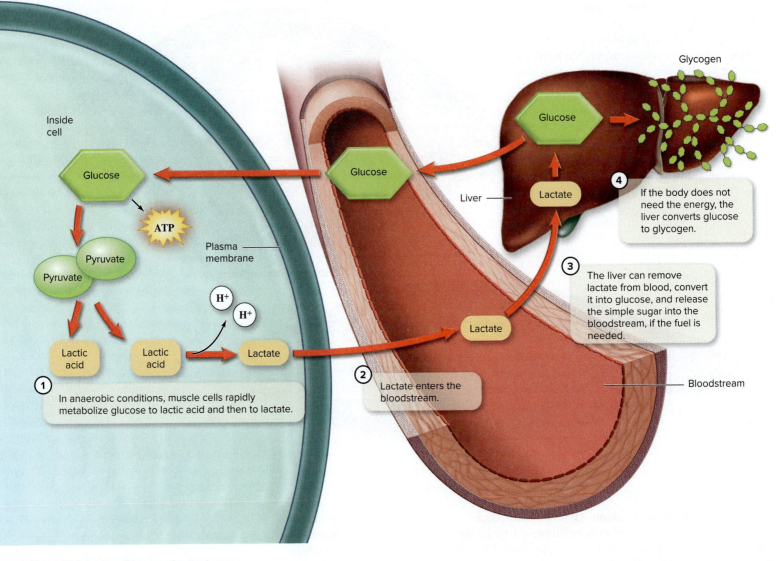

Figure 11.9 **Lactic acid conversion to glucose.**
This illustration summarizes basic steps in which lactic acid can be converted into glucose.

Inside cell

Glucose

ATP

Pyruvate

Pyruvate

Plasma membrane

H+

H+

Lactic acid

Lactic acid

Lactate

1 In anaerobic conditions, muscle cells rapidly metabolize glucose to lactic acid and then to lactate.

Glucose

Glucose

Glycogen

Liver

Lactate

Lactate

Lactate

Bloodstream

4 If the body does not need the energy, the liver converts glucose to glycogen.

3 The liver can remove lactate from blood, convert it into glucose, and release the simple sugar into the bloodstream, if the fuel is needed.

2 Lactate enters the bloodstream.

acid produces a small amount of ATP—only enough to sustain maximum physical exertion for 10 to 180 seconds.[7] Lactic acid accumulates in muscles and converts to a related substance, *lactate*. Although certain muscle cells can use lactate as a fuel, some of the compound enters the bloodstream (Fig. 11.9.2). The liver removes lactate from blood and can convert the compound into glucose (Fig. 11.9.3). The liver may then release the glucose into the bloodstream to help meet muscles' demand for fuel or use the simple sugar to make glycogen (Fig. 11.9.4).

Hydrogen ions (H+) form as a result of the conversion of lactic acid to lactate. The accumulation of H+ in muscle tissue contributes to muscle acidity, a condition that can lead to muscle fatigue and declining physical performance.

Oxygen (Aerobic) Energy System

You would not be able to enjoy activities such as walking at a fast pace, swimming laps, playing a game of soccer or basketball, or other continuous types of physical activity if your muscles depended only on the anaerobic energy systems. When muscle cells have plenty of oxygen, such as during low– to moderate–intensity

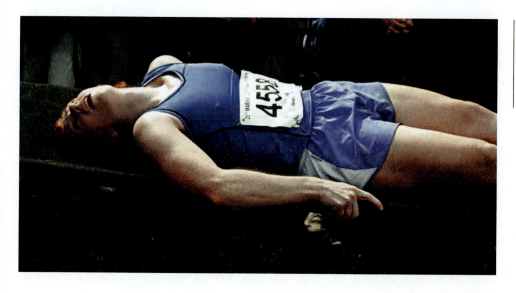

Even well-trained athletes experience muscle fatigue as the time they spend performing intense muscular exertion increases. This marathon runner collapsed as she crossed the finish line of the 28th Annual U.S. Marine Corps Marathon. Source: LCPL Richard A. Burkdall, USMC/DoD Media

exercise, they can metabolize glucose completely to CO_2 and H_2O. In fact, the availability of oxygen enables cells to produce about 18 times more ATP—energy than the amount produced by anaerobic systems.

The oxygen (aerobic) energy system enables muscles to continue working during intense physical activities that last for 2 minutes or longer.[7] The ability to obtain energy aerobically is useful for endurance athletes because it allows their muscle cells to contract repeatedly for hours. Table 11.1 presents various energy sources for resting and contracting muscles.

Aerobic Capacity The ability of your heart and lungs (sometimes referred to as the *cardiorespiratory system*) to deliver oxygen to muscles determines your capacity for intense aerobic physical activity. Scientists can use special equipment to estimate maximal oxygen intake (*aerobic capacity* or *VO_2max*) during vigorous physical exertion. A simple way to determine if you are nearing your aerobic capacity is to engage in vigorous exercise and note when your breathing rate increases to the point that you cannot carry on a conversation.

Did *YOU* Know?

As people grow older, their aerobic capacities decline with each passing decade. By being physically active, however, even elderly persons can maintain a higher degree of aerobic capacity than their sedentary counterparts. It is never too late to begin a training program to improve physical fitness. If you have existing health problems, you should have a complete medical checkup and obtain your physician's OK before beginning a moderate-intensity fitness program. Men older than 40 years and women older than 50 years who plan a vigorous-intensity program should also consult their physician for help designing a safe, effective program.

TABLE 11.1   Energy Sources for Muscles*

Source/System	When in Use	Examples of Activities
ATP	At all times	All types
Phosphocreatine (PCr)	All exercise initially; short bursts of exercise thereafter	Shot put, high jump, bench press
Carbohydrate		
Anaerobic	High-intensity exercise, especially lasting 10 to 180 seconds	200-yard sprint
Aerobic	Exercise lasting 2 minutes to 3 hours or more; the higher the intensity of exercise, the greater the use	Basketball, swimming, jogging
Fat	At rest	Sitting
	Exercise lasting more than a few minutes; low- to moderate-intensity physical activities	30-minute brisk walk
Protein	Low amounts during all exercise, slightly more during endurance exercise, especially when carbohydrate fuel is lacking	Long-distance running

* Note that at any given time, more than one energy system is operating.

Source: Adapted from Wardlaw GM, Smith AM, *Contemporary Nutrition*. 7th ed. New York: McGraw-Hill, 2009.

You can increase your aerobic exercise capacity by engaging in an endurance training program that gradually increases the intensity level of activities. Such training improves your muscle cells' ability to generate ATP rapidly. However, even highly trained athletes experience muscle fatigue after increasing the time they usually spend performing intense muscular exertion.

Fat or Carbohydrate for Fueling Exercise?

The intensity of a physical activity largely influences the relative amounts of fatty acids and glucose that muscles metabolize for energy. Glucose supplies only about 40% of the energy needed to sustain a person who is resting or engaged in very light to light activities, such as watching TV, typing, and walking. Fat is the primary fuel muscles use while resting or engaged in low- to moderate-intensity physical activities.[8] During high-intensity exercise, the rate of fat oxidation decreases while that of glucose oxidation increases. The chart in Figure 11.10 illustrates rough estimates of carbohydrate and fat metabolism during six forms of exercise.

An individual's level of training influences the ratio of glucose to fatty acids that his or her muscles use during exercise. Trained endurance athletes tend to oxidize more fat when exercising at the same intensity than untrained persons.[9] As a result, muscle cells of trained athletes "spare" glycogen; that is, they conserve their supply of glucose. By sparing their glycogen supplies, athletes can enhance their capacity to exercise longer.

Figure 11.10 **Rough estimates of** energy use during exercise. The intensity of an exercise largely influences the relative amounts of macronutrients that muscles metabolize for energy.

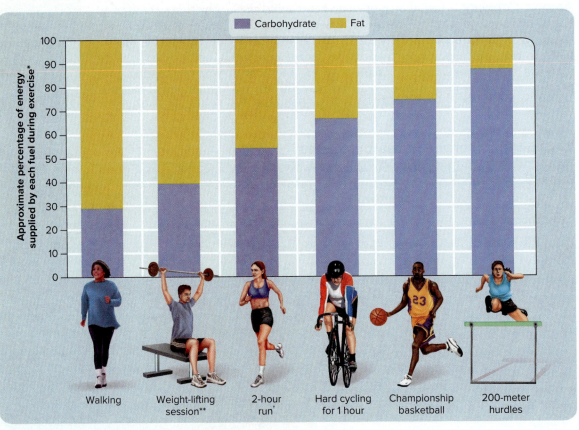

*Protein supplies a minor percentage of energy.
**Fat use generally is higher because much of the time spent weight lifting is for rest periods.
†The values shown are for a runner consuming carbohydrate during the run; more fat and less carbohydrate would be used if carbohydrate was not consumed.

Concept CHECKPOINT

7. How is glycogen used during exercise?

8. How is ATP formed? How do cells use ATP?

9. Explain how each energy system supplies ATP for muscles. Which energy systems operate under anaerobic conditions?

10. How can you improve your aerobic capacity?

11. When is fat a major source of energy for muscles?

See Appendix G for responses.

11.4 General Dietary Advice for Athletes

Learning Outcomes

1 Estimate an athlete's energy, protein, and other nutrient needs.

2 Explain the importance of optimal nutrition for athletes.

3 Identify high-carbohydrate/low-fat foods.

4 Discuss heat-related illnesses, including identification, prevention, and treatment of these conditions.

genetic endowment inherited physical characteristics that can affect physical performance

Athletes often manipulate their diets to lose or gain weight, increase their muscular strength, and prevent or delay fatigue during exercise. Although an athlete's diet plays a major role in determining if he or she finishes first or last in a competitive event, other factors, including genetic endowment and mental and physical training, also influence athletic performance. **Genetic endowment** refers to inherited physical characteristics that can affect an athlete's physical performance, such as body size, shape, and composition. Regardless of how well an athlete eats, if this person lacks the physical traits that are necessary for success in his or her chosen sport, the athlete will find it difficult to compete effectively. Athletes must also be highly motivated to compete and engage in a well-designed intensive training program to maximize their physical capabilities. Nevertheless, optimizing an athlete's diet may provide a competitive advantage, especially for sporting events in which hundredths of a second can mean the difference between finishing first and finishing second.

Athletes and coaches often believe misinformation concerning the value of dietary supplements, certain foods, and fad diets for optimizing physical health and performance. Such beliefs can lead to diet-related practices that are useless and a waste of money. In some cases, these practices are harmful or even deadly.

Sports nutrition focuses on applying nutrition principles and research findings to improving athletic performance. This section provides specific dietary recommendations that are appropriate for athletes and other physically active people. If you would like additional information on sports nutrition, contact a registered dietitian nutritionist. Other reliable sources of sports nutrition include websites of the American College of Sports Medicine (www.acsm.org) and *The American Journal of Sports Medicine*. If you are interested in studying sports nutrition, check with your academic advisor to determine whether your college or university offers sports nutrition courses.

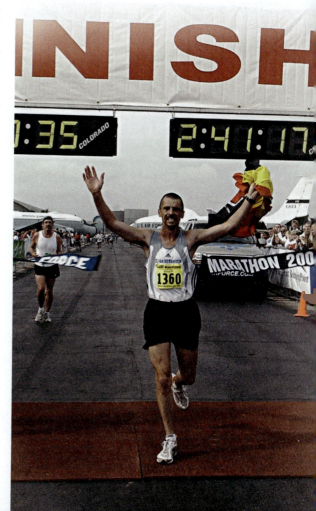

Optimizing an athlete's diet may provide a competitive advantage.
Source: U.S. Air Force photo by Tech. Sgt. Tracy L. DeMarco

TABLE 11.2 Sample Daily 5000 kcal Menu

5000 kcal 62% carbohydrate 21% fat 17% protein
Breakfast
Fat-free milk, 1 cup
Cheerios, 2 cups
Bran muffins, 2 medium
Orange, 1
Snack
Low-fat plain yogurt, 1 cup
Chopped dates, 1 cup
Lunch
Chicken enchilada, with beans and cheese, 2
Romaine lettuce, 2 cups
Garbanzo beans, 1 cup
Shredded carrots, ¾ cup
Chopped celery, ½ cup
Seasoned croutons, ½ cup
French dressing, 2 Tbsp
Whole-wheat bread, 2 slices
Soft margarine, 1 Tbsp
Snack
Banana, 1
Bagel, 1
Cream cheese, 1 Tbsp
Milk, 1%, 1 cup
Dinner
Lean beef, pot roast, 6 oz
Mashed potatoes, with milk, 2 cups
Soft margarine, 2 tsp
Spinach egg noodles, 1 ½ cups cooked
Grated parmesan cheese, ¼ cup
Green beans, 1 cup
Oatmeal-raisin cookies, 3, large
Milk, 1%, 1 cup
Snack
Whole-wheat bagel
Peanut butter, 1 Tbsp
Raisins, ½ cup
Cranberry juice, 1 ½ cups

Energy for Athletic Performance

Compared to nonathletes, athletes generally need more energy to support their physically active lifestyles. Athletes who do not consume enough food energy can lose muscle mass and bone density, experience fatigue and menstrual problems (females), and be at risk of injury.[7] Thus, low energy intakes can hinder an athlete's chances of performing well.

Male athletes who train or compete aerobically for more than 90 minutes daily need at least 50 kcal/kg/day; their female counterparts need at least 45 to 50 kcal/kg/day.[10] Thus, athletes may require 3000 kcal/day or more to support their energy needs and maintain their weight. Table 11.2 presents a sample daily menu that is nutritionally adequate, supplies approximately 5000 kcal/day, and provides ample amounts of carbohydrate.

How can athletes tell if they are consuming enough energy? One way is to have them keep accurate food records and use the information to estimate their daily calorie intakes. Athletes can also monitor their body weights and have their skinfold thicknesses measured regularly. If their weights were within the healthy BMI range before training and they start to lose weight during training, the individuals should consume more food until they regain their pretraining weights. Consuming an additional 500 to 700 kcal/day, especially by eating calorie- and nutrient-dense foods such as nuts and dried fruit, is a healthy way for anyone to boost his or her calorie intake. Athletes who gain too much body fat can increase their energy output by spending more time in training. Overfat athletes can also reduce their food intake by about 200 to 500 kcal/day until they are in the healthy BMI range. In general, a good way to reduce energy intake is to limit portions of fatty foods. Chapter 3 provides general information to help you plan nutritious menus.

For most physically active people, fat should supply 20 to 35% of energy, which is within the range recommended for the general population.[7] High-fat diets are not recommended for athletes. Furthermore, very-low-fat diets (< 20% of total energy from fat) are not beneficial for athletic performance.[7]

Focusing on Carbohydrate Intake

Recommended diets for athletes should supply adequate amounts of energy from carbohydrates. To maintain adequate muscle glycogen, athletes who perform moderate- to vigorous-intensity activity for 1 to 3 hours daily should consume 6 to 10 g of carbohydrate per kilogram of body weight each day.[7] Glycogen depletion is a major cause of fatigue during endurance exercise. By consuming several servings of grains, starchy vegetables, and fruits daily, an athlete can obtain enough carbohydrate to maintain adequate liver and muscle glycogen stores.

To calculate your recommended range of carbohydrate intake for endurance activities, multiply your weight in kilograms by 6 and then by 10. For example, a 145-pound (66 kg) female athlete (endurance) should consume between 396 and 660 g of carbohydrate each day. If she requires 3000 kcal/day to maintain her weight and physical activity level and she consumes 60% of her energy from carbohydrates, she will obtain about 450 g of carbohydrate, which is within the recommended range.

It is important to keep in mind that there is no "one size fits all" diet plan that specifies amounts of carbohydrate-rich foods for pre-event, event, or post-event meals and snacks. Diets for athletes should be individualized and based on factors such as the athlete's sex, body size and weight, sport and training level, and exposure to environmental conditions, as well as personal experiences and food preferences.[7] Furthermore, athletes should test any dietary strategies during practices or trials several days or weeks before a competitive event.

TABLE 11.3 High-Carbohydrate, Low-Fat Pre-Event Meals

Meal A	Meal B	Meal C
Instant oatmeal, cinnamon-flavored, 2 packets Fat-free milk, 8 oz	Pasta salad, 1½ cups French bread, 4 ounces Soft margarine, 1 Tbsp	Cornflakes, ready-to-eat cereal, 1½ cup Fat-free milk, 8 oz Banana, medium
Canned peaches, light syrup, sliced, 1 cup	Apple juice, 8 oz	Orange juice, 8 oz
Orange juice, 8 oz Raisin bread, toasted 2 slices Soft margarine Jelly, 2 Tbsp	Frozen yogurt, 1 cup	English muffin, toasted Soft margarine, 1 Tbsp Jelly, 2 Tbsp Nutty energy bar*

*See this chapter's "Recipe for Healthy Living."

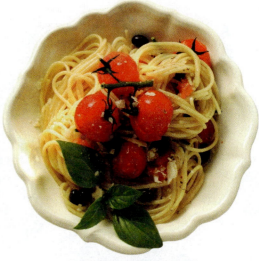

©FoodCollection/StockFood RF

Pre-Event Meals and Snacks

About 1 to 4 hours before competing in events lasting longer than 1 hour, athletes should consider eating a meal that supplies 1 to 4 g of carbohydrate per kg of body weight because such meals can improve performance.[7] Table 11.3 provides some menu ideas for high-carbohydrate, low-fat pre-event meals that supply approximately 200 g of carbohydrate. Eating fatty foods such as sausage, bacon, sauces, and gravies is not recommended because they may contribute to intestinal discomfort while competing.[7] Although some nutritionists advise athletes to exclude high-fiber foods from pre-event meals, there is a lack of scientific evidence to support this recommendation. Nevertheless, athletes can have different responses to eating high-fiber diets prior to events; individuals who react negatively may find it necessary to avoid eating high-fiber foods until after competing.

High-carbohydrate, low-fat food choices for pre-event meals or snacks include cereal with fat-free milk, bagels, dried fruit, pretzels and a sports drink, cooked oatmeal with fruit, pasta, baked potato topped with yogurt, and toasted bread with jelly. Table 11.4 presents commonly eaten foods that are high in

TABLE 11.4 Energy and Macronutrient Contents of Selected Foods

Food and Amount	kcal	Carbohydrate (g)	Protein (g)	Fat (g)
Macaroni, plain, cooked, 1 cup	220	42.95	8.06	1.29
Spaghetti with sauce, meatless, 1 cup	293	47.47	8.93	7.14
Rice, instant, white, cooked, 1 cup	204	44.22	4.22	0.44
Egg noodles, cooked, 1 cup	219	40.02	7.22	3.30
Baked potato, with peel, ½ large	138	31.40	3.71	0.19
Corn, canned, drained, 1 cup	140	23.52	3.79	5.42
Bagel, ½, regular	139	27.50	5.54	0.69
Banana, 1 med. (approx. 7" long)	105	26.95	1.29	0.39
Crackers, 6 rectangular saltines	150	26.66	3.41	3.11
Orange juice, unsweetened, 1 cup	104	24.90	1.69	0.17
Cornflakes, 1 cup	150	31.79	3.57	1.94
Pretzels, 1 cup	173	36.18	4.52	1.32

Source: U.S. Department of Agriculture, What's in the food you eat Search *Tool*, 2013–2014. https://www.ars.usda.gov /northeast-area/beltsville-md/beltsville-human-nutrition-research-center/food-surveys-research-group/docs/whats-in -the-foods-you-eat-emsearch-toolem/ Accessed: June 20, 2017.

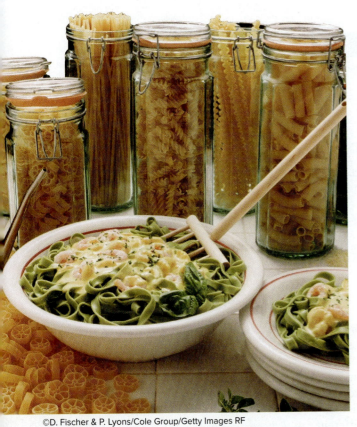

©D. Fischer & P. Lyons/Cole Group/Getty Images RF

carbohydrate and relatively low in fat. Food eaten about an hour before competing should be blended or liquid to promote rapid stomach emptying. Examples of such foods are low–fat smoothies or liquid meal–replacement formulas, such as "instant breakfast" products.

What Is Carbohydrate (Glycogen) Loading? A healthy person stores about 6 g of glycogen per kilogram of body weight. Therefore, an individual who weighs 165 pounds (75 kg) stores about 450 g of glycogen. This amount of glycogen supplies 1800 kcal, which is enough energy to enable the person to bicycle at 13 mph for about 4 hours and 15 minutes. Endurance athletes who have more muscle glycogen at the start of an event may be able to exercise longer than those who do not have as much muscle glycogen. **Carbohydrate (glycogen) loading** involves manipulating dietary and physical activity patterns 3 to 7 days before an event to increase muscle glycogen stores well above the normal range. The practice helps delay fatigue in athletes participating in events lasting more than 90 minutes.[7]

About 3 g of water are incorporated into muscle tissue along with each gram of glycogen. Thus, carbohydrate loading adds water to muscles. Although this fluid aids in maintaining proper hydration status, some individuals experience muscle stiffness and unwanted weight gain as a result of carbohydrate loading. Table 11.5 presents the classic 7–day method of carbohydrate loading and two modified versions. Athletes who would like to determine whether a carbohydrate–loading regimen helps their performance should try one of the regimens during training to

TABLE 11.5 Carbohydrate Loading: Comparing 7-Day Methods

Day	Classic Method	Modified Method 1	Modified Method 2
1	**Exercise:** Depletion **Diet:** Low carbohydrate	**Exercise:** Depletion **Diet:** High carbohydrate	**Exercise:** Tapering (reduced physical activity) **Diet:** Moderate carbohydrate
2	**Exercise:** Tapering **Diet:** Low carbohydrate	**Exercise:** Tapering followed by supplemental carbohydrate feeding **Diet:** High carbohydrate	**Exercise:** Tapering **Diet:** Moderate carbohydrate
3	**Exercise:** Tapering **Diet:** Low carbohydrate	**Exercise:** Tapering followed by supplemental carbohydrate feeding **Diet:** High carbohydrate	**Exercise:** Tapering **Diet:** Moderate carbohydrate
4	**Exercise:** Tapering **Diet:** Low carbohydrate	**Exercise:** Tapering followed by supplemental carbohydrate feeding **Diet:** Moderate carbohydrate	**Exercise:** Tapering **Diet:** Moderate carbohydrate
5	**Exercise:** Tapering **Diet:** High carbohydrate	**Exercise:** Tapering followed by supplemental carbohydrate feeding **Diet:** Moderate carbohydrate	**Exercise:** Tapering **Diet:** High carbohydrate
6	**Exercise:** Tapering or none (rest) **Diet:** High carbohydrate	**Exercise:** Tapering followed by supplemental carbohydrate feeding **Diet:** Moderate carbohydrate	**Exercise:** Tapering or rest **Diet:** High carbohydrate
7	**Exercise:** Tapering or rest **Diet:** High carbohydrate	**Exercise:** Tapering followed by supplemental carbohydrate feeding **Diet:** Moderate carbohydrate	**Exercise:** Tapering or rest **Diet:** High carbohydrate
8	Competitive event	Competitive event	Competitive event

Sources of data: Goforth HW Jr, "Effects of depletion exercise and light training on muscle glycogen supercompensation in men," *American Journal of Physiology, Endocrinology, & Metabolism* 285(6): E1304, 2003; Kreider RBet al., "ISSN exercise & sport review: Research & recommendations," *Journal of International Society of Sports Nutrition* 7: 7,2010. Published online February 2, 2010. doi: 10.1186/1550-2783-7-7; Williams MH and others: *Nutrition for Health, Fitness, & Sport.* 11th ed. New York: McGraw-Hill, 2017.

experience its effects. Rather than promote carbohydrate loading, many nutrition and human performance experts simply recommend that athletes routinely follow a high—carbohydrate diet and consume certain forms of carbohydrate during prolonged exercise.

Consuming Carbohydrate During Events

When athletes exercise vigorously for longer than 60 minutes, their glycogen supplies become depleted. At this point, athletes report they have "hit the wall"; that is, they feel unable to maintain a competitive pace. While performing prolonged physical activity, athletes can delay reaching "the wall" by consuming 30 to 60 g of carbohydrate per hour of activity.[7]

Sports drinks are a convenient way to obtain a source of glucose during lengthy and vigorous physical activities. Commercially available sports drinks are usually sweetened with nutritive sweeteners such as sucrose, glucose, fructose, or maltodextrin. Such beverages typically provide 15 to 27 g of carbohydrate per 12—ounce serving. Foods or drinks that are concentrated sources of fructose are not recommended because large amounts of this particular simple sugar may cause gastrointestinal upset. In addition to supplying carbohydrate, sports drinks contain water and electrolytes, such as sodium, that can benefit athletes during prolonged physical effort. Sports gels are also good sources of simple carbohydrate, but they generally supply very little fluid. Therefore, it is important for athletes who consume these products to drink enough water to maintain proper hydration during endurance events.

Consuming Carbohydrate During Exercise Recovery

After completing exhaustive physical activity, trained athletes can replenish nearly all of their glycogen stores within a few days, provided they rest and eat a high—carbohydrate diet. During a post—event meal, starchy foods such as whole—grain bread, mashed potatoes, rice, and pasta can be served to boost athletes' carbohydrate consumption.

During the exercise recovery period that occurs after an endurance event, athletes need to consume 6 to 12 g of carbohydrate/kg of body weight to replenish their muscle glycogen stores.[7] To restore their supply of muscle glycogen quickly after an event, athletes can consume sports drinks, candy, sugar—sweetened soft drinks, and fruit or fruit juices.

What About Protein?

The adult RDA for protein is 0.8 g/kg of body weight.[11] During prolonged physical activity, muscles lose some protein because they metabolize certain amino acids for energy. Furthermore, extra amino acids are needed to repair and increase muscle tissue after exercise (recovery).[12] According to a recent review, athletes generally need 1.2 to 2.0 g of protein/kg of body weight.[7]

An additional 0.3 of protein per kg of body weight per day should be consumed after exercising.[7] Consuming this amount of extra protein for recovery does not appear to be harmful for healthy physically active people. Recommended sources of protein include foods such as milk, chocolate milk, lean meats, and dietary supplements that contain whey, casein, soy, and egg proteins. Consuming excessive amounts of protein can be dangerous for people who cannot metabolize amino acids or ammonia properly (see Fig. 7.12).

Under normal conditions, carbohydrate and fat are the primary fuels for cellular activity. Protein is not a major biological fuel. To spare protein so the nutrient can be used for muscle tissue growth and repair during recovery, it is

carbohydrate (glycogen) loading practice of manipulating physical activity and dietary patterns to increase muscle glycogen stores

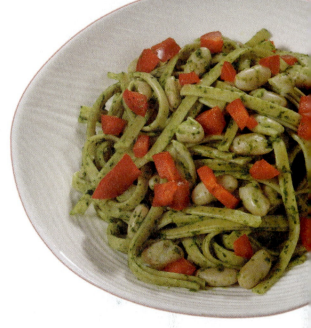

During a post-event meal, starchy foods, such as this spinach pesto pasta, can be served to boost an athlete's carbohydrate consumption. Source: Centers for Disease Control and Prevention

Did *YOU* Know?

Milk contains two major kinds of protein: casein and whey. *Whey proteins* can be isolated (separated) from the liquid that forms during cheese production. Whey protein is a source of essential amino acids, vitamins, and minerals.

Most dietary supplements that are made from whey are powders that contain *whey protein isolates*. The powder can be mixed with water, milk, or juice to form a drink; sprinkled on cereal; or incorporated into a smoothie. For healthy young adults engaged in heavy resistance training, whey protein supplementation can enhance exercise recovery and increase muscle protein production.[13,14]

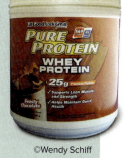

©Wendy Schiff

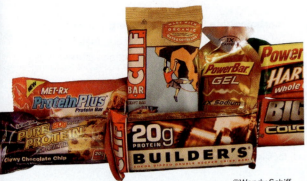

©Wendy Schiff

very important for physically active people to consume adequate amounts of carbohydrate and fat.

Raising the Bar?

"Lasting energy," "fast fuel," "optimal energy"—such claims are used to promote so—called "energy" bars, gels, and drinks. Energy or sports bars are essentially cookies made from soy and milk proteins that are fortified with vitamins, minerals, and fiber. Sugary syrups hold these ingredients together. *High—protein* energy bars may appeal to athletes who think proteins are a source of energy for physical activity. However, proteins are not a major biological fuel, and they are not "quick energy" sources because the liver must process amino acids before they can be used for energy.

Granola bars, fruit—filled cookies, and fresh or dried fruits are less expensive and more natural sources of energy and nutrients than energy or sports bars. You can make your own "energy" bars by following the recipe in the "Recipe for Healthy Living" feature. If you prefer to eat commercial energy bars, check the products' Nutrition Facts panels to determine amounts of carbohydrates and other nutrients that are in a serving. By eating several energy bars daily, you may ingest high amounts of iron, vitamin A, and other micronutrients. Therefore, consider energy bars as occasional snacks and not as meal replacements. Table 11.6 presents approximate energy and macronutrient contents per typical serving of various popular energy bars and gels.

caffeine naturally occurring stimulant drug

Energy drinks usually contain sugars and a lot of **caffeine,** a stimulant drug that is naturally in coffee and tea. When consumed in moderate amounts, caffeine can increase alertness and decrease fatigue. Some energy drinks also contain the amino acid *taurine* and herbal substances such as ginseng. Although the body uses taurine, the compound is not required by humans. At present, there is no scientific evidence that ginseng enhances the stimulating effects of caffeine.[15] The "Ergogenic Aids: Separating Fact from Fiction" section of this chapter provides more information about caffeine, ginseng, and some other substances that are promoted for enhancing physical performance.

TABLE 11.6 Popular Energy Bars and Gels: Energy and Macronutrient Contents/Serving

Product	Energy kcal	Carbohydrates g	Protein g	Fat g
PowerBar Protein Plus (chocolate peanut butter), 1 bar	210	23	20	6
PowerBar Protein (peanut butter caramel), 1 bar	200	23	12	9
PowerBar PowerGel (vanilla), 1 packet	110	27	0	0
Luna Protein Bar (chocolate peanut butter), 1 bar	190	19	12	8
Clif Bar (chocolate chip), 1 bar	250	45	10	5
Clif Shot (vanilla gel), 1 packet	100	24	0	0
Balance Bar (dark chocolate peanut), 1 bar	180	20	13	6
Balance Bar (caramel nut blast), 1 bar	210	23	15	7

Sources: Clif Bar & Company, www.clifbar.com/; Balance Bar Food Company, www.balance.com/; Power Bar, www.powerbar.com/ Accessed: July 27, 2016.

Focusing on Fluids

The Adequate Intake (AI) for total water intake is approximately 11 cups (2.7 L) and 15.5 cups (3.7 L) for young women and men, respectively. Athletes generally require more water than nonathletes to keep their bodies cool during muscular activity. Many factors, however, influence a person's hydration status. Among athletes in particular, differences in sports, fitness levels, and environmental conditions affect fluid needs. For example, sweating can cause runners to lose 3 to 8 cups (750 to 2000 ml) of water per hour.[16] Even a small degree of dehydration can lead to declines in an athlete's endurance, strength, and overall performance. Moreover, body temperature rises when dehydration occurs, increasing the risk of heat−related illness.

Heat-Related Illness

As the environmental temperature and humidity increase, the evaporation of sweat from skin slows, and the body has difficulty cooling itself by perspiring. Ineffective sweating contributes to fatigue, makes the heart work harder, and raises the risk of *heat−related illness*. Table 11.7 presents three major types of heat−related illness and their common signs and symptoms.

Heat cramps are the earliest symptoms of heat illness. These painful muscle *spasms* (involuntary contractions) can affect any muscle, but they usually occur in the abdominal or calf muscles. Other early signs and symptoms of heat illness include heavy sweating, tiredness, and thirst.[17] If heat cramps are not treated effectively, the person develops heat exhaustion.

Heat exhaustion can occur after heavy exercise in warm conditions, especially when fluid and salt intakes have been inadequate. A person suffering from heat exhaustion experiences weakness, nausea, and vomiting; complains of having a headache and feeling dizzy; and has dark urine and cool, moist skin.

To treat heat cramps or heat exhaustion, move the victim to a cool or shady place and have the person lie on his or her back with legs elevated 12 inches. To relieve leg cramps, massage the affected muscles until they relax. Cool the person by fanning, spraying with cool water, or giving a cool sponge bath. It is also very important to have the victim drink cool water or a sports drink, unless the person is vomiting or has lost consciousness. People with heat exhaustion should be monitored closely because the condition can rapidly develop into *heatstroke*.

Heatstroke is the most dangerous form of heat−related illness. Signs of heatstroke include dry, red, hot skin; elevated body temperature (often more than 104°F, measured rectally); rapid, shallow breathing; irrational and confused behavior; and loss of consciousness (coma).[17] Heatstroke is a medical emergency that needs to be treated by trained medical staff. If you suspect that a person has heatstroke, summon emergency medical assistance immediately (dial 911) and move the victim to a cool environment. While waiting for professional medical care to arrive, give the patient cool water to drink (if he or she is conscious and not vomiting) and spray the person's skin with cool water.

Replenishing Fluids

To reduce the risk of heat illnesses, athletes and other physically active people should avoid exercising under extremely hot, humid conditions and should replace fluid losses that occur during prolonged exertion. Athletes should drink fluids in response to becoming thirsty.[18] Experts no longer recommend drinking fluids even if you are not thirsty because this practice can lead to water intoxication (*hyponatremia*). However, athletes should avoid losing more than 2% of their body weight during exercise.[16]

TABLE 11.7 Heat-Related Illnesses: Signs and Symptoms

Heat cramps
- Painful muscle cramps, usually in legs or abdomen
- Very heavy sweating
- Tiredness
- Thirst

Heat exhaustion
- Dark urine
- Cool, moist skin
- Weakness
- Light-headedness or dizziness
- Headache
- Nausea and vomiting

Heatstroke
- Dry, hot, red skin
- High fever (over 104°F)
- Rapid, shallow breathing
- Confusion, irrational behavior
- Seizures, loss of consciousness

Source: National Library of Medicine: MedlinePlus: *Heat emergencies.* Updated November 2015. https://medlineplus.gov/ency/article/000056.htm Accessed: June 19, 2017.

heat cramps heat-related illness characterized by painful muscle contractions

heat exhaustion heat-related illness that can occur after intense exercise

heatstroke most dangerous form of heat-related illness

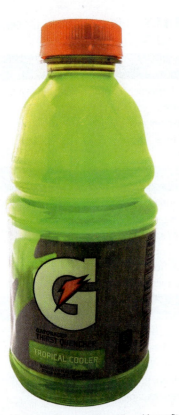

Sports drinks provide some nutritional benefits beyond those of plain water. ©Wendy Schiff

Food & Nutrition tips

Compared to commercially available sports drinks, dilute fruit juices with added sugar and salt are less expensive sources of water, sodium, and simple sugars. You can prepare your own "sports" drink by adding ¼ cup of orange juice, ¼ cup of sugar, and ⅛ tsp of table salt to 30 oz of water or club soda. Pour the beverage into a quart pitcher, stir, cover, and refrigerate until needed.

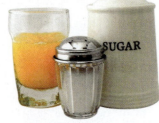

©Wendy Schiff

To estimate the amount of fluids needed to replace water loss during exercise (*rehydration*), athletes can weigh themselves prior to exercising and then calculate 2% of their body weight ($0.02 \times$ weight). After working out, athletes should weigh themselves again. If the difference between preexercise and postexercise body weights is more than 2%, fluid replacement is necessary during such activities. For example, if you weigh 150 pounds, 2% of that weight is 3 pounds (0.02×150). Therefore, you should drink enough watery fluids to avoid losing 3 or more pounds when you train or compete. In general, you can replace each pound that you lose during exercise by drinking 1 ¼ to 1 ½ pints (2 ½ to 3 cups) of water.[7] For example, if your usual weight is 150 pounds and you weigh 149 pounds immediately after exercising, you have lost 1 pound of body water during the activity. The next time you exercise under similar conditions, you can consume 3 cups of water during the activity to maintain your body's water balance. Why do you need to drink more fluids than you have lost in sweat? After exercise, rehydration may stimulate the kidneys to produce more urine than normal; thus, you need to drink the extra watery fluids to achieve proper hydration. As noted in Chapter 9, alcoholic beverages have a diuretic effect on the body and are not recommended for rehydration.

Do I Need a Sports Drink? Sports drinks provide some nutritional benefits beyond those of plain water. These beverages usually contain simple carbohydrates, a source of energy that can enhance performance during endurance activities. Recommended products contain about 21 g of carbohydrate per 12-ounce serving, or about 6% carbohydrate by weight. Drinks with sugar contents above 10%, such as soft drinks or fruit juices, are not recommended because they may cause intestinal discomfort. Sodium and other electrolytes in sports beverages help maintain blood volume, enhance the absorption of water and carbohydrate from the intestinal tract, and stimulate thirst.

Should you drink water or a sports drink during competition? According to the International Marathon Medical Directors Association (IMMDA), sports drinks are necessary when workouts are 10 kilometers or more.[18] Although electrolytes are lost in sweat, the quantities lost in shorter periods can be easily replaced by consuming foods and beverages, such as water or fruit juice, after the event.

It is possible to drink too much water and develop water intoxication (see Chapter 9). Endurance athletes, especially poorly trained individuals, may compete at relatively low exercise intensities for prolonged periods. Under these conditions, the athletes do not sweat as much; therefore, they do not need to replace as much water as better-trained athletes who exercise at higher intensities. Regardless of training level, athletes who drink too much water can dilute the level of sodium in their blood and develop serious and even deadly side effects. Although sports drinks generally contain sodium, these beverages are mostly water; therefore, consuming excessive amounts of sports drinks can contribute to fluid overload. To avoid water intoxication, athletes should drink water according to their thirst. If an athlete gains weight while exercising, he or she may be retaining too much fluid.

Antioxidant Vitamins

During aerobic physical activities, skeletal muscles use more oxygen and generate more free radicals than resting muscle tissue.[19] Exercise can produce a temporary imbalance between free radical generation and the ability of antioxidants to counteract them. Scientific evidence suggests that such *oxidative stress* may contribute to muscle fatigue and damage. Nevertheless, results of studies that examined whether antioxidant vitamin supplements enhanced athletic performance generally concluded that performance was not improved, unless there was a preexisting deficiency of those particular vitamins.

Findings of some scientific studies indicate that free radicals generated during intense exercise may stimulate the body's natural antioxidant defense system. Thus, the oxidative stress produced during exercise might have benefits, and blocking this process by taking antioxidant vitamin supplements may not be desirable.[7]

Athletes should be cautious about taking dietary supplements that contain antioxidants based on anecdotes or advertising claims because there is not enough scientific evidence concerning the long–term effects of using these products.[7] Rather than experiment on themselves with antioxidant supplements, athletes should follow diets that contain foods naturally rich in antioxidants, such as fruits, vegetables, whole–grain breads and cereals, and vegetable oils.

Iron

The body needs iron to produce red blood cells, transport oxygen, and obtain energy. Thus, iron deficiency can negatively affect athletic performance. Young female athletes are likely to develop iron deficiency because of their menstrual blood losses: Bleeding is a cause of iron deficiency. Athletes who follow low–calorie or vegetarian (especially vegan) diets are also at risk of iron deficiency because their food choices may be low in iron.

In the early phase of their training, endurance athletes often develop *sports anemia*, a temporary condition that results from an increase in the liquid portion of blood (*plasma*), rather than iron deficiency. This particular type of anemia does not appear to have negative effects on physical performance. Nevertheless, it can be difficult to differentiate between sports anemia and true iron deficiency anemia. It is a good idea for athletes, especially females, to have their iron status checked at the beginning of a training season and at least once during midseason. If an athlete is iron deficient, a physician needs to determine the cause and prescribe treatment.

Calcium

Athletes, especially those who are total vegetarians or restrict their consumption of dairy products to lose weight, can have marginal or low calcium intakes. This practice may result in weak bones that fracture easily, as well as in osteoporosis later in life. Additionally, female athletes who have irregular or no menstrual cycles may be deficient in the hormone estrogen. Although weight–bearing exercise, such as jogging, improves bone density, estrogen is also necessary for maintaining healthy bones. Female athletes who develop menstrual cycle abnormalities should consult a physician to determine the cause. Decreasing the amount of training or gaining weight may restore a regular menstrual pattern. For information about the *female athlete triad*, see the Chapter 10 "Nutrition Matters"; Chapter 9 provides information about osteoporosis.

Intense exercise may stimulate the body's natural antioxidant defense system. ©Javier Pierini/Getty Images RF

Concept CHECKPOINT

12. What are some practical ways to assess whether an athlete's energy intake is adequate?
13. Why should athletes be concerned about their carbohydrate intakes before, during, and after prolonged intense physical activity?
14. Identify at least five high-carbohydrate/low-fat foods.
15. Explain why athletes may need to consume more than the RDA for protein.
16. Why should athletes be concerned about their fluid status?
17. What are major signs and symptoms of heat cramps, heat exhaustion, and heatstroke?
18. When is consuming a sports drink a better choice than plain water for rehydration?
19. Explain why you would or would not recommend that an athlete take antioxidant supplements.
20. Explain why iron deficiency can impair an athlete's physical performance.
21. For young female athletes, what is the significance of having irregular or no menstrual cycles for bone health?

See Appendix G for responses.

11.5 Ergogenic Aids: Separating Fact from Fiction

Learning Outcomes

1 Discuss the pros and cons of using amino acid supplements and other ergogenic aids for athletic performance.

2 Identify three ergogenic aids that have been banned by at least one athletic association.

3 Identify rich sources of caffeine, and discuss the effects that the substance can have on the body.

ergogenic aids foods, devices, dietary supplements, or drugs used to improve physical performance

Athletes often use **ergogenic aids**—foods, devices, dietary supplements, and even drugs ("doping")—to improve their physical performance. Bee pollen, dried adrenal glands from cattle, seaweed, freeze-dried liver flakes, and ginseng are among the dietary supplements that athletes consume as they hope to gain the competitive edge over their rivals. However, no reliable scientific evidence supports the effectiveness of most dietary supplements purported to have ergogenic effects.[7] Nevertheless, many athletes firmly believe in the value of the performance-enhancing aids that they use. In many instances, the perceived benefits are more likely to result from the placebo effect than from actual physiological changes (see Chapter 2).

A few dietary substances and practices can enhance physical performance. These ergogenic aids include sufficient water and electrolytes, carbohydrates, and a balanced and varied diet consistent with MyPlate recommendations. For athletes, meeting carbohydrate and fluid needs—along with overall nutrient needs—is the most important ergogenic aid.

Athletes should be skeptical of claims made for any substance until its ergogenic effects and long-term safety have been determined by researchers who are not associated with the supplement industry. Rather than searching for a "magic bullet" to enhance their performance, athletes should concentrate their efforts on improving their dietary habits, training routines, and sports techniques. Nutrient supplements should be used for specific dietary deficiencies, such as preventing iron deficiency or boosting calcium intakes.

Table 11.8 summarizes science–based findings regarding caffeine, creatine, and some other dietary supplements and ergogenic aids that are popular among athletes. It is important to note that certain dietary supplements are known to be unsafe, and the use of others is restricted or banned by major athletic organizations. For example, in 2004, the U.S. Food and Drug Administration (FDA) banned the use of ephedrine–containing supplements. Ephedrine (ephedra, ma huang) increases central nervous system activity, but the drug can cause serious, even deadly side effects. The following section discusses the ergogenic properties of caffeine.

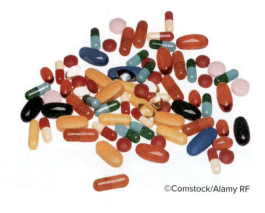
©Comstock/Alamy RF

Did *YOU* Know?

The human body makes DHEA, which certain cells convert to estrogen and testosterone, the "sex hormones." Testosterone stimulates muscle cells to remove amino acids from the bloodstream, which enables the cells to synthesize protein. As a result of this anabolic effect, muscular growth occurs. Anabolic steroids are synthetic substances that are chemically similar to testosterone. In the United States, a physician's prescription is needed to legally obtain anabolic steroids. When abused, such substances can cause serious side effects. Anabolic steroids, for example, can cause bloody liver cysts; increased risk of cardiovascular disease, hypertension, and reproductive problems; and aggressive behavior ("roid rage").

The body also synthesizes growth hormone (GH). As its name implies, GH stimulates muscle and bone growth, and it helps regulate metabolism. Long-term use of GH may increase the risk of cancer and have other potentially harmful side effects, such as elevated blood glucose levels. The FDA has few approved uses for medications that contain GH, including the treatment of GH deficiency in children.[20] Without access to the hormone, deficient children do not grow properly and, as adults, have heights that are much shorter than average. The National Collegiate Athletic Association, however, bans the use of GH as well as anabolic steroids by athletes.[21]

Caffeine

Worldwide, caffeine is the most widely used ergogenic aid. Caffeine raises the level of fatty acids in blood, and as a result, exercising muscles can use more fat for energy. Caffeine also enhances the ability of skeletal and heart muscles to contract and increases mental alertness. Although consuming even small amounts of caffeine may help endurance athletes, the National Collegiate Athletic Association bans the use of caffeine and limits the amount of caffeine that athletes can have in their bodies during competition.[21] Athletes who have more than 15 micrograms of caffeine per milliliter (mcg/ml) of their urine can be banned.[7] Nevertheless, the World Anti–Doping Agency does not prohibit the use of caffeine.[22]

People who are not regular caffeine consumers may experience shakiness, rapid heart rate, sleep disturbances, diarrhea, and frequent urination after ingesting relatively high amounts of the stimulant drug. Caffeine is addictive; discontinuing its use results in *withdrawal*, temporary unpleasant side effects, especially headache.

It is important to understand that the quick "energy" boost provided by "energy drinks" is a result of caffeine or other stimulants contained in the products. Nevertheless, energy drinks also provide calories if they are sweetened with

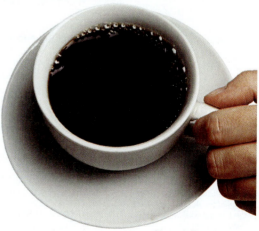
©bevrnja/Getty Images RF

added sugars. Table 11.9 compares the caffeine and calorie contents of popular beverages, including an energy drink (e.g., "Red Bull®"). "Stay awake" pills and chewing gums are concentrated sources of caffeine that can be purchased without a prescription. In September 2015, the FDA warned consumers to avoid "powdered" caffeine. At that time, the agency was aware of two deaths that were attributed to use of such products.[23]

TABLE 11.8 Evaluation of Some Popular Ergogenic Supplements/Aids

Substance	Claim	Current Evidence-Based Findings Concerning Claims	Side Effects
Beta-alanine	Enhances training capacity and improves performance during brief bouts of intense exercise	May be beneficial	May cause tingling sensations
Beta-hydroxy-beta-methylbutyrate (HMB)	Decreases protein metabolism, increasing muscle mass	May increase muscle mass, but evidence is weak	None reported, but results of long-term use are unknown
Branched-chain amino acids (BCAA)	Provide energy for muscles	May enhance muscle recovery after intense physical activity	None reported
Caffeine (guarana)	Enhances fat metabolism Delays depletion of muscle glycogen Increases alertness	Consuming 3 to 6 mg of caffeine/kg of body weight about 1 hour before exercise can benefit certain athletes.	High doses can cause nervousness, shakiness, and sleep disturbances; very high doses can be deadly. Intakes that cause the kidneys to eliminate more than 15 mcg of caffeine per ml of urine are banned by the National Collegiate Athletic Association.
Calcium pyruvate	Increases endurance and promotes weight loss	Not effective	Gastrointestinal upset May be harmful
Chromium	Increases lean mass	No benefit	Toxic intakes are above 400 mcg/day.
Creatine	Enhances muscular endurance and strength Increases lean muscle mass	Increases lean and total body mass, improves performance for intense activities that are not endurance activities, increases strength Such positive effects are not consistent among athletes.	May cause weight gain and gastrointestinal upset
Energy drinks	Increase alertness and focus Enhance anaerobic and endurance performance Increase fat metabolism	Results vary based on the composition of the energy drink. Some energy drinks may enhance the performance of athletes and promote a small amount of fat loss.	See "Caffeine." Elevated heart rate and blood pressure Increased likelihood of engaging in risky behaviors
Ginseng	Combats fatigue and improves stamina	Does not improve performance but may decrease muscle damage during exercise	May cause gastrointestinal upset, itching, sleeplessness, and, in rare cases, allergic reactions and liver damage
Nitrate	Improves exercise endurance and performance	Benefits are not evident in elite athletes.	Nitrate concentrates, such as beetroot juice, may cause intestinal upset and red urine.
Sodium bicarbonate (baking soda)	Reduces lactic acid accumulation	May enhance performance, particularly in exercises that rely primarily on the lactic acid energy system (e.g., 400-meter sprint)	May cause nausea, vomiting, and diarrhea

Sources: Position of the Academy of Nutrition and Dietetics, Dietitians of Canada, and the American College of Sports Medicine, "Nutrition and athletic performance," *Journal of the Academy of Nutrition and Dietetics* 116(3):501, 2016; Kreider RB et al., "ISSN exercise & sport nutrition review: research & recommendations," *Journal of the International Society of Sports Nutrition* 7 (7):1, 2010; NIH, Medline Plus, *American ginseng*. 2015. Accessed: June 20, 2017. https://medlineplus.gov/druginfo/natural/967.html

TABLE 11.9 Caffeine Content of Selected Beverages

Beverage and Amount	Approximate Energy (kcal)	Approximate Caffeine (mg)
Chocolate drink, milk based, 8 oz	120	2
Caffé Latte Starbucks 16 oz*	190	150
Coffee, brewed from grounds, unsweetened, 8 oz	2	95
Coffee, instant plain, prepared, 8 oz	5	62
Cola, with added sugar and caffeine, 12-oz can	155	33
5-Hour energy shot®, original, 1.9-oz bottle**	4	215
Monster® energy drink, 8-oz can**	100	92
Mountain Dew®, 12-oz can***	170	54
Red Bull®, 8.4-oz can**	110	83
Rockstar energy shot, 2.5-oz bottle**	10	229
Tea, black, brewed, unsweetened, 8 oz	2	47
Tea, sugar-sweetened, ready-to-drink, 12-oz can	183	37

Source: U.S. Department of Agriculture: *USDA national nutrient database for standard reference,* Release 26, May 2013.

*Starbucks Beverages: *Nutrition information.* www.starbucks.com Accessed: July 27, 2016.

**Consumer Reports:* The buzz on energy drink caffeine. December 2012. http://www.consumerreports.org/cro/magazine/2012/12/the-buzz-on-energy-drink-caffeine/index.htm Accessed: July 27, 2016.

***Pepsico: Facts about your favorite beverages. www.pepsicobeveragefacts.com Accessed: July 27, 2016

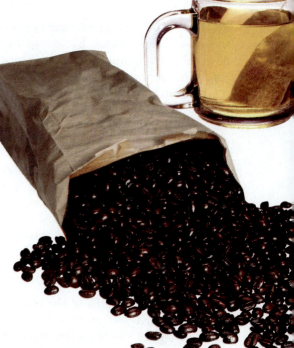

Tea and Coffee beans: ©John A. Rizzo/Getty Images RF

Concept CHECKPOINT

22. Why do many athletes use ergogenic aids?

23. Identify three ergogenic aids that have been banned by the FDA or an athletic association.

24. Identify at least three beverages that are rich sources of caffeine.

25. Discuss the ergogenic effects that caffeine can have on the body.

See Appendix G for responses.

11.6 Nutrition Matters: Developing a Personal Fitness Plan

Learning Outcomes

1 Identify the key components of an aerobic workout regimen.

2 Design a personal fitness program that suits your interests and lifestyle.

When developing your personal physical fitness plan, first consider your fitness goals. For example, if you want to lose weight, how much do you want to lose and how many weeks will it take to lose that amount? Do you want to focus more on strengthening your muscles or on improving your aerobic capacity? Then determine when you can work out and whether you'll need to join a fitness facility such as a gym or purchase special equipment, such as hand-held weights. For a comprehensive fitness program, make sure to include aerobic, resistance, and stretching activities in your weekly exercise regimen. The following fitness plan has three stages: initial, improvement, and maintenance phases.

Blueberries: ©PhotoAlto/Getty Images RF

Initiation

The first 3 to 6 weeks of your new exercise program is the *initiation* stage. Start by incorporating short periods of physical activity into your daily routine. For example, you can walk more often, take the stairs instead of the elevator, and do more housework, gardening, or other activities that cause you to "huff and puff" a bit. Furthermore, you can strive to reduce the time that you spend in sedentary activities.

The goal is to accumulate a total of 150 minutes of moderate—intensity types of activity each week. If necessary, the time that you spend engaging in the activity can occur in several short intervals, each lasting at least 10 minutes. If you do not have 150 minutes to spend on exercising, try increasing the intensity of the activities during shorter bouts of exercise to obtain some health benefits.

Improvement and Maintenance

The next 5 or 6 months of the program is the *improvement* stage, in which you increase the intensity and duration of exercises. When you begin the improvement phase, exercise at an intensity that is near the lower end of your target heart rate zone. As you progress and become more physically fit, you can increase the intensity by exercising at a higher heart rate.

By the end of the improvement stage, you may notice that you have reached your goals, and you do not seem to be making further gains in your fitness. This plateau marks the beginning of your *maintenance* stage. At this point, you can evaluate your personal fitness plan, and if you would like to make new goals, this is the time to develop them. If you are satisfied with your fitness level, continue with your present program. Discontinuing exercise gradually results in *detraining*, declining physical fitness.

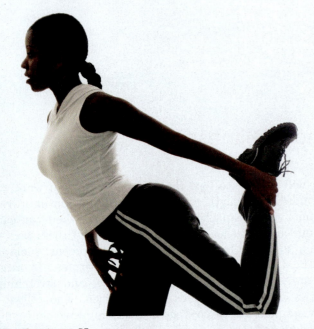

©Fuse/Getty Images RF

Components of an Aerobic Workout Regimen

Ideally, you should establish a regular time for exercising that fits into your daily routine. To be effective, your aerobic workout program needs to include the following components:

1. **Warm—up** Warming up muscles can increase your joints' range of motion (flexibility) and may decrease your risk of injury. Stretching for 5 to 10 minutes is a good way to warm up. Start with smaller muscle groups such as the arms and progressively work toward stretching larger muscle groups in the legs and abdomen. Hold your position in the stretch for 15 seconds and do not bounce. If stretching causes pain, stop immediately. "No pain, no gain" is not true: Pain is an indication of injury. Another way to warm up is to perform 5 to 10 minutes of the anticipated activity but at a low intensity. For example, if you walk for fitness, warm up by walking at a slower pace.

2. **Aerobic workout** To obtain substantial health benefits, you should engage in some form of aerobic activity regularly. A comprehensive aerobic workout emphasizes the *type, duration, frequency, intensity,* and *progression* of exercise.

   - **Type:** The kinds of exercise you choose should increase your heart and breathing rates and involve rhythmic movements of large muscle groups in the legs. Examples include brisk walking, running, swimming, and cycling. If you swim, add some *weight—bearing activities,* such as walking, to your comprehensive fitness plan. Weight—bearing exercises place stress on your bones, increasing their strength.
   - **Duration:** Duration is the amount of time spent in an exercise session. A session should generally last at least 20 to 30 minutes, depending on intensity, not including time spent warming up and cooling down. Ideally, the exercise session should be continuous (without stopping), but multiple 10—minute bouts of moderate to intense activity with rest periods in between are also acceptable.
   - **Frequency:** The frequency of exercise describes the number of times that the activity is performed, generally on a weekly basis. To derive significant health benefits, the frequency of aerobic exercise should be at least five times per week. By exercising daily, you can enjoy even greater benefits.
   - **Intensity:** Health benefits can occur when you achieve at least a moderate level of intensity during exercise.
   - **Progression:** Progression, the final component of a comprehensive fitness plan, refers to the gradual increase in the frequency, intensity, and duration of exercise that occurs over a period.

3. Cool—down To cool down, you can repeat the same stretches you performed during warming up. Stretch for 5 to 10 minutes. Cooling down may prevent injury and reduce muscle soreness.

What About Strength (Resistance) Training?

Strength training, such as weight lifting, is an important part of a comprehensive physical fitness plan. Strength training should be done at least 2 days per week. To start, warm up by stretching for 5 to 10 minutes. Then perform a group of 8 to 10 exercises that strengthen major muscle groups of the upper body and lower body. Cool down for 5 to 10 minutes at the end of each session.

Fitness centers have machines that provide resistance for various muscle groups. For resistance training outside of gymnasiums or fitness clubs, you can purchase simple elastic exercise cords designed to increase muscular strength (Fig. 11.11). For increasing upper arm strength, a set of inexpensive handheld weights can be kept in a convenient location for performing resistance exercise regularly, such as near the TV. The weights should allow you to perform at least one set of 8 to 15 repetitions. When you can do more than 15 repetitions with relative ease, consider increasing the weight slightly.

Mixing It Up

To make your exercise routine more enjoyable, include several types of physical activity in your weekly regimen. For example, jogging one day might be followed by swimming the

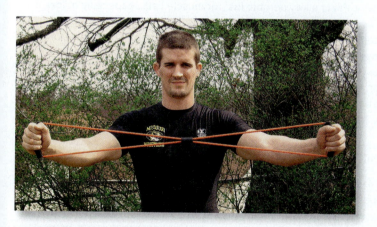

Figure 11.11 Increasing muscle strength. This individual is using a simple rubber exercise cord to increase muscular strength. ©Wendy Schiff

next day. Adding variety to a program not only keeps you from becoming bored with your workouts but also strength—ens different muscle groups in your body and reduces your risk of injury. Additionally, invite a friend or relative to be your exercise partner. Having an exercise partner may provide additional motivation and encouragement to exercise regularly.

Some overfat people do not experience significant weight loss while following an exercise regimen. However, they still benefit from regular physical activity. Initially, exercise programs for obese people should emphasize non—weight—bearing activities, such as swimming, water aerobics, and bicycling. As obese people lose weight and become more fit, they can add weight—bearing activities to their plans.

Whatever physical activities you choose to include in your fitness program, they should be enjoyable and easy to incorporate into your routine. You can apply the dietary principles of variety, balance, and moderation to your exercise routine:

- **Variety:** Perform several different activities to exercise different muscle groups.
- **Balance:** For overall fitness, balance your exercise regimen by including activities that build cardiovascular endurance, muscular strength, and flexibility.
- **Moderation:** Focus on exercising to keep fit without overdoing it and injuring yourself. You do not need to work out vigorously every day to become healthier.

To learn more about the health benefits of physical fitness, determine your level of fitness, or develop a personal fitness program, access the following websites:

https://www.cdc.gov/physicalactivity/
https://www.hhs.gov/fitness/index.html
https://www.hhs.gov/fitness/programs—and—awards
/presidents—challenge

Concept CHECKPOINT

26. List three key components of an aerobic workout regimen.

27. Develop a personal fitness regimen that you can follow for the rest of your life.

See Appendix G for responses.

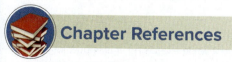

Chapter References

See Appendix H.

Stacked books: ©Stockbyte/Getty Images RF

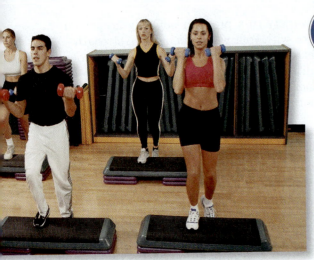

©Jeff Maloney/Getty Images RF

Summary

11.1 Introduction to Nutrition for Fitness and Sport

- Many Americans lead sedentary lives. People can manage their weight more effectively and reduce their risk of developing the major causes of death and disability by engaging in at least 150 minutes of moderate-intensity physical activity weekly. Furthermore, most people can achieve even greater health benefits by increasing the duration, frequency, and intensity of their physical activities.

11.2 Benefits of Regular Exercise

- Regular physical activity reduces the risk of dying prematurely and developing heart disease, diabetes, and high blood pressure. Additionally, regular exercise builds and maintains healthy bones, muscles, and joints; helps reduce blood pressure in people who have high blood pressure; reduces the risk of developing certain cancers; aids weight-control efforts; helps older adults become stronger and reduces their risk of falls; reduces risk of sleep disorders, depression, and anxiety; and promotes psychological well-being. Millions of Americans suffer from chronic illnesses that can be prevented or improved by exercising more often.

11.3 Energy for Muscular Work

- ATP is the major form of energy used by cells. Phosphocreatine (PCr) can rapidly reform ATP from its breakdown product ADP, but PCr supplies are limited. To generate ATP, muscle cells can metabolize carbohydrate, fat, and protein. In muscle cells, glucose molecules are broken down through a series of steps to yield lactic acid (in anaerobic conditions) or CO_2 plus H_2O (in aerobic conditions).

- The proportions of macronutrients used for energy largely depend on the intensity of the physical activity. Fat is a key aerobic fuel for muscle cells, especially at low-intensity exercise. At rest and during light activity, muscles burn primarily fat for energy needs. In comparison, little protein generally is used to fuel muscles. During brief bouts of intense physical effort, the cardiorespiratory system is unable to deliver adequate oxygen to muscles. Under such anaerobic conditions, muscle cells metabolize glucose rather than fat for energy, but their ability to sustain the release of energy for intense activity is limited. Muscle cells can obtain far more energy when in aerobic conditions.

11.4 General Dietary Advice for Athletes

- Sports nutrition focuses on applying nutrition principles and research findings to improving athletic performance. Athletes often manipulate their diets to enhance their body contours, increase their muscular strength, and prevent or delay fatigue during exercise. Although diet is important, genetic endowment, mental training, and physical training are crucial factors that influence athletic performance.

- A high-carbohydrate diet can be beneficial for athletes, and carbohydrate-rich foods should form the foundation of pre-event meals. Many athletes need more protein than the RDA.

- Physically active people need to be concerned about their fluid intakes. Fluid replacement should be based on thirst and loss of body weight while exercising. It is important to recognize signs and symptoms of heat illness. Consuming a source of electrolytes, such as a sports drink, can be helpful. It is important to avoid overconsumption of water because of the risk of water intoxication.

11.5 Ergogenic Aids: Separating Fact from Fiction

- Athletes often ingest certain substances, including herbal products, because they believe these substances have ergogenic effects. Scientific evidence, however, does not suggest that most of these substances are effective. Furthermore, long-term safety of many ergogenic aids has not been determined, and use of some substances is restricted or banned by various athletic organizations.

11.6 Nutrition Matters: Developing a Personal Fitness Plan

- The three components of an aerobic workout are warming up, performing the moderate or vigorous intensity activity, and cooling down.

Recipe for Healthy Living

Nutty Energy Bars

You can use the following recipe to make your own "energy bars." This recipe makes eight 4-by-2-inch bars. Each bar supplies approximately 253 kcal, 8 g protein, 13 g fat, 26 g digestible carbohydrates, 3 g fiber, and 4.9 mg iron.

©Wendy Schiff

INGREDIENTS:

Oil cooking spray
1 egg, large
1 ½ cups instant oats, dry
¼ cup almonds, slivered
¼ cup enriched wheat flour
½ cup smooth peanut butter
1 Tbsp vegetable oil
½ cup honey
½ tsp ground cinnamon
1 tsp vanilla

PREPARATION STEPS:

1. Preheat oven to 350°. Spray "nonstick" oil on the inside bottom and sides of an 8" × 8" pan.

2. Crack open the egg, drop the egg's contents into a medium-size bowl, and discard the shell. Using a fork, beat the egg until its yolk is completely mixed with the egg white.

3. Add remaining ingredients to the egg and stir until well blended. Mixture will be thick, like cookie dough. Using a large spoon, press dough into the bottom of the pan, covering the inside of the pan evenly.

4. Bake for 12 to 14 minutes. Cool completely before cutting into eight 4-by-2-inch bars.

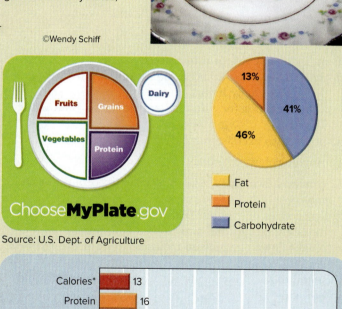

ChooseMyPlate.gov

Source: U.S. Dept. of Agriculture

- Fat — 46%
- Protein — 13%
- Carbohydrate — 41%

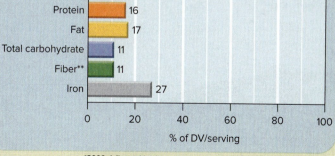

	% of DV/serving
Calories*	13
Protein	16
Fat	17
Total carbohydrate	11
Fiber**	11
Iron	27

*2000 daily total kcal
**Component of total carbohydrates

connect Further analyze this recipe or other recipes through activities located in Connect.

Critical Thinking

1. Analyze your weekly physical activity habits. Does your participation in various physical activities meet the minimum recommendations? If not, which physical activities are you willing to include in your weekly routine to improve your fitness level?

2. Calculate your target heart rate zone for moderate-intensity as well as vigorous-intensity activities.

3. Why do human cells rely far more on glucose and fat for energy than on protein?

4. What advice would you give a runner concerning fluid intake before and during a marathon?

5. One of your friends is a student athlete who uses ginseng, nitrate, and caffeine to enhance his physical performance. What would you tell your friend concerning the pros and cons of taking these substances?

6. Sunny is an athlete. According to the information in Section 11.4, calculate the recommended amount of protein (g) she should consume regularly.

Practice Test

Select the best answer.

1. Miranda is physically fit. She has
   a. an increased risk of osteoporosis.
   b. the strength, endurance, and flexibility to meet the demands of daily living.
   c. a greater need for vitamins and minerals than other women.
   d. no need to exercise regularly.

2. During glycolysis, the body
   a. converts two fatty acid molecules into one glucose molecule.
   b. synthesizes one amino acid molecule from one carbon dioxide molecule and two oxygen molecules.
   c. breaks down one glucose molecule to form two pyruvate molecules.
   d. metabolizes fatty acids into carbon monoxide and peroxide.

3. A _____ physical activity generally requires a high degree of exertion.
   a. vigorous   c. moderate
   b. basic   d. precise

4. Aerobic activities
   a. enable muscles to use less oxygen than normal.
   b. do not require voluntary muscular contractions.
   c. force muscle cells to use more vitamins and minerals for energy.
   d. involve sustained, rhythmic contractions of certain large skeletal muscles.

5. Which of the following statements is true?
   a. Resistance exercises do not help build bone mass.
   b. Sedentary activities do not require much energy to perform.
   c. Anaerobic energy systems need large quantities of oxygen to produce ATP.
   d. All of the above are correct.

6. Amy is studying quietly. Under these conditions, her muscles are using primarily _____ for energy.
   a. fat   c. amino acids
   b. glucose   d. ketone bodies

7. Carbohydrate loading
   a. provides a competitive edge for award-winning sprinters, bodybuilders, and weight lifters.
   b. involves manipulating dietary patterns and physical activities prior to an endurance event.
   c. often results in short-term weight loss and positive energy balance.
   d. is generally recommended for long-term weight control for athletes.

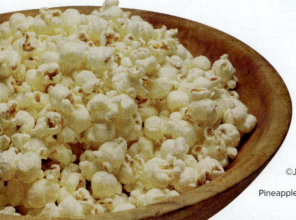

8. Which of the following foods is high carbohydrate and low fat?

   a. Roast chicken
   b. Swiss cheese
   c. Peanut butter
   d. Toast spread with strawberry jam

9. Caffeine

   a. is the most widely used ergogenic aid in the world.
   b. reduces the level of fatty acids in blood.
   c. is nonaddictive.
   d. decreases mental alertness.

10. Human cells release much of the energy stored in carbo–hydrates, fats, and amino acids as

    a. electricity.
    b. phosphocreatine.
    c. ATP.
    d. heat.

11. To obtain energy under aerobic conditions, cells need

    a. ribose.
    b. oxygen.
    c. methionine.
    d. alanine.

12. _____ is an immediate and direct source of energy for cells.

    a. LDP
    b. Glycogen
    c. ATP
    d. Phospholipid

13. Last August, Damien experienced heavy sweating, painful leg cramps, and fatigue, while exercising outdoors. Based on this information, he probably had

    a. heatstroke.
    b. heat cramps.
    c. hypothermia.
    d. hypothyroidism.

Answers to Quiz Yourself

1. People who exercise regularly can reduce their risk of type 2 diabetes. **True.** (Section 11.2)

2. Sports drinks are not useful for fluid replacement. **False.** (Section 11.4)

3. Protein is the body's preferred fuel for muscular activity. **False.** (Section 11.4)

4. Heatstroke is a serious illness that requires immediate professional medical treatment. **True.** (Section 11.4)

5. While at rest, skeletal muscles metabolize more glucose than fat for energy. **False.** (Section 11.3)

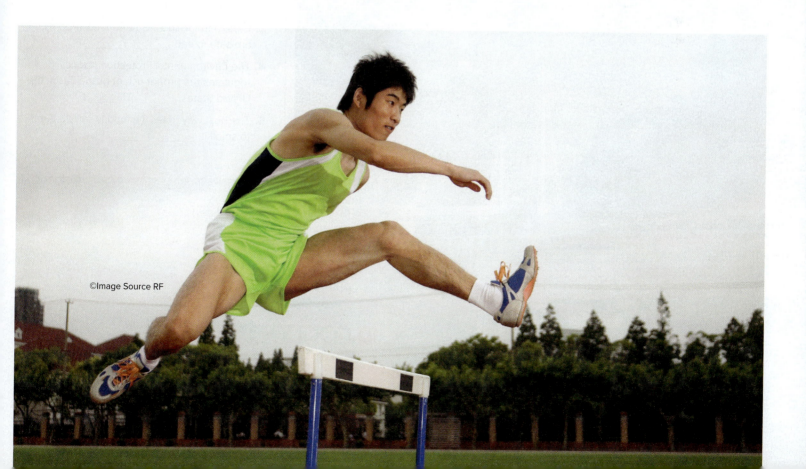
©Image Source RF

CHAPTER 12

Food Safety Concerns

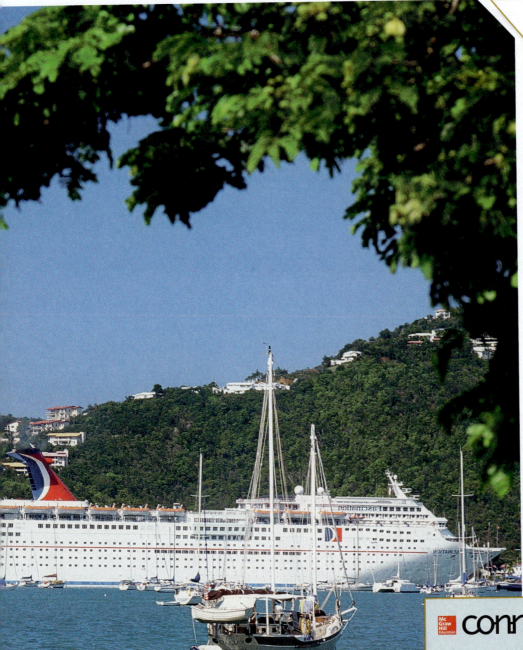

Quiz Yourself

Which foods are most likely to be responsible for food-borne illness? How can you reduce the risk of contracting one of these illnesses? Which government agencies monitor the safety of the U.S. food supply? By reading this chapter, you will learn answers to these questions. Test your knowledge of food safety by taking the following quiz. The answers are at the end of the chapter.

1. Aflatoxins are the most common sources of food-borne illness in the United States. _____ T _____ F

2. In case of emergency, it is not safe to drink the water that is in an undamaged water heater. _____ T _____ F

3. Certain fungi, such as button mushrooms, are safe to eat. _____ T _____ F

4. The Environmental Protection Agency regulates the proper use of pesticides in the United States. _____ T _____ F

5. The best way to tell if a food is safe to eat is to smell it. _____ T _____ F

Mc Graw Hill Education connect®

A wealth of proven resources are available on Connect® including SmartBook®, NutritionCalc Plus, and many other dynamic learning tools. Ask your instructor about Connect!

12.1 Introduction to Food Safety

Learning Outcomes

1 Identify the most common cause of food-borne disease outbreaks in the United States.

2 Explain the difference between a food-borne infection and a food-borne intoxication.

Most Americans look forward to taking vacations, and for many people, this involves boarding a cruise ship to visit tropical, Caribbean island destinations such as Montego Bay, the Bahamas, or Grand Cayman. The attractions of a cruise vacation include enjoyable activities for people of all ages, as well as dining opportunities that showcase plenty of delicious food. Every year, however, some people's dream vacation becomes a cruising nightmare, as hundreds of guests and crew members become miserably ill with stomach pain, diarrhea, and vomiting as a result of *norovirus* infection. In the United States, norovirus is the most common cause of **food—borne illness** outbreaks.[1]

People who are infected with norovirus will have the agent of infection in their vomit and feces. If people with the infection do not wash their hands thoroughly after vomiting or having bowel movements, they can spread the infection to others by handling food or ice cubes, shaking hands, or touching objects that other people touch. The infection spreads rapidly among people who are living in close quarters, such as on a cruise ship. To control the spread of the infection, sick passengers should be isolated from healthy people, and bathrooms, guest rooms, and any surface that may have been touched by ill persons should be disinfected with a strong bleach solution.[2]

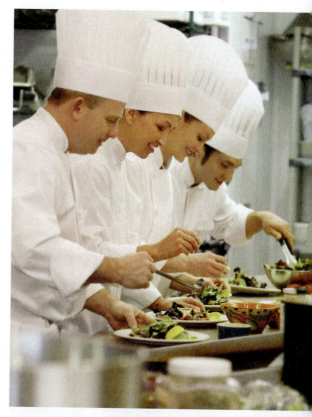

Food can become contaminated with pathogens or their toxins during production, processing, and preparation. ©Don Hammond/Design Pics RF

Pathogens

People develop food—borne illnesses when they consume foods or beverages that contain certain microbes, natural or human—made toxins (poisons), or other contaminants. Disease—causing agents, such as norovirus, are referred to as **pathogens.** When pathogens are in food, they can make the item unsafe to eat. Many kinds of food—borne pathogens infect the digestive tract, inflaming the tissues and causing an "upset stomach" within a few hours after being ingested. A few types of food—borne pathogens multiply in the human intestinal tract, enter the bloodstream, and cause general illness when they invade other tissues. Such illnesses are called **food—borne infections.** Other pathogens do not sicken humans directly, but these microbes contaminate food and secrete poisons. When the contaminated food is eaten, the toxins irritate the intestinal tract and cause a type of food—borne illness called **food intoxication** (or food poisoning).

Illnesses spread through the ingestion of food or water are common, debilitating, and sometimes life—threatening diseases for millions of people around the world. In the United States, water—borne disease—causing microbes are not major health threats because of the use of basic waste water and potable (drinkable) water treatment systems. Each year, an estimated 48 million Americans become sick from various food—borne illnesses.[3] Of those persons who contract such ailments, 128,000 require hospitalization and 3000 die. There are more than 250 food—borne illnesses; preventing these diseases is a major U.S. public health objective.[4]

food-borne illness disorder that is caused by consuming disease-causing agents in food or water

pathogens disease-causing agents

food-borne infection illness that results when a pathogen in food inflames the intestinal tract or other body tissues

food intoxication illness that results when poisons produced by certain microbes contaminate food and irritate the intestinal tract

This chapter focuses primarily on food—borne illness, including common sources of these infections in the United States. Additionally, this chapter pres—ents safe food handling practices.

Concept CHECKPOINT

1. Which agent of infection is responsible for most cases of food-borne illness in the United States?

2. Is the illness caused by norovirus the result of a food-borne infection or food intoxication?

See Appendix G for responses.

12.2 Protecting Our Food

Learning Outcomes

1 Identify government agencies that are responsible for ensuring the safety of the food supply in the United States.

2 Discuss the roles of the FDA, FSIS, and EPA.

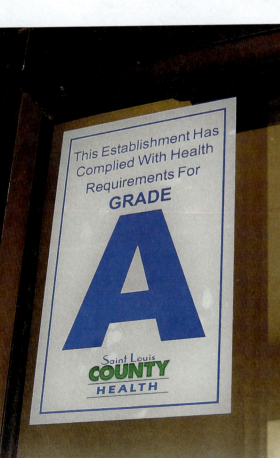

In many communities, restaurants must display their rating for sanitation where customers can easily see it. Local health departments can close restaurants that do not receive high enough ratings and not allow them to reopen until food safety hazards have been corrected.
©Wendy Schiff

The United States has one of the safest food supplies in the world, primarily the result of a team effort conducted by cooperating federal, state, and local agencies that regulate and monitor the production and distri—bution of food. The Food and Drug Administration (FDA) of the U.S. Department of Health and Human Services and the U.S. Department of Agriculture (USDA) are the key federal agencies that protect consumers by regulating the country's food industry. Other team members include the Environmental Protection Agency (EPA), the CDC, the Federal Trade Commission (FTC), and state and local governments.

To help protect our food supply, the FDA performs many important tasks, such as regulating nearly all domestic and imported food sold in inter—state commerce and enforcing federal food safety laws. Additionally, the FDA establishes standards for safe food manufacturing practices, such as Hazard Analysis and Critical Control Point (HACCP) programs. HACCP is a science—based, systematic approach to preventing food—borne illness by predicting which hazards are most likely to occur in a food produc—tion facility. When a hazard is identified, food manufacturers can then take appropriate measures to prevent the illness. If necessary, FDA officials can take certain enforcement actions, such as requesting that a food manufac—turer recall an unsafe item, so that it is removed from store shelves. Another important function of the FDA is educating the general public about safe food handling practices.

Although the FDA oversees the safety of most foods, the USDA's Food Safety and Inspection Service (FSIS) enforces food safety laws for domestic and imported meat and poultry products. FSIS staff inspect beef, poultry, and other food animals for diseases before and after slaughter, and the agency also ensures that meat and poultry processing plants meet federal standards. Addi—tionally, FSIS staff collect and analyze food samples to check for the presence of microbial and other unwanted and potentially harmful material in foods. If a food hazard is identified, FSIS officials can ask meat and poultry processors to recall their unsafe products. Additionally, food safety experts with FSIS conduct programs to educate people about proper food handling practices. For more information, visit the FSIS website at http://www.fsis.usda.gov/wps/portal/fsis/home.

The EPA oversees the quality of our drinking water. EPA staff establish safe drinking water standards and assist state officials in their efforts to monitor water quality. Furthermore, EPA staff regulate toxic substances and wastes to prevent their entry into foods and the environment.

State and local officials work with the FDA and other federal agency staff to implement national food safety standards for foods produced and sold within their state's borders. Local health departments, for example, are responsible for inspecting restaurants, grocery stores, dairy farms, and local food processing companies. In many communities, restaurants are required to post their sanitation rating where customers can easily see it. Local health departments can close restaurants that do not receive high enough ratings and prevent them from reopening until food safety hazards have been corrected.

After you obtain foods and bring them into your home, it becomes your responsibility to reduce the risk of food-borne illness by handling the items properly. However, if you suspect that something you consumed made you or a family member very sick, you should contact your physician for treatment. The physician may decide to report the case of food-borne illness to local public health officials so they can investigate and determine the source of your infection.

Concept CHECKPOINT

3. Discuss the roles of the FDA, FSIS, and EPA in protecting the U.S. food supply.

4. How do local health departments protect consumers from food-borne illness?

See Appendix G for responses.

12.3 Pathogens in Food

Learning Outcomes

1 Discuss ways that pathogens can contaminate human foods.

2 Explain how cross-contamination of food occurs.

3 Discuss the purpose of pasteurization.

4 Discuss conditions that favor the survival and multiplication of food-borne pathogens.

5 Identify foods that are high risk for supporting pathogens.

For thousands of years, people have used certain microbes to produce a variety of foods, including hard cheeses, raised breads, and alcoholic beverages. When microorganisms metabolize nutrients in food, they often secrete substances that alter the color, texture, taste, and other characteristics of the food in beneficial and desirable ways. Other kinds of microbes grow and multiply in

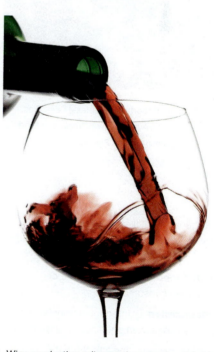

Wine production relies on the use of certain kinds of microbes. ©FoodCollection/StockFood RF

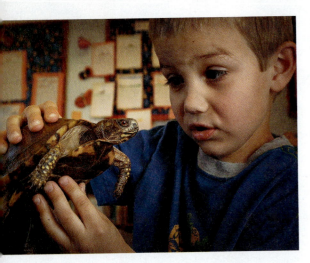

People who touch turtles or other potential *Salmonella* carriers should wash their hands thoroughly after handling the animals. Source: Centers for Disease Control and Prevention

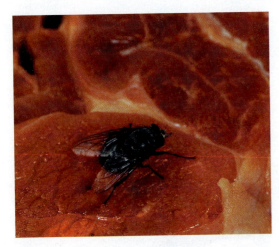

To reduce your risk of food-borne illness, keep flies, cockroaches, and other vermin away from your food.
©Dynamic Graphics Group/IT Stock Free/Alamy RF

parasite organism that lives in or on another organism, often deriving nourishment from its host

contaminated food item that is impure or unsafe for human consumption

cross-contamination unintentional transfer of pathogenic microbes from one food to another

pasteurization process that kills the pathogens in foods and beverages as well as many microbes responsible for spoilage

food, but their metabolic byproducts spoil the food, making it unfit for human consumption.

Some microorganisms are parasites. A **parasite** needs to live on or within a host organism to survive. Parasites often obtain their nourishment from the host's tissues, so the host's health suffers as a result of a parasitic infection.

A **contaminated food** (or beverage) is no longer wholesome—pure or safe for human consumption. Contamination generally occurs when something that may or may not be harmful enters food or beverages unintentionally. Such contaminants include pathogens, insect parts, residues of compounds used to kill insects that destroy food crops, and metal fragments from food processing equipment. The following section discusses how pathogens can contaminate our food.

Sources of Pathogens

The pathogens that cause food–borne illness can live practically anywhere—in air, water, soil, sewage, and on various surfaces. Our skin, nasal passages, and large intestines have vast colonies of various kinds of microbes, some of which can be pathogenic. Animals, including cats, dogs, reptiles, cattle, and poultry, can also harbor harmful microbes on and in their bodies, especially in their intestinal tracts. Because pathogens are found throughout your environment, there are numerous ways that the microbes can contaminate your food. To reduce your risk of food–borne illness, you need to be aware of how pathogens can enter foods. The "Preventing Food–Borne Illness" section of this chapter discusses specific steps you can take to reduce the chances of contracting or spreading food–borne illness.

Common Routes for Transmitting Pathogens

One common route for transmitting harmful microbes involves *vermin*, animals that often live around sewage or garbage, such as flies, cockroaches, mice, and rats. When vermin land on or crawl across filth, they pick up pathogens on their feet. When the vermin come in contact with food, they can transfer the pathogens to humans. To reduce your risk of food–borne illness, keep flies, cock–roaches, and other vermin away from your food.

Poor personal hygiene practices frequently transfer microbes to food. People can contaminate their hands with pathogens when they come in contact with feces, such as while using the toilet or changing a baby's soiled diaper. Furthermore, animals harbor pathogens in their feces as well as on their skin and fur. If children prepare or eat foods after stroking animals at petting zoos or playing with pets, they can transmit these microbes to themselves or others. Thus, it is important for people to wash their hands before preparing or eating foods. Children (and many adults) often need to be reminded to wash their hands.

Improper food handling frequently results in food–borne illness. A common practice is failing to wash cutting boards and food preparation utensils after they come in contact with raw meat or poultry. The contaminated boards and utensils are then used to prepare other foods. As a result of this practice, **cross–contamination** is likely to occur because the pathogens in one food are transferred to another food, contaminating it. If that food is eaten raw, such as carrots in a salad, it carries a high risk of food–borne illness. Failing to cook foods properly can also increase the likelihood of food–borne illness. **Pasteurization** is a special heating process used by many commercial food producers to destroy pathogens. In the United States, for example, most juices and milk have been pasteurized before they are marketed. The "Food Preservation" section of this chapter discusses other ways of preserving foods.

High-Risk Foods

Not all foods are likely to harbor pathogens. To survive and multiply, most microbes need warmth, moisture, and a source of nutrients, and some also require oxygen. In general, high-risk foods are warm, moist, and protein-rich, and they have a neutral or slightly acidic pH. Many of the foods we eat every day, such as meats, eggs, milk, and products made from milk, fit this description. Table 12.1 presents some high-risk foods and the primary food-borne pathogens they may contain. Figure 12.1 shows foods and beverages that were responsible for causing food-borne illnesses among Americans from 2009–2013.

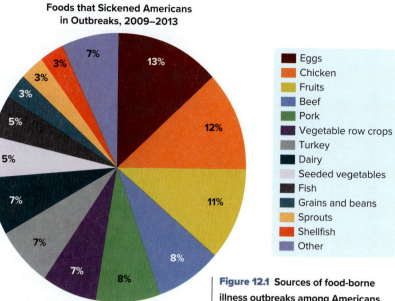

Foods that Sickened Americans in Outbreaks, 2009–2013

- Eggs
- Chicken
- Fruits
- Beef
- Pork
- Vegetable row crops
- Turkey
- Dairy
- Seeded vegetables
- Fish
- Grains and beans
- Sprouts
- Shellfish
- Other

Figure 12.1 Sources of food-borne illness outbreaks among Americans. Source: CDC National Outbreak Reporting System, 2009–2013.

TABLE 12.1 Some High-Risk Foods and Their Primary Pathogens

Raw or Undercooked Animal Food	Typical Menu Item	Common Pathogens
Beef	Rare hamburger	*Salmonella* species *E. coli* O157:H7
Pork	Undercooked pork (rarely in the United States)	*Trichinella*
Poultry	Chicken, turkey, duck	*Salmonella* species *Campylobacter jejuni*
Eggs	Salad dressings or sauces made with raw eggs, cream-filled desserts or toppings made with raw eggs	*Salmonella enteritidis*
Fresh produce	Tomatoes, peppers, cantaloupes, lettuce, spinach, sprouts	*Salmonella* species *E. coli* O157:H7
Raw fish/finfish	Sushi; lightly cooked fish	*Anisakis*
Shellfish	Oysters	*Vibrio vulnificus*
	Clams	*Vibrio* species Hepatitis A virus Norovirus
Milk and milk products	Raw or unpasteurized milk, some soft cheeses such as Camembert and Brie	*Listeria monocytogenes* *Salmonella* species *Campylobacter jejuni,* *E. coli* O157:H7 *Brucella* species

Source of data: Food and Drug Administration: *Bad bug book,* 2nd ed. 2012. http://www.fda.gov/Food /FoodborneIllnessContaminants/CausesOfIllnessBadBugBook/default.htm. Accessed June 26, 2017.

Oysters: ©lynx/iconotec.com/Glow Images RF; Cheese: ©J. Glenn/Cole Group/Getty Images RF

Concept CHECKPOINT

5. Discuss at least three ways pathogens can contaminate human foods.
6. With regard to food preparation, what is cross-contamination?
7. What is pasteurization?
8. List at least three conditions that favor the survival and multiplication of food-borne pathogens.
9. Identify at least four foods that are high risk for supporting pathogens.

See Appendix G for responses.

12.4 Food-Borne Illness

Learning Outcomes

1 Describe typical signs and symptoms of food-borne illness.

2 Explain when a person who has a food-borne illness should seek professional medical help.

3 Explain why it is incorrect to call a food-borne illness the "flu" or "stomach flu."

Signs and symptoms of food–borne (and water–borne) illnesses generally involve the digestive tract and include nausea, vomiting, diarrhea, and intestinal cramps. However, most pathogens have an *incubation period*, a length of time in which they grow and multiply in food or the digestive tract before they can cause illness. Thus, if you develop signs and symptoms of a food–borne illness, you might have difficulty identifying the source of the infection or intoxication. Was the vomiting and diarrhea that you experienced at 3 A.M. the result of eating soft–cooked eggs for breakfast 18 hours earlier or the sliced deli chicken you ate for lunch 2 days ago?

Various factors influence whether an individual becomes ill after consuming a food or beverage that has been contaminated with a pathogen or toxin. The number of pathogenic microbes in a food or the amount of toxin it contains can contribute to the risk and severity of a food–borne illness. Furthermore, individuals vary in their vulnerability to many food–borne pathogens. In general, high–risk groups are pregnant women, very young children, older adults, and persons who suffer from serious chronic illnesses or weakened immune systems.

In most cases, otherwise healthy individuals who suffer from common types of food–borne illness recover completely and without professional medical care within a few days.[5] However, vomiting, diarrhea, and other signs of illness can be so severe, the patient requires hospitalization. You should consult a physician when an intestinal disorder is accompanied by one or more of the signs and symptoms listed in Table 12.2.[6]

Many people mistakenly report that they have the "stomach *flu*" when they actually are suffering from a food– or water–borne illness. "Flu," or *influenza*, is an infectious disease caused by specific viruses that invade the respiratory tract. Influenza is characterized by coughing, fever, weakness, and body aches. On the other hand, food–borne illness primarily affects the digestive system and not the respiratory system. Intestinal cramps, diarrhea, and vomiting are *not* typical signs and symptoms of influenza, and coughing is not a usual sign of a food–borne illness. Thus, it is inaccurate to call a bout of diarrhea and intestinal cramps the "flu" or the "stomach flu."

TABLE 12.2 Serious Signs and Symptoms of Food-Borne Illness: When to See a Physician

Decreased urination and other signs of dehydration
Prolonged vomiting

Diarrhea for:
   more than 2 days in adults
   more than 24 hours in children

Severe intestinal pain
Fever exceeding 101°F
Stools containing blood or pus
Black, tarry stools
Trouble breathing, walking, or other signs of muscle weakness

Concept CHECKPOINT

10. Identify at least three typical signs and symptoms of food-borne illness.

11. When should a person suffering from a food-borne illness seek professional medical help?

12. Discuss the differences between a food-borne illness and the "flu."

See Appendix G for responses.

12.5 Common Food-Borne Pathogens

Learning Outcomes

1 Identify common pathogens that are sources of food-borne illness in the United States.

2 Discuss typical signs, symptoms, and incubation periods of food-borne illnesses that are caused by each major pathogen.

3 Identify high-risk foods that are often sources of pathogens or their toxins.

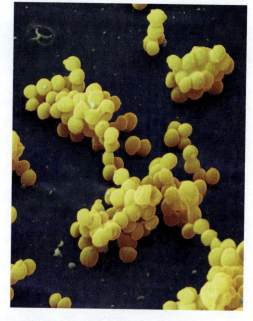

Improperly cooked or handled beef, poultry, eggs, and foods made with eggs are common sources of *Staphylococcus aureus.* ©Eye of Science/Science Source

The major kinds of pathogens are bacteria, viruses, protozoa, and fungi. In the United States, *bacteria* and *viruses* are responsible for most cases of food—borne illness. The following sections take a closer look at some of the major pathogens that can cause food—borne illness.

Bacteria

Bacteria are single—cell microorganisms that do not have the complex array of organelles that plant and animal cells contain. Some bacteria can live without oxygen, such as in canned or vacuum—packed foods. Other types of bacteria transform into inactive resistant forms called *spores* when living conditions are less than ideal. If the environment becomes more hospitable, the spores revert to the active bacterial state.

Many kinds of bacteria are pathogens that cause food—borne illness, includ—ing forms of *Campylobacter, Clostridium, Escherichia, Listeria, Salmonella* and *Staphylococcus (kam'—pih—low—bak'—ter, kloss—trid'—ee—um, esh'—er—ee'—she—ah, liss—tear'—ee—ah, sal'—mo—nell—ah, staff'—il—lo—cawk'—kiss).* Some types of pathogenic bacteria do not cause infections when they are con—sumed in food, but these microbes produce toxins that cause food intoxication. Table 12.3 summarizes some general information about common bacterial sources of food—borne illness in the United States.

bacteria simple single-celled microorganisms

virus microbe consisting of a piece of genetic material coated with protein

Viruses

Viruses are another common source of food—borne infection (Table 12.4). A **virus** is simply a piece of genetic material coated with protein (Fig. 12.2). Viruses must invade a living cell to produce more viruses. Unlike certain bacteria, viruses do not secrete toxins, and therefore, they do not cause food intoxication. Contaminated food or water, however, can transmit viruses to humans and cause food infection.

Vaccines that protect against hepatitis A virus and rotaviral infections are available. As of June 2017, a vaccine to prevent norovirus infections was in development.

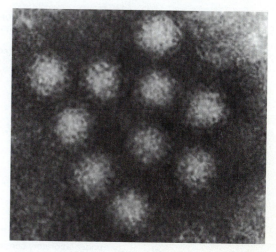

Figure 12.2 Norovirus. Source: F.P. Williams, U.S. EPA

TABLE 12.3   Common Sources of Food-Borne Illness: Bacteria

Bacterium	High-Risk Foods	Approx. Time of Onset	Typical Signs and Symptoms
Bacillus cereus (toxin)	Starchy foods (rice, potatoes, puddings, some soups)	6–15 hours	Abdominal cramps, watery diarrhea, nausea
Campylobacter jejuni	Raw, undercooked poultry; raw milk; contaminated water	2–5 days	Diarrhea (sometimes bloody), abdominal cramping, vomiting, fever
Clostridium botulinum (toxin)	Vacuum-packed foods, improperly canned foods, low-acid foods. Honey may contain spores.	18–36 hours	Vomiting, diarrhea, blurry or double vision, difficulty swallowing, muscular weakness. Can be fatal
Clostridium perfringens (toxin)	Cooked meat, poultry, casseroles, gravies	8–16 hours	Watery diarrhea (may be bloody), mild abdominal cramps
Escherichia coli O157:H7 (toxin)	Raw ground beef, raw seed sprouts, raw leafy greens, fresh fruit, raw milk, unpasteurized juices, foods contaminated with feces	3–4 days	Intestinal cramps, bloody diarrhea, kidney failure. Can be fatal
Listeria monocytogenes	Raw meat and poultry, raw milk, fresh soft cheese made from raw milk, liver paté, smoked seafood, deli meats, hot dogs, raw vegetables	Few hours to 3 days; 3 months for invasive disease	Fever, muscular aches, vomiting, diarrhea. In pregnant women, the infection can lead to stillbirth (birth of a dead fetus) or premature birth. Can be fatal
Salmonella species	Meat poultry, seafood, and eggs; raw seed sprouts; raw vegetables; unpasteurized juice	6 hours to 3 days	Nausea, vomiting, fever, headache, abdominal cramps, diarrhea. Can be fatal.
Shigella species	Unclean water; raw vegetables, herbs, and other foods that were contaminated with feces as a result of poor food handling and personal hygiene practices	8–50 hours	Abdominal cramps, fever, diarrhea that may contain blood and mucus. Can be fatal in infants, older adults, and people with a weak immune system
Staphylococcus aureus (toxin)	Meat and meat products, poultry, and eggs; foods made with eggs, such as potato, egg, macaroni, and tuna salads; custards, and cream-filled pastries	1–7 hours	Diarrhea, nausea, vomiting, abdominal cramps
Vibrio vulnificus	Raw oysters, clams, crabs and other raw or undercooked seafood; unclean water	12 hours to 3 weeks	Fever, vomiting, diarrhea, abdominal cramps. Can be fatal
Yersinia enterocolitica	Raw vegetables, undercooked pork, contaminated water, unpasteurized milk	1 day to 2 weeks	Diarrhea, high fever, abdominal pain, vomiting (in some cases)

Source of data: Food and Drug Administration: *Bad bug book,* 2nd ed. 2012. http://www.fda.gov/Food/FoodborneIllnessContaminants/CausesOfIllnessBadBugBook /default.htm. Accessed: June 26, 2017.

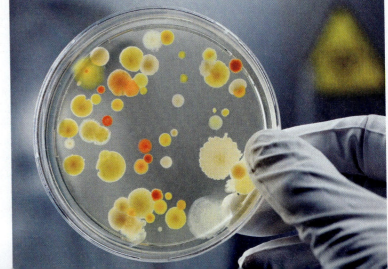

Scientists can often "grow" (culture) bacteria under laboratory conditions and identify them. ©Andreas Reh/Getty Images RF

TABLE 12.4 Common Sources of Food-Borne Illness: Viruses

Virus	High-Risk Foods	Approx. Time of Onset	Typical Signs and Symptoms
Norovirus	Food or water that has been contaminated with infected feces Virus can be spread person to person	12 hours to 2 days	"Explosive" vomiting; watery, nonbloody diarrhea; abdominal cramps; nausea; low-grade fever (occasionally)
Rotavirus	Food, water, or objects that have been contaminated with infected feces	2 days	Fever, abdominal pain, vomiting, watery diarrhea
Hepatitis A (HAV)	Food or water that has been contaminated with HAV from feces	2 to 4 weeks	Fever, loss of appetite, nausea, vomiting, diarrhea, muscle aches, general weakness May have signs of liver inflammation, such as jaundice, liver enlargement, and dark-colored urine

Source of data: Food and Drug Administration: *Bad bug book,* 2nd ed. 2012. http://www.fda.gov/Food/FoodborneIllnessContaminants/CausesOfIllnessBadBugBook/default.htm. Accessed: June 26, 2017.

Fungi

Fungi such as molds, yeast, and mushrooms are simple life forms that live on dead or decaying organic matter. Certain fungi, such as button mushrooms and the mold in blue cheese, are beneficial and edible. Other fungi are responsible for spoiling foods, such as bread molds, or causing respiratory problems or allergic reactions in sensitive people. A serious concern is the toxicity of several variet—ies of wild mushrooms. Cases of severe illness and death have been reported as a result of people picking and eating toxic wild mushrooms after mistaking them for edible varieties (Fig. 12.3). Nevertheless, fungi are not a major source of food—borne illness in the United States.

Certain molds produce *aflatoxins*, substances that can cause severe illness, particularly liver damage, and even death when consumed. Tree nuts, peanuts, rice, and corn that are stored under warm, humid conditions can become sources of aflatoxins. In some regions of the world, especially Africa and Southeast Asia, people often eat foods that are contaminated with aflatoxin—producing molds. Rates of liver cancer are high in these places. Thus, medical researchers think there is an association between exposure to aflatoxins and development of liver cancer. No outbreaks of food—borne intoxication caused by aflatoxins have been reported among the U.S. population.[5]

Protozoa and Parasitic Worms

Giardia (*jee—ar'—de—ah*) and *Cryptosporidium* (*krip'—toe—spo—rid'—ee—um*) are **protozoa** (*pro—toe—zoe'—ah*), single—celled microorganisms that have a more complex cell structure than bacteria. Table 12.5 lists some protozoa that often cause food—borne and water—borne illnesses in the United States. The "Nutrition Matters" section discusses traveler's diarrhea, which frequently results from a protozoal infection.

Certain types of worms such as *Trichinella* (*trick'—ah—nell'—ah*) and *Anisakis* (*ah'—ni—sa'—kis*) are parasites that can contaminate food or water (Fig. 12.4). A parasite is a life form that obtains its nourishment from another living thing (the host). Most Americans who become infected with parasitic worms that are found in the United States recover when they receive proper treatment. Nev—ertheless, some infected persons suffer long—term health problems and even die as a result of the illnesses. Table 12.5 provides information about the kinds of parasitic worms that can infect people.

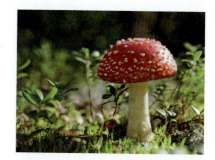
Figure 12.3 Deadly mushrooms. Severe illness and even death can occur if people pick and eat toxic mushrooms, such as this *Amanita* mushroom.
©Jorgen Bausager/Getty Images RF

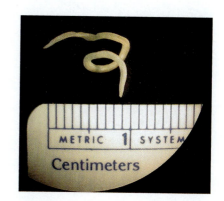
Figure 12.4 *Anisakis.* Source: Centers for Disease Control and Prevention, DPDx

fungi simple organisms that live on dead or decaying organic matter

protozoa single-celled microorganisms that have complex cell structures

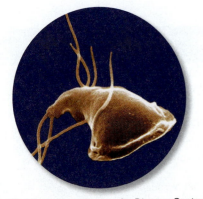

Giardia. Source: Centers for Disease Control and Prevention

TABLE 12.5 Common Sources of Food-Borne Illness: Protozoa and Parasitic Worms

Pathogen	High-Risk Foods	Approx. Time of Onset	Typical Signs and Symptoms
Protozoa			
Cryptosporidium	Foods prepared by people whose hands were contaminated with infected feces; fresh juices, produce, and milk	7–10 days	Profuse, watery diarrhea; abdominal pain; fever; nausea; vomiting
Giardia	Consumption of contaminated water, including water from lakes, streams, swimming pools Travelers to certain countries, hikers, and people who swim in or camp by lakes and streams.	1–2 weeks	Diarrhea, abdominal pain, weight loss
Toxoplasma	Raw or partially cooked wild game (especially bear and wild pig), clams, oysters Accidentally ingesting infected cat feces	5–23 days	Fever, headache, muscle aches, rash Pregnant women should avoid contact with cat feces because the parasite can infect their unborn offspring, causing eye or brain damage and even fetal death.
Parasitic Worms			
Trichinella	Raw or undercooked infected meat, especially pork, bear, seal, and walrus meat	1 to 4 weeks	Nausea; vomiting; diarrhea; fatigue; fever; abdominal discomfort; facial swelling, especially around the eyes; muscle pain Death can occur in severe cases.
Anisakis	Raw or undercooked infected seafood	1 day to 2 weeks	Abdominal pain, nausea, vomiting, diarrhea

Source of data: Food and Drug Administration: *Bad bug book,* 2nd ed. 2012. http://www.fda.gov/Food/FoodborneIllnessContaminants/CausesOfIllnessBadBugBook/default.htm. Accessed: June 26, 2017.

Certain fungi, such as button mushrooms and the mold in blue cheese, are beneficial and edible.
Mushrooms: ©McGraw-Hill Education/Stephen P. Lynch, photographer; Blue cheese: ©Stockbyte/Getty Images RF

Concept CHECKPOINT

13. Identify at least three bacterial sources of food-borne illness in the United States.

14. Identify three viruses that are sources of food-borne illness in the United States.

15. What are aflatoxins?

16. Identify a parasitic worm and a parasitic protozoan that can cause food- or water-borne illness in the United States.

See Appendix G for responses.

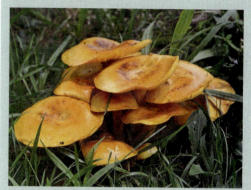
12.6 Preventing Food-Borne Illness

Learning Outcomes

1 Explain how to reduce the risk of food-borne illness when purchasing, preparing, cooking, and storing foods and beverages.

2 Explain why ground meat and poultry often are sources of food-borne illness.

3 Identify the temperature range that encourages rapid multiplication of pathogens.

4 Discuss the federal government's simple actions for reducing the risk of food-borne illness.

While you cannot control the safety of foods that are prepared in restaurants or other places outside your home, you can greatly reduce your risk of food–borne illness by following some important rules, most of which require changing risky food selection, preparation, and storage practices.

Purchasing Food

The following tips can help reduce your risk of food–borne illness:

- When shopping in a supermarket, select frozen foods and highly perishable foods, such as meat, poultry, or fish, last.

- Check "best by" dates on packaged perishable foods. Choose meats and other animal products with the latest dates.

- Do not buy food in damaged containers; for example, avoid containers that leak, bulge, or are severely dented, or jars that are cracked or have loose or bulging lids.

- Open egg cartons and examine eggs; do not buy cartons that have cracked eggs.

- Purchase only pasteurized milk, cheese, and fruit and vegetable juices (check the label).

- Pack meat, fish, and poultry in separate plastic bags, so their drippings do not contaminate each other and your other groceries.

- After shopping for food, take groceries home immediately. Refrigerate or freeze meat, fish, egg, and dairy products promptly.

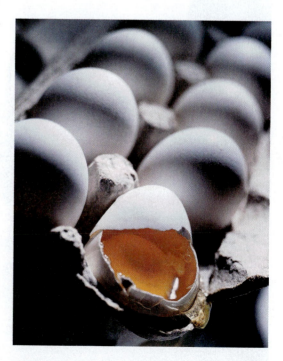

Before purchasing eggs, open the carton and check the eggs. Do not buy cartons that have any cracked eggs.
©evitaphoto/Getty Images RF

- Store whole eggs in their cartons, even if your refrigerator has a place for storing eggs. Egg cartons are designed to keep eggs fresh longer than a refrigerator's egg compartment.

Setting the Stage for Food Preparation

Contaminated hands and food preparation surfaces spread pathogens. The following tips can help reduce the risk of food—borne illness:

- Wash hands thoroughly with very warm, soapy water for at least 20 seconds before and after touching food. If clean water for handwashing is not available, use sanitizing hand wipes.

- Before preparing food, clean food preparation surfaces, including kitchen counters, cutting boards, dishes, knives, and other food preparation equipment with hot, soapy water. You can destroy most pathogens when you clean and *sanitize* food preparation surfaces with a solution made by adding a tablespoon of bleach to 1 gallon of water.

- The FDA recommends cutting boards with unmarred surfaces made of easy—to—clean, nonporous materials, such as plastic, marble, or glass. If you prefer to use wooden cutting boards, make sure they are made of a nonabsorbent hardwood, such as oak or maple, and have no obvious seams or cracks.

- Replace cutting boards when they become streaked with cuts because these grooves can be difficult to clean thoroughly and may harbor bacteria.

- If possible, have a cutting board reserved for meats, fish, and poultry; have another cutting board for fruits and vegetables; and have a third board for breads. Clean all cutting boards in the dishwasher or with hot, soapy water. You can also sanitize cutting boards with a dilute bleach solution.

Wash hands thoroughly with hot, soapy water for at least 20 seconds before and after touching food. ©McGraw-Hill Education/Rick Brady, photographer

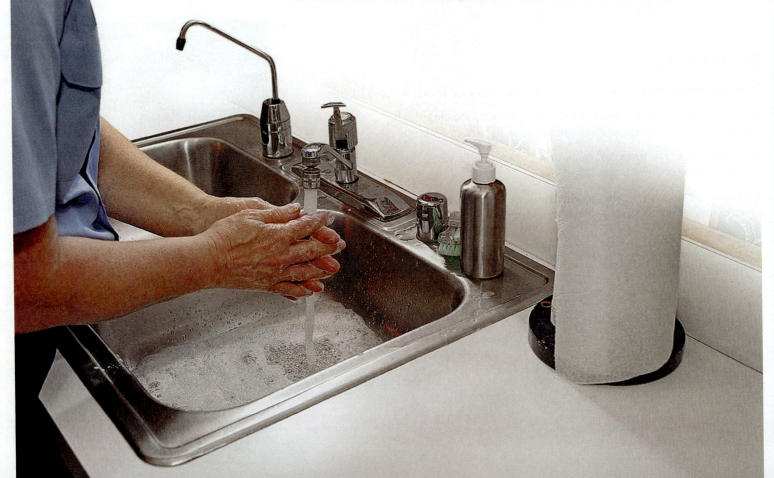

- Sanitize food preparation surfaces and equipment that have come in contact with raw meat, fish, poultry, and eggs as soon as possible to destroy pathogens that may be present. In addition, sanitize damp kitchen sponges by heating them in a microwave oven for 60 seconds and machine–wash and –dry kitchen towels frequently.

Preparing Food

The following tips can help reduce your risk of food–borne illness:

- Do not use foods from containers that leak, bulge, or are severely dented or from jars that are cracked or have loose or bulging lids.

- Do not use foods from containers that have damaged safety seals because the food they contain may have been contaminated.

- Do not taste or use food that spurts liquid or has a bad odor when the can is opened.

- Read product labels to determine whether foods need to be refrigerated after their packages are opened.

- Before preparing fresh produce, carefully wash the foods under running water to remove dirt and bacteria clinging to the surface. Bacteria can be sticky, so scrub the peel with a vegetable brush if it is to be eaten. Even if you plan to remove the skin or peel, wash the produce before you cut it.

- Avoid eating moldy foods. Mold does not grow well on low–moisture foods. Thus, small amounts of mold on hard cheeses and on firm fruits and vegetables can be removed by cutting away the mold along with at least 1 inch of food that surrounds the moldy area.[7]

- **When in doubt, throw the food out.**

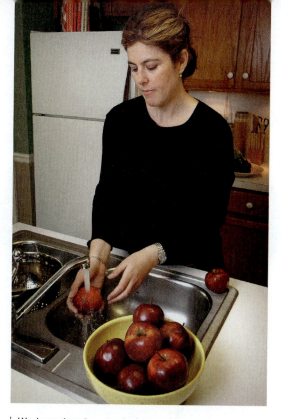

Wash produce in water before eating or preparing it.
Source: Centers for Disease Control and Prevention/ James Gathany

Maintaining the Proper Temperature of Foods

Most microbes grow well when the temperature of a high–risk food is between 40°F and 140°F—the "danger zone" (Fig. 12.5).[8] Cooking foods to the proper tem–perature destroys food–borne viruses and bacteria, such as *Norovirus* and *E. coli* O157:H7. To be safe, a product must be cooked to an internal temperature that is high enough to destroy harmful pathogens and bacterial toxins. Using a meat thermometer is a reliable way to ensure that meat, poultry, thick pieces of fish, and egg–containing dishes have reached the proper internal temperature without overcooking. Table 12.6 indicates recommended minimum internal temperatures for cooking these foods.

Meat thermometers must be used properly. In general, the thermometer should be placed in the thickest part of the muscle tissue, away from bone, fat, or gristle (Fig. 12.6). If the thermometer is inserted incorrectly or placed in the wrong area, the reading may not accurately reflect the internal temperature of the product.

Microwave cooking can result in uneven heating that does not destroy microbes in the cool spots. While cooking a food in a microwave oven, keep the dish covered, and stop the oven occasionally to stir the food. Stirring the food reduces uneven heating. Cook the food until it reaches 165°F. Microwave cooking is not recommended for stuffed foods because during cooking, the temperature of the stuffing may not be high enough to eliminate pathogens.[9]

Chilling food slows the growth of microbes in the items, but some bacteria can grow even at proper refrigeration temperatures. Freezing does not destroy

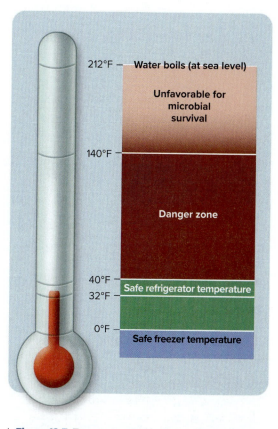

Figure 12.5 Temperature guide for food safety. Most pathogenic microbes grow well when the temperature of risky food is between 40°F and 140°F—the "danger zone."

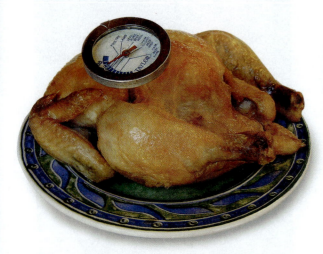

Figure 12.6 Use of a meat thermometer.
©Wendy Schiff

TABLE 12.6 USDA Recommended Safe Minimum Internal Temperatures

Food	Safe Minimum Internal Temperature (°F)
Beef steaks and roasts	145
Fish	145
Pork	145
Ground beef, pork, lamb, and veal	160
Egg dishes	160
Poultry products	165

Source: U.S. Department of Health and Human Services, *Safe minimum cooking temperatures*. ND. Accessed: July 30, 2016. https://www.foodsafety.gov/keep/charts/mintemp.html

bacteria or inactivate viruses in food; the process just halts the microbes' ability to multiply. As frozen food thaws, the bacteria and viruses resume their activities and can cause illness.

A major challenge for food handlers involves keeping large amounts of high-risk foods at safe temperatures when they are served from a single container. Food that is near the sides of the container may stay hotter or colder than food that is near or in the center of the container. As shown in Figure 12.7, chilled foods should be kept covered and served from a shallow container filled with ice. Hot foods should be kept covered and be served from shallow, heated pans. The best simple advice to follow: "Keep hot foods hot and cold foods cold."

The following tips can help reduce your risk of food-borne illness:

- Always thaw high-risk foods in the refrigerator, under cold running water, or in a microwave oven.

- Cook foods immediately after thawing.

- Marinate food in the refrigerator, and if marinating meat, fish, or poultry, discard the marinade.

- Do not remove cold foods from the refrigerator or hot foods from the stove until it is time to serve them.

Raw Fish

Eating raw fish, such as sushi, can be safe for most healthy people if the fish is very fresh before being commercially frozen and then thawed. While frozen, the fish must maintain an internal temperature of 10°F for 7 days. The freezing step is important because very cold temperatures can kill parasites that are often in fish tissues. If you choose to eat uncooked fish, purchase it from reputable establishments that have high standards for quality and sanitation. Nevertheless, it is prudent to not eat any raw animal products, including fish.

Ground Meats, Poultry, and Fish

Ground meats, poultry, and fish are highly perishable and must be thoroughly cooked to avoid being a source of food-borne illness. The interior portion of an intact piece of raw animal flesh is free of bacteria because the tissues are not exposed to air. However, ground meats, fish, and poultry products are often

Did *YOU* Know?

Have you heard about the "5-second rule"? Supposedly, food that drops on the floor will not pick up microbes if it is picked up within 5 seconds. A study determined that this is a food-related myth. As soon as food touches a contaminated surface such as a floor, some microbes adhere to it.[10]

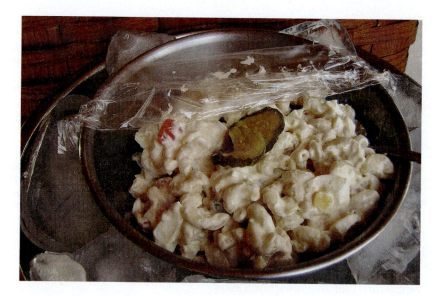

contaminated with microbes. Prior to being ground up, the surface of a chunk of meat, fish, or poultry may contain relatively harmless concentrations of pathogens. The grinding process, however, mixes the pathogens throughout the meat. At the same time, grinding the meat greatly increases its surface area, exposing more of the protein–rich tissues to microbes in air. Furthermore, the meat grinder can be a source of pathogens and spread them to the food product, especially if the machine was not properly cleaned after its last use. The particles of food that remained in the grinder can provide food for pathogenic microorganisms. Therefore, surfaces that touch ground meats should be cleaned carefully.

The following tips can help reduce your risk of food–borne illness:

- Cook beef, poultry, pork, thick pieces of fish, and egg–containing dishes thoroughly, using a meat thermometer to check for doneness.

- Cook eggs until the yolk and white have solidified and no "runniness" remains.

- Bake stuffing separately from poultry, or wash the poultry cavity thoroughly and stuff the bird immediately before cooking. Make sure the temperature of the stuffing reaches 165°F. After cooking, transfer the stuffing to a clean bowl for serving or storage.

- Serve meat, poultry, and fish on a clean plate. Never use the same plate that held the raw product. For example, when grilling hamburgers, do not put cooked items on the plate that was used to carry the raw meat to the grill.

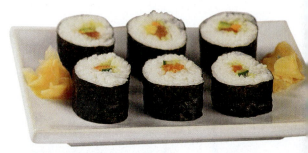

Eating raw fish, such as some forms of sushi, can be safe for most healthy people if the fish is very fresh before being commercially frozen and then thawed. ©Steve Lupton/Getty Images RF

The grinding process mixes pathogens throughout the raw meat. Source: U.S. Department of Agriculture, Food Safety and Inspection Service

Storing and Reheating Food

After food is cooked, careless food handling continues to set the stage for the growth of pathogens. Food–borne pathogens thrive at "room temperature," temperatures that are between 60°F and 110°F. A common practice is to let hot or cold foods remain on the table at room temperature for a few hours. Although you may not feel like clearing the table after eating, it is a good idea to cover leftovers and refrigerate or freeze them as soon as you have finished eating, or within 2 hours. If environmental temperatures are above 90°F, refrigerate the leftovers within 1 hour.[11] There is no need to let hot foods cool before chilling or freezing them.

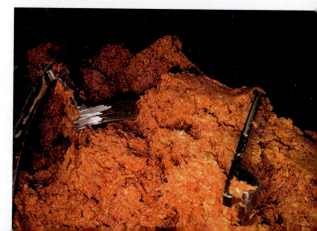

Did *YOU* Know?

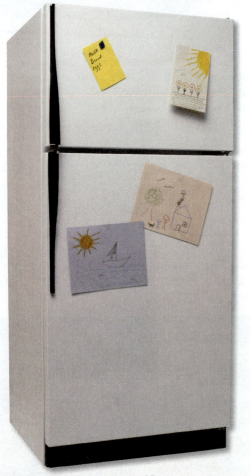

©C Squared Studios/Getty Images RF

To reduce your risk of food—borne illness, follow these food storage tips:

- Check your refrigerator's temperature regularly to make sure it stays below 41°F. Keep the refrigerator as cold as possible without freezing milk and lettuce.

- Cook ground meats and poultry soon after purchasing. If this is not possible, freeze the ground items.

- Note that raw fish, shellfish, and poultry are highly perishable. It is best to cook these foods or freeze them the day they are purchased.

- Use refrigerated ground meat and patties within 1 to 2 days, and use frozen meat and patties within 3 to 4 months after purchasing them. Table 12.7 presents recommended time limits for refrigeration and freezer storage of foods. Foods that are stored in the freezer for longer than recommended periods are safe to eat after being thawed properly, but they often develop unappealing flavors.[11] Note that ground meats are more perishable than intact cuts of meat.

- Use refrigerated leftovers within 4 days.

Cross—contamination is a threat not only during food preparation; it can also become a problem during food storage. Therefore, keep all foods, including leftovers, covered while they are in the refrigerator. This practice can prevent drippings from foods that are often contaminated, such as raw chicken, from tainting other foods. Furthermore, store raw meats, fish, poultry, and shellfish on

TABLE 12.7 Cold Storage Time Limits for Perishable Foods

Product	Storage Period in Refrigerator (40°F)	Storage Period in Freezer (0°F)
Fresh meat		
Ground meat	1–2 days	3–4 months
Steaks and roasts	3–5 days	4–12 months
Fresh pork		
Chops	3–5 days	4–6 months
Ground	1–2 days	3–4 months
Cured meats		
Luncheon meat, deli sliced or open package	3–5 days	1–2 months
Unopened package	2 weeks	1–2 months
Fresh fish	1–2 days	—
Fresh chicken or turkey (whole)	1–2 days	12 months
Parts	1–2 days	9 months
Eggs		
Fresh, in shell	3–5 weeks	—
Hard-cooked	1 week	—

Source: U.S. Department of Agriculture, Food Safety and Inspection Service, *Basics of handling foods safely: Cold storage chart.* Modified 2015. http://www.fsis.usda.gov/wps/portal/fsis/topics/food-safety-education/get-answers /food-safety-fact-sheets/safe-food-handling/basics-for-handling-food-safely/ct_index/ ; *Refrigeration and food safety.* Modified 2015. http://www.fsis.usda.gov/wps/portal/fsis/topics/food-safety-education/get-answers/food-safety -fact-sheets/safe-food-handling/refrigeration-and-food-safety/ct_index. Accessed: June 26, 2017.

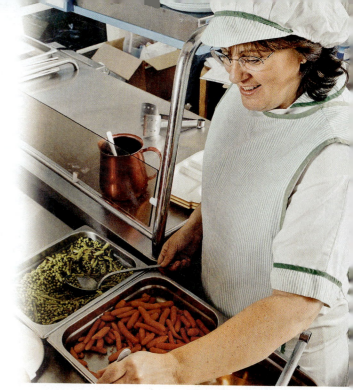
lower shelves of the refrigerator, so they are separated from foods that are to be eaten raw. Examine Figure 12.8. Can you find two examples of improperly stored refrigerated foods?

Food safety educators with the federal government condensed these rules into four simple actions as a part of their Check Your Steps program:

1. **CLEAN.** Wash hands and surfaces often.

2. **SEPARATE.** Do not cross—contaminate.

3. **COOK.** Cook to proper temperatures.

4. **CHILL.** Refrigerate promptly.

You can find reliable information about food—borne illness at www.foodsafety.gov. For general food safety questions, you can call the FDA's food safety hotline at 1—888—723—3366.

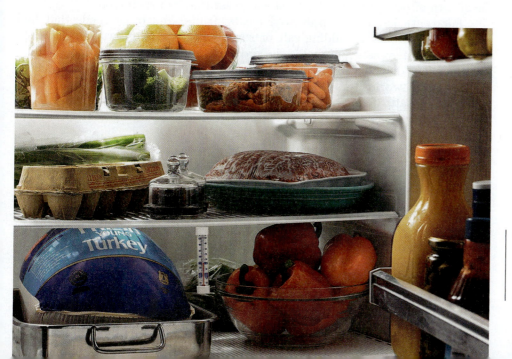

Figure 12.8 Storing risky foods in the refrigerator.
In this photograph, can you identify two risky foods that are improperly stored? What can be done to store the foods safely? Source: U.S. Department of Agriculture, Food Safety and Inspection Service

Concept CHECKPOINT

17. List at least four rules for reducing the risk of food-borne illness when you purchase foods and beverages.

18. List at least five rules for reducing the risk of food-borne illness when you prepare and cook foods.

19. List at least three rules for reducing the risk of food-borne illness when you store cooked foods.

20. Explain why ground meat and poultry often are sources of food-borne illness.

21. What preparation step can be taken to make fish safer to eat raw?

22. What temperature range encourages rapid multiplication of pathogens?

23. What are the federal government's four simplified actions for reducing the risk of food-borne illness?

See Appendix G for responses.

12.7 Food Preservation

Learning Outcomes

1 Discuss food preservation methods, including how each method extends the shelf life of foods.

2 Explain how to prepare home-canned, low-acid foods that are safe to eat.

shelf life period of time that a food can be stored before it spoils

fermentation process used to preserve or produce a variety of foods, including pickles and wine

sterilization process that kills or destroys all microorganisms and viruses

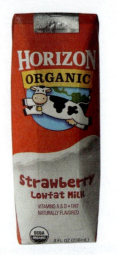

This package contains fluid milk that has been pasteurized and placed into a sterilized container. As long as the package remains sealed, the milk does not need to be refrigerated. ©Wendy Schiff

If nothing is done to preserve a fresh food, the item soon undergoes various chemical changes that eventually result in spoilage. Preserving food extends its shelf life. **Shelf life** refers to the period of time that a food can be stored before it spoils. Heating is one of the oldest ways to preserve foods. Heat can kill or deactivate pathogens, and the process also destroys naturally occurring enzymes in foods that can contribute to food spoilage.

Fermentation is an ancient method of food preservation that is still used to produce a variety of foods, including yogurt, wine, pickles, and sauerkraut. The fermentation process involves adding certain bacteria or yeast to food. These microbes use sugars in the food to make acids and alcohol, chemicals that hinder the growth of other types of bacteria and yeast that can spoil food.

For centuries, people preserved meats, fruits, and other foods that had high water contents by adding salt or sugar to them. To grow, bacteria need plenty of water; yeasts and molds can grow when less water is available. Adding sugar or salt to foods draws water out of cells, including bacteria, fungi, protozoa, and worms. As a result, these pathogens are less likely to survive in sugary or salty foods. Drying reduces a food's water content. Dried fruits such as raisins, for example, have a longer shelf life than grapes, their natural counterparts.

Today, we can add pasteurization, refrigeration, freezing, canning, irradiation, additives, and *aseptic* processing to the list of food preservation techniques (Table 12.8). Aseptic processing involves sterilizing a food and its package separately, before the food enters the package. The **sterilization** process destroys all microorganisms and viruses. After undergoing aseptic packaging, boxes of sterile foods and beverages, such as milk or juices, can remain free of microbial growth for several years while sitting on store or pantry shelves. However, once the containers of these products are opened, the foods or beverages have the same shelf life as their counterparts that have not undergone aseptic processing.

TABLE 12.8 Summary of Food Preservation Methods

Method	Means of Effectiveness	Examples of Foods
Heating (cooking, pasteurization, aseptic processing)	Kills or deactivates spoilage and pathogenic microbes, destroys enzymes that result in food spoilage	Most foods
Adding salt/sugar	Binds water, decreasing the amount available for microbes	Ham, bacon, fish, pickled foods
Smoking	Kills spoilage microbes, destroys enzymes that result in food spoilage Smoking is a method of heating. The process involves salting food before smoking and refrigerating or freezing the food after smoking.	Meats, fish
Curing	Retards the growth of *C. botulinum* and stabilizes the flavor of the food Additives such as sodium nitrate and nitrite are used to cure meat, fish, or poultry.	Luncheon meats, smoked fish
Chilling/freezing	Slows molecular movement, retarding microbial and enzymatic activity	Most foods
Drying (dehydration)	Removes much of the moisture in food that microbes need to survive	Fruit, herbs, meat jerkies, seeds
Fermenting	Produces acids and alcohol that interfere with the survival of unwanted microbes	Alcoholic beverages, yogurt, cheeses, soy sauce
Canning	Kills spoilage microbes, destroys enzymes in food that result in spoilage, removes oxygen that certain microbes need to survive	Meat, fish, poultry, fruits, vegetables, milk
Irradiating	Destroys most pathogens, delays sprouting (potatoes)	Spices, raw meat and poultry, fresh fruits and vegetables

Source: *Complete Guide to Home Canning*, 2015 revision. http://nchfp.uga.edu/publications /publications_usda.html. Dried fruit: ©C Squared Studios/Getty Images RF; Pickles: ©Kevin Sanchez/Cole Group/Getty Images RF; Spam: ©McGraw-Hill Education/Elite Images, photographer; Cheese: ©Brand X Pictures/Getty Images RF

Home-Canned Foods

When food is canned, commercial food production methods require heating the food to certain temperatures for specified times. Thus, unless the can or jar has been damaged, properly processed canned foods should be free of pathogens. Certain home—canned foods, however, may contain the micro—organism *Clostridium botulinum* (*C. botulinum*) that causes *botulism* or its toxin. The home—canning process may kill *C. botulinum* bacteria in the food, but their spores or toxin may remain. That is why home—canned, *low—acid* foods such as beans and corn should be boiled for 10 min-utes before eating. Foods made with vinegar, tomatoes, or citrus juices are usually high—acid foods, and as a result, such items are not likely to be sources of *C. botulinum*. The botulinum toxin is highly poisonous; never taste a home—canned, low—acid food before boiling it. For more informa-tion about proper home canning of foods, obtain a copy of the U.S. Depart-ment of Agriculture's *Complete Guide to Home Canning, 2015 revision* (http://nchfp.uga.edu/publications/publications_usda.html) or contact a food and nutrition specialist at your community's university extension office.

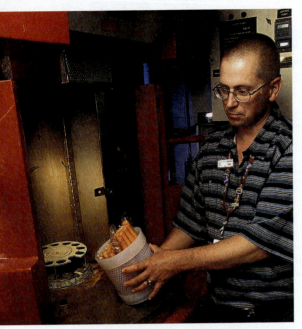

Figure 12.9 Irradiating food. U.S. Department of Agriculture microbiologist Glenn Boyd places a batch of hot dogs into the gamma radiation source to rid them of food-borne pathogens. Source: Stephen Ausmus/ARS/USDA

Irradiation

The process of food irradiation preserves food by using a high amount of energy to kill pathogens such as *Salmonella* and *E. coli* O157:H7 (Fig. 12.9). The processes used to irradiate foods do not make the items radioactive. The energy passes through the food, as in microwave cooking, and no radioactive material is left behind. The energy is strong enough to destroy the genetic material as well as cell membranes or cell walls of insects and microbes. As a result, irradiation is a highly effective way of destroying insects and microorganisms that may be in foods. However, irradiation is not always an effective way to destroy viruses.[13] It is important to recognize that even when foods, especially meats, have been irradiated, once their packaging has been opened, the foods can still become contaminated.

Irradiation extends the shelf life of spices, dry vegetable seasonings, meats, seeds, shell eggs, and fresh fruits and vegetables. Except for dried seasonings, packages that contain irradiated foods must be labeled with the international food irradiation symbol, the Radura, and include a statement indicating the product has been treated by irradiation (Fig. 12.10).

According to medical experts with the World Health Organization, FDA, and CDC, irradiated foods are safe to eat.[13] Furthermore, irradiation causes few or no nutritive losses. Despite such assurances, many Americans are skeptical about the safety of irradiated foods, and they avoid purchasing such products.

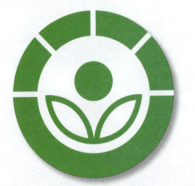

Figure 12.10 Radura symbol. The Radura symbol indicates the food in this package has been irradiated. Source: U.S. Department of Agriculture, Food Safety and Inspection Service

Concept CHECKPOINT

24. Define *shelf life*.
25. Identify four methods of food preservation and explain how each method extends the shelf life of foods.
26. What preparation step can be taken to make home-canned, low-acid foods safe to eat?
27. List three foods that may undergo irradiation to extend their shelf life.

See Appendix G for responses.

12.8 Preparing for Disasters

Learning Outcomes

 Explain actions people in households can take to have safe food and water available after a disaster.

2 Discuss ways to safely prepare food when a power outage occurs.

On October 29, 2012, Hurricane Sandy moved onto land in New Jersey and proceeded to batter much of the East Coast of the United States with high winds and severe flooding. The hurricane took the lives of 117 Americans and caused billions of dollars in property damage.[14] Immediately after the storm struck, millions of utility customers in the affected region lost power.[15] What steps can you take to have enough water and food available to survive hurricanes, earth-quakes, or other serious emergency situations?

A supply of clean water and wholesome food is necessary for surviving disasters such as hurricanes and earthquakes. This chapter's "Nutrition Matters" provides instructions for sanitizing water. The following recommendations may help sustain you and your loved ones for several days:

- Store at least 1 gallon of water per person per day. Ideally, you should have at least a 3– to 5–day supply of drinking water, or at least 5 gallons of water for each person in a household. Children and breastfeeding women may need more than 1 gallon of water per day. Also, more water may be necessary for people living in warm climates. Furthermore, store extra water for food preparation, personal hygiene, dishwashing, and pets.

- Water should be maintained in a cool place and in sturdy plastic bottles with tight–fitting lids.

- Change stored water every 6 months.

- Drink only bottled, boiled, or treated water until you are certain the public water supply is safe.

- If you have time to prepare, fill a bathtub with water to use if it becomes necessary. The water, however, will need to be sanitized before being consumed.

- If you drink bottled water, make sure the seal has not been broken.

If your emergency water supply is inadequate, you can consume melted ice cubes from the freezer, canned fruit juices, and water drained from an undam-aged water heater. Water stored in the tank of the toilet (not the bowl) is also fit to drink. Water in swimming pools and spas can be used for personal hygiene needs but not for drinking. Never drink water from car radiators, home heat-ing systems, or water beds. Alcoholic beverages contribute to dehydration and therefore should be avoided.

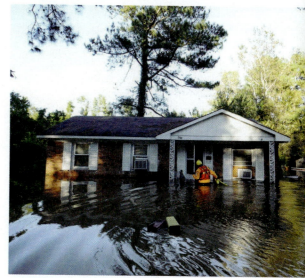

Flooding in North Carolina that was associated with Hurricane Matthew (2016). Source: Photo by Jocelyn Augustino/FEMA

Emergency Food Supply

A disaster can easily disrupt your access to safe food; therefore, you should store at least a 3–day supply of food for emergency use. Choose foods that have a long storage life, require no refrigeration, and can be eaten without cooking, such as canned meats, fruits, and vegetables. Table 12.9 lists foods that can be included in your emergency food supply. Also store a manual can opener, paper plates, and eating utensils.

If stored under proper conditions, unopened canned or boxed foods will remain fresh for about 2 years. Before storing food, use a permanent marking pen to write the date on the package. You should use and replace foods before they lose their freshness or reach their expiration dates. An ideal food storage location is a cool, dry, dark place. Do not store foods near gasoline, oil, paints, or petroleum–based solvents, because some food products absorb their odors. You can protect foods from rodents and insects by storing them in airtight containers or plastic storage bins.

If you have no electricity, consume perishable food in your refrigerator or freezer before using your emergency food supply. However, discard cooked foods after they have been at room temperature for 2 hours. Do not eat food that appears spoiled or is from cans that are leaking or bulging.

TABLE 12.9 Foods to Store for Emergency Situations

- Canned meats, fish, fruits, and vegetables
- Canned fruit juices
- Unopened boxes of cereal, low-salt crackers, and trail mix
- Prewrapped fruit-filled granola bars
- Peanut or other nut butters
- Raisins and other dried fruit
- Dry milk powder
- Baby foods

To prepare meals safely after a disaster, you will need to store:

- a camp stove or charcoal grill.
- fuel for cooking, such as charcoal. **Never** cook food on a camp stove or charcoal grill indoors. The fumes contain *carbon monoxide*, an odorless gas that can be deadly when it accumulates in a closed space.
- matches.
- cooking and eating utensils.
- paper plates, cups, and towels.

For more information about emergency preparedness, visit http://www.cdc.gov/healthywater/emergency/preparedness/index.html and http://www.fda.gov/Food/RecallsOutbreaksEmergencies/Emergencies/ucm2006925.htm.

Concept CHECKPOINT

28. Develop an emergency food and water supply plan for your home. Identify at least five foods that are appropriate for an emergency food supply.

29. In case public water supplies are disrupted, identify at least three sources of drinking water in homes that are safe for humans. Identify at least two sources of water that are unsafe to drink.

See Appendix G for responses.

12.9 Food Additives

Learning Outcomes

1 Explain the difference between direct and indirect food additives, and provide examples of each type of additive.

2 Discuss the impact of the GRAS list and the Delaney Clause on the use of food additives.

3 Identify unintentional food additives.

4 Discuss pesticides, including the pros and cons of their use.

5 Explain the usefulness of integrated pest management.

A **food additive** is any substance that becomes incorporated into food during production, packaging, transport, or storage. Food manufacturers incorporate *direct* or *intentional additives* into their products for various reasons. Such additives may make food easier to process, more nutritious, able to stay fresh longer, or better tasting. Most additives are added to influence a food's sensory characteristics, including taste or color.

Many direct food additives help maintain the safety of foods by limiting the growth of bacteria that cause food—borne illness. Other additives protect against the action of enzymes that can lead to undesirable changes in the food's color and taste. Such unwanted chemical changes occur when enzymes that are naturally in certain foods are exposed to the oxygen in air. *Antioxidant additives*, including vitamins E and C and a variety of *sulfites*, can prevent oxygen from reacting with these enzymes. **Color additives** are dyes, pigments, or other substances that provide color to foods, drugs, or cosmetics, such as beta—carotene in margarine and FD&C (Food, Drug, & Cosmetic) Red No. 40 in cherry—flavored

food additive any substance that becomes incorporated into food during production, packaging, transport, or storage

color additives dyes, pigments, or other substances that provide color to food

Food Additives Amendment U.S. legislation that requires evidence that a new food additive is safe before it can be marketed for use

Generally Recognized as Safe (GRAS) ingredients considered to be safe

TABLE 12.10   Common Types of Direct Food Additives

Type of Additive	Functions	Typical Products	Examples of Specific Ingredients
Preservatives	Prevent food spoilage	Jellies, beverages, baked goods, cured meats, cereals, snack foods	Ascorbic acid, citric acid, sodium benzoate, calcium propionate, sodium erythorbate, BHA, BHT, EDTA, sodium nitrite
Sweeteners	Add sweetness	Processed foods, beverages, baked goods, sugar substitutes	Sucrose, glucose, mannitol, corn syrup, aspartame, sucralose
Flavors and spices	Add specific flavors	Puddings, pie fillings, gelatins, cake mixes, candies, soft drinks	Natural flavorings, artificial flavorings, spices
Flavor enhancers	Enhance flavors already present	Many processed foods	Monosodium glutamate (MSG), hydrolyzed soy protein
Nutrients	Replace nutrients lost during processing, boost levels of nutrients naturally in food	Flour, cereals, margarine, fruit beverages, energy bars	Thiamin hydrochloride, riboflavin, niacin, niacinamide, folic acid, beta-carotene, ascorbic acid
Emulsifiers	Keep oily and watery ingredients from separating	Salad dressings, peanut butter, chocolate, frozen desserts	Soy lecithin, mono- and diglycerides, polysorbates
Leavening agents	Promote rising of certain baked goods	Baked goods	Baking soda, monocalcium phosphate, calcium carbonate
Stabilizers, thickeners, binders	Provide uniform texture and improve "mouth feel"	Frozen desserts, puddings, sauces	Gelatin, pectin, guar gum, carrageenan, whey
Color additives	Enhance natural colors, provide color to colorless and "fun" foods as well as medications and cosmetics	Processed foods, including candies, snack foods, margarine, cheese, soft drinks, gelatin	FD&C Blue No. 1, FD&C Red No. 40, beta-carotene, caramel color

Source: Modified from International Food Information Council and U.S. Food and Drug Administration: *Food: Overview of food ingredients, additives & colors.* 2014. http://www.fda.gov/food/ingredientspackaginglabeling/foodadditivesingredients/ucm094211.htm. Accessed: June 26, 2017.

cough syrup. Table 12.10 lists common types of direct food additives (including color additives), their uses, examples of products that contain the additives, and names of specific additives.

Indirect additives, such as compounds from a food's wrapper or container, can enter food as it is packaged, transported, or stored. Indirect additives, however, have no purpose. The FDA and certain international organizations regulate all food additives to ensure that processed foods and their packaging are safe.[16]

Food Safety Legislation: Food Additives

By the 1950s, hundreds of ingredients were being added to foods during processing. Many of these substances had long histories of being safe; others were deemed safe after undergoing scientific testing. In 1958, the U.S. Congress enacted the **Food Additives Amendment.** According to this amendment, an ingredient that had been in use prior to 1958 was **Generally Recognized as Safe (GRAS)** when qualified experts generally agreed that the substance was safe for its intended use. The Food Additives Amendment excluded GRAS substances from being defined as food additives.[16] Thus, modern food manufacturers can include substances on the GRAS list

Color additives are dyes, pigments, or other substances that provide color to foods, drugs, or cosmetics. ©Wendy Schiff

Delaney Clause component of the 1958 Food Additives Amendment that prevents manufacturers from adding carcinogenic compounds to food

unintentional food additives substances that are accidentally in foods

Common biological and physical food contaminants include rodent feces or urine. ©Image Source RF

as ingredients without testing them for safety or getting prior approval from the FDA.

As a result of the 1958 Food Additives Amendment, the manufacturer of a *new* food additive (one developed after 1958) must provide evidence of the substance's safety to the FDA before the additive can be used.[16] When evaluating the safety of a newly developed food additive, FDA experts consider the chemical composition and characteristics of the substance, the amount of the substance that Americans would typically ingest, and the additive's effects on the body. If the additive is safe in amounts that people are likely to consume, FDA experts establish a level of the substance that can be added to foods.

According to the **Delaney Clause** of the Food Additives Amendment, food manufacturers cannot add a new compound that causes cancer at *any* level of intake. Thus, if an additive causes cancer, even though very high doses may be necessary to cause the disease, no amount of the additive is considered to be safe, and none is allowed in food. Evidence for cancer risk could come from either laboratory animal or human studies. The FDA allows very few exceptions to this clause.

The FDA cannot ban **unintentional food additives**—various industrial chemicals, pesticide residues, and mold toxins—from foods, even though some of these contaminants may be carcinogenic. The Food Quality Protection Act of 1996 established the safety standard of "a reasonable certainty of no harm" for pesticide residues in foods.[17] As a result of this act, the "no risk" provision of the Delaney Clause does not apply to pesticide residues. However, the Delaney Clause remains in effect for food additives. The following section discusses chemical contaminants and other unintentional food additives.

Other Substances in Foods

Various substances can accidentally enter food during processing. Although such contaminants can blend into a food, they are not food additives. Common biological and physical food contaminants are insect parts, rodent feces or urine, dust and dirt, and bits of metal or glass from machinery used to process food. Although some of these substances may not be harmful to health, most people find it unappealing to have filth and other unintentional ingredients in their foods.

According to the Federal Food, Drug, and Cosmetic Act, adulterated food contains objectionable and unsanitary material, and it cannot be distributed. However, the FDA permits very small amounts of unavoidable, naturally occurring substances such as dirt and insect parts in foods, because they are not harmful when consumed in minute amounts. The FDA established guidelines concerning amounts (*action levels*) of certain materials that are permitted in specific foods, such as mold and rodent hairs in paprika or insect eggs in canned orange juice. According to the FDA, "...it is economically impractical to grow, harvest, or process raw products that are totally free of non−hazardous, naturally occurring, unavoidable defects. Products harmful to consumers are subject to regulatory action whether or not they exceed the action levels."[18]

Chemical contaminants also enter foods unintentionally. Toxic metals, such as lead, cadmium, and mercury, are naturally in our environment, and these elements may also be in our food. Poisonous human−made compounds such as *benzene* and *polychlorinated biphenols* (*PCBs*) are in the environment as well. Toxic metals or poisonous compounds resulting from human manufacturing practices can pollute sources of water used by consumers (well water, for example). Americans who drink water from municipal supplies can be assured that the water is analyzed regularly to determine its concentrations of toxic substances. However, people who rely on privately owned wells should have the water tested routinely.

What Are Pesticides?

A **pesticide** is any substance that people use to control or kill unwanted insects, weeds, rodents, fungi, or other harmful organisms. There are several different kinds of pesticides. **Insecticides** control or kill insects; **rodenticides** kill mice and rats; **herbicides** destroy weeds; and **fungicides** limit the spread of fungi, such as mold and mildew.

Pesticide Residue Tolerances The use of pesticides in modern farming practices has helped increase crop yields, reduce food costs, and protect the quality of many agricultural products. However, many pesticides leave small amounts (*pesticide residues*) in or on treated crops, including fruits, vegetables, and grains, even when they are applied correctly. Concentrations of pesticide residues often decrease as food crops are washed, stored, processed, and prepared. Nevertheless, some of these substances may remain in fresh produce, such as apples or peaches, as well as in processed foods, such as canned applesauce or peaches.

The EPA regulates the proper use of pesticides. The agency can limit the amount of a pesticide that is applied on crops, restrict the frequency or location of the pesticide's application, or require the substance be used only by specially trained, certified persons. The EPA also sets pesticide **tolerances,** which are the maximum amounts of pesticide residues that can be in or on each treated food crop.

Nonchemical Methods of Pest Management Although the EPA focuses on chemical methods of managing pests, the agency also promotes nonchemical pest management techniques that may be safer for humans and the environment. Integrated pest management (IPM) involves using a variety of methods for controlling pests while limiting damage to the environment. IPM methods include growing pest–resistant crops, using predatory wasps to control crop–destroying insects, and trapping adult insect pests before they can reproduce. Biologically based pesticides, such as sex hormones (*pheromones*) that attract pesky insects to predators or traps and viruses that infect insects and weeds, are becoming increasingly popular among farmers (Figure 12.11). Such methods are often safer for humans than traditional chemical pesticides.

Fruits and vegetables grown without use of pesticides are available and may bear an "organic" label (see Chapter 3 for information about organic foods). These products generally are more expensive than those grown using pesticides, and they are not necessarily safer or more nutritious than conventionally produced foods.

How Safe Are Pesticides? Pesticides used in agriculture have both beneficial and unwanted effects. Pesticides help protect the food supply and make food crops available at reasonable cost. Nevertheless, pesticides have the potential to harm humans, animals, or the environment because they are designed to kill or otherwise negatively affect organisms. If a pesticide is applied improperly to cropland, it may remain in the soil, be taken up by plant roots, decompose to other compounds, or enter groundwater and waterways. Winds may carry

---

pesticide substance that people use to kill or control unwanted insects, weeds, or other harmful organisms

insecticides substances used to control or kill insects

rodenticides substances used to kill mice and rats

herbicides substances used to destroy weeds

fungicides substances used to limit the spread of fungi

tolerances maximum amounts of pesticide residues that can be in or on each treated food crop

Did *YOU* Know?

Lead is a highly toxic mineral that may be in candies imported from Mexico and traditional ethnic folk remedies, especially *greta, azarcon, ghasard,* and *ba-baw-san.* Therefore, it is prudent to avoid ingesting these candies or folk remedies.

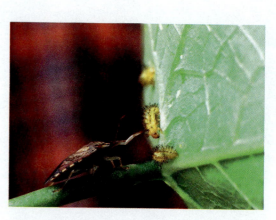

Figure 12.11 Helpful insect. The spined soldier bug (*left*) makes a meal of a Mexican bean beetle larva. Bean beetle larvae are devastating pests of snap beans and soybeans. The spined soldier bug's pheromone may help farmers control many insects that eat crops. Source: ARS/USDA

pesticides in air and dust to distant locations. Each path can be a route to the human food chain (Fig. 12.12).

The potential harmful effects of a pesticide in food depend on the particular chemical and how effectively the body can eliminate it, its concentration in the food, how much and how often it is eaten, and the consumer's vulnerability to the substance. Tolerable amounts of pesticide residues on or in foods are extremely small. However, it is possible that regular exposure to small amounts of these chemicals may enable the substances to accumulate in the body and produce toxicity or initiate cancer.[19] Health experts have studied rates of cancers among people who have close contact with pesticides, such as farmers and pesticide applicators. People who are exposed to certain pesticides have a greater risk of developing specific cancers, particularly bladder and colon cancer, than people who have not been exposed to the chemicals.[20] More research is needed to confirm these findings and explain how exposure to pesticides influence cancer risk. Thus, environmental health experts continue to monitor the effects of pesticides on humans.

Figure 12.12 Pesticide pathways. If a pesticide is applied improperly to cropland, it may remain in the soil, be taken up by plant roots, decompose to other compounds, or enter groundwater and waterways. Winds may carry pesticides in air and dust to distant locations. Each path can be a route to the human food chain.

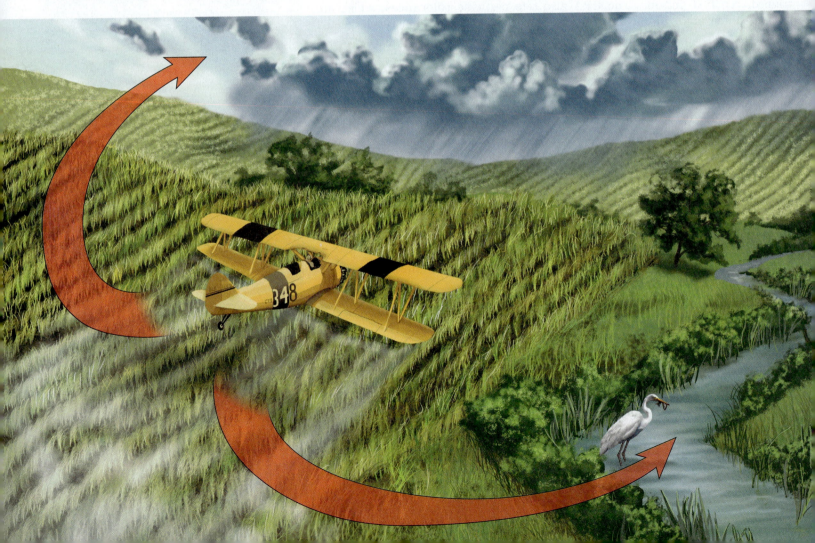

Concept CHECKPOINT

30. What is a food additive? What is the difference between direct and indirect food additives?

31. What is a color additive?

32. What is the GRAS list?

33. Explain the role of the Delaney Clause in protecting the U.S. food supply.

34. What is an unintentional food additive? Provide at least three examples of such additives.

35. What is a pesticide? Provide at least three examples of types of pesticides.

36. Define *integrated pest management,* and provide an example of this method.

37. Which U.S. agency regulates the use of pesticides?

38. What is a pesticide tolerance?

39. Explain how pesticides can enter the human food chain.

See Appendix G for responses.

12.10 Nutrition Matters: Avoiding "The Revenge"

Learning Outcomes

1 Discuss ways to prevent traveler's diarrhea.

2 Identify nations where visitors are most likely to develop traveler's diarrhea.

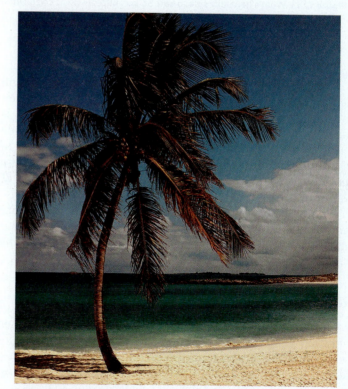
©Steve Allen/Getty Images RF

If you like traveling to foreign countries and enjoy sampling exotic cuisines in these places, one thing you do not need to encounter is *travelers' diarrhea (TD)*. Also referred to as "Montezuma's Revenge" and "Tut's Tummy," TD can ruin your vacation. By taking some precautions, however, your digestive system can stay healthy while you travel abroad.

TD results from consuming food or water contaminated with pathogens. The illness is characterized by the abrupt onset of abdominal cramps and loose or watery bowel movements. Additional symptoms may include nausea, vomiting, intestinal bloating, and fever. TD generally lasts 3 to 5 days without treatment, but signs and symptoms may persist in a small percentage of infected travelers.

Unless precautions are taken, TD is likely to occur during or shortly after traveling in regions where sanitary water supplies are not always available, people who prepare food have less than ideal personal hygiene practices, and untreated human feces are used for fertilizer. Health experts estimate that bacterial pathogens are responsible for 80 to 90% of cases of TD.[21] Protozoa such as *Giardia* account for

about 10% of TD cases. When travelers suffer from persistent symptoms, the illness is likely to be the result of a protozoal rather than a bacterial infection.

Blueberries: ©PhotoAlto/Getty Images RF

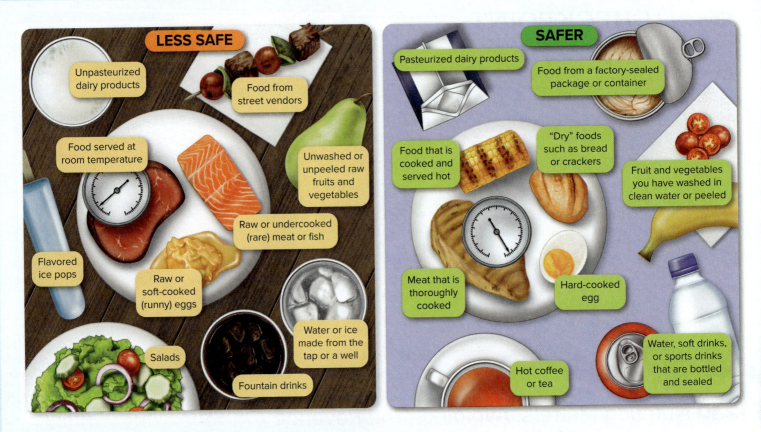

| **Figure 12.13** **What's generally safe to eat?** Source: https://wwwnc.cdc.gov/travel/page/infographic-food-water-whats-safer

Thirty to 70 percent of travelers to international places will develop TD, depending on their destinations and the season in which they travel.[21] A trip to every foreign destination is likely to include some risk of TD. Low–risk countries include the United States, Canada, Australia, Japan, and countries in Northern and Western Europe. Intermediate–risk countries include those in Eastern Europe, South Africa, and some of the Caribbean islands. High–risk areas generally have high–density populations, widespread pollution, and inadequate water treatment systems. These regions include Mexico and other Central American countries, and most of Asia, the Middle East, Africa, and South America.

Reducing Your Risk of TD

Experts at the CDC recommend several approaches for reducing your risk of TD. These include following instructions regarding food and beverage selection, avoiding contact with contaminated waterways, sanitizing drinking water, and using medications that may prevent TD.

Carry a small container of an alcohol–based (at least 60% alcohol) hand cleaner with you. Before you eat, wash your hands with the hand cleaner. When you visit places where risk of contracting TD is moderate to high, avoid consuming food or beverages purchased from street vendors. Before you eat meat or other high–risk foods, make sure they are fully cooked and served hot. Avoid raw foods that have been washed in water, such as fresh fruits, raw vegetables, and salads. Do not eat fresh fruit without peeling it first. Avoid water, ice, and beverages diluted with water or ice, such as reconstituted fruit juices and iced drinks. Do not drink fresh fluid milk or milk products that have not been pasteurized. Safe beverages include those that are bottled and sealed; bottled beer and wine may also be safe to drink. If boiled water is used to make tea and coffee, these beverages may be safe to consume. Use bottled water to wash hands, brush teeth, and take medication. Figure 12.13 shows foods and beverages that can be eaten and menu items that should be avoided because they are too risky to eat.

TD can be spread when pathogens from human or animal feces are in sources of water, including swimming pools, lakes, rivers, and other bodies of water. Accidentally swallowing even small amounts of contaminated water can cause illness. Swimming pools that contain chlorinated water may be safe places to swim, if the disinfectant and pH levels are properly maintained. However, some pathogens are resistant to levels of chlorine commonly used to disinfect swimming pools. Thus, you should also avoid swallowing chlorinated swimming pool water.

How Can I Sanitize Drinking Water?

Boiling is the most reliable method to make impure water safe to drink.[22] Water should be boiled for 1 minute, covered, and allowed to cool to room temperature without adding ice.

Chemical Disinfection Disinfection methods destroy large numbers of microorganisms, reducing the likelihood of infection. Chemical disinfection with chlorine (in house—hold bleach) or iodine is an alternative method of sanitizing water when boiling water is not practical. Iodine and chlorine are available in tablets and drops. To reduce the risk of TD, follow the manufacturer's instructions for sanitizing water with these chemicals.

Filtering Water Microstrainer filters can remove bacteria and protozoa from drinking water, but they may not remove viruses (Fig. 12.14). To destroy viruses by chemical means, you should disinfect the water with iodine or chlorine after using microstrainer filters. "Hollow—fiber" strainers remove bacteria as well as viruses from water.[22]

Filters collect organisms from water, so wash your hands with sanitized water after handling used filters. For more information about water filters and other water disinfection methods, visit http://wwwnc.cdc.gov/travel/page/water —disinfection.

Preventive Medications Before you leave the United States to enter a high—risk region, see your physician for his or her recommendations for preventing TD. You can also take medications that contain bismuth subsalicylate (BSS), the active ingredient in Pepto—Bismol, to reduce the risk of TD. Side effects of BSS commonly include nausea, constipation, and blackening of the tongue and bowel movements. BSS is not recommended for children under 12 years of age, and the medication should be avoided by people who are allergic to aspirin or have certain chronic conditions. Therefore, check with your physician before taking BBS along when you travel to other countries.

Treating TD

Because pathogenic bacteria are often the cause of TD, antibiotics are the primary method of treating the condition. In the United States, physicians often prescribe

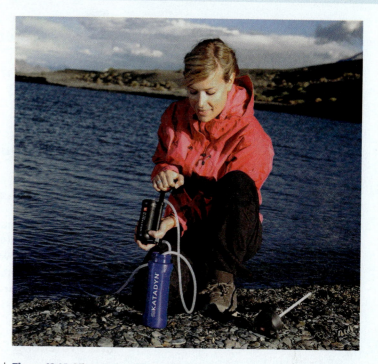

Figure 12.14 Microstrainer filters. Microstrainer filters can remove bacteria and protozoa from drinking water. Source: Courtesy of Katadyn North America

antibiotics for their patients to bring with them when they travel out of the country. When used in combination with antibiotics, *antimotility* agents can be helpful. These medications, such as loperamide, the active ingredient in Imodium, slow the muscular activity of the digestive tract and can provide relief from the diarrhea associated with TD.

Dehydration can be a serious complication of TD. To prevent dehydration, it is important for people suffering from TD to replace fluids and electrolytes lost by vomiting and diarrhea. However, travelers should remember to use only beverages that are in sealed containers, including car—bonated soft drinks. If fluid loss is severe, it is best to obtain professional medical treatment.

Concept CHECKPOINT

40. List three ways to reduce the risk of traveler's diarrhea.

41. List three foods that are generally safe to eat while traveling in Africa, India, and Central America, according to Figure 12.13.

See Appendix G for responses.

Chapter References

See Appendix H.

Summary

12.1 Introduction to Food Safety

- In the United States, millions of people become ill from various food-borne illnesses each year. Food-borne illness occurs when microscopic pathogens or their toxic by-products enter food (or beverages) and are consumed. Many kinds of pathogens infect the digestive tract; other types of food-borne pathogens do not sicken humans directly, but these microbes secrete toxins into food. When the food is eaten, the toxins irritate the intestinal tract and cause food intoxication.

12.2 Protecting Our Food

- The United States has one of the safest food supplies in the world, primarily the result of a team effort conducted by cooperating federal, state, and local agencies that regulate and monitor the production and distribution of food. The FDA and the USDA are the key federal agencies that protect consumers by regulating the country's food industry.

12.3 Microbes in Food

- When certain microorganisms metabolize nutrients in food, they often secrete substances that alter the color, texture, taste, and other characteristics of the food in beneficial and desirable ways. When pathogens are in food, they can make the item unsafe to eat. Food contaminants include pathogens, insect parts, residues of compounds used to kill insects that destroy food crops, and metal fragments from food processing equipment.

- The microbes that cause food-borne illness can live practically anywhere. Common routes for transmitting harmful microbes to food involve vermin, poor personal hygiene practices, and improper food preparation and storage practices.

- To grow, most microbes need warmth, moisture, and a source of nutrients, and some microorganisms also need oxygen. In general, high-risk foods are warm, moist, and protein-rich, and they have a neutral or slightly acidic pH. Such foods include meat, poultry, milk and milk products, and eggs.

12.4 Food-borne Illness

- Many factors influence whether an individual becomes ill after eating food or drinking a beverage that has been contaminated with a pathogen. The number of pathogens in a food or the amount of toxin it contains can contribute to the risk and severity of a food-borne illness. In general, high-risk groups are pregnant women, very young children, older adults, and persons who suffer from serious chronic illnesses or weakened immune systems.

- Signs and symptoms of food- or water-borne illnesses primarily involve the digestive tract and include nausea, vomiting, diarrhea, and intestinal cramps. Medical treatment

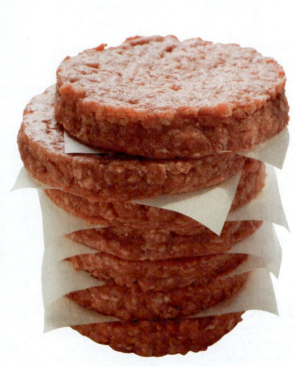

©FoodCollection/StockFood RF

should be obtained when an intestinal disorder is accompanied by fever, bloody bowel movements, prolonged vomiting and diarrhea, and/or dehydration.

12.5 Common Food-Borne Pathogens

- The major kinds of pathogens are bacteria, viruses, protozoa, and fungi. In the United States, bacteria and viruses are responsible for most cases of food-borne illness.

12.6 Preventing Food-Borne Illness

- People can reduce their risk of food-borne illness by following some important rules, most of which require changing risky food selection, preparation, and storage practices. Cooking foods is an effective way to destroy pathogens. After food is cooked, however, careless food handling sets the stage for the growth of pathogens. A simple rule to follow is this: "Keep hot foods hot and cold foods cold." Other simple rules include these: Wash hands and surfaces often, do not cross-contaminate, heat foods to proper temperatures, and chill foods promptly.

12.7 Food Preservation

- Modern methods of food preservation include pasteurization, refrigeration, freezing, canning, aseptic processing, using preservative additives, and irradiation.

12.8 Preparing for Disasters

- It is important to have a supply of clean water and wholesome food on hand to survive disasters.

12.9 Food Additives

- Direct food additives can make food easier to process, more nutritious, able to stay fresh longer, better tasting, or more attractive in appearance. An indirect food additive is a substance that becomes incorporated into food during production, packaging, transport, or storage. The 1958 Food Additives Amendment established the GRAS list and requires the manufacturer of a new food additive to provide evidence of the substance's safety to the FDA before the additive can be marketed for use. According to the Delaney Clause of the Food Additives Amendment, food manufacturers cannot add a new compound that causes cancer at *any* level of exposure.

- Unintentional food additives are substances that accidentally are in foods. A pesticide is any substance that people use to kill or control unwanted insects, weeds, rodents, or other organisms. The EPA regulates the proper use of pesticides and sets pesticide tolerances. IPM methods control agricultural pests while limiting damage to the environment.

- Agricultural pesticides have both beneficial and unwanted effects. Pesticides help protect the food supply and make food crops available at reasonable cost. Nevertheless, these substances may harm humans, animals, or the environment. Environmental health experts continually monitor the effects of pesticides on humans.

12.10 Nutrition Matters: Avoiding "The Revenge"

- Traveler's diarrhea (TD) results from consuming food or water contaminated with pathogens. TD is likely to occur during or shortly after travel in regions where sanitary water supplies are lacking, people who prepare food have less than ideal personal hygiene practices, and untreated human feces are used for fertilizer. To reduce the risk of TD, follow instructions regarding safe food and beverage selection, avoid contact with contaminated waterways, sanitize drinking water, and use medications that may prevent the condition.

Recipe for Healthy Living

Very Easy Chicken Salad

Chicken that is properly prepared, cooked, and stored is a safe, nutritious, economical food. A good way to use up day-old cooked chicken is to make chicken salad. This recipe is unusual because it includes seedless grapes and sunflower seeds. (You can substitute day-old cooked turkey for the chicken and chopped apple or dried apricots for the grapes.)

The chicken salad recipe makes approximately three 1-cup servings. A serving of this salad supplies approximately 320 kcal, 23 g protein, 19 g fat, 3.3 g fiber, and 190 mg sodium.

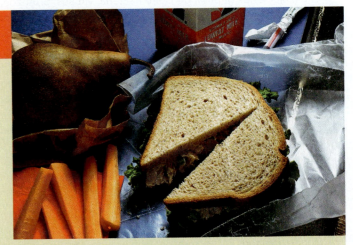

Source: Courtesy of National Cancer Institute

INGREDIENTS:

1 ¼ cups cooked and chilled, skinless, boneless chicken meat (approximately 1 whole chicken breast)
1 medium stalk celery, washed and chopped
½ cup raw onion, skinned and finely chopped
½ cup washed seedless red or green grapes, halved
½ cup unsalted roasted sunflower seeds
⅛ tsp curry powder
⅛ tsp ground black pepper
¼ cup low-fat mayonnaise-type salad dressing

PREPARATION STEPS:

1. Cut chicken into small pieces and place in a large bowl.

2. Add the rest of the ingredients to the chicken and gently mix until well blended.

3. Serve on a bed of washed leaf lettuce or as a sandwich filling.

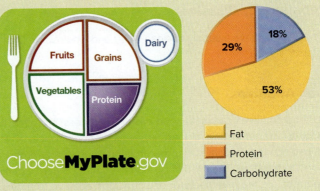

ChooseMyPlate.gov

Source: U.S. Dept. of Agriculture

18%
29%
53%

Fat
Protein
Carbohydrate

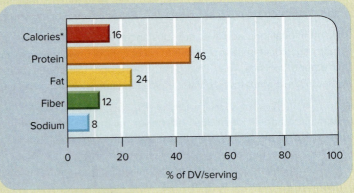

Calories* 16
Protein 46
Fat 24
Fiber 12
Sodium 8

% of DV/serving

*2000 daily total kcal

Further analyze this recipe or other recipes through activities located in Connect.

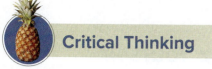

Critical Thinking

1. Consider your usual food preparation practices. After having read this chapter, list any food preparation practices you have that are unsafe.

2. Consider your usual food storage practices. After having read this chapter, list any of your food storage practices that are unsafe.

3. For lunch on Monday, you visited a restaurant and ordered a hamburger, French fries, baked beans, and a sealed container of pasteurized orange juice. Two days later, you developed nausea, vomiting, fever, chills, headache, abdominal cramps, and diarrhea. You suspect Monday's lunch made you sick. Considering the foods that you ate for lunch on Monday, which one was the most likely source of your infection? Why? Which food—borne pathogen was the most likely suspect for causing the intestinal disorder? In the future, what steps can you take to reduce the likelihood that the food will make you sick again?

4. One of your friends plans to vacation in Mexico next week. What practical advice can you provide to help him avoid traveler's diarrhea?

5. Develop a pamphlet to educate consumers about food—borne illness, including ways to reduce the risk of such illnesses.

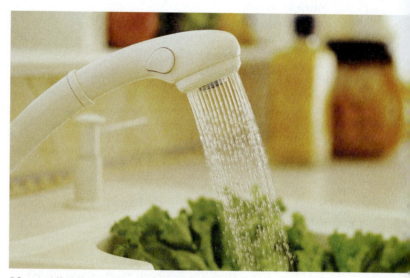

©Comstock/Getty Images RF

Practice Test

Select the best answer.

1. _____ are disease—causing microbes.

   a. Pathogens
   b. Toxins
   c. Teratogens
   d. Oxidants

2. The _____ is the primary government agency that oversees the safety of most foods in the United States.

   a. Food and Drug Administration (FDA)
   b. Agricultural Research Service (ARS)
   c. Centers for Disease Control and Prevention (CDC)
   d. Environmental Protection Agency (EPA)

3. Which of the following foods is most likely to support the growth of pathogens?

   a. Overripe bananas
   b. Pasteurized milk
   c. Raw ground meat
   d. Commercially canned tomato soup

4. Food—borne illnesses are usually characterized by

   a. flulike signs and symptoms.
   b. coughing, sneezing, and respiratory inflammation.
   c. megaloblastic anemia and nervous system defects.
   d. abdominal cramps, diarrhea, and vomiting.

5. In the United States, common sources of food—borne illness include all of the following, except

   a. norovirus.
   b. *Staphylococcus aureus*.
   c. fungi.
   d. *Salmonella*.

6. Aflatoxins are

   a. responsible for 30% of food—borne illnesses in the United States.
   b. harmful compounds produced by certain molds.
   c. a type of parasitic worm.
   d. medications that are effective against viral toxins.

7. Which of the following practices can help reduce the growth of food—borne pathogens?

   a. Washing hands before preparing food
   b. Keeping cold foods cold and hot foods hot
   c. Cooking foods to proper internal temperatures
   d. All of the above are correct.

Pineapple, Radish: ©Stockbyte/Getty Images RF

8. Which of the following substances are *not* direct food additives?

   a. Sulfites
   b. Enrichment nutrients
   c. Pesticide residues
   d. Emulsifiers

9. Irradiation of food is

   a. an untested technology.
   b. not recommended, because the process increases nutrient losses.
   c. considered to be a safe process by the FDA.
   d. a widely accepted method of food preservation in the United States.

10. Which of the following food preservation processes effectively destroys microbes?

    a. Freezing
    b. Sterilization
    c. Smoking
    d. Chilling

11. _____ is the commercial heating process that destroys harmful bacteria in milk and fruit juices.

    a. Sporulation
    b. Sedimentation
    c. Detoxification
    d. Pasteurization

12. When you travel to countries outside the United States, you can reduce your risk of "traveler's diarrhea" by

    a. eating whole fresh fruits and vegetables.
    b. avoiding water that has not been bottled and sealed.
    c. purchasing foods from street vendors.
    d. consuming ice with beverages.

13. In the United States, _____ is responsible for most out—breaks of food—borne illness.

    a. norovirus
    b. *Clostridium botulinum*
    c. aflatoxin
    d. *E. coli*

Answers to Quiz Yourself

1. Aflatoxins are the most common sources of food-borne illness in the United States. **False.** (Section 12.5)

2. In case of emergency, it is not safe to drink the water that is in an undamaged water heater. **False.** (Section 12.8)

3. Certain fungi, such as button mushrooms, are safe to eat. **True.** (Section 12.5)

4. The Environmental Protection Agency (EPA) regulates the proper use of pesticides in the United States. **True.** (Section 12.9)

5. The best way to tell if a food is safe to eat is to smell it. **False.** (Section 12.3)

©Kevin Sanchez/Cole Group/Getty Images RF

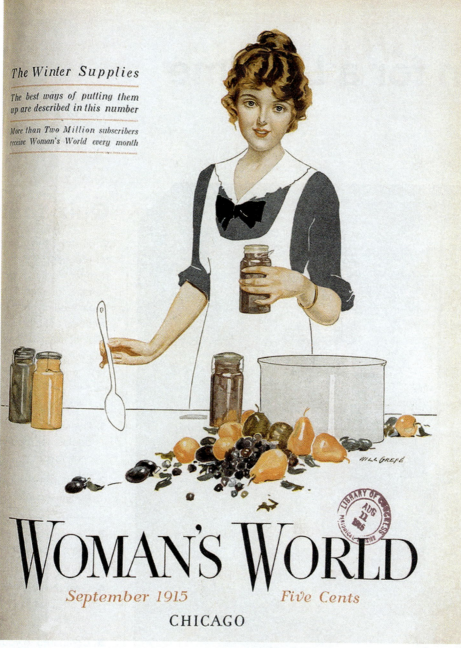

Source: Historicus/Library of Congress

CHAPTER 13

Nutrition for a Lifetime

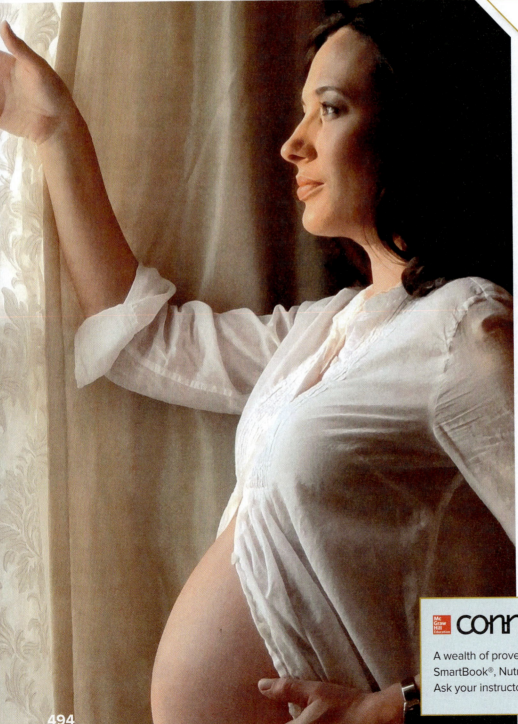

Quiz Yourself

What steps can young women take to prepare for pregnancy? Compared to breast milk, do infant formulas provide the same health benefits for infants? When is the best time to begin feeding solid foods to infants? Which nutrients are most likely to be deficient in diets of older adults? While reading this chapter, you will learn answers to these questions. Test your knowledge of nutrition during various life stages by taking the following quiz. The answers are at the end of the chapter.

1. During pregnancy, a mother-to-be should double her food intake because she's "eating for two." _____ T _____ F

2. Infant formulas provide the same health benefits to infants as breast milk. _____ T _____ F

3. Caregivers should add solid foods to an infant's diet within the first month after the baby is born. _____ T _____ F

4. Over the past few decades, the prevalence of obesity has increased among American children. _____ T _____ F

5. Compared to younger persons, older adults have lower risks of nutritional deficiencies. _____ T _____ F

Mc Graw Hill Education connect®

A wealth of proven resources are available on Connect® including SmartBook®, NutritionCalc Plus, and many other dynamic learning tools. Ask your instructor about Connect!

©Karena Rigby

13.1 Introduction to Nutrition for a Lifetime

Learning Outcomes:

1 Identify the life stages.

2 Explain why it is important to learn about nutrition concerns for pregnancy, lactation, childhood, and the older adult years.

The chapter opening portrait features a young woman during her eighth month of pregnancy, looking forward to a bright future. Thanks to technological and medical advances that occurred during the 21st century, her baby has an excellent chance of enjoying a long, healthy life.

If you are a woman, are you pregnant? Do you already have children? If you have children, were they breastfed or formula-fed? Do you live with and help care for an elderly parent or grandparent? These may seem to be personal questions, but many undergraduate college students do not fit the stereotype of being 18 to 22 years of age, having no children, and residing away from home.

Most of the nutrition recommendations presented in this textbook apply to people who are "adults"—loosely defined as the period when a person is 19 to 70 years of age.[1] This chapter focuses on the differing nutrition needs and health concerns of people who are in specific *life stages*. These particular life stages are the **prenatal period** or pregnancy, the time between conception and birth; **lactation** (milk production for breastfeeding); infancy; childhood; adolescence; and the older adult period that generally spans from about 70 years of age until death.

Why is it necessary to learn some basic information about nutrition-related concerns during various life stages? If you do not have children, you may become a parent in the future. If your parents and grandparents are relatively young and vigorous now, you can expect them to experience declining physical functioning as they grow older. Finally, you need to recognize that most of these changes are normal and will affect you as well.

Today in the United States, many of the leading causes of death are chronic diseases, such as heart disease and cancer. Long-term health-related practices, including dietary and physical activity habits, often contribute to the development of these diseases. Whether you enjoy overall good health or suffer from one or more disabling physical ailments as you grow older depends not only on your lifestyle choices but also on several other factors, including your heredity, relationships, environment, income, education level, and access to health care. Achieving and maintaining a healthy body weight is critical to enjoying good health throughout life. This chapter also includes information about obesity during childhood and adolescence.

prenatal period time between conception and birth; pregnancy

lactation milk production

Concept CHECKPOINT

1. John is 79 years of age. He is in the _____ life stage.
2. For women, which life stage involves milk production for breastfeeding?

See Appendix G for responses.

©Elyse Lewin/Getty Images RF

conception moment when a sperm enters an egg (fertilization)

uterus female reproductive organ that protects the developing organism during pregnancy

embryo human organism from 14 days to 8 weeks after conception

fetus human organism from 8 weeks after conception until birth

13.2 Pregnancy

Learning Outcomes

1 Discuss the roles of the placenta and uterus during pregnancy.

2 Explain why an infant's birth weight is an important aspect of the baby's health during its first year of life.

3 List major physiological changes that occur during pregnancy, and identify typical nutrition-related discomforts associated with this stage of life.

4 Discuss the importance of appropriate weight gain during pregnancy, and identify recommended ranges of weight that pregnant women should gain.

5 Explain why prenatal care and a nutritious diet are important for the health of the pregnant woman and her unborn offspring.

"It's positive!" Each day, the results of pregnancy testing are a source of excitement, relief, or concern for thousands of women. About 50% of pregnancies are unplanned in the United States.[2] Therefore, all sexually active women of childbearing age should be aware of their likelihood of becoming pregnant. Regardless of whether a pregnancy is planned or not, dietary practices before and during pregnancy play a major role in the course of the pregnancy and the primary outcome—a healthy infant.

The prenatal period (*gestation*) encompasses the time from **conception,** the moment a male sperm cell enters a female egg cell, until the birth of a *full-term* infant, about 38 to 42 weeks later. During the first 2 weeks after conception, the fertilized egg (*ovum*) divides repeatedly, forming a mass of cells that enters the woman's **uterus,** the female reproductive organ that protects the developing organism. The mass of cells buries itself into the nutrient-rich lining of the uterus (implantation) and continues to develop. For the next 6 weeks, the rapidly dividing mass of cells, called an **embryo,** increases in size and forms organs. Eight weeks after conception, the developing human being is referred to as a **fetus** (Fig. 13.1).

Figure 13.1 Prenatal development: Conception to fetus. During the first 2 weeks after conception, the fertilized egg divides repeatedly, forming a mass of cells that eventually enters the uterus and buries itself into the organ's nutrient-rich lining. From 14 days through 8 weeks after conception, the rapidly dividing mass of cells is called an embryo. Eight weeks after conception and until its birth, the developing human being is referred to as a fetus.

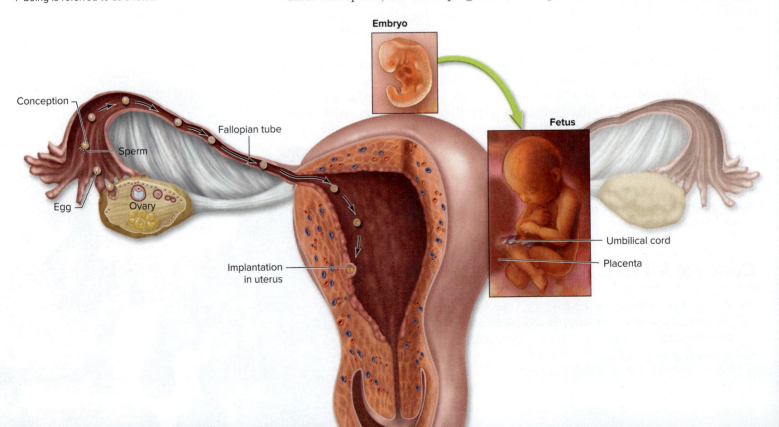

The prenatal period is often divided into three stages or *trimesters*. During the first trimester, the embryo/fetus develops most of its organs, and by the end of this period, the fetus can move. The first trimester is a critical stage in human development because nutrient deficiencies or excesses and exposure to toxic compounds, such as alcohol, are most likely to have devastating effects on the embryo/fetus. However, many women who are in their first trimester do not realize they are pregnant.

As the second trimester begins, the fetus is still very tiny, about 2½ to 3 inches in length, and weighs only about an ounce. However, the fetus is beginning to look more like a human infant: It has fully formed arms, hands, fingers, legs, feet, and toes. The fetus's organs continue to grow and mature in their ability to function. As the fetus moves around, its mother becomes increasingly aware of its presence within her body.

By the beginning of the third trimester, the fetus is approximately 10 inches long (from crown to rump) and weighs about 2 pounds. During this trimester, the fetus will nearly double in length and multiply its weight by three to four times. Thus, a healthy fetus usually weighs about 6 to 8 pounds and is 19 to 21 inches long by the time it is full–term and ready to be born.

Throughout the prenatal period, the embryo/fetus depends entirely on its mother for survival. During most of the pregnancy, the expectant mother nourishes her embryo/fetus through the **placenta,** the organ of pregnancy that connects the uterus to the embryo/fetus via the *umbilical cord* (see Fig. 13.1). The role of the placenta is to transfer nutrients and oxygen from the mother's bloodstream to the embryo/fetus. Additionally, the placenta transfers wastes from the embryo/fetus to the mother's bloodstream, so her body can eliminate them. Unfortunately, the placenta does not filter many microbes and toxic substances, such as alcohol and nicotine, from the mother's blood. Thus, agents of infection and harmful chemicals can pass through the placenta, enter the embryo/fetus, and cause disease, birth defects, or embryonic/fetal death.

A fetus generally needs to spend at least 37 weeks developing within the uterus for its organs to be physiologically mature enough to survive after birth without the need for special care. A fetus's weight depends on the supply of nutrients that it receives through the placenta.[3] If the placenta fails to grow properly, the developing fetus is likely to be born too soon and be lighter than average at birth.

Birth Weight

Birth weight is a major factor that determines whether a baby is healthy and survives his or her first year of life. **Low–birth–weight (LBW)** infants generally weigh less than 5½ pounds at birth. LBW is the second leading cause of death among American infants (birth defects are the leading cause).[4] In 2015, 8% of infants born in the United States were low birth weight.[5] Pregnant females who are under 15 years of age or 45 to 54 years of age are more likely to give birth to LBW infants than women in other age groups. Additionally, women who smoke during pregnancy are at risk to have LBW babies.[6] Low birth weight is often associated with premature or preterm births. In 2015, about 10% of births in the United States were preterm; that is, they occurred before the 37th week of pregnancy.[5]

Very preterm infants are born before 32 weeks of gestation. In 2015, 1.6% of babies born in the United States were very preterm infants.[5] Such infants are more likely to have serious health problems or die soon after birth than babies delivered after 34 weeks of pregnancy.[7] A very preterm infant who is born after about 26 weeks of pregnancy may survive if cared for in a hospital nursery for high–risk newborns (Fig. 13.2). However, the tiny infant's body will not

placenta organ of pregnancy that connects the uterus to the embryo/fetus via the umbilical cord

low-birth-weight (LBW) describes baby generally weighing less than 5½ pounds at birth

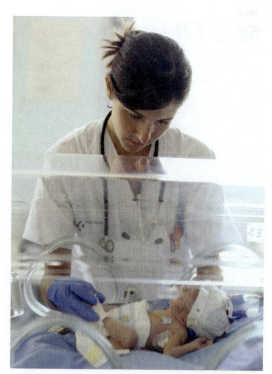

Figure 13.2 Preterm infant.
©Javier Larrea/age fotostock/Alamy

have stores of fat and certain minerals that normally accumulate during the last month of pregnancy. Additionally, very preterm babies are likely to have conditions that complicate their medical care and food intake, such as breathing difficulties and weak sucking and swallowing abilities.

Nutrition-Related Signs of Pregnancy

During pregnancy, a woman's body undergoes major physiological changes, such as increased blood volume, breast size, and levels of several hormones. These adaptations enable her body to nourish and maintain the developing embryo/fetus, as well as produce milk for her infant after its birth. However, some of the physical changes cause discomfort for the pregnant woman.

In the first trimester, most women experience physical signs that they are pregnant, such as enlarged breasts and "morning sickness." Other common nutrition—related signs as well as complaints of pregnancy include extreme tiredness, swollen feet, constipation, and heartburn. In most cases, such discomforts do not create serious complications, and they resolve within a few months.

Breast Changes

During pregnancy, hormones signal the breasts to increase in size in preparation for lactation. The mother's pituitary gland in the brain produces **prolactin,** a hormone that stimulates the development of milk—producing tissue in the breasts. However, a pregnant woman's breasts do not form milk because high levels of progesterone, a hormone that helps maintain pregnancy, inhibit milk production.[8] After birth, the level of progesterone drops rapidly, essentially removing the "brakes" from the breasts' ability to produce milk.

Morning Sickness

A common sign of pregnancy is **morning sickness,** nausea that is sometimes accompanied by vomiting. The name "morning sickness" is misleading because the queasy feeling can occur at any time of the day. The cause of this unpleasant condition is unclear, but it may be the result of the pregnant woman's body adapting to higher levels of female hormones. Additionally, emotional stress and certain foods can contribute to nausea. The condition generally begins early in the first trimester, and most women are no longer affected by the 16th week of pregnancy.[9] However, some women experience nausea and vomiting occasionally throughout their pregnancies.

To help control mild morning sickness, pregnant women can avoid odors and foods, such as fried or greasy foods, that trigger nausea. Some women find that eating crackers and drinking some water helps reduce the likelihood of feeling nauseated, especially before they get out of bed in the morning. Furthermore, eating smaller but more frequent meals and nutritious snacks can be helpful. Products that contain ginger, such as ginger tea, can also help relieve the nausea of morning sickness.[9]

If the nausea and vomiting occur more than 3 times a day or contribute to weight loss of more than 2 pounds, the pregnant woman should contact her physician for treatment.[9] Morning sickness that persists beyond the fourth month of pregnancy should also be brought to the attention of a physician. During pregnancy, excessive vomiting is harmful because it can lead to dehydration, weight loss and electrolyte imbalances.[10]

Fatigue in Pregnancy

Early in pregnancy, the mother's blood volume expands to approximately 150% of normal. The number of red blood cells, however, increases by only 20 to 30%,

prolactin hormone that stimulates milk production after delivery

morning sickness nausea and vomiting associated with pregnancy

Did *YOU* Know?

In 2012, Kate Middleton, wife of Great Britain's Prince William, was hospitalized for 3 days because of excessive vomiting during early pregnancy. She recovered and gave birth to a healthy baby boy on July 22, 2013. Although she experienced severe morning sickness with her second pregnancy, she delivered a healthy baby girl on May 2, 2015. In September of 2017, news media reported that Kate Middleton was expecting her third child and experiencing another bout of severe excessive vomiting associated with pregnancy.

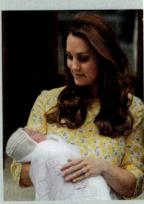

©Samir Hussein/WireImage/ Getty Images

and this change occurs more gradually. As a result, the pregnant woman develops *physiological anemia*, a condition characterized by a lower concentration of red blood cells in the bloodstream. This form of anemia is a normal response to pregnancy, rather than the result of inadequate nutrient intake. Nevertheless, physiological anemia may be responsible for the extreme tiredness experienced by pregnant women during their first trimester. As their red blood cell numbers increase, expectant mothers report having more energy, especially during the second trimester. By the third trimester, however, most pregnant women are easily fatigued again, possibly because carrying a rapidly growing fetus is physically demanding.

What Is Edema?

High levels of certain hormones can cause various tissues to retain fluid during pregnancy. Although the extra fluid causes some minor swelling (edema), especially in the hands and feet, the condition is normal. In most cases, mild edema does not require treatment such as restricting salt intake or taking diuretics. Edema, however, can be a sign of trouble if hypertension and the appearance of protein in the urine accompany the swelling. The "Importance of Prenatal Care" section of this chapter discusses hypertension during pregnancy.

Digestive Tract Discomforts

During pregnancy, certain hormones produced by the placenta relax muscles of the digestive tract. As a result, intestinal movements slow down and digested material takes longer to pass through the tract, increasing the likelihood of constipation (see the "Fiber and Health" section of Chapter 5). To help prevent constipation, pregnant women should consume adequate amounts of fiber and fluids. During pregnancy, the Adequate Intake (AI) for fiber is 28 g/day, and the AI for total water is 3 L/day.[1] If constipation still persists after making these dietary changes, the pregnant woman should discuss this concern with her physician.

Heartburn is another common complaint of pregnant women. As the fetus grows, the uterus pushes upward in the mother's abdominal cavity and applies pressure on her stomach. When this occurs, stomach acid can enter the esophagus, causing heartburn (see the Chapter 4 "Nutrition Matters"). To help avoid heartburn, the pregnant woman can consume smaller meals, avoid lying down after eating, eat less fatty foods, and learn to identify and avoid foods that seem to contribute to heartburn. If heartburn continues to be bothersome, the woman should consult her physician and discuss other ways to treat the condition.

Pregnancy: General Dietary Recommendations

Ideally, women of childbearing age should take steps to ensure good health before becoming pregnant. For example, women can analyze the nutritional adequacy of their diets and choose to eat foods that correct any marginal or deficient intakes. Prior to pregnancy, sedentary women can begin an exercise regimen; overweight or obese women can lose some excess weight; and women who smoke can join smoking cessation programs. The time to remedy faulty lifestyle practices and increase chances of having a healthy pregnancy and baby is long before pregnancy occurs.

During pregnancy, the mother-to-be should follow a diet that meets her own nutritional needs as well as those of her developing offspring. Depending on the trimester, an expectant woman's requirements for energy (calories), protein, and many other nutrients are greater than her needs prior to pregnancy. Nevertheless, a pregnant woman does not need to double her usual food intake just because she is "eating for two." Table 13.1 compares Recommended Dietary Allowances (RDAs) for energy and selected nutrients that apply to healthy 25-year-old nonpregnant and pregnant women.

TABLE 13.1 Comparing Selected DRIs: 25-Year-Old Nonpregnant and Pregnant Women

Energy/ Nutrient*	Nonpregnant	Pregnant
Kilocalories	Estimated Energy Requirement (EER)	First trimester = EER + 0
		Second trimester = EER + 340
		Third trimester = EER + 452
Protein	46 g/day	71 g/day
Vitamin C	75 mg/day	85 mg/day
Thiamin	1.1 mg/day	1.4 mg/day
Niacin	14 mg/day	18 mg/day
Folate	400 mcg/day	600 mcg/day
Vitamin D	15 mcg/day	15 mcg/day
Calcium	1000 mg/day	1000 mg/day
Iron	18 mg/day	27 mg/day
Iodine	150 mcg/day	220 mcg/day

* RDA

Source: Data from Institute of Medicine: *Dietary Reference Intakes.*

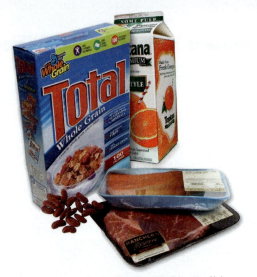

Cereal box and other foods: ©McGraw-Hill Education/John Flournoy photographer; Orange juice: ©McGraw-Hill Education/ Emily & David Tietz, photographers; Kidney beans: ©Wendy Schiff

TABLE 13.2 Sample Menu for a 25-Year-Old Pregnant Woman (Second Trimester)

Breakfast
¾ cup cooked oatmeal, made with ½ cup fat-free milk and sprinkled with ¼ cup raisins
½ cup calcium-fortified orange juice
Mid-morning snack
½ cup calcium-fortified orange juice
1 rectangular graham cracker
2 Tbsp peanut butter
Lunch
Cheese sandwich
2 slices whole-grain bread
1 slice American cheese
2 slices tomato
¼ cup leaf lettuce
2 tsp mayonnaise-type low-calorie salad dressing
1 cup apple slices
1 cup fat-free milk
½ cup orange sherbet
Mid-afternoon snack
1 whole-grain English muffin, toasted
1 Tbsp soft margarine
2 tsp jelly
½ cup fat-free milk
Dinner
Broiled salmon filet, 5 oz
1¼ cups mixed salad greens
1 Tbsp low-calorie Italian dressing
½ cup enriched white rice
1 cup steamed broccoli
2 small dinner rolls
1 Tbsp soft margarine
Evening snack
1 cup frozen yogurt

Energy Needs

In the first trimester, a pregnant woman's daily energy requirement (*Estimated Energy Requirement* or *EER*) is essentially the same as a nonpregnant woman's, because the embryo/fetus is quite small (see Table 13.1). However, the fetus grows rapidly during the second and third trimesters, and the pregnant woman requires more energy and nutrients to support its growth as well as her own body's needs. During the second trimester, the expectant mother should consume approximately 340 more kilocalories per day than her prepregnancy EER. Throughout the third trimester, she should add about 450 kcal per day to her prepregnancy EER (see Table 13.1). If a woman is physically active during her pregnancy, she may need to increase her kilocalorie intake by even more than these levels. Why? As the pregnant woman gains weight, her muscles require more energy to move her body. The average expectant mother, however, reduces her physical activity level during the third trimester, conserving energy.

Folate and Iron Needs

A pregnant woman's requirements for folate and iron are 50% higher than those of a nonpregnant woman. It is important for women to enter pregnancy with adequate folate status because embryos need the vitamin to support rapid cell division. As discussed in Chapter 8, pregnant women who are folate deficient have high risk of giving birth to infants with neural tube defects, such as spina bifida (see Fig. 8.26). To obtain adequate folate, women of childbearing age as well as pregnant women should include rich food sources of folate in their diets, such as green leafy vegetables, and take a multivitamin/mineral supplement that supplies at least 400 mcg of folic acid, a form of folate.

As the pregnant woman's blood volume expands, her need for iron increases because her body must make more hemoglobin for the extra red blood cells. Additionally, the woman's body transfers iron to the fetus to build its stores of the mineral. If women fail to meet their iron needs during pregnancy, their iron stores can be severely depleted, and they can develop iron deficiency anemia. Pregnant women who are iron deficient have high risk of giving birth prematurely and having low-birth-weight infants.[11] As mentioned in Chapter 3, iron is a nutrient of public health concern for pregnant women.

Even when their diets include good sources of iron such as red meats and enriched cereals, pregnant women often need a supplemental source of iron. Thus, most physicians recommend special prenatal multivitamin/mineral supplements that contain iron for their pregnant patients.

Menu Planning for Pregnant Women

Rather than view pregnancy as a time to splurge by eating foods that are high in empty calories, the mother-to-be should obtain the extra energy from nutrient-dense foods. For example, drinking an additional cup of fat-free milk, eating a bowl of an enriched whole-grain cereal, and taking a prenatal supplement each day can supply extra kilocalories as well as protein, fiber, and micronutrients. Table 13.2 presents a day's meals and snacks for a sedentary 25-year-old woman who is in her second trimester of pregnancy. Her prepregnancy EER was 2000 kcal, so her sample menu is based on MyPlate recommendations for 2400 kcal, enough to cover her increased EER during this trimester.

Is Fish Safe to Eat During Pregnancy? Fish and shellfish (e.g., clams, shrimp, and crabs) are excellent sources of many minerals, omega-3 fatty acids, and high-quality protein. However, most fish and shellfish contain very small amounts of methylmercury, a compound that contains the toxic mineral mercury.[12] Certain kinds of fish, however, contain higher levels of methylmercury than others. Therefore, pregnant and breastfeeding women should avoid eating swordfish, shark, king mackerel, tilefish from the Gulf of Mexico, marlin, orange roughy, and bigeye tuna.[12] When a pregnant woman eats these foods, the methylmercury in them can eventually reach the developing fetus and damage its nervous system. Chapter 3 provides recommendations for safe levels of fish consumption by pregnant women.

What About Cravings?

The stereotype of a pregnant woman who craves pickles and ice cream is not simply a myth. Cravings are common during this stage of life. However, ask pregnant women to identify the foods they crave, and you are likely to get a variety of responses. The causes of cravings are unknown, but they may be responses to the hormonal changes associated with pregnancy or to the emotional state of the mother–to–be. In other instances, specific food cravings may simply reflect the pregnant woman's family traditions. Unless food cravings contribute to excess weight gain, they are generally harmless.

Some women develop **pica,** the practice of eating nonfood items such as laundry starch, chalk, cigarette ashes, and soil. Some studies have linked pica with iron and zinc deficiency, but it is not clear if pica is the result or the cause of such deficiencies. Pregnant women should refrain from practicing pica, especially eating clay or soil. Soil may contain substances that interfere with the absorp–tion of minerals in the intestinal tract. Furthermore, eating soil can be harmful because the dirt may be contaminated with toxic substances, such as lead and pesticides, and pathogenic microbes.

pica practice of eating nonfood items

Weight Gain During Pregnancy

Nearly all pregnant women experience weight gain. In fact, gaining an appro–priate amount of weight is crucial during pregnancy. How much weight a woman should gain depends on her prepregnancy weight (Table 13.3). Women who were underweight prior to pregnancy should gain 28 to 40 pounds; women whose prepregnancy weights were within the healthy range can expect to gain 25 to 35 pounds.[13] Women who were overweight before they became pregnant should gain 15 to 25 pounds, and obese women should gain 11 to 20 pounds during pregnancy. The recommendations are higher for women who are pregnant with more than one fetus. For example, a healthy woman who is carrying twins may gain as much as 54 pounds during pregnancy.[13]

In 2015, 48% of women in the United States who were pregnant with one fetus gained more than the recommended amount of weight during pregnancy.[13] Women who gain excess weight during pregnancy are likely to retain the extra pounds long after their babies are born. Furthermore, expectant mothers who gain excessive amounts of weight are more likely to give birth to high–birth–weight (HBW) babies, which may be referred to as large for gestational age infants. A HBW baby weighs more than 8.8 pounds at birth. When compared to newborns with healthy weights, HBW infants have higher risk of being injured during the birth process. Furthermore, HBW infants may be more likely to develop obesity, diabetes, and hypertension at some point in their lives.[14] In 2015, 8% of babies born in the United States were HBW.[5]

Underweight women who do not gain enough weight during pregnancy are at risk of having preterm or low–birth–weight infants. Underweight pregnant women should try to reach healthy weights by the end of the first trimester and then meet the recommended weight–gain goals. Obese women have a greater risk of developing hypertension as well as type 2 diabetes during pregnancy. Obese pregnant women are also at risk of giving birth to HBW babies. However, women should not try to lose weight while they are pregnant because calorie restriction may harm the fetus.

TABLE 13.3 Recommended Weight Gain During Pregnancy*

Weight Classification Before Pregnancy (BMI)	Range of Weight Gain During Pregnancy (pounds)
Underweight (< 18.5)	28–40
Healthy weight (18.5–24.9)	25–35
Overweight (25.0–29.9)	15–25
Obese (30.0 or more)	11–20

*Pregnant with one fetus

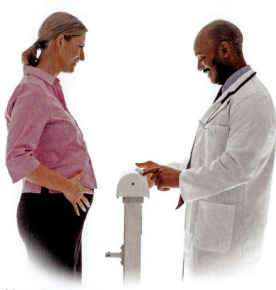

©George Doyle/Getty Images RF

TABLE 13.4   Distribution of Weight Gain During Pregnancy

Tissue	Approximate Pounds
Maternal	
Blood	3
Breasts	2
Uterus	2
Fat, protein, and retained fluid	11
Fetus	7.5
Placenta	1.5
Amniotic fluid*	2.0

* Protective fluid that surrounds fetus.

Source: March of Dimes, *Weight gain during pregnancy*. ND. Accessed: July 2, 2017. http://www.marchofdimes.org/pregnancy /weight-gain-during-pregnancy.aspx

Accounting for the Weight Gain

It is important to understand that much of the weight a woman gains during a healthy pregnancy is not body fat. By the end of a full–term pregnancy, the average fetus weighs about 7½ pounds, and the placenta and *amniotic fluid* that surrounds the fetus account for about 3½ pounds. The remaining weight is comprised of tissues and fluids the mother's body gains during pregnancy (*maternal weight* gain). Table 13.4 indicates the typical distribution of weight that is gained during this life stage.

Rate of Weight Gain

For an expectant mother, the rate of weight gain is important, as well as the amount of weight gained. Most pregnant women add up to 4 pounds of weight during the first trimester.[15] Throughout the rest of their pregnancies, healthy women typically gain at a faster rate, 3 to 4 pounds *each* month. Figure 13.3 charts the course of weight gain in a healthy pregnancy. Note how the rate reaches a steady pace of about 1 pound/week during the second and third trimesters. During the second and third trimesters, recommended weight gains are higher for underweight women and lower for overweight or obese women.

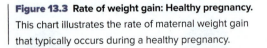

Figure 13.3   Rate of weight gain: Healthy pregnancy. This chart illustrates the rate of maternal weight gain that typically occurs during a healthy pregnancy.

The Importance of Prenatal Care

Ideally, women of childbearing age should plan for pregnancy and receive dietary advice before becoming pregnant. If this is not possible, *prenatal care* should begin early in pregnancy because many medical problems that may occur during this life stage can be diagnosed and treated before the health of the mother or her fetus are threatened. **Prenatal care** is specialized to meet the health care needs of pregnant women. Routine prenatal health care includes measuring and monitoring the pregnant woman's weight, blood pressure, blood glucose level, and uterine growth. The prenatal health care provider may also discuss various con-cerns with the expectant mother, such as morning sickness, safe types of physical activity, what to expect during the birth pro-cess, and basic infant care skills. Additionally, the health care provider can advise the pregnant woman to make appropriate lifestyle choices, such as avoiding the use of tobacco, alcohol, and illegal sub-stances. Women who receive adequate prenatal care are more likely to have good pregnancy outcomes, including babies who have healthy birth weights, than women who do not receive such care.[16]

During pregnancy, it is important for a woman to decide whether she will breastfeed her baby. Pregnant women who decide to breastfeed their babies should inform their physicians and learn as much as they can about breastfeeding early in their pregnancy.

Gestational Diabetes

According to estimates, as many as 9% of pregnant women in the United States develop type 2 diabetes during pregnancy (*gestational diabetes*).[17] When a woman has gestational diabetes, her fetus receives too much glucose and converts the excess into fat. Thus, women with this form of diabetes often give birth to HBW babies. After birth, these infants often have difficulty controlling their own blood glucose levels and are at risk of becoming overweight as children.

Gestational diabetes can be detected during routine prenatal care. For more information about diabetes during pregnancy, see Chapter 5.

prenatal care specialized health care for pregnant women

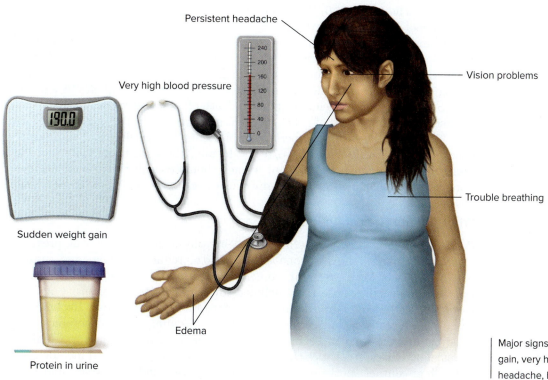

Persistent headache

Very high blood pressure

Vision problems

Trouble breathing

Sudden weight gain

Edema

Protein in urine

Major signs of preeclampsia include sudden weight gain, very high blood pressure, edema, persistent headache, breathing problems, and protein in urine.

Gestational Hypertension

Some women who had normal blood pressure values before they became pregnant develop hypertension during pregnancy. This condition is called **gestational hypertension** (formerly called "pregnancy–induced" hypertension). Approximately 15 to 25% of women with gestational hypertension develop a more severe form of the condition, called *preeclampsia (pre—e—klamp'—see—a)*.[18] Preeclampsia is characterized by sudden, dramatic increase in weight that is due to edema, particu—larly of the hands and face; severe hypertension; persistent headache; vision prob—lems; trouble breathing; and protein in urine.

Pregnant women who have high risk of preeclampsia are those who are under 20 or over 35 years of age, are obese, have a history of diabetes or hypertension, are African American, and are carrying more than one fetus.[18] If a woman suffering from preeclampsia develops convulsions, her condition is called *eclampsia (e—klamp'—see—a)*. In the United States, eclampsia is the second leading cause of death among pregnant women.[19]

At present, the only effective treatment for preeclampsia and eclampsia is delivering the fetus, but infants born before the 24th week of pregnancy are unlikely to survive. If the fetus is older than 24 weeks, its mother may be hospi—talized for treatment. This practice helps physicians monitor the mother's condi—tion and enables the fetus to mature until it has a better chance of surviving after a premature birth.

Drug Use

Exposure to alcohol and tobacco is harmful to the embryo/fetus. Women who drink alcohol during pregnancy are at risk of having a child with a fetal alcohol spectrum disorder such as FAS (see Fig. 6.27). Scientists do not know if there is a "safe" amount of alcohol that pregnant women can consume; therefore, women of childbearing age who are sexually active or pregnant should avoid alcoholic

gestational hypertension type of hypertension that can develop during pregnancy

Did *YOU* Know?

Caffeine is a stimulant drug that can pass through the placenta and enter the embryo/fetus. The drug may depress the flow of blood in the placenta, which may be harmful to the developing offspring. At present, there is no clear scientific evidence that a pregnant woman's consumption of caffeinated beverages contributes to *miscarriage*. A miscarriage is the death of an embryo or fetus that occurs before the 20th week of gestation. Nevertheless, pregnant women should avoid drinking concentrated sources of caffeine, especially "energy shots," and limit their caffeine consumption to 200 mg/day.[20] This is approximately the amount of caffeine in 1.5 cups of regular brewed coffee.

beverages. The Chapter 6 "Nutrition Matters" provides more information about fetal alcohol spectrum disorder.

Compared to pregnant women who do not smoke cigarettes, expectant mothers who smoke have higher risk of giving birth too early and having LBW babies. Furthermore, expectant mothers who smoke cigarettes may increase the risk of having babies with birth defects or that die of *sudden infant death syndrome* (*SIDS*). SIDS is the sudden, unexplained death of an infant younger than 1 year of age and the leading cause of death for babies between 1 month and 1 year of age.[21]

The use of illegal drugs, herbal supplements, and medications during pregnancy can also harm the embryo/fetus. Ideally, the time to quit abusing illegal drugs is before pregnancy. Pregnant women should consult their physicians before using herbal supplements or taking any drugs, even over-the-counter medications.

What About Physical Activity?

Women can derive many benefits from being physically active during pregnancy, including enhanced muscle tone and strength, reduced edema, and improved mood and sleep. Most pregnant women can continue their prepregnancy exercise regimens, especially those that included low- or moderate-intensity activities. However, the exercise routine should not result in weight loss. Recommended activities generally include walking, cycling, swimming, or light aerobics. Pregnancy is not the time to begin an intense fitness regimen or perform high-risk physical activities. Activities that are risky and should be avoided include downhill skiing; contact sports such as volleyball, soccer, and basketball; and horseback riding.[22] Pregnant women should discuss their physical activity practices and needs with their physicians. Some expectant women, such as those experiencing hypertension or premature labor contractions, may need to restrict their physical activity.

Most pregnant women can continue their prepregnancy exercise regimens, especially those that included low- or moderate-intensity activities.
©Ascent/PKS Media Inc./Getty Images RF

Concept CHECKPOINT

3. When is an embryo referred to as a fetus?
4. What is the role of the placenta?
5. What is a major factor that determines whether a newborn baby is healthy and survives its first year of life?
6. Why can gestational hypertension be dangerous?
7. Identify at least three different nutrition-related signs of pregnancy.
8. How much weight should a woman at a healthy weight gain during pregnancy? How much weight should she gain if she was underweight before becoming pregnant? How much weight should she gain if she was overweight or obese before pregnancy?
9. Why is having adequate folate and iron status important for pregnant women?
10. Discuss the harmful effects that a pregnant woman's alcohol consumption and cigarette smoking can have on her embryo/fetus.

See Appendix G for responses.

13.3 Infant Nutrition

Learning Outcomes

1 Discuss the physiological processes of lactation and breastfeeding.

2 Discuss the nutrient and energy needs of a lactating woman.

3 Describe benefits that women derive from breastfeeding and infants derive from consuming their mother's milk.

4 Compare the energy and nutrient contents of human milk, cow's milk, and infant formulas.

5 Describe signs that an infant is ready to eat solid foods, and identify appropriate foods for infants.

6 Discuss a healthy infant's rate of growth.

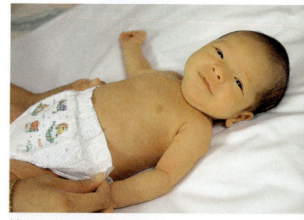
(a)

Rapid physical growth characterizes infancy, the life stage that extends from birth to about 2 years of age. During the first 4 to 6 months of life, a healthy baby doubles its birth weight, and by 1 year of age, an infant's birth weight has tripled. Additionally, an infant's length increases by 50% during its first year of life. Thus, if a baby girl weighs 7 pounds and is 20 inches long at birth, you would expect her to weigh 21 pounds and be 30 inches long by her first birthday (Fig. 13.4).

Compared to older children, an infant needs more energy and nutrients per pound of body weight to support its rapid growth.[1] If an infant's diet lacks adequate energy and nutrients, the baby's growth may slow or even stop. The following sections take a closer look at infant nutrition, including breastfeeding and other infant feeding practices.

Breast Milk Is Best Milk

Two hundred years ago, if a new mother was unable to breastfeed her baby, the child faced certain death—unless a woman who was producing breast milk could be located to suckle (*nurse*) the infant. Today, a new mother can choose to nurse her baby or feed the child an **infant formula,** a synthetic food that simulates human milk. Although both foods provide adequate nutrition for young babies, breastfeeding provides benefits beyond nutrition for the new mother as well as her infant.

Human milk is uniquely formulated to meet the nutrient needs of a newborn baby. During the first couple of days after giving birth, the new mother's breasts produce **colostrum** (*co−loss'−trum*), a yellowish fluid that does not look like milk. By the end of the first week of lactation, colostrum has undergone a transition to *mature milk*. If you compare the appearance of mature human milk to cow's milk, you will notice that breast milk is more watery than cow's milk and may have a slightly bluish color.

Colostrum is a very important first food for babies because the fluid contains antibodies and immune system cells that can be absorbed by the infant's immature digestive tract. Colostrum also contains substances (prebiotics) that encourage the growth of beneficial bacteria in the infant's GI tract. The biologically active substances in colostrum help an infant's body fight infections and hasten the maturation of the baby's immune and digestive systems.[23] Thus, breastfed infants have lower risks of allergies and gastrointestinal, respiratory, and ear infections than formula−fed infants.[24] Furthermore, breastfed babies may be less likely to develop childhood asthma, leukemia, obesity, sudden infant death syndrome, and type 1 diabetes than infants who are not breastfed.

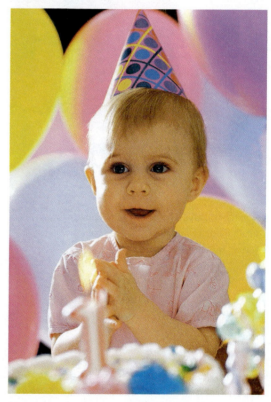
(b)

Figure 13.4 Growth rates during infancy. A healthy newborn baby (*a*) grows rapidly during its first year. During the first 4 to 6 months of life, a baby doubles its birth weight, and by 1 year of age, an infant's birth weight has tripled (*b*). Additionally, an infant's length increases by 50% during its first year of life.

Newborn: ©Diane Macdonald/Getty Images RF; Birthday baby: ©Elyse Lewin/Getty Images RF

infant formula synthetic food that simulates human milk

colostrum initial form of breast milk that contains anti-infective properties

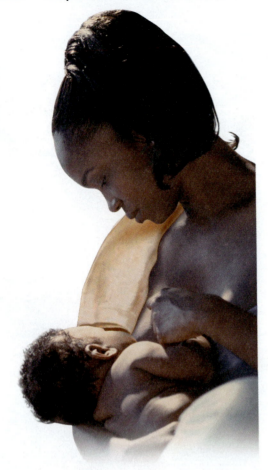

American infants who are breastfed have a lower infant mortality rate than American babies who are not.
©Jiang Jin/Purestock/SuperStock RF

Human milk is a rich source of lipids, including cholesterol, and fatty acids such as linoleic acid, *arachidonic acid* (*AA*), and *docosahexaenoic acid* (*DHA*). An infant's nervous system, especially the brain and eyes, depends on AA and DHA for proper development. Furthermore, the fat in breast milk helps supply the energy needed to maintain the infant's overall growth.

The practice of breastfeeding also provides some important advantages for parents, particularly the new mother. Breastfeeding is more convenient and economical than using infant formula. Human milk is readily available; there is no need to purchase cans of infant formula and have them on hand. As milk leaves the breast, it is always fresh, free of bacteria, and ready to feed without mixing, bottling, or warming. Because human milk production requires a considerable amount of energy, lactating women can lose the extra body fat gained during pregnancy faster than mothers who use infant formula. Additionally, women who breastfeed their babies have lower risks of breast cancer (before menopause) and ovarian cancer than women who do not breastfeed. Some of these benefits depend on whether a woman breastfeeds exclusively, that is, provides no other foods, and the number of months the mother nurses her infant. Table 13.5 lists these and several other advantages of breastfeeding.

The Milk Production Process: Lactation

When an infant suckles, nerves in the mother's nipple signal her brain to release prolactin and **oxytocin** (*ox–e–tose′–in*) into her bloodstream. Prolactin stimulates specialized cells in breasts to form milk. These cells carry out the lactation process by synthesizing some nutrients and removing others from the mother's bloodstream and adding them to her milk. Oxytocin plays a different role in establishing successful lactation. This hormone signals breast tissue to "let down" milk. The *let–down reflex* enables milk to travel in several tubes (ducts) to the nipple area. A reflex is a physical response that is automatic and not under conscious control. When let–down occurs, the infant removes the milk by continued sucking (Fig. 13.5). Shortly before the flow of milk begins,

oxytocin hormone that elicits the "let-down" response and causes the uterus to contract

Did *YOU* Know?

When a new mother breastfeeds her newborn immediately after delivery, oxytocin signals her uterus to contract, reducing the risk of excessive uterine bleeding.

TABLE 13.5 Advantages of Breastfeeding

Advantages for Infants
Human milk • Is free of bacteria as it leaves the breast. • Supplies antibodies and immune cells. • Is easily digested. • Reduces risk of food allergies, especially to proteins in infant formulas and cow's milk. • Changes in composition over time to meet the changing needs of a growing infant. • Contains zinc, iron, and other minerals in highly absorbable forms. • Decreases risks of ear, intestinal, and respiratory infections. • May reduce the risk of asthma, obesity, and type 1 diabetes in childhood.
Advantages for New Mothers
Breastfeeding • Reduces uterine bleeding after delivery. • Promotes shrinkage of the uterus to its prepregnancy size. • Decreases the risk of breast cancer (before menopause) and ovarian cancer. • May promote maternal weight loss. • May enhance bonding with the infant. • Is less expensive and more convenient than feeding infant formula.

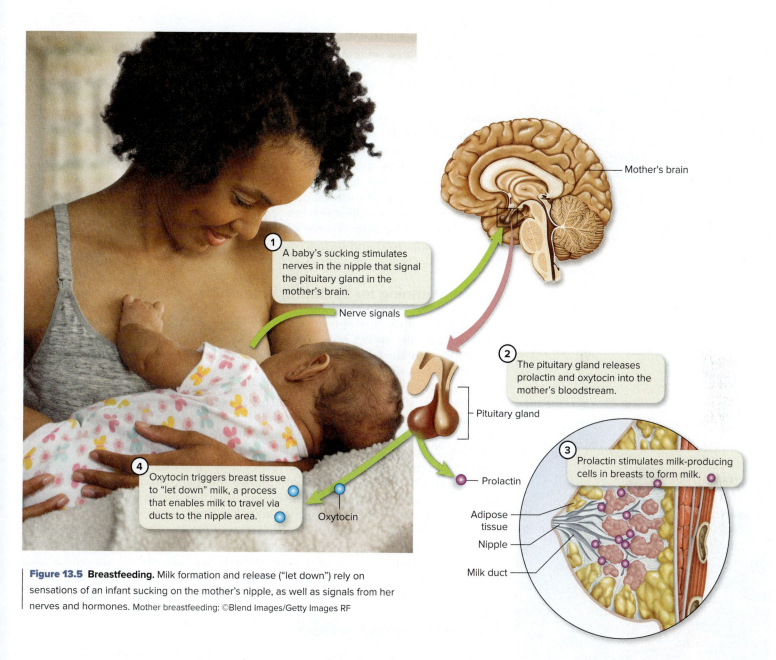

1 A baby's sucking stimulates nerves in the nipple that signal the pituitary gland in the mother's brain.

Nerve signals

Mother's brain

2 The pituitary gland releases prolactin and oxytocin into the mother's bloodstream.

Pituitary gland

4 Oxytocin triggers breast tissue to "let down" milk, a process that enables milk to travel via ducts to the nipple area.

Oxytocin

Prolactin

3 Prolactin stimulates milk-producing cells in breasts to form milk.

Adipose tissue

Nipple

Milk duct

Figure 13.5 Breastfeeding. Milk formation and release ("let down") rely on sensations of an infant sucking on the mother's nipple, as well as signals from her nerves and hormones. Mother breastfeeding: ©Blend Images/Getty Images RF

the lactating woman often feels a tingling sensation in her nipples, a signal that let–down is occurring.

Embarrassment, emotional stress and tension, pain, and fatigue can easily block the let–down reflex. For example, if a lactating mother is tense or upset, let–down does not occur, and her infant will not be able to obtain milk when it suckles. When this happens, the hungry infant becomes frustrated and angry, and the mother may respond by becoming even more tense and upset, setting up a vicious cycle. At this point, new mothers often give up breast–feeding, reporting that they tried to suckle their babies but were unable to "produce" milk.

Lactating women need to be aware of the connection between their emo–tional state and failure to let down. To smooth the path to successful lactation, it helps if new mothers are in a comfortable, relaxed environment when they

Did *YOU* Know?

The size of a woman's breasts does not influence her ability to breastfeed her infant. However, certain surgical procedures used to enlarge or decrease breast size can disrupt the nerves and milk-producing tissue in the breasts.[25] Women who had surgery to alter their breasts may be able to produce milk after giving birth, but their infants' growth rates should be monitored to make sure the babies are obtaining enough milk.

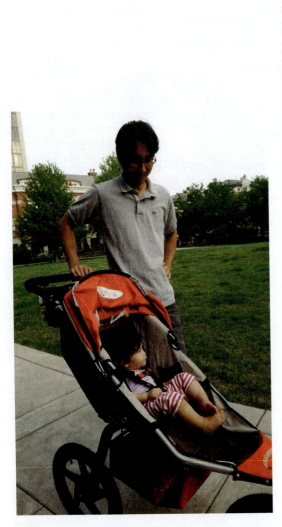

Figure 13.6 Vitamin D and infants. Exposing an infant's skin to some direct sunlight enables the baby's body to form vitamin D. ©Keith Eng 2007 RF

breastfeed their babies. When lactation and breastfeeding are well established, the let−down response often occurs without the need for suckling. For example, the mother's let−down reflex may be triggered just by thinking about nursing her infant or hearing it cry.

Breastfeeding is a skill, and like other skills, it takes some practice to fully master. Thus, it may take a few weeks for the new mother to feel comfortable with the process. By persevering, she and her baby are likely to become a suc−cessful breastfeeding team.

Typically, a lactating woman produces over 3 cups of milk per day.[8] It is important to recognize that milk production relies on "supply and demand." The more the infant suckles (demand), the more milk its mother's breasts produce (supply). However, if milk is not fully removed from the breasts, milk production soon ceases. This is likely to occur when infants are not hungry because they have been given baby food and formula to supplement breast milk feedings.

Dietary Planning for Lactating Women

Milk production requires approximately 800 kcal every day. However, the lactat−ing woman's daily energy needs can be met by adding only about 300 to 400 kcal to her prepregnancy EER. The difference between the energy needed for milk production and the recommended energy intake can enable the new mother to lose the extra body fat she accumulated during pregnancy. This loss is more likely to occur if she continues breastfeeding her baby for 6 months or more and increases her physical activity level. A woman, for example, who needed 2000 kcal before becoming pregnant would require about 2300 to 2400 kcal daily during lactation. To help plan meals and snacks that are nutritionally adequate, she can follow MyPlate recommendations at www.choosemyplate.gov.

No special foods are necessary to sustain milk production. However, a lactating woman should drink fluids every time her infant suckles to help her maintain adequate milk volume and keep her body properly hydrated. For as long as she breastfeeds her baby, the lactating mother should limit her intake of alcohol− and caffeine−containing beverages because her body secretes these drugs into her milk. A woman who breastfeeds her baby should also check with her physician before using any medications, even over−the−counter and herbal products, because such substances may also end up in her breast milk.

Is Breast Milk a Complete Food?

Registered dietitian nutritionists (RDNs) and pediatricians generally recom−mend that new mothers breastfeed their healthy infants exclusively for about 6 months.[24,26] It is not necessary to supplement healthy young infants' diets with other fluids, such as water and infant formula.[26] After an infant reaches 4 to 6 months of age, the breastfed infant should also be given some appropriate solid foods. Breastfeeding may be combined with infant foods until the child's first birthday. However, there is no reason why children cannot be breastfed for longer periods. Throughout the world, many mothers continue to nurse their babies well past the babies' first birthdays, but in the United States, this prac−tice is uncommon.

Although breast milk is highly nutritious, it is not a complete food for all infants. Human milk may contain inadequate amounts of vitamins D and B−12 and the minerals iron and fluoride. The American Academy of Pediatrics (AAP) rec−ommends all breastfed infants be given a supplement that supplies 400 IU of vitamin D per day until they are consuming that amount of the vitamin from food or infant formula. Exposing the infant to some sun can also help meet part of the child's vitamin D needs (Fig. 13.6). If a lactating woman is a total vegetarian and she does not consume a source of vitamin B−12, she should consult her physician concerning the need for vitamin B−12 supplementation. When breastfed infants are about 6 months old, they should also be consuming some iron−containing solid foods because the amount of iron in their mother's milk may no longer meet their needs. Furthermore, a fluoride supplement may be necessary for breastfed babies. Before giving any dietary supplements to their baby, parents or caregivers should discuss their infant's nutritional needs with the child's physician.

Quitting Too Soon

Nearly all healthy women are physically capable of breastfeeding their infants. In 2013, 81% of American women started breastfeeding their babies soon after birth.[27] Within 2 days of birth, 17% of the breastfed babies were also consum−ing formula. By the time the infants were 6 months old, about 52% continued to be breastfed. By their first birthday, approximately 31% of the babies were still consuming their mother's milk.

Women who breastfeed their newborns often stop the practice within 6 months. There are many reasons why women discontinue nursing their infants too soon. New mothers often quit because they lack information about and support for breastfeed−ing their babies. Some women discontinue breastfeeding because of uncertainty over how much milk their babies are consuming. Baby bottles are marked to indicate ounces, so a mother who bottle−feeds her infant can easily measure the amount of formula consumed. A lactating mother, however, has to observe her baby for cues indicating the child is full. When a breastfeeding baby is no longer interested in nursing and stops, its mother has to assume the infant is satisfied with the feeding. A well−nourished breastfed infant will gain weight normally and generally have six or more wet diapers as well as one or two bowel movements that have soft stools per day. Parents or caregivers who are concerned about their infants' food intake or nutritional status should consult their physician immediately.

Many new mothers discontinue breastfeeding before their babies are 6 months old because they need to return to work and have caregivers feed their babies. Although lactating women can learn to express milk from their breasts and preserve it for later feedings, many workplaces do not have comfortable, private facilities for women to express milk and then store it safely.

To enhance the likelihood that a nursing mother continues to breastfeed, it is helpful to enlist the support of a female relative or friend who has successfully breastfed her children. Furthermore, the woman's partner needs to understand and appreciate the function of the human breast as a source of nearly perfect nourishment for infants. New mothers are unlikely to begin and continue nursing their babies without their partners' support. La Leche League is an international organization dedicated to providing education and support for breastfeeding women (1−877−4−LALECHE or www.llli.org). Also, hospitals may employ lac−tation consultants or specialists. Lactation consultants are often nurses who are trained to provide information and advice about breastfeeding. For more infor−mation about breastfeeding, visit http://www.cdc.gov/breastfeeding/.

Infant Formula Feeding

Not every woman wants or is able to breastfeed her baby. Infant formulas are a safe and nutritionally adequate source of nutrients for babies who are not breast−fed. To produce artificial milk for babies, infant formula manufacturers alter cow's milk to improve its digestibility and nutrient content. Infant formulas generally contain heat−treated proteins from cow's milk, lactose and/or sucrose, and veg−etable oil. Infant formulas generally lack cholesterol, but some of these products

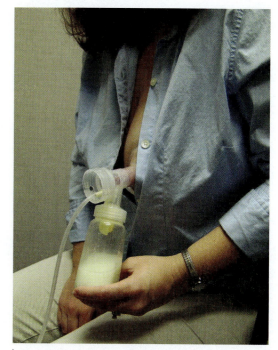

This mother is using an electric device to express milk in a private room at her workplace. She will chill the milk and give it to her baby's caregiver for bottle-feeding. ©Wendy Schiff

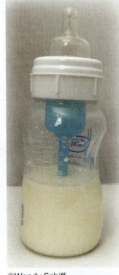

Do not heat infant formula or human milk in a microwave oven. The heat can destroy immune factors in human milk and create hot spots that can scald an infant's tongue.

©Wendy Schiff

casein major protein in cow's milk

have prebiotics and the fatty acids DHA and AA added to them. Vitamins and minerals are added to the product, and in some instances, infant formula contains higher levels of micronutrients than human milk. Although infant formulas mimic the water, macronutrient, and micronutrient content of human milk, their compositions are not identical to human milk (Table 13.6). Formula manufacturers have been unable to duplicate human antibodies and other unique immune system factors that are in breast milk.

An interesting feature of human milk is that its fat content changes during each feeding, which usually lasts about 20 minutes. In the beginning of the session, the mother's milk is low in fat, but as her infant continues to suckle, the fat content of her milk gradually increases.[28] The higher fat content of the "hind milk" may make the baby feel satisfied and, as a result, discontinue feeding. Infant formulas, however, have uniform composition; that is, they do not change their fat content during a feeding session. Thus, the mother or infant caregiver is more likely to control the amount of formula the baby consumes, possibly leading to overfeeding. Nevertheless, the overall energy content of human milk is about the same as that of infant formulas (about 20 kcal per ounce).

Experts with the AAP recommend that caregivers provide an iron-fortified infant formula for babies who are not breastfed. Not all infant formulas contain iron, so it is important to read the product's label before purchasing it. Formula-fed babies may also need a source of fluoride, but caregivers should check with their infants' physicians before providing a supplement containing the mineral. For babies who are allergic to infant formulas made from cow's milk proteins, similar products made with soy or other proteins are available.

What About Cow's Milk?

Why not feed fresh fluid cow's milk to an infant? Cow's milk is too high in minerals and protein and does not contain enough carbohydrate to meet an infant's nutrient needs (see Table 13.6). In addition, infants have more difficulty digesting **casein** (*kay'–seen*), the major protein in cow's milk, than the major proteins in human milk.

TABLE 13.6 Comparing Approximate Compositions of Human Milk, Cow's Milk, and Iron-Fortified Infant Formulas (per Ounce)

Milk or Iron-Fortified Formula	Energy (kcal/oz)	Protein (g/oz)	Carbo-hydrate (g/oz)	Fat (g/oz)	Choles-terol (mg/oz)	Iron (mg/oz)	Calcium (mg/oz)
Human milk	22.0	0.32	2.12	1.35	4.00	0.01	10.0
Cow's milk, whole	19.0	0.96	1.46	0.99	3.00	0.01	34.0
Cow's milk, fat-free	10.0	1.03	1.51	0.02	1.00	0.01	37.0
Cow's milk protein-based formulas							
Similac Advance®	20.0	0.41	2.10	1.06	1.12	0.36	16.0
Enfamil Premium Newborn®	20.0	0.42	2.25	1.06	0.00	0.36	16.0
Soy protein-based formulas							
ProSobee Lipil®	19.0	0.50	1.86	1.07	0.00	0.36	21.0
Similac Isomil Advance®	20.0	0.49	2.04	1.09	0.00	0.36	21.0

Source: Data from U.S. Department of Agriculture, Agricultural Research Service: *What's in the foods you eat search tool, 2013–2014.* Accessed July 2, 2017. https://www.ars.usda.gov/northeast-area/beltsville-md/beltsville -human-nutrition-research-center/food-surveys-research-group/docs/whats-in-the-foods-you-eat-emsearch-toolem/

Milks and infant formulas: ©Wendy Schiff

Cow's milk can also contribute to intestinal bleeding and iron deficiency.[29] Thus, whole cow's milk should not be fed to infants until they are 1 year of age.[30]

Whole milk is major source of saturated fat in young children's diets. According to the AAP, reduced−fat forms of milk can be given to children who are between 1 and 2 years of age, but only as part of a diet that supplies 30% of total calories from fat.[30] To reduce the risk of developing cardiovascular disease later in life, children over age 2 years should consume low−fat or fat−free dairy products.[30]

Allergies   Allergies are immune system responses to the presence of foreign pro−teins in the body. Allergies to proteins in foods, especially cow's milk proteins, often begin in infancy and may persist through childhood. Signs and symptoms of food allergies typically include the following:

- Vomiting, diarrhea, intestinal gas and pain, bloating, or constipation
- Skin rash called eczema (*ek'−zeh−mah*)
- Runny nose and breathing difficulties, such as asthma

Compared to breastfed infants, formula−fed babies have a greater risk of food allergies. When a woman has a personal or family history of food aller−gies, she may be able to prevent her children from developing such allergies if she breastfeeds her babies exclusively for 4 months.[31]

Introducing Solid Foods

Before about 6 months of age, babies' nutritional needs can generally be met with human milk and/or infant formula. Solid ("complementary" or "baby") foods should not be introduced to infants until they are about 4 to 6 months of age.[31] At this age, many infants need the additional calories supplied by solid foods. Breastfed babies may also need a dietary source of iron because their stores of the mineral are usually exhausted about 6 months after birth. Nevertheless, caregivers should continue to provide human milk or iron−fortified infant formula as the foundation of the baby's diet for the first year.

Many new parents are anxious to start feeding their young infants solid food. However, babies are not physically mature enough to consume solids before they are 4 to 6 months of age. For example, a baby's kidney functions are quite limited until the child is about 4 to 6 weeks of age. Additionally, an infant's digestive tract cannot readily digest starch before the child is about 3 months old.

Infants are born with the **extrusion reflex,** an involuntary response that occurs when a solid or semisolid object is placed in an infant's mouth. As a result of this reflex, a young baby thrusts its tongue forward, pushing the object out of its mouth. Thus, trying to feed the infant solid foods is a messy, frustrat−ing process, as the child automatically pushes the food out of its mouth. Liquid foods, such as breast milk or infant formula, do not elicit the extrusion reflex, so the baby swallows fluids.

As the infant reaches 4 to 6 months of age, the extrusion reflex disappears, and the child has developed the physiological abilities to digest, metabolize, and excrete a wider range of foods. Moreover, a 6−month−old infant can usually sit up with back support and coordinate muscular control over his or her mouth and neck movements. These signs indicate the baby is ready physically to eat solid foods, is less likely to choke on such foods, and can turn his or her head away from food when full. **Weaning** is the gradual process of shifting an infant from breastfeeding or bottle−feeding to drinking from a cup and eating solid foods.

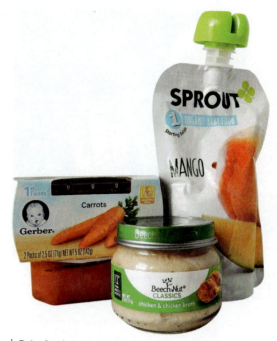

Baby foods are available in a variety of forms and packaging. ©Wendy Schiff

extrusion reflex involuntary response in which a young infant thrusts its tongue forward when a solid or semisolid object is placed in its mouth

weaning gradual process of shifting from breastfeeding or bottle-feeding to drinking from a cup and eating solid foods

Did *YOU* Know?

Many parents think adding solid foods to infants' diets helps babies sleep through the night. Actually, this developmental milestone generally occurs around 3 to 4 months of age, regardless of what infants are eating.

©Sky View/Getty Images RF

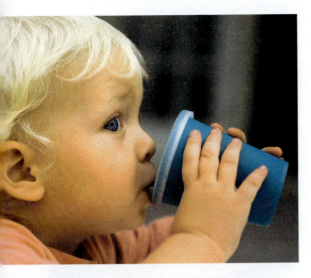

Figure 13.7 Learning to drink from a "sippy" cup.
©Arthur Tilley/Getty Images RF

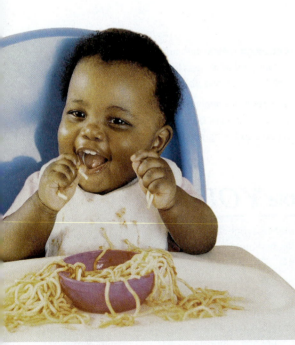

Babies need to practice self-feeding skills, even if it means playing with food and creating messes.
©Nancy Ney/Getty Images RF

Typical first foods include "baby cereal," ground meat or chicken mixed with breast milk or formula, pureed green beans or squash ("baby vegetables"), and mashed bananas. Each new food should be introduced into a baby's diet one at a time. If the child consumes the food for about 3 to 5 days and does not show signs of an allergic response, such as diarrhea, vomiting, eczema, or runny nose, the caregiver can consider that food safe for the child to eat. The caregiver should continue to introduce a single new food into the infant's diet over a period of several days and watch the baby for signs of allergic reactions.

In the past, highly allergenic foods, such as peanut butter, fish, and eggs, were not introduced into a baby's diet until the child was at least 1 year of age. However, results of current studies indicate that *delaying* such foods may *increase* the child's risk of food allergies. According to experts with the National Institutes of Health, infants who have severe eczema, egg allergy, or both conditions are at high risk of developing peanut allergy. Such high-risk infants should be fed a small amount of a peanut-containing food (such as a mixture of smooth peanut butter and water) when they are 4 to 6 months of age.[32] This practice has been shown to prevent the infants from developing peanut allergy later in childhood.

Foods that are likely to be allergenic can be introduced to a healthy baby in very small amounts after the typical first foods have been consumed without causing allergic responses. If the infant does not show signs of an allergic reaction to the food, the child can be fed higher amounts of the item. Caregivers should always check with the infant's physician for advice on when to start feeding a new food to the child.

Many varieties of strained baby food are available. Single-food items, such as carrots or peas, are more nutrient-dense choices for feeding infants than mixed dinners and desserts. It is a good idea to avoid giving mixed foods such as casseroles or commercially prepared baby food "dinners" to young infants. If the baby has an allergic reaction after eating a food mixture, it will be difficult to determine which ingredient was responsible. Serving mixed foods is acceptable when the child has eaten each ingredient individually without having an allergic response. Section 7.9 of Chapter 7 has more information about food allergies.

Most brands of baby food have no added salt, but some fruit desserts contain a lot of added sugar. As an alternative, caregivers can prepare their own baby food by taking plain, unseasoned cooked foods and pureeing them in a blender. If a large amount of the item is blended, the pureed food can be poured into an ice cube tray, covered with a plastic bag, and frozen. When it is feeding time, an ice cube portion of the baby food can be popped out of the tray and warmed.

At about 6 to 8 months of age, the baby's first set of teeth, the "primary teeth," begin to appear. These teeth are important for proper nutrition because they help the child bite and chew food. By 8 to 12 months of age, most infants can use their fingers to pick up and chew finger foods such as crackers, toast, and cooked string beans. Babies can also hold a bottle and practice drinking from a special cup ("sippy cup") that has a lid with a spout (Fig. 13.7). Babies need to practice self-feeding skills, even if it means playing with food and creating messes. By about 10 months of age, many infants are mastering self-feeding and making the transition from baby foods to healthy menu items that the rest of the family enjoys.

What Not to Feed an Infant

By the end of the first year, an infant should be consuming many different foods—grain products, meats, fruits, and vegetables—along with breast milk or infant formula. Introducing a baby to various foods helps the child learn about

Food & Nutrition tips

When feeding solid foods to an infant:

- Use a baby-sized spoon—a small spoon with a broad handle.

- Hold the infant comfortably on your lap, as for breastfeeding or bottle-feeding, but in a more upright position to ease swallowing.

- Add some breast milk or infant formula to the food, and place a small dab of the semisolid food on the spoon's tip. Gently place the spoon on the infant's tongue and tilt it so the food slides onto the tongue. If the infant spits it out, the baby is not ready to eat solid foods, so do not continue with the feeding.

- When the infant accepts and swallows the food, expect the child to take only two or three bites during these early feeding sessions.

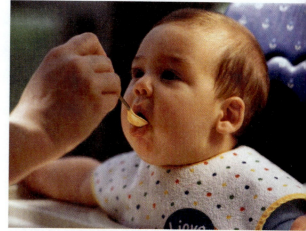
©Arthur Tilley/Getty Images RF

different tastes, odors, and textures. However, certain foods and beverages are not appropriate for infants. Avoid feeding an infant these things:

- **Honey.** This product may contain spores of *Clostridium botulinum* that can produce a potentially fatal toxin in children who are under 1 year old (see Chapter 5).

- **Excessive infant formula or human milk.** Depending on their age, most infants need less than 30 ounces of human milk or infant formula daily. A child who drinks too much milk may not eat enough solid foods that contain nutrients lacking in milk.

- **Semisolid baby cereal in a baby bottle that has the nipple opening enlarged.** This practice contributes to overfeeding and does not help the child learn self–feeding skills.

- **Candy, flavored gelatin water, or soft drinks.** These items provide few micronutrients.

- **Small pieces of hard or coarse foods.** Foods such as hot dogs (unless finely cut into sticks, not coin shapes), whole nuts, grapes, chunks of cooked meat, raw carrots, and popcorn can cause choking. Caregivers should supervise meals to keep young children from stuffing too much food in their mouths.

- **Fruit juice.** Babies should not be given fruit juices before they are 1 year of age. Fruit juice lacks the fiber content of whole or mashed fruit, and children may consume the beverages instead of more nutritious foods. Also, the fructose and sorbitol (a sugar alcohol) in pear, apple, and prune juice may cause diarrhea, gas, and abdominal pain.

- **Unpasteurized (raw) milk.** Raw milk may be contaminated with bacteria or viruses.

- **Goat's milk.** Goat's milk is low in iron, folate, and vitamins C and D.

Baby Bottle Caries

At bedtime, many caregivers place infants in their cribs with a baby bottle containing formula, juice, or a sugar–sweetened drink. This practice is not recommended because the sleepy infant sucks slowly, allowing the carbohydrate–containing fluid to bathe the child's teeth and provide a source of nutrients for bacteria that stick to teeth. These bacteria produce acids that dissolve tooth enamel, causing cavities to form in the teeth (*dental caries*). Dentists often refer to this condition as "baby bottle caries." To reduce the risk of baby bottle caries, infants should be given only water in their bedtime bottles.

Concept CHECKPOINT

11. What is the "let-down reflex"?
12. How does lactation affect a new mother's energy needs?
13. What is colostrum, and why is it a valuable first food for breastfed babies?
14. RDNs recommend that healthy infants be breastfed exclusively during their first _____ months of life.
15. List at least five benefits that infants derive from breastfeeding.
16. Identify at least three benefits that women derive from breastfeeding their babies.
17. Compare the energy, macronutrient, and calcium contents of an ounce of human milk with those of an ounce of cow's milk.
18. Identify at least three physiological indications that an infant is ready to eat solid foods.
19. How much should a healthy infant's weight increase during its first year of life?

See Appendix G for responses.

13.4 The Preschool Years

Learning Outcomes

1 Identify some major nutrition-related health concerns facing American preschool children.

2 Summarize practical suggestions for encouraging healthy eating habits among preschool children.

3 Describe steps caregivers can take to improve the nutritional status of preschool children.

Childhood can be divided into the preschool period (2 to 5 years of age), the school—age period (6 to 11 years of age), and adolescence (12 to 19 years of age). In this section, we focus on some major nutrition concerns of preschool children. The rapid growth rate that characterizes the first 12 months of life tapers off quickly during the preschool years and proceeds at a slow but steady rate until the end of childhood. If an average infant's growth rate did not slow down, he or she might weigh about 190 pounds and be about 5 feet, 7 inches tall by 3 years of age! However, the average 3—year—old weighs about 32 pounds and is about 3 feet in height.

As the growth rate slows after infancy, preschoolers' appetites decrease because they do not need as much food. Parents and other caregivers must recognize that a 3—year—old child should not be expected to eat as eagerly as he or she did as an infant. Furthermore, children do not have the stomach capacity to eat adult—size portions of foods (Fig. 13.8).

When planning meals and snacks for children, caregivers should emphasize nutrient—dense foods, such as lean meats, low—fat dairy products, whole—grain cereals, fruits, nuts, and vegetables. Although many ready—to—eat cereals are sweetened with sugar, it is not necessary to eliminate such foods. Caregivers, however, should read product labels and choose varieties with less added sugar. Additionally, it is important to monitor children's intake of sweets because

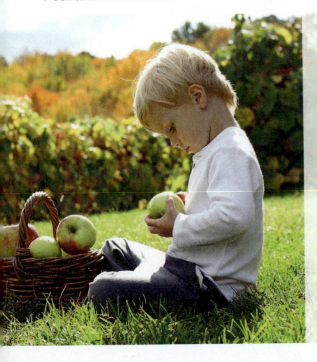

Figure 13.8 Age-appropriate portion sizes. Healthy young children should not be expected to eat adult-size portions of food. A few apple slices would be an appropriate snack for this toddler.
©Christin Lola/Shutterstock RF

TABLE 13.7 Preschool Children: Daily Food Plan Based on MyPlate Recommendations

Energy/Food Group	2 Years	3 to 5 Years
*Kilocalories**	1000	1200 to 1400
Grains	3 oz	4 to 5 oz
Vegetables	1 cup	1½ cups
Fruits	1 cup	1 to 1½ cups
Dairy	2 cups	2½ cups
Protein foods	2 oz	3 to 4 oz

* Kilocalorie estimates are based on age and 30 to 60 minutes of physical activity.

Source: U.S. Department of Agriculture: *MyPlate checklist calculator.* Accessed: July 1, 2017. https://www.choosemyplate.gov /MyPlate-Daily-Checklist-input

sugary items can crowd out more nutritious foods from their diets. Table 13.7 presents a day's food group selections, based on MyPlate recommendations, that are appropriate for children who are 2 to 5 years of age.

Snacks

Snacking is not necessarily a bad habit, especially if snacks are nutrient dense and fit into the child's overall diet. Nutritious snacks can be offered at midmorning or midafternoon, when the child is likely to become hungry between meals. A healthy 4– or 5–year–old child can safely eat raw vegetables without fear of choking. Nutritious dips, such as the yogurt dip in this chapter's "Recipe for Healthy Living," may make raw vegetables more appealing to children. Table 13.8 lists some nutritious snacks that children tend to like.

TABLE 13.8 Nutritious Snacks

- Peanut butter spread on graham crackers
- Fruit smoothies (see Chapter 4 "Recipe for Healthy Living")
- Fruit salad (or cut-up fruit)
- Mini-pizzas (half an English muffin, topped with tomato sauce and mozzarella cheese, and heated in toaster oven or microwave oven)
- Plain, low-fat yogurt topped with granola or fresh fruit
- Peanuts, cashews, or sunflower seeds
- Cheese melted on whole-wheat crackers
- Dried fruit
- Trail mix
- Ready-to-eat cereal
- Vegetable sticks dipped in hummus

Fostering Positive Eating Behaviors

Parents often refer to their preschool children as "picky eaters" because the youngsters do not eat everything offered to them. Furthermore, it is not unusual for children to have "food jags," periods in which they refuse to eat a food that they liked in the past or want to eat only a particular food, such as peanut butter and jelly sandwiches or cereal and milk. Picky eating and food jags may be expressions of a child's growing need for independence. Caregivers should avoid nagging, forcing, and bribing children to eat. Instead, caregivers can offer the children a variety of healthy foods each day and allow the youngsters to choose which items and how much to eat.

Many children, especially preschool children, resist eating new foods. The temperature, appearance, texture, and taste of a food influence whether children will sample it. For example, young children often reject lumpy or hot–temperature foods. Sometimes children object to having foods mixed together such as in stews and casseroles, even though they like the ingredients when served separately. It is not unusual for young children to dislike vegetables that have strong flavors or odors, such as broccoli, onions, and asparagus.

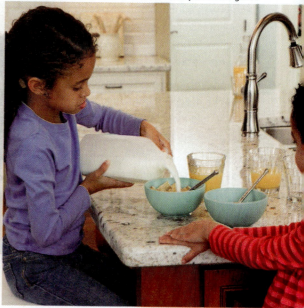
©Ariel Skelley/Blend Images RF

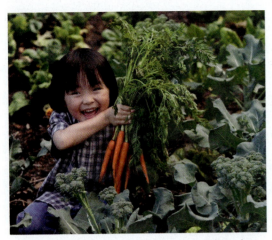

Eating vegetables may become more appealing when children help grow, select, or prepare fresh produce.

©Blend Images/Image Source RF

The idea of eating vegetables may become more appealing when children help grow, select, or prepare fresh produce. Nevertheless, it is important to recognize that everyone, including a child, is entitled to dislike certain foods.

The social atmosphere can make mealtimes enjoyable or unbearable, which in turn influences a child's desire to eat. Mealtimes should be happy, social occasions to enjoy healthful foods with parents or other caregivers. The kitchen table should not become a battleground in which adults use threats or bribes to force children to eat unfamiliar foods. For example, avoid telling a child, "You'll just sit there until you clean your plate" or "You can have a cupcake if you eat your peas." When a child refuses to eat, have the youngster remain at the table for a while. If the child continues to be disinterested in eating, remove the food and wait until the next scheduled meal or snack.

Healthy children are not in danger of starving if they skip a meal. A child who is not hungry at mealtimes may have eaten a snack before the meal at a friend's home. If a child's lack of appetite persists, caretakers should consult the child's physician to rule out illness.

Common Food-Related Concerns

Nutrition—related problems that often affect preschool children are iron deficiency, dental caries, food allergies, and obesity. Section 13.7 focuses on obesity during childhood and adolescence.

Iron Deficiency

Iron deficiency can lead to decreased physical stamina, learning ability, and resistance to infection. The best way to prevent iron deficiency in children is to provide foods that are good sources of iron, such as lean meat and enriched breads and cereals. Milk and other dairy products are poor sources of iron, so caregivers may need to limit daily servings of foods from this food group. Preschool children should consume 2 to 2.5 cups/day of fat—free or low—fat milk or equivalent dairy products (see Table 13.7). Chapter 9 provides more information about iron deficiency.

Dental Caries

Many preschool children have had one or more dental caries by the time they enter school. If dental caries are not treated, jaw pain, gum infection, and tooth loss can occur. The following tips can help reduce the risk of dental caries in children:

- Brush teeth with a pea—sized amount of fluoride—containing toothpaste twice daily.

- Provide routine pediatric dental care and fluoridated drinking water.

- Any carbohydrate can contribute to dental caries, so reduce the number of snacks the child eats. Also, provide the child with more nutrient—dense snacks, such as raw fruits and vegetables or pieces of cheese.

- If preschoolers want to chew gum, have them chew sugarless gum to reduce the risk of dental caries.[33]

Concept CHECKPOINT

20. What is a "food jag"?

21. Discuss effects that iron deficiency can have on children.

22. List at least three steps caregivers can take to reduce the risk of dental caries in children.

See Appendix G for responses.

Food & Nutrition *tips*

- Foods with bright colors, crisp textures, and sweet or mild flavors usually appeal to children. When planning meals, consider including foods with these attractive characteristics.

- As a parent, you may want to consider having the "one bite policy." According to this policy, your child should try at least one bite of each new food provided at mealtimes.

- To stimulate your child's appetite, try serving food on a small colorful plate that is designed to appeal to young children.

- Keep in mind that you are your children's role model for food choices and physical activity habits. If you eat a variety of nutrient-dense foods and are physically active, your children are likely to eat such foods and be active as well.

13.5 School-Age Children

Learning Outcomes

1 Compare the typical eating patterns of school-age children with those of preschool children.

2 Identify some major nutrition-related health concerns facing American school-age children.

3 Summarize practical suggestions for encouraging healthy eating habits among school-age children.

Many school–age children adopt diets that are nutritionally inadequate.[34] Compared to preschoolers, older children often skip breakfast. Furthermore, school–age children typically consume more foods away from home and more fried items and sugar–sweetened beverages than younger children. Diets of school–age children tend to provide excessive amounts of solid fat, added sugars, and sodium.[34] Excessive intakes of fat and sugar contribute to the development of obesity, and high intake of sodium may contribute to hypertension among children.

School–age children often do not eat recommended amounts of fruits and vegetables, and the youngsters typically consume less than recommended amounts of dietary fiber. Low fiber intake contributes to constipation; as many as 10% of American children suffer from chronic constipation.[35]

Table 13.9 presents a day's MyPlate food recommendations for healthy school–age children, who are 6 to 11 years of age. The www.choosemyplate.gov website has a special series of web pages for children who are 6 to 11 years of age. Children can visit the "MyPlate Kids' Place" website and play the interactive "Blast Off Game." To test the game, visit http://www.choosemyplate.gov/kids/index.html.

Caregivers can help improve children's diets by encouraging youngsters to eat breakfast regularly. Children who routinely eat breakfast are more likely to have better diets and healthier body weights than children who skip this meal.[36] Break–fast menus do not need to feature traditional fare such as bacon, eggs, waffles, or pancakes. For example, leftovers from the previous night's dinner can be eaten for breakfast. Convenient "fast breakfasts" that school–age children can prepare quickly include ready–to–eat cereal with milk and fruit, cottage cheese and fruit, a peanut butter and jelly sandwich, or yogurt topped with trail mix or pieces of fresh fruit.

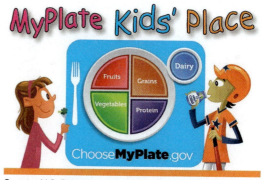

Source: U.S. Department of Agriculture, Center for Nutrition Policy and Promotion

TABLE 13.9 Six- to 11-Year-Old Children: Daily Food Plan Based on MyPlate Recommendations

Energy/Food Group	Age/Sex 6 Years		Age 7–8 Years	Age/Sex 9 Years		Age 10–11 Years	
	Girls	Boys	Both	Girls	Boys	Girls	Boys
Kilocalories*	1400	1600	1600	1600	1800	1800	2000
Grains	5 oz	5 oz	5 oz	5 oz	6 oz	6 oz	6 oz
Vegetables	1.5 cups	2 cups	2 cups	2 cups	2.5 cups	2.5 cups	2.5 cups
Fruits	1.5 cups	1.5 cups	1.5 cups	1.5 cups	1.5 cups	1.5 cups	2 cups
Dairy	2.5 cups	2.5 cups	2.5 cups	3 cups	3 cups	3 cups	3 cups
Protein foods	4 oz	5 oz	5 oz	5 oz	5 oz	5 oz	5.5 oz

* Kilocalorie estimates are based on age, sex, and 30 to 60 minutes of physical activity.

Source: U.S. Department of Agriculture: *MyPlate checklist calculator.* https://www.choosemyplate.gov/MyPlate-Daily-Checklist-input. Accessed: July 1, 2017.

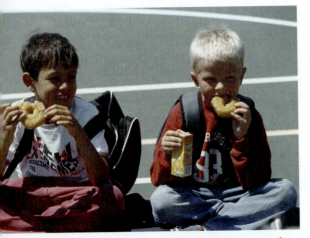

Parents and other caregivers need to be concerned about their children's food choices, especially while they are at school. ©Pixtal/age fotostock RF

Parents and other caregivers need to be concerned about foods that are available at school and obtain answers to the following questions: What kinds of foods are offered for school breakfasts and lunches? Does the school have vending machines accessible to youngsters? If so, what kinds of foods and beverages are sold from these machines? Do vending machines offer competitively priced, nutrient–dense foods? What can be done to ensure that the machines and the school's cafeteria provide nutritious foods that children will eat? Furthermore, what efforts are being made to teach children about proper nutrition while they are in school?

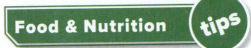

The following tips can help you improve your child's diet:

- Guide your family's food choices instead of dictating what they eat.
- Eat meals together as a family as often as possible.
- If necessary, reduce the amount of fat, especially saturated and trans fat, in your family's diet.
- Do not place your child on a restrictive diet unless the diet is recommended by the child's physician.
- Avoid using food as a reward or punishment.
- Encourage the child to drink water instead of sugar-sweetened beverages.
- Keep healthy snacks (such as fat-free or low-fat milk, fresh fruit, and vegetables) on hand.
- Serve at least 5 servings of fruits and vegetables each day.
- Discourage eating meals or snacks while watching TV or playing electronic games.
- Encourage the child to eat a nutrient-dense breakfast daily.

Concept CHECKPOINT

23. Discuss how young children's eating patterns often change when they enter school.
24. List at least three tips for improving diets of school-age children.

See Appendix G for responses.

13.6 Adolescence

Learning Outcomes

1 Discuss puberty and how it affects an adolescent's energy and nutrient needs.
2 Discuss some major nutrition-related health concerns facing American adolescents.

adolescence life stage in which a child matures physically into an adult

Adolescence is the life stage in which a child matures physically into an adult. During adolescence, the reproductive organs increase in size and begin functioning properly. Furthermore, individuals typically attain their full height by the end of adolescence. During this life stage, youth also develop emotionally, intellectually, and socially as they prepare for their adult roles.

Healthy adolescents learn to function independently of their adult caregivers. Thus, youths face a variety of lifestyle choices, including decisions regarding eating and physical activity habits. Such decisions often set the stage for the quality of their health in adulthood. For many teens, however, pressure to con—form to fads and be influenced by other adolescents ("peer pressure") negatively affects their diets and overall health.

Puberty signals the end of childhood. Most boys begin puberty when they are between 10 and 12 years of age; most girls begin puberty between 8 and 10 years of age.[37] Puberty is a period characterized by dramatic physical changes, including increases in height and weight, known as the adolescent "growth spurt."

Most girls begin their growth spurt between 10 and 13 years of age. Boys begin their growth spurt later than girls—generally when they are between 12 and 15 years of age. Girls usually begin menstruating during their growth spurt. A girl's skeletal growth is almost complete about 2 years after her first menstrual period, whereas boys typically continue to gain stature until they are in their early twenties. The timing of puberty and growth spurts can vary widely, primarily due to genetic, environmental, and nutritional factors. Figure 13.9 shows a group of adolescents who are about the same age but are at different stages of physical maturity.

The amount of energy and nutrients required during adolescence reflects the individual's stage of growth and physical activity level. Early in adolescence, when a girl is at the peak of her growth spurt, she typically consumes more energy than a boy of the same age, especially if she is active in sports. By the age of 13 or 14 years, girls' growth rate slows and boys' growth spurt begins. As a result, adolescent boys' food intake generally surpasses that of adolescent girls. If maturing boys and girls choose to eat nutritious foods and maintain a high level of physical activity, they can take advantage of their increased hunger and gain lean body mass without gaining excess body fat.

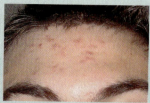
Nutrition-Related Concerns of Adolescents

People generally establish their future eating habits and physical activity practices when they are teenagers. According to results of a nationwide survey, many youth are not following healthy diets or getting enough exercise. In 2015, 21.5% of the high school students had not consumed milk during the week before they were questioned about their eating habits.[39] Almost 64% of the students had skipped breakfast each day during the same period of time. According to findings of this survey, only about 27% of the high school students met recommended levels of physical activity during each of the 7 days before the survey.

Adolescents who are physically inactive and whose diets rely heavily on unhealthy foods purchased at fast—food restaurants or vending machines may be setting the stage for the development of obesity, type 2 diabetes, heart disease, and other serious chronic diseases later in life. Obesity, eating disorders, and low iron and calcium intakes are major

Figure 13.9 Different rates of physical maturity. Although these adolescents are about the same age, they are in different stages of physical maturity.
©Purestock/Getty Images RF

nutrition—related concerns of adolescents. Youth, especially teenage girls, are at risk of developing disordered eating practices and eating disorders. You can learn more about eating disorders by reading the Chapter 10 "Nutrition Matters." In this chapter, Section 13.7 discusses adolescent obesity.

Iron and Calcium Intakes

Adolescent boys may become iron deficient during their growth spurt because their iron intakes do not keep up with their bodies' needs for the mineral. Adolescent girls are also at risk of iron deficiency, especially if their diets lack iron—rich foods and they have heavy menstrual blood losses. Iron deficiency leads to increased fatigue and decreased ability to concentrate and learn. Teenagers need to understand why iron is important for good health and incorporate reliable food sources of the mineral in their diets (see Chapter 9).

Over the last 20 years, many adolescents have switched from drinking milk to drinking soft drinks. RDNs and other nutrition experts are concerned that these adolescents have inadequate calcium intakes because of this practice. Inadequate calcium intake during adolescence is associated with decreased bone mass and increased likelihood of bone fractures later in life. To encourage youth to consume recommended amounts of calcium, parents or other caregivers should explain the importance of the mineral to bone health and provide calcium—rich foods and beverages during meals and snacks. Adolescents should consume 3 cups/day of fat—free or low—fat milk or equivalent dairy products. Furthermore, teenagers need to be aware that physical activity can strengthen bones, whereas smoking cigarettes is a risk factor for *osteoporosis*, a condition characterized by loss of bone density. To learn more about this condition, see the "Major Minerals" section of Chapter 9.

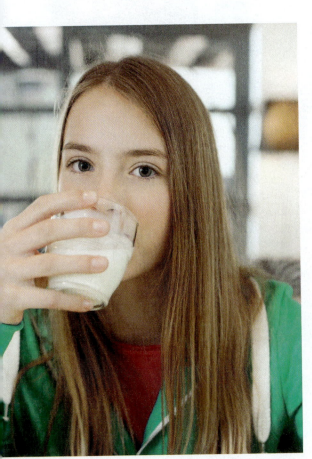
Adolescents should consume 3 cups/day of fat-free or low-fat milk or equivalent dairy products. ©Fabrice Lerouge/Onoky/Corbis RF

Vegetarianism

Some teenagers adopt vegetarian diets as a way of defining their identity and asserting independence from their caregivers. Although vegetarian diets can be healthy alternatives to the typical American diet, some youth use vegetarianism to mask disordered eating behaviors (see Chapter 10's "Nutrition Matters").[40] When planning their diets, teenage vegans need to include foods that supply adequate amounts of calcium, iron, and zinc, and vitamins D and B—12. For information to help plan well—balanced, nutritionally adequate diets, teens can use the recommendations of the MyPlate food guide that are appropriate for their age, sex, and physical activity level. Chapter 7 discusses vegetarianism in more detail.

Concept CHECKPOINT

25. At what age does the adolescent growth spurt usually occur in boys? At what age does the growth spurt generally occur in girls?

26. Why are intakes of iron and calcium important during adolescence?

See Appendix G for responses.

13.7 Childhood Obesity

Learning Outcomes

1 Provide definitions for *overweight, obesity,* and *extreme obesity* in childhood and adolescence.

2 Identify health consequences of childhood obesity.

3 Discuss the prevalence of and factors that contribute to childhood obesity.

4 Discuss strategies for preventing and treating childhood obesity.

Over the past few decades, U.S. public health officials became concerned about the increasing prevalence of obesity among children and adolescents ("childhood obesity"). Approximately 17% of American children who are between the ages of 2 and 19 years are obese.[41] Between 1988–1994 and 2013–2014, the prevalence of obesity among American children who are between 6 and 19 has increased dramatically (Fig. 13.10). There is some good news: Obesity rates among preschoolers are declining.[41]

Defining Obesity in Children

Health care professionals use BMI–for–age charts that are available from the Centers of Disease Control and Prevention to determine children's and adolescents' weight status. The BMI for children is calculated in the same way as for adults, but BMIs for children are plotted on sex–specific growth charts (see Appendix F). Children and adolescents whose BMI–for–age is greater than or equal to ($\geq$) the 85th percentile and less than ($<$) the 95th percentile are overweight, and youngsters who are at or above the 95th percentile are obese (Table 13.10). There is no generally accepted definition for extreme obesity among children. However, a BMI at or above 120% the 95th percentile may be used to identify children who have extreme obesity.[42]

Health Problems Associated with Childhood Obesity

Compared to children who have healthy body weights, obese children and adolescents are more likely to have elevated blood pressure, cholesterol, and glucose levels.[43] These chronic conditions are risk factors for cardiovascular disease (CVD). Obesity also affects children's psychological and social health. Obese children, for example, are more likely to experience weight–based bullying and teasing than children who are not obese.[43] Table 13.11 lists serious health problems that obese children are more likely to have than children who have healthy body weights.

Many obese children and adolescents do not "grow out" of their excess body fat. Obese children are more likely than children who have healthy weights to be obese as adults.[43]

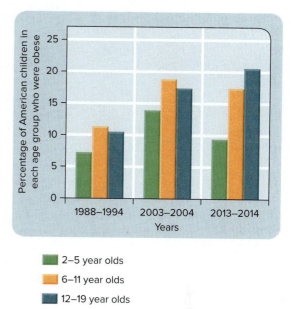

Figure 13.10 Prevalence of obesity among American children aged 2 to 19 years, for selected years 1988–1994 through 2013–2014.

Legend:
- 2–5 year olds
- 6–11 year olds
- 12–19 year olds

TABLE 13.10 Weight Status Classifications: Children and Adolescents (Ages 2 to 19)

Age	BMI-for-Age Percentile
Desirable weight	> 5th to < 85th
Overweight	≥ 85th to < 95th
Obese	≥ 95th

TABLE 13.11 Serious Health Problems Associated with Childhood Obesity

- Impaired glucose tolerance, insulin resistance, and type 2 diabetes
- Elevated blood lipids
- Breathing problems, including sleep apnea and asthma
- Musculoskeletal problems, including joint discomfort
- Fatty liver disease, gallstones, and gastroesophageal reflux (heartburn)
- Social and psychological problems, such as discrimination and poor self-esteem

Source: Centers for Disease Control and Prevention, Overweight & obesity: *Childhood obesity causes & consequences.* Updated December 2016. Accessed: June 2, 2017. https://www.cdc.gov/obesity/childhood/causes.html

Childhood Obesity: Contributing Factors

There is no single cause of excess body fat in children, but researchers have identified multiple factors that are associated with the development of the condition. As in cases of adult obesity, the development of childhood obesity results from complex interactions among multiple factors (see Chapter 10). The following sections examine the roles of genetic, biological, and environmental factors that contribute to childhood obesity.

Genetic and Other Biological Factors

Scientific evidence supports the role of inherited (genetic) and other biological factors in the development of childhood obesity, especially in cases of obesity that begin early in life.[44] Some of the biological factors that contribute to obesity include:

- **Having overfat parents.** Children of overfat parents have a greater risk of obesity than children whose parents have healthy weights. If both parents are obese, the child has 10 times the risk of obesity as a child who has only one obese parent.

- **Having a mother who was overfat during pregnancy.** A mother's weight during pregnancy is a more important predictor of childhood obesity than the father's body weight. When compared to children whose mothers have a healthy body weight during pregnancy, babies born to overweight mothers are nearly three times as likely to be overweight. Furthermore, obese women are more likely than women who have healthy body weights to have large babies, and such infants have a high risk of childhood obesity.

- **Having a mother who gained too much weight and/or had diabetes during pregnancy.** Women who gain too much weight during pregnancy or have diabetes are more likely to give birth to high-birth-weight babies. Such children are also at risk of developing excess body fat in childhood.

- **Having a mother who smoked during pregnancy.** Although the reasons are unclear, women who smoke during pregnancy set the stage for the future development of overweight and obesity in their babies.

- **Being undernourished during prenatal development.** Poor nutrition (undernutrition) during pregnancy contributes to delivery of a low-birth-weight infant. Such infants are more likely to develop hypertension, CVD, and type 2 diabetes later in life, which are chronic diseases associated with obesity. At this point, scientists have been unable to explain why prenatal undernutrition contributes to hypertension, CVD, and type 2 in adulthood.

Biological factors, however, are not entirely responsible for the current obesity epidemic. In many cases, it is difficult to determine whether genes play a more important role than environmental factors in the development of childhood obesity. Is a child obese because the youngster inherited genes from his or her parents that "program" for obesity? Or is a child obese because his or her caregivers provide an excess of empty calories and do not encourage the child to be physically active?

Impact of the Child's Environment

In the United States, many children are exposed to an environment that encourages overeating and consumption of foods that supply a lot of empty calories. Additionally, the environment often does not provide children with opportunities to participate in enough physical activity. Table 13.12 lists these and other environmental factors that contribute to childhood obesity.

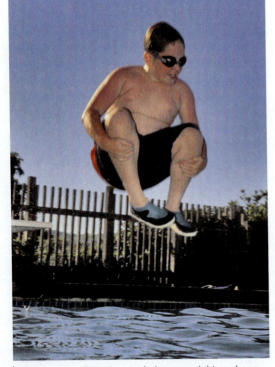

Being physically active can help overweight or obese children lose excess body fat. ©Ingram Publishing/SuperStock RF

TABLE 13.12 Environmental Factors That Contribute to Childhood Obesity

- Easy access to foods and drinks that are high in empty calories at or near schools
- Limited access to healthy and affordable foods, particularly in areas that have many convenience stores and fast-food restaurants
- Advertising of unhealthy foods that targets youth
- Lack of set periods for daily physical activity in schools and safe places to be active in many communities
- Large portion sizes of foods sold from vending machines and in restaurants and grocery stores
- Excess exposure to digital media, including television. Such exposure contributes to childhood obesity because the sedentary activities can reduce the time children spend being physically active.

Source: Centers for Disease Control and Prevention, *Childhood obesity causes & consequences.* Updated December 2016. Accessed: June 2, 2017. https://www.cdc.gov/obesity/childhood/causes.html

Preventing Childhood Obesity

Recommendations that may reduce the likelihood of obesity among children include:

- New mothers of healthy infants should breastfeed their babies exclusively for about the first 6 months of life and continue breastfeeding along with introducing appropriate foods until the children are old enough to drink cow's milk safely.

- Child care providers and schools should provide opportunities for children to be physically active throughout the day.

- Caregivers should limit children's exposure to video games, smartphones, tablets, computers, and TV ("screen time"). For specific recommendations concerning such limits, visit https://www.healthychildren.org/.

- Community leaders can support ways to increase physical activity for children and adults. Such efforts may include creating safe parks, playgrounds, and bicycling and walking trails as well as organizing and promoting supervised recreational sports activities.

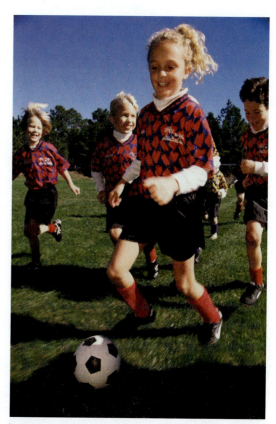

To help reduce the prevalence of childhood obesity, community leaders can organize and promote supervised recreational sports activities for children.
©Purestock/SuperStock

Treating Childhood Obesity

The treatment goal for managing childhood obesity is maintaining weight rather than losing weight.[45] As the obese child grows taller, his or her BMI may fall into the healthy range. To ensure the child's growth rate is not slowed, caregivers need to balance the calories children consume with the calories they use for physical activity and need for growth. Encouraging more physical activity, especially for sedentary children, is also recommended.

Caregivers should not place a child or youth on a weight reduction diet without consulting the child's physician. For severely obese adolescents, treatment approaches that go beyond dietary changes and increased physical activity are often necessary. Such interventions may include prescription medication and weight loss surgery (see Chapter 10).

Bariatric Surgery for Youth

Bariatric (weight loss) surgery can improve the health of adolescents with extreme obesity.[46] According to a review of bariatric surgery outcomes in the United States, the surgeries are safe for adolescents. At this time, however, the adjustable gastric banding procedure has not been approved for use with patients who are under 18 years of age.

To qualify for bariatric surgery, an adolescent should have:

- extreme obesity (BMI>40);

- failed to lose weight after 6 months of trying to reduce his or her weight;

- attained his or her adult height (skeletal maturity), which is generally at 13 years of age for girls and 15 years of age for boys; and

- developed serious chronic conditions that are associated with obesity, such as type 2 diabetes or sleep apnea, which may improve after surgery.[46]

Regardless of one's age, bariatric surgery is a drastic measure to lose excess body weight and involves some risks. Thus, caregivers and health care providers should carefully determine whether an extremely obese adolescent is a suitable candidate for bariatric surgery. For example, is the adolescent emotionally ready to handle the surgery and make the necessary lifestyle changes to achieve good health and well—being after the procedure?

Concept CHECKPOINT

27. Define *overweight* and *obese* for children as defined by the Centers for Disease Control and Prevention.

28. List at least three health consequences of childhood obesity.

29. List at least three factors that contribute to the development of childhood obesity.

30. What information is used to determine whether an obese adolescent qualifies for bariatric surgery?

See Appendix G for responses.

13.8 Nutrition for Older Adults

Learning Outcomes

1 Explain the difference between life expectancy and life span.

2 Identify physiological changes that are associated with the normal aging process.

3 Discuss nutrient needs for older adults.

4 Identify nutrients that are often lacking in diets of older adults.

5 Discuss steps caregivers can take to improve nutrient intakes of older persons.

In 1900, the life expectancy of a baby born in the United States was only 47 years. **Life expectancy** is the length of time a person born in a specific year, such as 1900, can expect to live. One hundred years ago, the top three leading causes of death for Americans were pneumonia, influenza, and other infectious diseases. By 2015, life expectancy in the United States rose to almost 79 years.[47] Major factors that contributed to increased life expectancy during the past century include improved diets, housing conditions, and public sanitation, as well as advances in medicine.

According to the U.S. Census Bureau, almost 15% of the U.S. population were 65 years of age or older in 2015 (Fig. 13.11).[48] By 2050, government experts estimate that 22% of Americans will be in this age group. Americans who are the "oldest old," 85 years of age or older, comprise one of the fastest—growing segments of the U.S. population. In 2015, almost 2% of Americans were in that age group. By 2050, over 4.7% of Americans will be 85 years of age or older.[49]

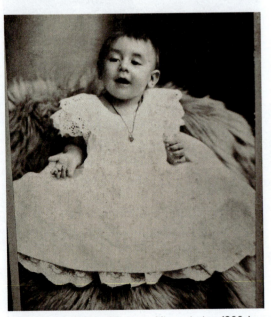

George John Blum of St. Louis, Missouri, circa 1900. In 1900, the life expectancy of a baby born in the United States was only 47 years. ©Wendy Schiff

life expectancy length of time an average person born in a specific year can expect to live

Although more Americans are living longer than their ancestors, they are not necessarily living well. Chronic diseases are among the leading causes of death in the United States (see Figure 1.2). These diseases are associated with lifestyles that include smoking, eating a poor diet, and being physically inactive.[50]

The Aging Process

The aging process begins at conception and is characterized by numerous predictable physical changes. By the time you are about 70 years of age, you will have reached the final life stage, *older adulthood*. What causes people to age is unclear. Scientists who study the aging process have learned that cell structure and function inevitably decline with time, leading to many of the physiological changes shown in Table 13.13. Eventually, most cells lose the ability to regenerate their internal parts, and they die. As more and more cells in an organ die, the organ loses its functional capacity, and as a result, other organs fail and body systems are adversely affected. When this happens, the person soon dies. **Senescence** (*se−ness'−enz*) refers to declining organ functioning and increased vulnerability to disease that occur after a person reaches physical maturity.

Extending the Human Life Span

Life span refers to the maximum number of years an organism such as a human can live. To date, a Frenchwoman, Jeanne Calment, had the longest documented human life span—122 years. Some scientists think the human life span can be lengthened considerably just by making certain dietary changes. This chapter's "Nutrition Matters" takes a closer look at the role of diet and longevity.

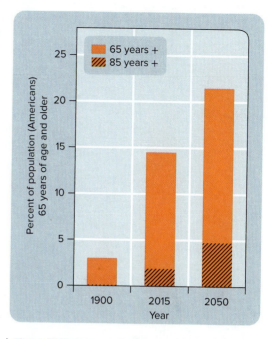

Figure 13.11 Older adult population of the United States: 1900, 2015, and projection for 2050.

senescence declining organ functioning and increased vulnerability

life span maximum number of years an organism can live

TABLE 13.13   Aging: Normal Physiological Changes

Body System	Changes
Digestive	Reduced saliva, gastric acid, and intrinsic factor secretion; increased heartburn and constipation
Skin, hair, and nails (integument)	Graying hair; drier skin and hair; skin loses elasticity and forms wrinkles; skin bruises easily
Musculoskeletal	Bone-forming cells become less active, resulting in bone loss that can lead to tooth loss and bones that fracture easily; fractures heal more slowly; joints become stiff and painful; muscle mass declines, resulting in loss of strength and stamina
Nervous	Decreased brain weight, reduced production of neurotransmitters, delayed transmission of nervous impulses, loss of short-term memory, and reduced sensory abilities (e.g., vision, hearing, smell, and taste)
Lymphatic (immune)	Reduced functioning resulting in increased vulnerability to cancer and infections
Circulatory	Hardening of the arteries, reduced cardiac output, increased risk of blood clots
Endocrine	Decreased production of reproductive, growth, and thyroid hormones
Respiratory	Reduced lung capacity, increased vulnerability to respiratory infections
Urinary	Increased loss of functional kidney cells, resulting in decreased blood filtration rate; loss of bladder control
Reproductive	Men: Decreased male hormone production and sperm count Women: Declining female hormone production, cessation of menstrual cycles, and loss of fertility

Growing old is a normal and natural process. Your body ages, regardless of dietary and other health—related practices you follow. Nevertheless, scientists have found a strong genetic component to human longevity. If you have ancestors who are very old or lived to be 90 years of age or more, you may have inherited "longevity genes." If your ancestors were not so fortunate, to some extent, you can control the rate at which you age. How? By making responsible healthy lifestyle decisions while you are still young, such as selecting a nutritious diet, exercising regularly, and avoiding tobacco. Your focus should not be simply on living longer but on living longer *and* healthier.

Common Nutrition-Related Concerns

Compared to younger persons, older adults have greater risk of nutritional deficiencies because of physiological changes associated with the normal aging process. An older adult's food intake tends to decrease as his or her metabolic rate and physical activity level decline. Despite having lower energy needs, older adults need the same or even higher amounts of vitamins and minerals. Meeting micronutrient needs while eating less food can be difficult for older adults to accomplish. Other factors that can influence an older person's nutritional status include illnesses, medications, low income, and lack of social support.

Critical nutrients for older adults are protein, omega—3 fats, fiber, calcium, magnesium, potassium, and the vitamins folate, B—12, B—6, D, E, and K.[51] Older adults tend to consume more than recommended amounts of sodium, saturated fat, and added sugars. Their diets, however, generally do not provide enough fiber, calcium, magnesium, potassium, zinc, folate, and vitamins A, B—6, C, D, and E.[52] Table 13.14 shows results of a study that focused on the food choices of older American adults. According to these findings, many men and women ages 71 years and older did not meet the recommendations concerning amounts of foods from MyPlate food groups.[53] Intakes of vegetables, dairy foods, and fruits were low compared to intakes of grains and protein foods. The following sections discuss some of the major health concerns that often affect the nutritional status of older adults. Some of these conditions have been discussed in previous chapters.

Changes in Body Weight

As the human body ages, its need for energy decreases. In senescence, muscle mass declines as some muscle cells shrink or die (*sarcopenia*). The loss of muscle mass leads to a decrease in muscular strength and basal metabolism. The aging body

TABLE 13.14 Percentages of American Adults Ages 71 Years and Older Who Follow USDA Dietary Recommendations

Food Group	MyPlate Recommendations for Older Adult Men*	Older Adult Men Who Meet the Recommendations (%)	MyPlate Recommendations for Older Adult Women*	Older Adult Women Who Meet the Recommendations (%)
Fruit (cups)	2	23	1.5	34.5
Vegetables (cups)	2.5	12	2	13.0
Grains (oz equivalents)	6	55	5	53.0
Dairy (cups)	3	7	3	3.6
Protein (oz equivalents)	5.5	46	5	40.0

*Amounts are for people who obtain fewer than 30 minutes/day of moderate physical activity, beyond their normal daily activities.

Source: Adapted from Krebs-Smith SM and others: "Americans do not meet federal dietary recommendations," *Journal of Nutrition* 140(10): 1832, 2010.

typically loses lean tissue and gains some fat tissue. Increased body fat results from overeating and lack of physical activity, but even athletic men and lean women usually gain some central body fat after they are 50 years of age. Being overfat may protect the older adult from being injured in falls, but having too much body fat increases the risk of type 2 diabetes, hypertension, cardiovascular disease, and osteoarthritis. For more information about overweight and obesity, see Chapter 10.

Older people may develop *sarcopenic obesity*—the loss of skeletal muscle mass and strength combined with an excessive increase in body fat. Eating too many calories and being physically inactive contribute to the development of sarcopenic obesity. People with this form of obesity are more likely to experience mobility problems and other physical limitations than people who do not have the condition.[54]

Older adults, especially those who are over 75 years of age, may unintentionally lose weight. Several factors can contribute to weight loss among older adults (Table 13.15). Older adults may eat less because they have lost the ability to taste and smell food. Loss of teeth and difficulty swallowing (*dysphagia* [*diss−fay′−jee−ah*]) can also result in decreased food consumption. Declines in normal *cognitive* functioning (thought processes) resulting from conditions such as Alzheimer's disease or reduced blood flow to the brain can contribute to poor nutritional status. People who lack normal cognitive functioning may be unable to make decisions regarding planning nutritious meals, as well as to shop for and prepare food. Conditions that interfere with mobility and flexibility, such as arthritis and osteoporosis, can also interfere with food shopping and preparation activities. Social and economic factors often play a role in reduced food intake. Many older people live alone and on fixed incomes, circumstances that are associated with depression and inability to afford adequate amounts of nutritious food. In many instances, very old people refuse to eat and, as a result, lose considerable amounts of weight, a situation that hastens their death.

For older adults who find that food no longer tastes "good," adding more spices may improve the taste of food and, as a result, stimulate weak appetites. Efforts to make mealtimes social events, such as inviting friends to share potluck meals together, can enhance older adults' mental outlooks and spark their interest in eating. Older adults can increase or maintain their weight by consuming energy−dense snacks between meals, such as cheese, milkshakes, nuts, or oatmeal cookies. If weight loss becomes significant, a physician should be consulted to determine the cause.

Physical Inactivity

Many of the undesirable physical changes we associate with growing old are the result of a lifetime of physical inactivity. Regardless of a person's age, a physically active lifestyle increases muscle strength and mobility, improves balance, slows bone loss, and boosts emotional well−being. Most older adults can benefit from performing aerobic and strength−training activities regularly. Before embarking on a program to increase physical fitness, however, sedentary older adults should consult their physicians concerning appropriate activities. The "Real People, Real Stories" feature in this section is about Paul Appelbaum, a 90−year−old who works out regularly and is physically fit.

Digestive System Problems

Constipation is a major complaint of older adults. By increasing their intakes of fiber−rich foods, such as whole−grain products and vegetables, older adults may be able to have more regular bowel movements (see the "Fiber" section of Chapter 5). Dehydration contributes to constipation, so older persons should make sure their fluid intake is adequate.

TABLE 13.15 Reduced Food Intake Among Older Adults: Contributing Factors

- Reduced ability to taste and smell food
- Difficulty swallowing
- Loss of teeth
- Loss of normal cognitive function
- Lack of income
- Depression
- Reduced mobility and flexibility

Did *YOU* Know?

You are never too old to gain some benefits from exercise. Any form of physical activity, from swimming to performing household chores, can help extend an older adult's longevity.

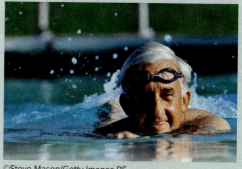

©Steve Mason/Getty Images RF

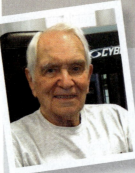

©Wendy Schiff

Paul Appelbaum

Paul Appelbaum is a 90-year-old father of three children, grandfather of two and great-grandfather of one. He's been married for over 50 years. Several years ago, he retired from working as a businessman, but he has not retired from taking excellent care of himself.

Some clues to Paul's good health are in his lifestyle—past and present. "I grew up during the Great Depression. I paid no attention to my diet, but I never went hungry. I ate a lot of home-cooked foods . . . vegetables, fruits, dairy foods, meat, seafood, chicken. . . . I ate a 'balanced' diet. I wasn't fond of sweets . . . things that were too sweet were distasteful to me. I've never been overweight." Paul's height is 5 feet, 8 inches, and his weight is 160 pounds.

"I've always been physically active. When I was a boy, my friends and I didn't have sports teams or youth organizations. We just found empty spaces and played sandlot baseball and football. In high school, I was on the track team—I was a good runner."

"I never had desk job. . . . I was always on my feet, moving around . . . that's partially what I owe my longevity and health to." Compared to the average person who is Paul's age, he *is* very active. For over 20 years, he has maintained an impressive workout regimen. Six days a week, he walks for an hour and a half at a nearby community gymnasium. When Paul does not walk, he rides a stationary bike for 20 minutes, at an average speed of 12 miles per hour. In addition to his aerobic activity routine, he performs resistance exercises that focus on the muscles of his upper body three days a week. On three alternating days, he focuses on doing exercises that strengthen his lower body muscles. "I like working out! But I also like to keep my brain well-stimulated. . . . I read books and play bridge [a complex card game]."

"I had no serious health problems until I was in my early 80s. When I was 82, I had to have a triple bypass [surgery to restore blood flow to areas of the heart that were supplied by three blocked arteries]. My doctors are all very happy with me!" According to Paul, "Longevity is fine, but quality of life is more important. Keep physically fit and follow a healthy diet, and you'll have it all."

As a person ages, his or her stomach secretes less hydrochloric acid and intrinsic factor. These changes can contribute to poor absorption of vitamin B−12 and the development of vitamin B−12 deficiency and pernicious anemia. Older adults may be able to meet their vitamin B−12 needs by eating foods fortified with the micronutrient or taking vitamin B−12 supplements. Some older adults, however, must take injections of the B vitamin to prevent pernicious anemia (see Chapter 8). Older persons are also at risk of iron deficiency because reduced stomach acid production may hinder iron absorption. Furthermore, many older adults take aspirin regularly, and this practice can cause intestinal bleeding that can lead to iron deficiency anemia. Intestinal ulcers and cancer can also cause blood loss from the digestive tract. The discovery of blood in bowel movements needs to be reported to a physician—regardless of one's age.

Many older adults take one or more prescription drugs daily. Although such medications can improve health and quality of life of older adults, some drugs interfere with the body's absorption and/or use of certain nutrients. Additionally, older adults often take one or more dietary supplements regularly.

Certain dietary supplements, including herbal products, can reduce or amplify the effects of prescribed medications. Therefore, older adults should notify their physicians about their use of all dietary supplements. A few foods also interfere with prescribed drugs. Grapefruit juice, for example, can alter the potency of certain medications that are used to lower blood pressure or cholesterol.

Tooth Loss In the 1950s, surveys of Americans indicated that the majority of older adults had lost all their natural teeth. Since then, the percentage of older adults who retain all or most of their teeth has increased in the United States. Adults should have 28 natural teeth. In 2011–2012, 19% of Americans who were 65 years of age or older had lost all of their teeth.[55] Tooth loss is related to long–term poor dental hygiene, cigarette smoking, and poor dietary practices. By following recommended dental hygiene practices, obtaining regular dental care, and avoiding tobacco use, you can greatly increase your chances of keeping most of your teeth as you age.

Excessive tooth loss can lead to faulty eating habits. People who lack teeth often avoid crisp or chewy foods, such as fresh fruits, vegetables, whole–grain cereals, and meat. According to results of a study involving over 300 older adults, subjects who had 10 or fewer teeth consumed considerably less than the recommended amounts of fruits, vegetables, meat and beans, and oils when compared to older adults who had more than 10 teeth.[56] Although dentures that replace natural teeth can enable some people to chew normally, many older adults do not like to wear them because they can be uncomfortable. When a person has difficulty chewing food, serving soft foods such as ground meats, cooked vegetables, pureed fruits, and puddings can stimulate the individual's appetite.

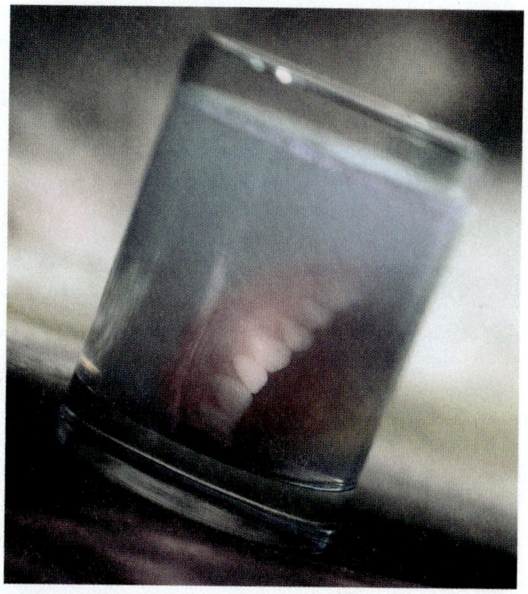

Many older adults do not like to wear dentures because they can be uncomfortable. ©Steve Cole/Getty Images RF

Depression in Older Adults

In 2014, 15% of women and 10% of men age 65 and over reported having symptoms of depression.[57] Situations that contribute to depression among the older adult population include coping with chronic illness or loss of mobility, and isolation and loneliness as family members and friends move away or die. If the depressed person loses interest in cooking and eating, weight loss and nutrient deficiencies are likely to occur. In many instances, depression can be managed with medication, but social support and psychological counseling may be necessary as well. Without proper treatment, depressed persons, especially males, are at risk of alcoholism and suicide. Nevertheless, suicide is not a leading cause of death among older adults.[58]

Dietary Planning in Older Adulthood

MyPlate can provide the basis for planning nutritionally adequate meals and snacks for healthy older adults. However, amounts of foods recommended in these diet plans may not provide enough vitamin D and calcium for older adults. By regularly consuming fortified and/or enriched foods, older adults can increase their intakes of these micronutrients. In many instances, older adults can also benefit from taking a daily multiple vitamin/mineral supplement.

Friends, relatives, and health care personnel should be alert for indications of poor nutrient intakes among older people, especially those who are at risk and live in nursing homes or other long–term care facilities. For example, family members can make sure the older adult's nutrient needs are met by visiting the person's residence during mealtimes, observing the foods that are offered, and, if necessary, helping the older adult eat. Additionally, monitoring the older person's weight can indicate whether long–term food intake has been adequate. Older adults who live at home may need help planning nutritionally adequate diets. In these instances, registered dietitian nutritionists can be consulted to provide personalized dietary advice.

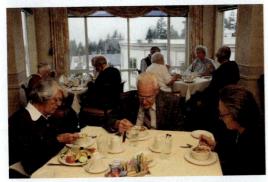

People enjoying the social benefits of dining together at a community center for independent older adults.
©Kieth Brofsky/Getty Images RF

Food & Nutrition tips

The following suggestions can help caregivers improve nutrient intakes of older adults:

- Emphasize nutrient-dense foods when planning daily menus.
- Try new foods, seasonings, and ways of preparing foods.
- Have easy-to-prepare, nutrient-dense foods on hand for times when the older person is too tired to cook large meals.
- Serve meals in well-lit or sunny areas, and plan appealing meals by using foods with different flavors, colors, shapes, textures, and smells.
- Plan occasions for the older adult to share cooking responsibilities and eat meals with friends or relatives.
- Encourage the older person to eat at a senior center whenever possible. Investigate community resources for helping the older adult obtain groceries, cook, or manage other daily care needs.
- If biting and chewing are difficult for an older adult, chop, grind, or blend tough or crisp foods.
- Prepare extra amounts of soup, stew, or casserole, so leftovers can be frozen for future meals.

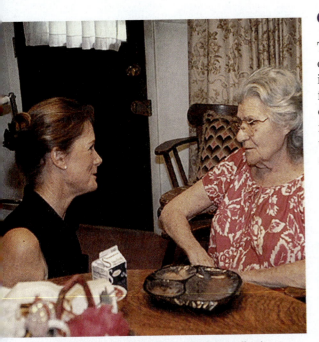

Many communities in the United States offer the Meals on Wheels program in which volunteers deliver nutritious meals prepared at a senior center to qualified, homebound older adults. Source: USDA Photo by Ken Hammond

Community Nutrition Services for Older Adults

The Chapter 1 "Nutrition Matters" provides information about popular community–based nutrition services for American older adults. You can obtain information regarding locally available nutrition services for older people from medical clinics, private practitioners, hospitals, and health maintenance organizations in your area. To learn more about nutrition–related programs for older adults, visit the following websites: National Institute on Aging, www.nia.nih.gov/; American Geriatrics Society, www.americangeriatrics.org/; and Administration for Community Living, https://www.acl.gov/.

Concept CHECKPOINT

31. What is the difference between *life expectancy* and *life span*?
32. Identify at least five physiological changes that are associated with the normal aging process.
33. Explain why nutrient needs for older adults are often higher than those for younger persons.
34. List at least four nutrients that are often lacking in diets of older adults.
35. Suggest at least three ways caregivers can improve nutrient intakes of older persons.

See Appendix G for responses.

13.9 Nutrition Matters: In Search of the Fountain

Learning Outcomes

1 Discuss at least two aging theories.

2 Explain the effects of calorie restriction on the aging process.

3 Identify steps people can take to extend their life expectancy.

In 1513, Spanish explorer Juan Ponce de León sailed to the southeastern coastal region of North America and discovered an area he named "Land of Flowers" (Florida). Ponce de León was on a mission to find gold, but he was also eager to locate a natural spring that supposedly had magical powers. According to Native Americans in the area, elderly people who drank the spring's water regained their youthful looks and vigor. Unfortunately, Ponce de León never found gold or the mythical "fountain of youth" in Florida. Nevertheless, many older adults still seek ways to combat aging, especially by taking certain hormones and dietary supplements promoted as having age—defying properties. Older Americans spend considerable amounts of money on such products, some of which may be harmful in the long run. Promoters of antiaging formulas or therapies claim their treatments can stop, and even reverse, the process of aging. Is there any reliable scientific evidence to support claims that you can take something to stay young longer?

Claims that a nutritional fountain of youth exists are simply not true. Currently, scientific evidence does not support the use of antiaging therapies that include taking antioxidants and hormones.[59] Scientists have determined that consuming a nutritious diet and obtaining adequate amounts of physical activity can promote good health as one ages.[59] Nevertheless, researchers are conducting experiments to better understand the process of aging and the keys to longevity.

Biogerontologists are scientists who study the biology of aging. Biogerontologists have proposed several theories to explain why aging occurs and why some people live longer than others. According to one of these theories, longevity results from the body's ability to maintain and repair the damage done by a lifetime of exposure to the environment and the effects of everyday wear and tear. Some multicellular organisms are able to live longer when they can improve their abilities to repair damage to their DNA, reduce the toxicity of free radicals, and replace nonfunctioning cells. Antioxidants reduce the toxic effects of free radicals (see Chapter 8), and organisms produce a variety of antioxidants to control free radical production. Scientific

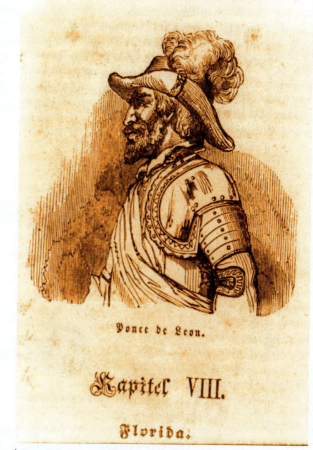

Ponce de León. Source: Library of Congress, Prints and Photographs Division

studies, however, provide little evidence that increasing one's intake of antioxidants slows the aging process.[59]

One area of biogerontological research that shows some promise is the use of *calorie restriction (CR)* to extend longevity. Although CR provides fewer calories than an organism's usual diet, the dietary pattern supplies all essential nutrients. Since the 1930s, scientists have studied the effects of CR on the health and life spans of various species of multicellular organisms. According to some research findings, CR can increase life spans of various organisms, including some kinds of rodents, fruit flies, and yeast.[59] Results of other studies, however, were not so promising, because the calorie—restricted animals either had the same or shorter life spans when compared to controls.

Blueberries: ©PhotoAlto/Getty Images RF

Even if scientists provide evidence that any form of CR adds some years to the human life span, would you be interested in reducing your food intake considerably to extend your life? How enjoyable would your life be if you ate only 900 kcal daily? What is important to you: how long you can live, or how *well* you live?

The science of biogerontology is still in its beginning stages; researchers have much to learn about the aging process before they can develop safe ways to enhance longevity. We already know that you can reduce your risk of dying prematurely from chronic diseases such as heart disease, hypertension, type 2 diabetes, and many forms of cancer by adopting healthy lifestyles. Rather than wait until the fountain of youth becomes a reality, you can take charge of your health now by consuming a nutritionally

adequate diet, obtaining regular moderate– to vigorous–intensity physical activity, maintaining a healthy weight, avoiding tobacco products, limiting your alcohol consumption, and having regular physical checkups.

Concept CHECKPOINT

36. According to scientific evidence, which dietary modification may extend the life expectancies of organisms that include fruit flies and rodents?

37. List three steps you can take that may extend your life expectancy.

See Appendix G for responses.

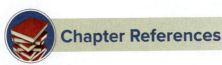

Chapter References

See Appendix H.

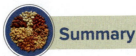

Summary

13.1 Introduction to Nutrition for a Lifetime

- The leading causes of death for Americans are chronic diseases: heart disease, cancer, and stroke. Lifestyles, especially dietary practices and physical activity patterns, contribute to the development of these chronic conditions. Other factors that influence a person's overall health include heredity, relationships, environment, income, education level, and access to health care.

13.2 Pregnancy

- Embryonic/fetal life is characterized by rapid rates of cell division, resulting in a dramatic increase in cell numbers. The first trimester of pregnancy is a critical stage in human development because inadequate or excessive nutrient intakes as well as exposure to toxic compounds can have devastating effects on the embryo/fetus during this period. The placenta is the organ of pregnancy that transfers nutrients and oxygen from the mother's bloodstream to her embryo/fetus. The placenta also transfers wastes from the embryo/fetus to the mother's bloodstream so her body can eliminate them.

- Women of childbearing age should take steps to ensure they are in good health prior to becoming pregnant. During pregnancy, the woman's body undergoes various physiological changes. These changes enable her body to nourish and maintain the developing fetus, as well as to produce milk for her infant after its birth. A pregnant woman should follow a diet that meets her own nutritional needs as well as those of her developing offspring. The mother-to-be can use MyPlate to develop nutritionally adequate daily menus, but she may also need to take a prenatal vitamin/mineral supplement.

- Women whose prepregnancy weights were within the healthy range can expect to gain 25 to 35 pounds during pregnancy. Women who gain excess weight during pregnancy may retain the extra weight long after delivery.

- Monitoring weight gain is an important aspect of prenatal care. Underweight women who do not gain enough weight during pregnancy are at risk of having preterm or low-birth-weight infants. Obese women have a greater risk of developing hypertension and type 2 diabetes during pregnancy.

13.3 Infant Nutrition

- Breast milk is the best first food for infants. Compared to babies who are not breastfed, breastfed infants have lower risks of allergies and of gastrointestinal, respiratory tract, and ear infections. Women who breastfeed their babies can also derive some important benefits from the practice, such as losing extra fat gained during pregnancy.

- When an infant suckles, nerves in the nipple signal the mother's brain to release prolactin and oxytocin into her bloodstream. Oxytocin is necessary for the let-down reflex and causes the uterus to contract. Milk production relies on "supply and demand." If the breasts are not emptied fully, milk production soon ceases. To support milk production, the lactating mother needs about 400 to 500 extra kilocalories daily.

- Growth is very rapid during infancy. Health care practitioners can assess growth in infants and children by measuring body weight, height (or length), and head circumference over time. For about the first 6 months, a healthy infant's nutrient needs can be met by human milk or iron-fortified infant formula. Breastfed babies need vitamin D and possibly iron and fluoride supplements.

- Most infants do not need solid foods before 4 to 6 months of age. The first solid food offered to babies should be an iron-containing food such as an iron-fortified infant cereal, meat, or poultry. New foods should be added one at a time, and the child should be observed for allergy signs and symptoms. Whole cow's milk should not be fed to babies until they are 1 year of age.

13.4 The Preschool Years

- It is normal for a preschooler's appetite to decline as the child's growth rate tapers off. Additionally, it is not unusual for preschool children to be "picky eaters" or embark on "food jags." Caregivers should avoid nagging, forcing, and bribing children to eat but instead offer a variety of healthy food choices and allow the child to choose what and how much to eat. Nutrition-related problems that often affect preschool children are iron deficiency, dental caries, obesity, and food allergies.

©Corbis/VCG/Getty Images RF

13.5 School-Age Children

- School-age children often skip breakfast, and they tend to consume more foods away from home, larger portions of food, and more fried foods and sweetened beverages. Children who eat breakfast are more likely to have better diets and healthier body weights than children who skip this meal. Diets of many school-age children fail to supply recommended amounts of calcium and potassium while providing too much sodium.

13.6 Adolescence

- A child matures physically into an adult during adolescence. For many teens, pressure to conform to fads and be influenced by other adolescents negatively affects their diets and overall health. Obesity, eating disorders, and low iron and calcium intakes are major nutrition-related concerns of adolescents.

13.7 Childhood Obesity

- Public health experts are very concerned about the increasing prevalence of obesity among children in the United States. Overfat children have higher risks of elevated blood pressure, cholesterol, and glucose levels than children whose weights are within the healthy range. Overfat children may also have higher risk of hypertension, heart disease, and type 2 diabetes later in life. Such children are also more likely to have low self-esteem and become obese as adults.

13.8 Nutrition for Older Adults

- The aging process is characterized by numerous predictable physical changes. Senescence refers to declining organ functioning and increased vulnerability to disease that occurs after a person reaches physical maturity. Although genetics play a role in determining longevity, lifestyle practices and environmental conditions influence a person's rate of aging. People may be able to live longer and healthier by making responsible healthy lifestyle decisions while they are still young.

- Factors that can influence an older person's nutritional status include illnesses, tooth loss, medications, low income, depression, and lack of social support. Diets of older adults often provide inadequate amounts of fiber, calcium, magnesium, potassium, zinc, folate, and vitamins A, B-6, C, D, and E. Friends, relatives, and health care personnel should be alert for indications of poor nutrient intakes among older people, especially those who live in nursing homes or other long-term care facilities.

13.9 Nutrition Matters: In Search of the Fountain

- According to biogerontologists, longevity results from the body's ability to maintain and repair the damage done by a lifetime of exposure to the environment and the effects of everyday wear and tear. Little credible scientific evidence exists to support the use of antiaging therapies that include taking hormones or megadoses of vitamins and antioxidants. Researchers are conducting experiments to better understand the process of aging and determine whether calorie restriction is a key to longevity.

Recipe for Healthy Living

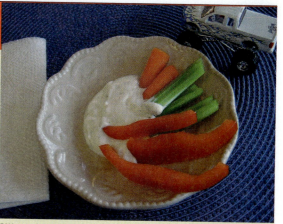

Vegetable Dip

You can make low-fat versions of fruit or vegetable dips by replacing sour cream or mayonnaise in recipes with plain, low-fat yogurt. This vegetable dip recipe makes approximately five ¼-cup servings of dip. Each serving provides approximately 46 kcal, 3 g protein, 2 g fat, 90 mg calcium, 160 mg sodium, and 120 mg potassium.

©Wendy Schiff

INGREDIENTS:

1 cup plain, low-fat yogurt
3 Tbsp calorie-reduced ranch dressing
¼ tsp curry powder (optional)

PREPARATION STEPS:

1. In a small bowl, combine yogurt with the dressing and stir until well blended.

2. Refrigerate until ready to serve.

3. Serve chilled in a bowl that is surrounded with fresh pieces of raw vegetables.

4. Discard any remaining dip.

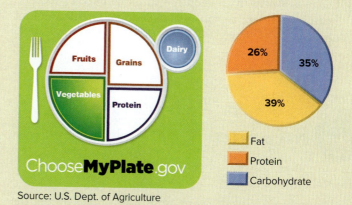

Source: U.S. Dept. of Agriculture

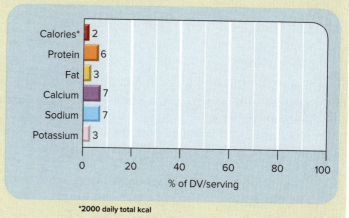

*2000 daily total kcal

connect Further analyze this recipe or other recipes through activities located in Connect.

Critical Thinking

1. One of your friends just found out that she is pregnant. Although her BMI is within the healthy range, she is concerned about gaining too much weight during pregnancy. What advice would you provide concerning the need to gain some weight during this life stage? If your friend's prepregnancy weight was 125 pounds, how much weight would be appropriate for her to gain during pregnancy?

2. Your pregnant friend wants your advice concerning whether she should breastfeed or formula-feed her baby. After reading Chapter 13, what information would you provide to help your friend decide to breastfeed?

3. Olivia is a healthy 2-month-old baby. Olivia's mother, Kara, wants to replace Olivia's iron-fortified infant formula with the same fresh fluid 2% milk that she drinks. What advice would you give to Kara concerning the appropriateness of making such a decision?

4. Marcus is 8 years old, and his weight is in the overweight range. His caregivers are also overweight, but they seem to be concerned about Marcus's excess body weight. What advice would you provide his caregivers to help Marcus achieve a healthy body weight?

5. Are your parents, grandparents, and great-grandparents still alive? If any of your ancestors died before they were 60 years of age, can you identify their causes of death and factors that contributed to their deaths? What lifestyle changes can you make now that can help you achieve a longer, healthier lifetime?

Practice Test

Select the best answer.

1. The embryo/fetus develops most of its organs during the
   a. preconception period.
   b. first trimester.
   c. second trimester.
   d. third trimester.

2. The placenta cannot
   a. transfer nutrients from the mother's bloodstream to the embryo/fetus.
   b. eliminate waste products from the embryo/fetus.
   c. prevent all toxic substances from reaching the embryo/fetus.
   d. transfer oxygen from the mother's bloodstream to the embryo/fetus.

3. During the first trimester, a pregnant woman's daily energy requirement is _____ her daily energy needs before she became pregnant.
   a. 300 kcal lower than
   b. about the same as
   c. 300 kcal higher than
   d. 500 kcal higher than

4. Obese women who are pregnant with one fetus should gain _____ pounds during pregnancy.
   a. 11-20
   b. 20-25
   c. 25-35
   d. 35-50

5. Preeclampsia is a form of _____ that can develop during pregnancy.
   a. hypertension
   b. diabetes
   c. cancer
   d. anemia

6. Which of the following statements is true?
   a. A woman's energy needs are higher during the first trimester than at any other time in pregnancy.
   b. Using infant formula to bottle-feed a baby is more convenient and less expensive than breastfeeding a baby.
   c. Oxytocin is necessary for the "let-down" reflex to occur.
   d. The American Pediatric Association recommends feeding fresh whole milk to infants when they are 6 months of age.

7. A healthy infant who weighs 8.2 pounds at birth can be expected to weigh _____ pounds by her first birthday.

a. 13.0
b. 16.4
c. 19.5
d. 24.6

8. Breastfed infants are _____ than babies who are fed infant formula.

a. more likely to have diarrhea
b. less likely to have cystic fibrosis
c. more likely to have respiratory infections
d. less likely to have ear infections

9. Which of the following factors is associated with increased risk of obesity during childhood?

a. Having a family history of obesity
b. Eating 3 to 5 servings of fresh fruit daily
c. Being a full−term infant
d. Taking dietary supplements that contain zinc and vitamin C

10. Which of the following practices has been scientifically shown to extend the life spans of certain flies and rodents?

a. Taking antioxidant supplements
b. Eating a high−protein diet
c. Performing vigorous physical exercise
d. Consuming a calorie−restricted diet

11. Which of the following characteristics is not associated with the normal aging process?

a. Increased risk of blood clots
b. Increased brain weight
c. Reduced saliva production
d. Reduced immunity to infectious diseases

Answers to Quiz Yourself

1. During pregnancy, a mother-to-be should double her food intake because she's "eating for two." **False.** (Section 13.2)

2. Infant formulas provide the same health benefits to infants as breast milk. **False.** (Section 13.3)

3. Caregivers should add solid foods to an infant's diet within the first month after the baby is born. **False.** (Section 13.3)

4. Over the past few decades, the prevalence of obesity has increased among American children. **True.** (Section 13.7)

5. Compared to younger persons, older adults have lower risks of nutritional deficiencies. **False.** (Section 13.8)

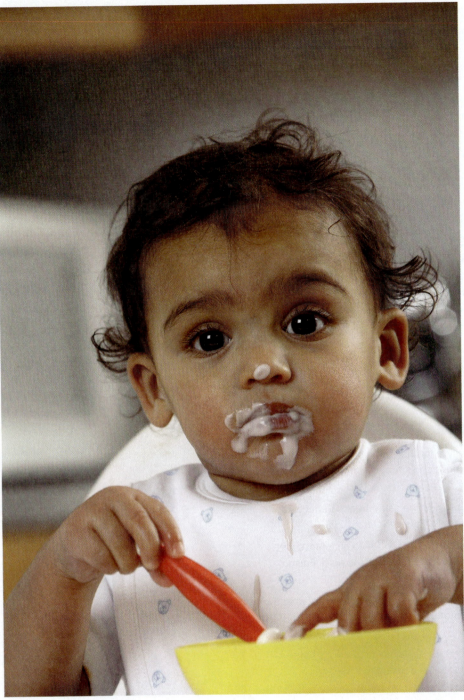

©Andrew Olney/age fotostock RF

Appendix A

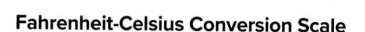

English-Metric Conversions and Metric-to-Household Units

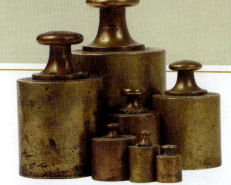

©Hermera Technologies/Alamy RF

English-Metric Conversions

Length

English (USA)	Metric
inch (in)	= 2.54 cm, 25.4 mm
foot (ft)	= 0.30 m, 30.48 cm
yard (yd)	= 0.91 m, 91.4 cm

Metric	English (USA)
millimeter (mm)	= 0.039 in (thickness of a dime)
centimeter (cm)	= 0.39 in
meter (m)	= 3.28 ft, 39.4 in
kilometer (km)	= 0.62 mi, 1091 yd, 3273 ft

Weight

English (USA)	Metric
ounce (oz)	= 28.35 g
pound (lb)	= 453.60 g, 0.45 kg

Metric	English (USA)
milligram (mg)	= 0.000035 oz
gram (g)	= 0.04 oz ($\frac{1}{28}$ of an oz)
kilogram (kg)	= 35.27 oz, 2.20 lb

Volume

English (USA)	Metric
teaspoon (tsp)	= 5 ml
tablespoon (Tbsp)	= 15 ml
fluid ounce	= 0.03 liter (30 ml)
cup (c)	= 237 ml
pint (pt)	= 0.47 liter
quart (qt)	= 0.95 liter
gallon (gal)	= 3.79 liters

Metric	English (USA)
milliliter (ml)	= 0.03 oz
liter	= 1.06 qt
liter	= 0.27 gal

Metric and Other Common Units

Unit/Abbreviation	Other Equivalent Measure
milligram/mg	$\frac{1}{1000}$ of a gram
microgram/mcg	$\frac{1}{1,000,000}$ of a gram
deciliter/dl	$\frac{1}{10}$ of a liter (about ½ cup)
milliliter/ml	$\frac{1}{1000}$ of a liter (5 ml is about 1 tsp)

Fahrenheit-Celsius Conversion Scale

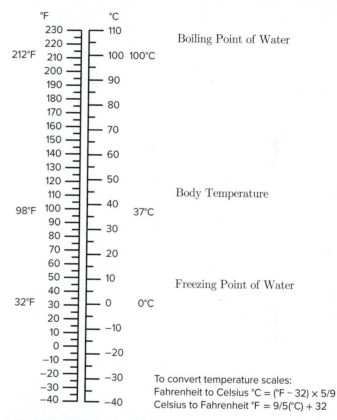

To convert temperature scales:
Fahrenheit to Celsius °C = (°F − 32) × 5/9
Celsius to Fahrenheit °F = 9/5(°C) + 32

Household Units

3 teaspoons	= 1 tablespoon
4 tablespoons	= ¼ cup
5⅓ tablespoons	= ⅓ cup
8 tablespoons	= ½ cup
10⅔ tablespoons	= ⅔ cup
16 tablespoons	= 1 cup
1 tablespoon	= ½ fluid ounce
1 cup	= 8 fluid ounces
1 cup	= ½ pint
2 cups	= 1 pint
4 cups	= 1 quart
2 pints	= 1 quart
4 quarts	= 1 gallon

Appendix B

Daily Values Table

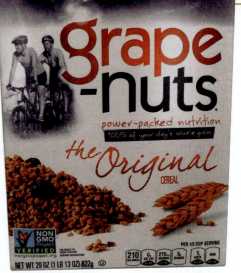

©Wendy Schiff

Dietary Constituent	Unit of Measure	Daily Values for People Over 4 Years of Age
Total fat	g	78
Saturated fatty acids	"	20
Protein	"	50
Cholesterol	mg	300
Total carbohydrate	g	275
Added sugars	g	50
Fiber	"	28
Vitamin A	μg (RAEs)	900
Vitamin D	μg	20
Vitamin E	mg	15
Vitamin K	μg	120
Vitamin C	mg	90
Folate	μg	400
Thiamin	mg	1.2
Riboflavin	"	1.3
Niacin	"	16
Vitamin B-6	"	1.7
Vitamin B-12	μg	2.4
Biotin	μg	30
Pantothenic acid	mg	5
Choline	mg	550
Calcium	"	1300
Phosphorus	"	1250
Iodine	μg	150
Iron	mg	18
Magnesium	"	420
Copper	"	0.9
Zinc	"	11
Sodium	"	2300
Potassium	"	4700
Chloride	"	2300
Manganese	"	2.3
Selenium	μg	55
Chromium	"	35
Molybdenum	"	45

Abbreviations: g = gram, mg = milligram, μg = microgram, RAEs = retinol activity equivalents

Energy Metabolism

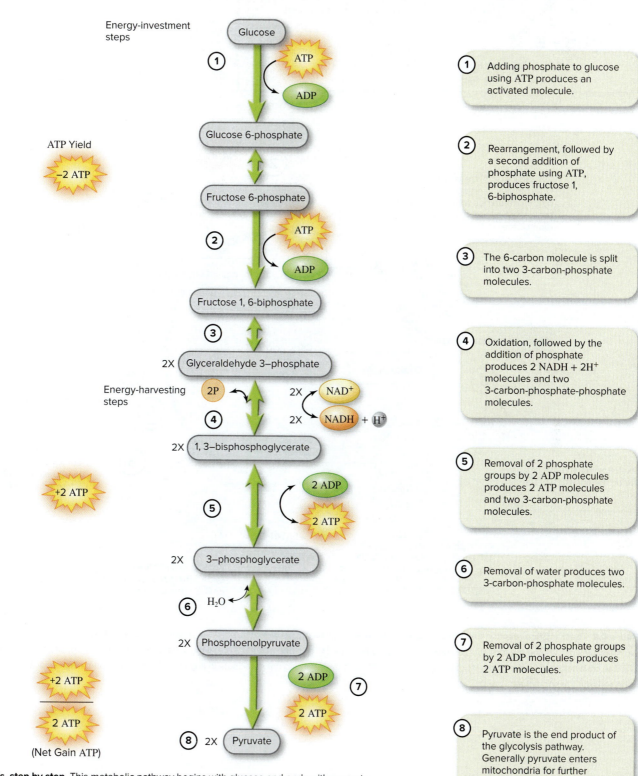

Energy-investment steps

① Adding phosphate to glucose using ATP produces an activated molecule.

ATP Yield

−2 ATP

Glucose

ATP → ADP

Glucose 6-phosphate

② Rearrangement, followed by a second addition of phosphate using ATP, produces fructose 1, 6-biphosphate.

Fructose 6-phosphate

ATP → ADP

Fructose 1, 6-biphosphate

③ The 6-carbon molecule is split into two 3-carbon-phosphate molecules.

2X Glyceraldehyde 3–phosphate

Energy-harvesting steps

2P

2X NAD+

2X NADH + H+

④ Oxidation, followed by the addition of phosphate produces 2 NADH + 2H+ molecules and two 3-carbon-phosphate-phosphate molecules.

2X 1, 3–bisphosphoglycerate

+2 ATP

2 ADP → 2 ATP

⑤ Removal of 2 phosphate groups by 2 ADP molecules produces 2 ATP molecules and two 3-carbon-phosphate molecules.

2X 3–phosphoglycerate

⑥ H₂O

⑥ Removal of water produces two 3-carbon-phosphate molecules.

2X Phosphoenolpyruvate

+2 ATP
_____
2 ATP

2 ADP → 2 ATP

⑦ Removal of 2 phosphate groups by 2 ADP molecules produces 2 ATP molecules.

⑧ 2X Pyruvate

(Net Gain ATP)

⑧ Pyruvate is the end product of the glycolysis pathway. Generally pyruvate enters mitochondria for further breakdown.

Figure C.1 Glycolysis, step by step. This metabolic pathway begins with glucose and ends with pyruvate. Net gain of two ATP molecules can be calculated by subtracting those used during the energy-investment steps from those produced during the energy-harvesting steps. Text in boxes explains the reactions.

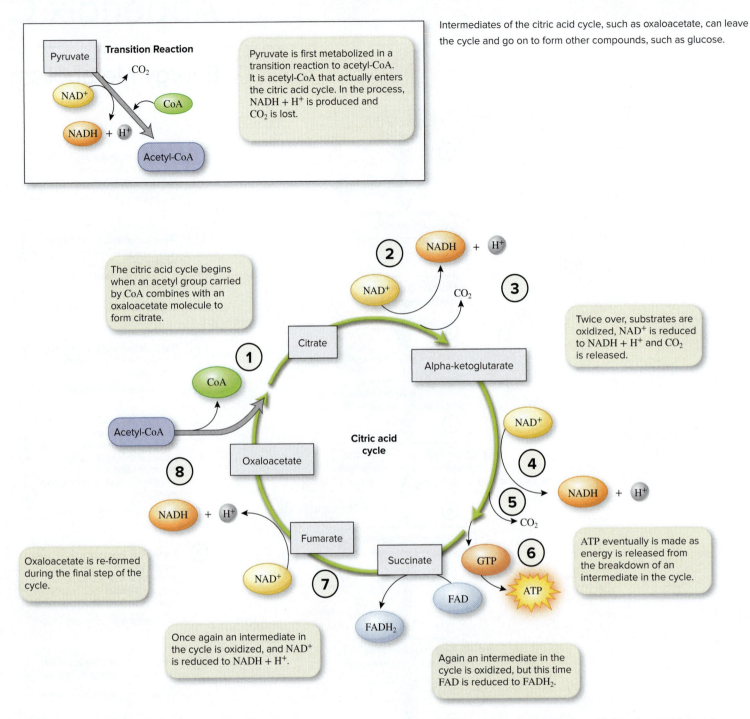

Intermediates of the citric acid cycle, such as oxaloacetate, can leave the cycle and go on to form other compounds, such as glucose.

Transition Reaction

Pyruvate is first metabolized in a transition reaction to acetyl-CoA. It is acetyl-CoA that actually enters the citric acid cycle. In the process, NADH + H$^+$ is produced and CO$_2$ is lost.

The citric acid cycle begins when an acetyl group carried by CoA combines with an oxaloacetate molecule to form citrate.

Twice over, substrates are oxidized, NAD$^+$ is reduced to NADH + H$^+$ and CO$_2$ is released.

Oxaloacetate is re-formed during the final step of the cycle.

ATP eventually is made as energy is released from the breakdown of an intermediate in the cycle.

Once again an intermediate in the cycle is oxidized, and NAD$^+$ is reduced to NADH + H$^+$.

Again an intermediate in the cycle is oxidized, but this time FAD is reduced to FADH$_2$.

Figure C.2 The transition reaction and the citric acid cycle. The net result of one turn of this cycle of reactions (steps 1–8) is the oxidation of an acetyl group to two molecules of CO$_2$ and the formation of three molecules of NADH + H$^+$ and one molecule of FADH$_2$. One GTP molecule also results, which eventually forms ATP. The citric acid cycle turns twice per glucose molecule. Note that oxygen does not participate in any of the steps in the citric acid cycle. It instead participates in the electron transport chain.

Figure C.3 Simplified depiction of electron transfer in energy metabolism. High-energy compounds, such as glucose, give up electrons and hydrogen ions to NAD$^+$ and FAD. The NADH + H$^+$ and FADH$_2$ that are formed transfer these electrons and hydrogen ions, using specialized electron carriers, to oxygen to form water (H$_2$O). The energy yielded by the entire process is used to generate ATP from ADP and Pi.

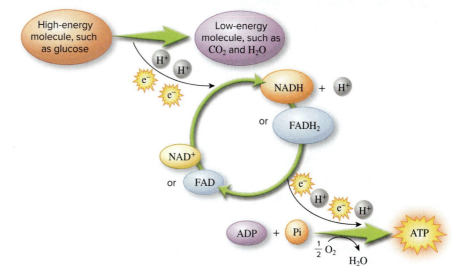

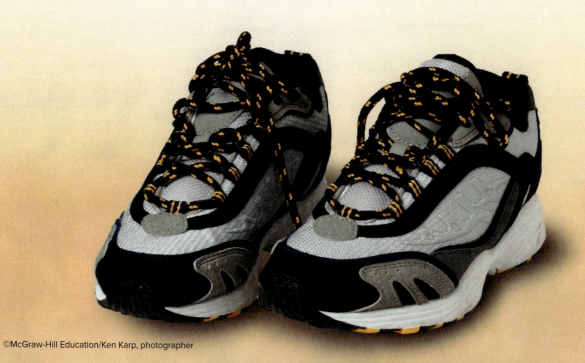

Appendix D

Amino Acids

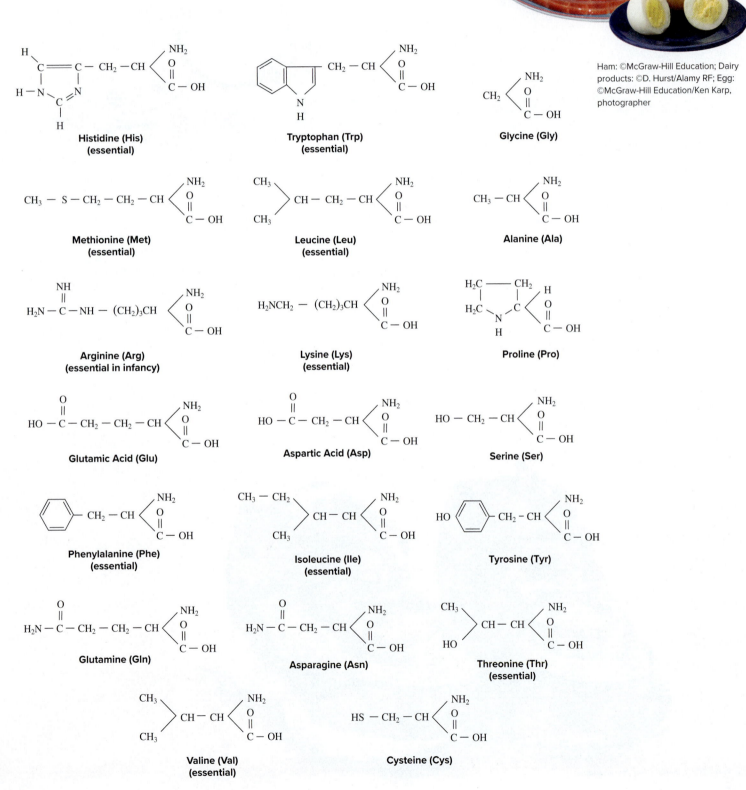

Histidine (His)
(essential)

Tryptophan (Trp)
(essential)

Glycine (Gly)

Methionine (Met)
(essential)

Leucine (Leu)
(essential)

Alanine (Ala)

Arginine (Arg)
(essential in infancy)

Lysine (Lys)
(essential)

Proline (Pro)

Glutamic Acid (Glu)

Aspartic Acid (Asp)

Serine (Ser)

Phenylalanine (Phe)
(essential)

Isoleucine (Ile)
(essential)

Tyrosine (Tyr)

Glutamine (Gln)

Asparagine (Asn)

Threonine (Thr)
(essential)

Valine (Val)
(essential)

Cysteine (Cys)

Vitamins Involved in Energy Metabolism

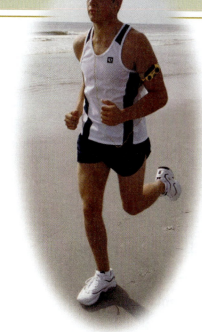

©Purestock/SuperStock RF

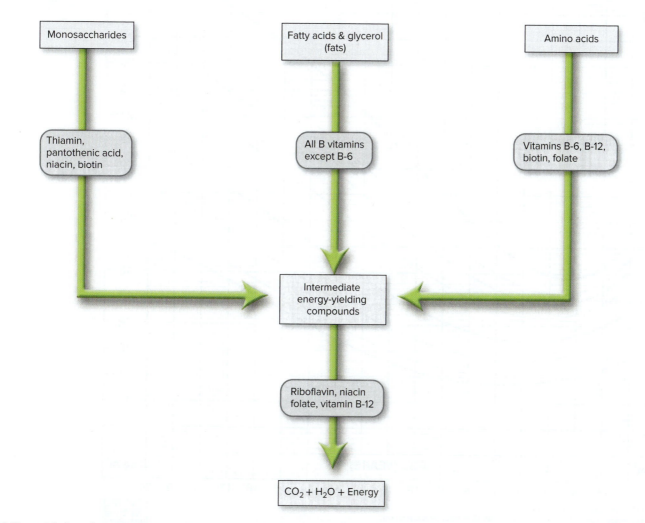

| Monosaccharides | Fatty acids & glycerol (fats) | Amino acids |

Thiamin, pantothenic acid, niacin, biotin

All B vitamins except B-6

Vitamins B-6, B-12, biotin, folate

Intermediate energy-yielding compounds

Riboflavin, niacin folate, vitamin B-12

$CO_2 + H_2O + Energy$

| **Figure E.1** The metabolism of monosaccharides, fats, and amino acids for energy requires several vitamins.

Body Mass Index-for-Age Percentiles

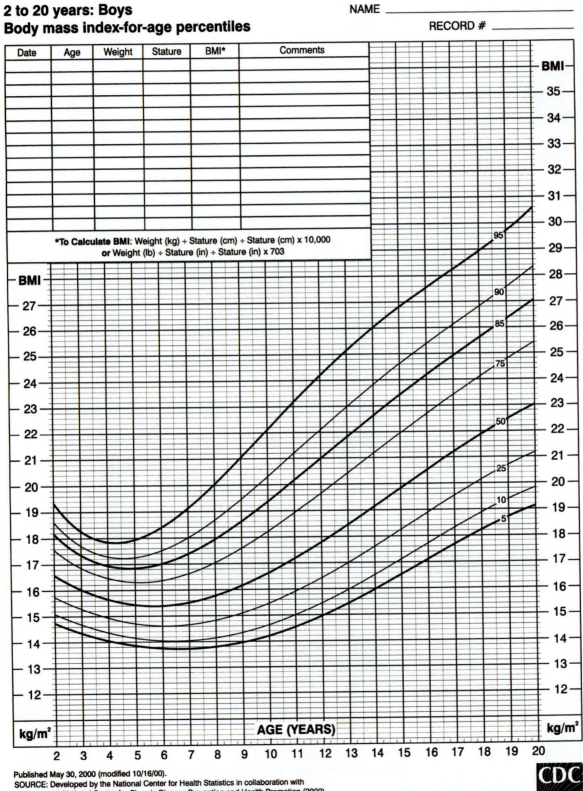

2 to 20 years: Boys
Body mass index-for-age percentiles

NAME _____

RECORD # _____

Date	Age	Weight	Stature	BMI*	Comments

*To Calculate BMI: Weight (kg) ÷ Stature (cm) ÷ Stature (cm) x 10,000
or Weight (lb) ÷ Stature (in) ÷ Stature (in) x 703

AGE (YEARS)

Published May 30, 2000 (modified 10/16/00).
SOURCE: Developed by the National Center for Health Statistics in collaboration with
the National Center for Chronic Disease Prevention and Health Promotion (2000).

CDC

2 to 20 years: Girls
Body mass index-for-age percentiles

NAME _____

RECORD # _____

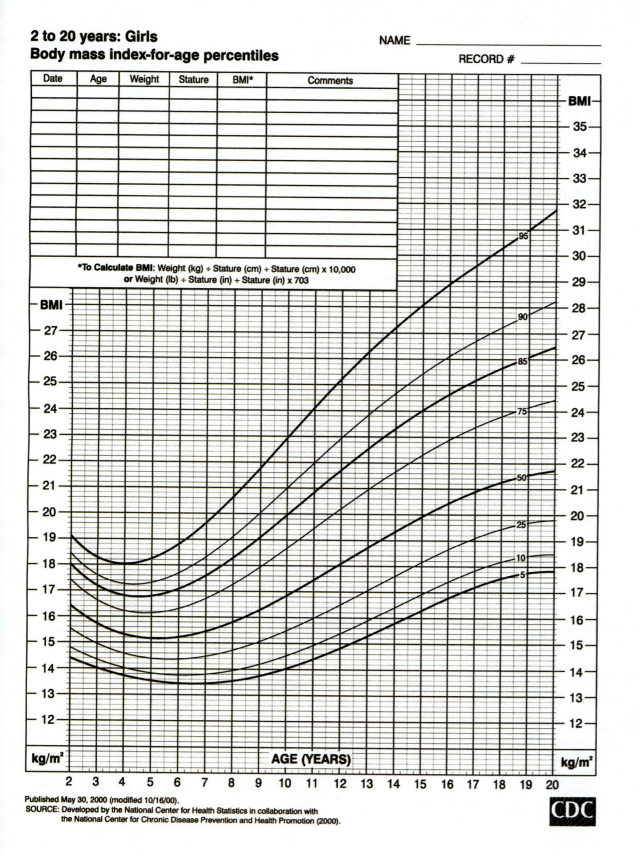

Date	Age	Weight	Stature	BMI*	Comments

*To Calculate BMI: Weight (kg) ÷ Stature (cm) ÷ Stature (cm) x 10,000
or Weight (lb) ÷ Stature (in) ÷ Stature (in) x 703

AGE (YEARS)

kg/m²

Published May 30, 2000 (modified 10/16/00).
SOURCE: Developed by the National Center for Health Statistics in collaboration with
the National Center for Chronic Disease Prevention and Health Promotion (2000).

CDC

Appendix G

Answers to Concept Checkpoint Questions and Practice Test Questions

Concept Checkpoint Answers

Chapter 1

1. Heart disease, some types of cancer, stroke, and type 2 diabetes are among the 10 leading causes of death that are diet related.

2. Answers will vary but should include factors shown in Figure 1.1.

3. The six major classes of nutrients are carbohydrates, fats and other lipids, proteins, vitamins, minerals, and water.

4. The key features that indicate a substance is an essential nutrient include the following: a deficiency disease results when the substance is missing from the diet; the deficiency disease is corrected when the missing substance is added to the diet; and scientists can identify the nutrient's specific roles in the body and explain why abnormalities occurred when the substance was missing from the diet.

5. A phytochemical is a substance made by plants. According to the DSHEA, a dietary supplement is a product (excluding tobacco) that contains a vitamin, a mineral, an herb or other plant product, an amino acid, or a dietary substance that is taken by mouth to supplement the diet by increasing total intake.

6. A risk factor is a personal characteristic that increases chances of developing a chronic disease.

7. Answers will vary but should include lifestyle factors such as diet; alcohol, tobacco, and other drug use; and physical activity patterns.

8. Americans eat less red meat, milk and yogurt, and eggs, and more fish and shellfish, cheese, and chicken and turkey, than in 1970. The diet supplies more grain and cereal products, but refined grain foods make up the majority of these products. Americans are eating additional servings of fruit, but not enough to meet recommended amounts. Today, Americans eat higher amounts of fruits and vegetables than in the past, but choices tend to lack variety. Over the past 40 years, Americans' intake of calories, added sugars, and added fat has increased.

9. The main nutrition–related goal of *Healthy People* 2020 is to promote good health and reduce the risk of chronic disease by consuming healthful diets and achieving and maintaining healthy body weights.

10. Scientists generally use liters, grams, and meters to report volume, weight, and length.

11. A 187–pound person weighs 85 kg. To obtain the answer, divide 187 by 2.2 (85 kg).

12. To estimate the number of kilocalories in the slice of bread, add the number of kilocalories contributed by carbohydrate (12 g × 4 kcal = 48 kcal), fat (2 g × 9 kcal = 18 kcal), and protein (3 g × 4 kcal = 12 kcal). The answer is 78 kcal/slice.

13. Carbohydrates, fats, and proteins are macronutrients; vitamins and minerals are micronutrients.

14. Answers will vary but should be taken from the key nutrition–related concepts listed in Table 1.7.

15. A food that contains a lot of empty calories supplies excessive amounts of solid fat, added sugars, and/or alcohol. A nutrient–dense food contains more key beneficial nutrients (such as protein, fiber, calcium, and iron) in relation to its total calories per serving.

16. The physiological dose of a nutrient is the amount that is within the range of safe intake and enables the body to function optimally. A megadose is generally defined as an amount of a vitamin or mineral that is much greater than the recommended amount of the nutrient. Megadose amounts of certain nutrients can be toxic.

17. Unfavorable environmental conditions that contribute to poor health in developing countries include lack of access to clean water for drinking and preparing foods. Disruptive political conditions, including wars and civil unrest, contribute to poverty and food shortages.

18. Undernutrition increases the risk of death among pregnant women and children. Children who survive undernutrition often have stunted and delayed physical growth, blindness, and impaired intellectual development.

19. WIC is the Women, Infants, and Children feeding program, which is federally subsidized. WIC provides access to specific nutritious foods to improve the diets of low–income infants, children under the age of 5 years, and pregnant or breast–feeding women who are at nutritional risk.

20. Conventional farming methods require considerable amounts of water and pesticides that can harm the environment. Sustainable agriculture involves farming methods that provide food without depleting natural resources or harming the environment.

21. A genetically modified organism is a living thing that results from genetic engineering.

Chapter 2

1. Epidemiology is the study of the occurrence, distribution, and causes of health problems in a population.

2. A control group is used to compare results of having a treatment against those of not having a treatment.

3. A prospective study follows a large group of healthy people over time to determine whether those with a certain characteristic develop a disease and those without that characteristic remain disease free. A retrospective study follows a group of people who already suffer from a disease and compares them to a group of people with similar characteristics who do not have the disease.

4. A placebo is a fake treatment, such as a sham pill, injection, or medical procedure. Providing placebos to members of the control group enables scientists to compare the extent of the treatment's response with that of the placebo.

5. In a double—blind study, both the investigators and the subjects are unaware of the subjects' assignments in treatment or control groups.

6. A peer—reviewed article is one that has been critically analyzed by a group of "peers." If peers agree that a study was well conducted, its results are fairly represented, and the research is of interest to the journal's readers, these scientists are likely to recommend that the journal's editors publish the article.

7. Conflicting research findings often result from differences in the ways various studies are designed and results analyzed. For example, the numbers, ages, and physical conditions of subjects; the type and length of the study; the amount of the treatment provided; and the statistical tests used to analyze results typically vary among studies. Other factors, such as genetic and lifestyle differences among human subjects, can influence the results of nutrition research.

8. A testimonial is a personal endorsement of a product. Anecdotes are reports or personal experiences.

9. Answers will vary but should be clues that indicate a source of nutrition information is unreliable.

10. Answers will vary but should include points presented in Table 2.1.

11. Although some states regulate and license people who call themselves nutritionists, consumers cannot always rely on someone who refers to him— or herself as a "nutritionist" because there are no standard legal definitions and registered dietitian nutritionists for this descriptor. Registered dietitians and registered dietitian nutritionists are college—trained professionals who have extensive knowledge of foods, nutrition, and dietetics, the application of nutrition and food information to treat many health—related conditions. The titles "registered dietitian" and "registered dietitian nutritionist" are legally protected.

12. Consumers may find reliable nutrition experts, including registered dietitians, among faculty members in universities or colleges. Other ways to find registered dietitians include contacting the local dietetic association, calling the dietary department of a local hospital, or visiting the Academy of Nutrition and Dietetics website (www.eatright.org) or the Dietitians of Canada website (www.dietitians.ca).

13. Answers may vary but can include chiropractic manipulations, homeopathy, naturopathy, massage therapy, and use of herbal remedies and nonvitamin, nonmineral products.

14. According to the FDA, a drug is a substance, natural or human—made, that alters body functions. Although many dietary supplements act as drugs in the body, the FDA regulates dietary supplements as foods, not medications. Therefore, consumers do not need to obtain a physician's prescription to purchase a dietary supplement.

15. Answers will vary but can include the dietary supplements listed in Table 2.2. Responses should not include vitamins or minerals.

Chapter 3

1. RDAs are standards for recommending daily intakes of several nutrients. RDAs meet the nutrient needs of nearly all healthy individuals (about 98%) in a particular life stage/sex group. In some instances, scientists set AIs for certain nutrients because they do not have enough information to establish RDAs for them. An AI represents a group's average daily intake that appears to be adequate for health.

2. To establish an RDA for a nutrient, nutrition scientists first determine its estimated average requirement. Then scientists add a "margin of safety" amount to the EAR that allows for individual variations in nutrient needs and helps maintain tissue stores.

3. The EER is more specific than RDAs or AIs because it takes into account the person's physical activity level, height, and weight, as well as sex and life stage. Furthermore, the EER does not include an additional number of kilocalories to serve as a margin of safety.

4. Dietitians refer to DRIs as standards for planning nutritious diets for groups of people and evaluating the nutritional adequacy of a population's diet. Pharmaceutical companies refer to DRIs when developing formulas that replace breast milk or regular foods. For nutrition labeling purposes, the FDA uses RDAs to develop Daily Values (DVs).

5. Answers will vary but should include grains, such as products made from wheat, rice, and oats. Pasta, noodles, and flour tortillas are grains because wheat flour is their main ingredient. Corn is a type of grain; therefore, cornmeal and popcorn are usually grouped with grains.

6. Enrichment is the replacement of some nutrients that were lost during processing. Fortification is the addition of nutrients to food to boost its nutritional value.

7. Foods generally classified as dairy include forms of fluid milk, yogurt, hard cheese, cottage cheese, ice cream, pudding, and frozen yogurt.

8. Dry beans are protein–rich foods that can substitute for meats.

9. According to the USDA, one–half cup of dried fruit is nutritionally equivalent to 1 cup of fresh fruit. Therefore, 1 cup of dried apricots is nutritionally equivalent to 2 cups of fresh apricots.

10. Eggs and nuts are protein–rich foods that can substitute for meats.

11. Solid fats are usually hard at room temperature, such as beef fat, butter, lard, and shortening. Cream and coconut oil are also considered solid fats.

12. Answers will vary but should include the guidelines listed in Table 3.3.

13. A healthy person should limit his or her sodium intake to less than 2300 mg/day.

14. Answers will vary but should include the recommendations listed in Table 3.4.

15. Replace solid fats with oils.

16. Your diet should have less than 10% of total calories from saturated fat.

17. Limit added sugars intake to less than 10% of total calories.

18. At least one–half of your grains should be whole grains.

19. Adult men who drink alcohol should limit their intake to no more than two drinks/day.

20. Women who drink alcohol and are not pregnant should limit their intake to no more than one drink/day.

21. Calcium, vitamin D, potassium, and dietary fiber are nutrients that Americans tend to consume in limited amounts.

22. Answers are fruit, dairy, or vegetables.

23. Answers may vary but should include comparing dietary intakes against recommended amounts of foods and beverages within one's diet pattern. Furthermore, a response can involve using the interactive tracking features at the www.choosemyplate.gov website to monitor food and nutrient intakes.

24. Answers may vary but should be either grains or meat.

25. The Exchange System focuses on the energy, protein, carbohydrate, and fat content of foods. Unlike the MyPlate food groupings, classification of foods into exchange lists is based on energy and macronutrient contribution.

26. Answers may vary but should discuss how %DVs are percentages instead of specific quantities, such as grams or milligrams of nutrients. Also, fresh or raw foods generally do not have labels indicating %DVs. Therefore, people may underestimate their intakes of nutrients if they rely on nutrition labels for the information.

27. Information provided on food labels and dietary supplements can be used to compare ingredients as well as energy and nutrient contributions of similar products.

28. A health claim describes the relationship between a food, food ingredient, or dietary supplement and the reduced risk of a nutrition–related condition. Examples of health claims can vary, but students can use the ones listed in Table 3.8. A structure/function claim describes the role a nutrient or dietary supplement plays in maintaining a structure, such as "calcium strengthens bone," or in promoting a normal function, such as "fiber aids bowel regularity." Examples of nutrient claims can vary, but students can use the ones listed in Table 3.9.

29. The FDA does not permit manufacturers to market a dietary supplement product as a treatment or cure for a disease, or to relieve signs or symptoms of a disease. If FDA officials question the safety of a dietary supplement or the truthfulness of claims that appear on supplement labels, manufacturers are responsible for providing the agency with evidence that their products are safe and the claims on labels are honest and not misleading. The FDA requires dietary supplement manufacturers to evaluate the purity, quality, strength, and composition of their products before marketing them.

30. The organic milk would be from cattle that were fed 95–100% organic feed and not given antibiotics or hormones.

31. The USDA permits food processors to use the organic seal on packaging when the food contains at least 95% organic ingredients.

32. The Nutrition Facts panels on food labels, nutrient analysis software programs, and government websites can be reliable sources of information about the energy and nutrient contents of foods and beverages.

33. Many Americans enjoy Mexican and Chinese foods, but traditional dishes are often modified to appeal to consumers who do not have Mexican or Chinese ancestry. Authentic Mexican meals are based primarily on rice, tortillas, and beans, depending on the region. To appeal to many non–Mexican Americans, "Mexican" fast–food restaurants in the United States often serve dishes that contain large portions of high-fat beef topped with sour cream and cheese. Although Chinese food is popular among Americans, many non–Asian members of the population do not like dishes that feature seafood and contain large portions of vegetables and grains. To appeal to these individuals, many North American Chinese restaurants offer menu items that contain much larger portions of beef and chicken than authentic dishes. Furthermore, American–Chinese foods are often prepared with more fat than is used in true Chinese cooking.

34. Answers will vary but should include information from Table 3.12.

Chapter 4

1. Electrons are negatively charged particles that surround the nucleus; protons are positively charged particles in the nucleus of an atom. An element is a substance that cannot be broken down into distinctive components under usual conditions. A chemical bond is an attraction that forms when atoms interact. A molecule results from the formation of chemical bonds. A compound is a molecule that contains two or more different elements. A solution is an evenly distributed mixture of two compounds. The solvent is the primary compound of a solution, and the solute is the substance dissolved in the solvent.

2. An ion is an atom or group of atoms that has an electrical charge because it has gained or lost one or more electrons.

3. Acids are substances that lose H^+ when dissolved in water; bases are substances that remove and accept H^+ when dissolved in water.

4. The pH of a watery solution refers to its hydrogen ion concentration.

5. A chemical reaction is a process that changes the arrangement of atoms in molecules.

6. Enzymes are proteins that initiate or facilitate (catalyze) chemical reactions.

7. Enzymes are sensitive to environmental conditions, including pH, temperature, and the presence of certain vitamins and minerals.

8. A cell is the smallest living functional unit in an organism. An organelle is a structure within the cell that has specific functions. DNA is a molecule that provides coded instructions for synthesizing proteins. A tissue is comprised of cells usually joined together that have similar characteristics and functions.

9. Homeostasis is an internal chemical and physical environment that supports life and good health.

10. Answers will vary but should include information from Table 4.2.

11. Answers will vary but should relate to Figure 4.21 and begin with the mouth and end with the anus.

12. Examples of mechanical digestion include the biting and grinding actions of teeth and the muscular contractions of the GI tract. Chemical digestion includes actions of enzymes and HCl.

13. Answers may vary but should include four of the following known tastes for humans: sweet, salty, bitter, sour, and umami.

14. Choking can occur while eating if the epiglottis does not function properly and food enters the windpipe (trachea).

15. Peristalsis and segmentation, normal muscular movements of the digestive tract, keep food and chyme from becoming stuck in the tract.

16. The gastroesophageal sphincter keeps stomach contents from backing up into the esophagus.

17. The three sections of the small intestine are the duodenum, jejunum, and ileum. Most nutrient digestion and absorption takes place in the upper portion of the small intestine, primarily in the jejunum.

18. Removal of the pancreas would reduce nutrient digestion because the pancreas produces digestive enzymes.

19. Answers will vary but should include transport proteins or pumping mechanisms within the absorptive cell's plasma membrane, diffusion, or plasma membrane "swallowing" large substances.

20. Vomiting and diarrhea can cause dehydration, which can be dangerous.

21. Answers will vary but should include the information in Table 4.4.

22. Answers will vary but should include avoid smoking, heavy consumption of alcohol, and use of NSAIDs.

23. Common signs and symptoms of irritable bowel syndrome are intestinal cramps, diarrhea, constipation, or alternating episodes of both diarrhea and constipation. Loose stools are often accompanied with mucus, and after bowel movements, the affected person feels as though elimination of stools was incomplete.

Chapter 5

1. Plants use carbon dioxide and water to make carbohydrates.

2. Plants use sunlight to obtain energy they need to live.

3. A human cell needs glucose to obtain energy.

4. The three most important dietary monosaccharides are glucose, fructose, and galactose.

5. Glucose is blood sugar; sucrose is table sugar; lactose is milk sugar; and maltose is malt sugar. Maltose is comprised of two glucose molecules; glucose and galactose comprise lactose; and glucose and fructose comprise sucrose.

6. A nutritive sweetener provides energy, whereas a nonnutritive sweetener does not provide energy in the amounts typically used to sweeten foods.

7. The parents should give their child the beverage sweetened with sucralose because the sweetener does not provide phenylalanine.

8. Starch and glycogen are both storage forms of polysaccharides, but starch is in plant foods and glycogen is primarily in liver and muscle tissue.

9. Most forms of dietary fiber are nondigestible carbohydrates. Oat bran and oatmeal, beans, apples, carrots, oranges and other citrus fruits, and psyllium seeds are rich sources of soluble fiber; whole-grain products, including brown rice, contain high amounts of insoluble fiber.

10. A minor amount of starch is digested in the mouth by the action of salivary amylase. Starch digestion stops soon after the food enters the acid environment of the stomach. In the small intestine, pancreatic amylase breaks down remaining

starch molecules into maltose molecules. The enzyme maltase splits each maltose molecule into two glucose molecules. The glucose molecules are absorbed by small intestinal cells; they enter the bloodstream and travel to the liver via the portal vein. In the small intestine, sucrase splits the sucrose molecules in the grape jelly into glucose and fructose molecules. These monosaccharides are absorbed by small intestinal cells and eventually enter the hepatic portal vein and travel to the liver. The fiber in the crackers was not digested. The fiber moves through her intestinal tract and may be fermented by bacteria in her large intestine or contribute to her feces.

11. Insulin helps regulate blood glucose levels because the hormone enables glucose to enter most cells. The hormone enhances energy storage by promoting fat, glycogen, and protein production. Glucagon opposes insulin's effects by promoting the breakdown of glycogen. This process releases glucose into the bloodstream and, as a result, boosts the blood glucose level back to normal. Glucagon also stimulates liver and kidney cells to produce glucose from certain amino acids, the basic molecules that make up proteins. Furthermore, glucagon stimulates the breakdown of triglyceride into glycerol and fatty acids. As a result, glycerol and fatty acids rapidly enter into the bloodstream.

12. A ketone body is a chemical that results from the incomplete breakdown of fat. Cells form ketone bodies when they must use greater-than-normal amounts of fat for energy. Under these conditions, there is not enough glucose available for cells to metabolize the fat efficiently, and excessive ketone bodies form as a result.

13. Sugar-sweetened beverages, sugary snacks, and sweets are the main sources of added sugars in Americans' diets.

14. Fruit juice is a better choice because juice is a natural product that contains nutrients and phytochemicals in fruit. "Orange-Ade" is not a nutritionally equivalent substitute for orange juice, because it may contain only 10% fruit juice.

15. To estimate the grams of starch in the serving of the cereal, subtract the amount of starch and total sugars in a serving (20 grams) from the amount of total carbohydrates (44 grams), and the remainder is the amount of starch (24 grams).

16. Answers will vary but should be the signs and symptoms listed in Table 5.9.

17. To reduce her risk of developing type 2 diabetes, Lata should avoid overweight, be physically active, and eat a healthy diet.

18. Answers may vary but should include signs presented in Table 5.11.

19. Lactose intolerance is a condition characterized by the inability to digest lactose completely.

20. Answers will vary but should include increasing one's intake of plant foods, especially whole-grain breads and cereals.

21. Eating soluble fiber can reduce the risk of cardiovascular disease by reducing blood cholesterol levels. The liver recycles the cholesterol from bile that is absorbed by the intestinal tract to make new bile. Soluble fiber interferes with the absorption of bile salts in the intestinal tract. As a result, the liver must use other sources of cholesterol, such as blood cholesterol, to produce bile. The fiber in food attracts water and swells in the digestive tract, forming a large soft mass that applies pressure to the inner muscular walls of the large intestine, stimulating the muscles to push the residue quickly through the tract. As a result, people who eat adequate amounts of fiber are less likely to strain while having bowel movements than people whose diets lack fiber.

22. Of this group of foods, raw apple has the lowest glycemic index.

Chapter 6

1. Rose's excess body fat can provide a source of energy for her, if she is ill and cannot eat. Also, the fat provides some insulation against cold temperatures and may protect her bones from breaking if she falls.

2. The cake is likely to taste better and have a more desirable texture, because the fat in the milk contributes to flavor and "mouth feel."

3. Major lipids include fatty acids, triglycerides, phospholipids, and sterols, particularly cholesterol.

4. A saturated fatty acid has each carbon within the fatty acid chain completely filled with hydrogen atoms. An unsaturated fatty acid has two neighboring carbons within the chain that are missing two hydrogen atoms. Monounsaturated fatty acids have one double bond within the carbon chain; polyunsaturated fatty acids have two or more double bonds within the carbon chain.

5. Answers will vary but will relate to Table 6.2.

6. Alpha-linolenic acid and linoleic acid are essential fatty acids.

7. Phospholipids have a hydrophylic region that contains phosphorus and a hydrophobic region with two fatty acids. A triglyceride has three fatty acids attached to a glycerol "backbone."

8. An omega-3 fatty acid has the first double bond in the polyunsaturated fatty acid's carbon chain appearing at the third carbon, when you start counting carbons at the omega end of the molecule. Alpha-linolenic acid, eicosapentaenoic acid (EPA), and docosahexaenoic acid (DHA) are omega-3 fatty acids.

9. Egg yolk or whole egg would keep the oil and milk emulsified.

10. Cholesterol is found only in animal foods. Egg yolk, liver, meat, poultry, whole milk, cheese, and ice cream are rich sources of cholesterol. Cholesterol is a component of every cell membrane; cells use cholesterol to synthesize vitamin D, bile, and steroid hormones.

11. Answers will vary but should follow the steps outlined in Figure 6.9 and the summary of lipid digestion and absorption presented in Figure 6.11.

12. Plants contain substances that interfere with enterohepatic circulation. This interference can reduce blood cholesterol levels, because the liver must remove cholesterol from the bloodstream to make new bile salts.

13. The body needs energy to survive. The triglycerides stored in fat cells can be used for energy. Thus, a person with excessive body fat has more energy stored in his or her body than a slim person.

14. On average, fat contributes almost 35% of the typical American diet's total energy intake.

15. The AMDR for fat is 20 to 35% of total calories.

16. According to the Dietary Guidelines, people should consume less than 10% of their total calories from saturated fatty acids.

17. The serving of chips provides 9 g of fat. Each gram of fat supplies 9 kcal. Thus, fat contributes 81 of the 150 kcal in a serving of the chips (9 g × 9 kcal/g).

18. Atherosclerosis is a long-term disease process in which plaques build up inside arterial walls. Arteriosclerosis is a condition that results from atherosclerosis and is characterized by loss of arterial flexibility. A thrombus is a fixed bunch of clots that remains in place. An embolus is a thrombus or part of a plaque that breaks free and travels through the bloodstream. Atherosclerosis can occur when something in the bloodstream irritates the lining of an artery. The body's immune system responds by producing inflammation within the artery. Inflammation can stimulate healing, but the process can also trigger certain cells within the arterial wall to deposit cholesterol and other substances under the artery's lining. As a result, arterial plaque forms. Plaque interferes with or blocks circulation in the affected area. Plaque also roughens the normally smooth surface that lines the artery. The rough lining slows blood flow in the area and makes clots more likely to form. If a plaque ruptures, repairing the damage also involves clot formation, and such blood clots can be life threatening.

19. Answers will vary but should include king mackerel, marlin, swordfish, or shark.

20. Answers will vary but should relate to information about risk factors presented in Table 6.4.

21. According to this information, Bernard has a low risk of CVD because his HDL cholesterol level is high.

22. The liver releases high-sensitivity C-reactive protein in response to infection and inflammation. Elevated CRP may be a marker for atherosclerosis, which means it may be an early warning sign for the condition. A lipoprotein profile can provide information about blood levels of HDL, LDL, and triglycerides.

23. Answers will vary but should include reducing intakes of meats; foods made from whole milk; and crackers, cakes, cookies, pies, and other high-fat processed foods. Increasing intakes of most nuts, fatty fish, and sources of polyunsaturated oils can increase intakes of unsaturated fats.

24. A statin is a prescription drug that reduces elevated blood lipid levels. Statins interfere with the liver's metabolism of cholesterol, effectively reducing LDL cholesterol and/ or triglyceride levels as a result.

25. Answers will vary but should include points in Figure 6.25.

26. BAC is "blood alcohol concentration." In June 2017, the legal limit for BAC was 0.8 for people who are 21 years of age or older.

27. Samuel is a heavy drinker.

Chapter 7

1. The amino acid is the chemical unit that makes up a protein.

2. Answers may vary but may include cell development and maintenance, and the production of enzymes, antibodies, certain hormones, structural and contractile components, and blood-clotting factors. Additionally, proteins transport nutrients and oxygen in the bloodstream, help maintain acid-base and fluid balance, and can be used for energy.

3. The three groups that make up an amino acid are the amino or nitrogen-containing group, R group, and acid group.

4. A carbon skeleton is the part of an amino acid that remains after the amino group is removed.

5. Twenty amino acids are needed to make human proteins. Nine of these amino acids are essential.

6. A high-quality or complete protein contains all essential amino acids in amounts that will support protein deposition in muscles and other tissues or support a young child's growth. A low-quality protein lacks one or more essential amino acids.

7. Most animal proteins are sources of high-quality proteins. Quinoa and processed soy proteins are also good sources of high-quality protein. Other plant foods, particularly fruits and vegetables, are sources of low-quality proteins.

8. Tryptophan, threonine, lysine, methionine, and cysteine are often the limiting amino acids in foods.

9. Answers will vary but should include key steps noted in Figure 7.6.

10. A protein undergoes denaturation when it is exposed to various conditions that alter the macronutrient's natural folded and coiled shape. Deamination is the removal of the nitrogen-containing group from an amino acid. Transamination is the transfer of an amino group from an amino acid to a receiving compound such as a carbon skeleton.

11. Negative balance occurs during starvation, serious illnesses, and severe injuries. Positive balance occurs during periods of rapid growth such as pregnancy, infancy, and puberty, and when people are recovering from illness or injury. Performing weight-training activities also leads to nitrogen retention.

12. To calculate the answer, convert the woman's weight to kilograms by dividing 143 pounds by 2.2 (65 kg). Multiply her weight in kilograms (65) by 0.8 grams of protein/kg to calculate her RDA for protein (52 g).

13. Answers will vary but should follow the path illustrated in Figure 7.10.

14. The AMDR for adult protein intake is 10 to 35% of energy from protein.

15. Americans generally eat about the same percentage of total calories from protein that they did in the early 1900s. Americans, however, now consume more protein from meat, fish, and poultry than from grains.

16. Answers will vary based on individual food intakes.

17. To calculate the answer, divide the amount of protein/serving (5 g) by the Daily Value for protein, which is 50 g (5/50 = .10). Then, convert .10 to a percentage by moving the decimal point two spaces to the right and replacing it with a percent symbol. The answer is 10%.

18. Foods that substitute for meat include fish, poultry, eggs, soy products, or protein–rich dairy products such as cheese and yogurt. Extending high–quality protein refers to preparing dishes that incorporate small amounts of animal proteins with much larger amounts of plant proteins. Spaghetti with meat sauce is an example of a dish that extends high-quality protein in meat with more low–quality proteins in pasta.

19. The recipe does not provide a complementary mixture of proteins because fruit is not a good source of plant proteins to combine with peanuts.

20. Answers will vary but should include quinoa or legumes to complement or improve the cereal protein.

21. Semivegetarians consume small amounts of meat, fish, or poultry, whereas other vegetarians do not eat animal flesh.

22. Plant–based diets may not contain enough energy, high-quality protein, omega–3 fatty acids, vitamins B–12 and D, and minerals zinc, iron, and calcium to meet a person's nutritional needs.

23. Children have higher protein and energy needs per pound of body weight than adults do. Since plant foods add bulk to the diet, vegan children are more likely to eat far less food than adult vegans because they become full sooner during meals. Thus, very young vegans may be unable to eat enough plant foods to meet their protein and energy needs.

24. People suffering from alcoholism, anorexia nervosa, or certain intestinal tract disorders are at risk of protein undernutrition. People with low incomes, especially older adults, are also at risk of protein deficiency.

25. Children with PEM do not have enough protein and energy to grow properly and fight infections.

26. According to this information, the child probably suffers from severe protein–energy malnutrition because of the parental neglect and presence of muscular wasting.

27. Common signs and symptoms of food allergy are hives, swollen or itchy lips, skin flushing, eczema, difficulty swallowing, wheezing and difficulty breathing, and abdominal pain, vomiting, and diarrhea. Common signs and symptoms of celiac disease are abdominal bloating, chronic diarrhea, weight loss, and poor growth in children.

28. They must provide their children with a special diet that is very low in phenylalanine.

29. Information about a patient's genetic makeup could enable physicians to prescribe more effective treatments, including special diets.

30. Answers will vary but may include the points in the "Food & Nutrition Tips" feature in this section.

31. Answers may vary, depending on the person's living situation. The 3.5–pound bag of frozen peaches cost $7.99; the fresh peaches cost $2.49/lb, so 3.5 pounds of the peaches would cost about $8.72. So, people can save about $0.73 by purchasing the frozen peaches. However, they need to have access to a large freezer if they intend to store the fruit. Buying smaller quantities of the fresh fruit may be a better option for people who do not have a way of storing the frozen fruit.

Chapter 8

1. Vitamins are complex organic compounds that regulate metabolic reactions. The body cannot synthesize most vitamins; vitamins naturally occur in commonly eaten foods; signs and symptoms of deficiency disease eventually occur when a vitamin is missing from the diet; if the deficiency disorder is treated early, good health is restored by supplying the missing vitamin.

2. Foods generally contain much smaller amounts of vitamins than of macronutrients; the body requires vitamins in much smaller amounts than macronutrients; and the body does not use vitamins directly for energy.

3. A provitamin is a vitamin precursor—a substance that does not function as a vitamin until the body converts it into an active form. An antioxidant is a substance that protects other compounds from oxidizing agents. A radical is a substance with an unpaired electron; radicals are highly reactive.

4. The federally regulated grain enrichment program specifies amounts of thiamin, riboflavin, niacin, and folic acid that manufacturers must add to their refined flour and other milled grain products.

5. Answers will vary but should relate to information concerning food preparation, such as cooking methods, and food storage practices.

6. Answers will vary, but the table should include vitamins A, D, E, and K and conform to information provided in Table 8.2.

7. Answers will vary, but the table should include all B vitamins, vitamin C, and choline, and conform to information provided in Table 8.7.

8. Taking megadoses of vitamins can produce druglike effects in the body, including unpleasant and even dangerous side effects.

9. Liver damage is one of most serious side effects of taking megadoses of niacin (see Table 8.7).

10. High doses of vitamin B–6 have been associated with sensory nerve damage. The damage is usually reversible—after affected people stop taking excessive amounts of the vitamin.

11. Routine vitamin C supplementation does not protect against infection by common cold viruses, but the practice may shorten the duration of cold symptoms.

12. There is no scientific evidence that taking beta–carotene prevents healthy people from developing macular degeneration.

13. Lung cancer is the leading cause of cancer deaths in the United States.

14. *Metastasize* means "spread," so Margaret's breast cancer has spread to her lungs.

15. Answers will vary but should include intakes of alcohol; processed and red meats; fried, grilled, and broiled meats; salted fish; and moldy nuts (see Table 8.15).

16. Answers will vary but should include not smoking, limiting alcohol consumption, and maintaining a healthy body weight.

Chapter 9

1. A mineral nutrient is classified as a major mineral if humans require 100 mg or more per day or a trace mineral if humans require less than 100 mg/day.

2. List should include at least five of the minerals in the trace minerals column of Table 9.1.

3. List should include at least five of the minerals in the major minerals column of Table 9.1.

4. Water is a major solvent, and the nutrient often participates directly in chemical reactions. Water's other physiological roles include transporting substances, removing waste products, lubricating tissues, and regulating body temperature and acid–base balance. Additionally, water is a major component of blood, saliva, sweat, tears, mucus, and the fluid in joints.

5. Osmosis is the diffusion of a solvent, usually water, through a selectively permeable membrane.

6. Extracellular water contains higher concentrations of sodium and chloride ions than intracellular water. Intracellular water contains higher concentrations of potassium and phosphate ions than extracellular water.

7. The body obtains water by consuming various foods and liquids, such as fruit juice, milk, soup, coffee, tea, soft drinks, tap water, and plain or flavored bottled water. Cells also form some water as a metabolic by–product of metabolism. The body loses water in urine, perspiration, exhaled air, feces, vomit, and insensible perspiration.

8. If the body cannot regulate its water balance, cells can shrink, swell, and even die.

9. In response to dehydration, the posterior pituitary gland releases antidiuretic hormone that stimulates kidneys to conserve water. Additionally, the adrenal glands secrete aldosterone, a hormone that signals kidneys to reduce the elimination of sodium in urine. As a result, the kidneys return the mineral to the general circulation. Because water follows sodium, it is conserved as well.

10. The AI for total water intake is approximately 11 cups (2.7 L) for young women and approximately 15.5 cups (3.7 L) for young men.

11. A diuretic is a substance that increases urine production. Alcohol and caffeine have diuretic effects on the body.

12. Signs and symptoms of dehydration include weight loss, fatigue, thirst, loss of muscular strength and endurance, severe weakness, and coma.

13. Signs and symptoms of water intoxication may include drowsiness, nausea and vomiting, confusion, inability to coordinate muscular movements, and weight gain. If not treated early, overhydration can result in death.

14. Answers may vary, but may include inorganic structural components of tissues, such as calcium and phosphorus in bones and teeth. Minerals may also function as inorganic ions, such as calcium ions (Ca^{++}) that participate in blood clotting and sodium ions (Na^+) that help maintain fluid balance. Some ions, such as magnesium (Mg^{++}) and copper (Cu^{++}), are cofactors for chemical reactions. Many minerals are components of various enzymes, hormones, or other organic molecules, such as cobalt in vitamin B–12, iron in hemoglobin, and sulfur in the amino acids methionine and cysteine.

15. Refining foods can result in mineral losses. Minerals are water soluble and can be lost by leaching into watery cooking fluids.

16. The bioavailability of minerals depends largely on the body's need for the micronutrient. Additionally, minerals from animal foods are often better absorbed than minerals in plant foods.

17. The enrichment program for grains requires the addition of iron to grain products.

18. Osteoporosis is a chronic disease characterized by low bone mass and reduced bone structure. People with osteoporosis have weak bones that are susceptible to fractures that can be costly to treat and result in disability and death, particularly among older adults.

19. Answers may vary, but should relate to risk factors listed in Table 9.7.

20. Prehypertension is a condition characterized by persistent systolic blood pressure readings of 120 to 139 mm Hg and diastolic readings of 80 to 89 mm Hg. Hypertension is characterized by persistent systolic values ≥140 mm Hg and diastolic values ≥90 mm Hg. Risk factors for hypertension include advanced age, African–American ancestry, obesity, physical inactivity, smoking cigarettes, and excess alcohol and sodium intakes. Table 9.11 presents major risk factors for hypertension.

21. The Dietary Approaches to Stop Hypertension (DASH) diet is low in sodium, total fat, and saturated fat; and high in fruits, vegetables, and low—fat dairy products. Other lifestyle changes that can reduce blood pressure include losing excess body fat and increasing physical activity.

22. Answers should conform to information in Table 9.5.

23. Iron deficiency is a condition characterized by low blood iron levels that are not low enough to result in severe health problems. Iron deficiency anemia occurs when oxygen transport in blood is impaired, generally because there are not enough red blood cells to carry the oxygen or because red blood cells do not contain enough hemoglobin. Signs and symptoms of iron deficiency anemia include conditions listed in Table 9.17. People who are likely to develop iron deficiency include those who have lost substantial amounts of blood and young women who exclude meat and enriched bread and cereal products from their diets. Additionally, others at risk of iron deficiency are women of childbearing age (who generally lose some iron during menstruation), pregnant women, and infants born to women who are iron deficient.

24. Hemochromatosis is an inherited disorder in which the body absorbs too much iron. Signs and symptoms include joint pain, fatigue, lack of energy, abdominal pain, loss of sex drive, abnormal bronze skin color, and heart problems. The condition is treated by avoiding iron supplements and periodically having blood removed.

25. Goiter is an enlarged thyroid gland. Cretinism occurs in infants born to women who were iodine deficient during pregnancy. The condition is characterized by permanent brain damage, reduced intellectual functioning, and growth retardation. Cretinism can be prevented by including a source of iodine in diets of pregnant women.

26. Answers will vary but should conform to information presented in Table 9.15.

27. Answers will vary but should include arsenic, boron, lithium, nickel, silicon, or vanadium.

28. Answers will vary but should conform to information provided in Table 9.22.

29. In the United States, most tap water undergoes a thorough purification process and is constantly tested for safety.

30. Answers will vary but should include avoiding containers that have the symbol that is shown in Figure 9.25.

Chapter 10

1. Calvin can be "overweight" if he has more muscle and less body fat than other people who are his height.

2. In 2013–2014, almost 38% of adult Americans were obese.

3. Total body fat includes adipose cells and fat in cell membranes, nervous tissue, and certain bones. Fat—free mass is comprised of body water; mineral—rich tissues such as bones and teeth; and protein—rich tissues, including muscles and organs.

4. Body fat stores energy. Additionally, fat cells secrete numerous proteins, some of which have roles in regulating food intake, glucose metabolism, and immune responses.

5. Subcutaneous fat helps insulate the body against cold temperatures and protects muscles and bones from bumps and bruises. Subcutaneous fat also provides body contours.

6. Answers will vary but may include "underwater weighing" and measuring dual—energy x—ray absorptiometry, air displacement, bioelectrical impedance, and skinfold thicknesses. For many of the techniques, drawbacks include cost and size of equipment needed to measure body fat.

7. He is overweight.

8. To estimate daily basal metabolic needs of a 185—pound woman, first convert the woman's weight to kilograms by dividing 185 pounds by 2.2 (approximately 84 kg). Then multiply 84 kg by 0.9 kcal to determine the amount of energy expended for metabolism in an hour (approximately 76 kcal/hr). Multiply 76 kcal/hour by 24 hours to obtain the amount of energy expended for basal metabolic needs in a day (1824 kcal).

9. The three major ways the body uses energy are basal metabolism, physical activity, and TEF. Energy needs for physical activity can be easily altered.

10. For most people, basal metabolism uses the most energy each day.

11. Answers will vary but may include body composition, thyroid hormone level, sex, body surface area, age, calorie intake, fever, stimulants, pregnancy, milk production after childbirth, and recovery after exercise.

12. A person gains weight when in positive energy balance.

13. Positive energy balance is desirable for pregnant women and during periods of growth, such as during fetal development, infancy, childhood, and puberty.

14. Weight loss is characterized by negative energy balance.

15. This woman is likely to be obese.

16. Answers will vary but should include conditions listed in Table 10.5.

17. The stigma of obesity is the negative attitude that many people have toward obese persons, such as characterizing overfat people as lazy, stupid, and sloppy.

18. Central—body obesity ("apple shape") is more likely to pose serious health risks than having excess fat below the waist, or a pear—shaped fat distribution. Central—body fat distribution is associated with increased risks of type 2 diabetes and CVD.

19. Measuring a person's waist circumference is a quick and easy way to determine whether body fat distribution is likely to result in serious chronic health problems.

20. Hunger is an uncomfortable feeling that drives a person to consume food. Satiety is the sense that enough food or beverages have been consumed to satisfy hunger.

21. Adipose cells secrete leptin, a hormone that reduces hunger and inhibits fat storage in the body. The stomach secretes ghrelin that stimulates eating behavior.

22. Thrifty genes could benefit people during periods of food deprivation, such as famine.

23. According to the set–point theory, the body's fat content (and, therefore, body weight) is genetically predetermined. The set point acts like a home thermostat, except that it regulates body weight instead of temperature.

24. Hunger is a drive to eat food, whereas appetite is a desire to eat appealing food.

25. Answers will vary but should include food marketing and sensory appeal, such as appearance, taste, and odor. Our work and home environments influence whether we are sedentary or physically active by providing opportunities to be active.

26. Answers will vary but should include genetics, occupations that do not provide enough physical activity, and psychological factors, such as mood and self–esteem.

27. Four key elements necessary for weight loss and maintenance are motivation, calorie reduction, regular physical activity, and behavior modification.

28. Answers will vary but should include points listed in Table 10.6.

29. Before joining a weight–loss group or plan, consumers should find out how much the program costs and how often they will need to pay for the program. Consumers should ask whether they need to sign a contract and the length of the contract. Do special foods or supplements need to be purchased? If nutrition counseling is provided, what are the credentials of the persons providing nutrition counseling and information? Furthermore, does the plan emphasize the importance of making lifestyle changes? Does the program's advertising include questionable weight–loss claims and deceptive testimonials?

30. Answers will vary but should include these: eat a low–calorie diet; eat regular meals, including breakfast almost every day; weigh themselves at least once a week; exercise for an average of 60 minutes daily; and limit television watching.

31. Weight–loss medications may suppress appetite or interfere with fat digestion and absorption.

32. Roux–en–Y gastric bypass and gastric banding procedures are common forms of bariatric surgery performed in the United States. Bariatric surgeries are effective because they reduce the size of the stomach. As a result, patients can consume only small portions of food at a time. Gastric banding is easier to perform, safer than other types of bariatric surgery, and relatively easy to reverse.

33. A fad diet is a trendy dietary practice that has widespread appeal among a population; after a period, people lose interest in the practice and it becomes no longer fashionable. Fad diets typically promote rapid weight loss without calorie restriction and increased physical activity; limit food selections to be from only a few food groups and dictate specific diet rituals; require buying a book or various gimmicks; use outlandish and unscientific claims to support their usefulness; rely on testimonials from famous people; connect the diet to trendy places; and do not emphasize the need to change eating habits and physical activity patterns.

34. Many overweight and obese people are attracted to fad diets and dietary supplements for weight loss because they believe promoters' claims that the diets or products are "magic bullets" for shedding unwanted weight quickly and effortlessly.

35. Answers will vary but should include supplements presented in Table 10.7.

36. Answers will vary but should include features or claims that the product or service causes rapid and extreme weight loss; requires no need to change dietary patterns or physical activity; results in permanent weight loss; is scientifically proven or doctor endorsed; includes a money–back guarantee; is safe; is supported by satisfied customers; displays before–and–after photos; and provides disclaimers in small print, such as "Results not typical" at the bottom of the ad or with an "after" photo.

37. Chronic diseases such as cancer, tuberculosis, AIDS, inflammatory bowel disease, depression, and hormonal imbalances can result in severe weight loss that is difficult to treat.

38. To gain weight, underweight adults can gradually increase their consumption of calorie–dense foods, especially those high in healthy fats. Eating regular meals and snacks also aids in weight gain and maintenance. If excess physical activity habits contribute to the inability to gain weight, underweight people can find ways to be less active. Furthermore, underweight individuals can add muscle mass by following resistance–training programs regularly, but their calorie intake must support extra energy demands of those programs.

39. Skipping breakfast regularly is a sign of disordered eating, not an eating disorder.

40. The three major types of eating disorders are anorexia nervosa (AN), bulimia nervosa (BN), and binge–eating disorder (BED). Major signs of AN are severely restricted food intake and maintenance of an unhealthy low body weight. People with BN are difficult to recognize, but characteristic signs of the condition are bite marks and scars on the knuckles that result from self–induced vomiting. The major sign of BED is consuming a much larger amount of food than most people would eat under similar circumstances in a brief period of time.

41. Answers will vary but should include the risk factors shown in Table 10.8.

42. Answers will vary but should include the health consequences listed in Table 10.9, as well as death.

Chapter 11

1. Physical activity is any movement that results from skeletal muscle contraction. Exercise refers to physical activities that are usually planned and structured for a particular purpose.

2. A physically fit person can perform moderate– to vigorous–intensity activities, for a reasonable amount of time, without becoming excessively fatigued.

3. Healthy adults under 65 years of age should engage in at least 150 minutes of moderate–intensity physical activity a week or 75 minutes of vigorous–intensity physical activity a week. Additionally, adults should include eight to 10 strengthening exercises at least twice a week.

4. Answers will vary but should include benefits indicated in Figure 11.1.

5. Performing resistance exercises regularly can increase muscle mass, strength, and flexibility. Resistance exercises can also increase bone mass.

6. To calculate the target heart rate range of a 24–year–old person performing moderate–intensity activity, subtract the person's age (24) from 220 to obtain 196, the age–related maximum heart rate. Moderate–intensity activity raises the heart rate to 50 to 70% of the age; therefore, multiply $196 \times .50$ to obtain the lower limit of the range (98 bpm), and $196 \times .70$ to obtain the upper limit of the range (approximately 137 bpm). Thus, the heart rate range for this individual is 98 to 137 bpm.

7. Muscle cells break down glycogen to provide a source of glucose during exercise.

8. ATP is formed as a result of glycolysis and aerobic respiration. Some ATP is also formed by the breakdown of triglycerides, amino acids, and alcohol. Muscle cells also use phosphocreatine to produce ATP quickly under anaerobic conditions.

9. Muscle cells rely on the PCr–ATP, lactic acid, and oxygen systems to obtain energy. The PCr–ATP system forms ATP by breaking down PCr into creatine and P_i. The energy that is released helps synthesize ATP from ADP and P_i. In anaerobic conditions, muscle cells metabolize glucose to pyruvate and then convert pyruvate to lactic acid. The degradation of glucose to lactic acid produces a small amount of ATP. Lactic acid accumulates in muscles and converts to a related substance, lactate. Although certain muscle cells can use lactate as a fuel, some of the compound enters the bloodstream. The liver removes lactate from blood and can convert the compound into glucose. The oxygen system metabolizes glucose completely to CO_2 and H_2O, resulting in the production of far more ATP–energy than the amount produced by anaerobic systems. The PCr–ATP and lactic acid systems do not need oxygen to produce ATP.

10. Individuals can increase their aerobic exercise capacity by engaging in endurance–training programs that gradually increase the intensity level of activities. Such training improves muscle cells' ability to generate ATP rapidly.

11. Fat is a major energy source for muscles while one is resting or engaged in low– to moderate–intensity physical activities.

12. Practical ways to assess whether an athlete's energy intake is adequate include having the athlete keep accurate food records and use the information to estimate his or her daily calorie intakes. An athlete can also monitor his or her body weight and have skinfold thicknesses measured regularly.

13. Carbohydrate intake contributes to glycogen stores; glycogen depletion is a major cause of fatigue during endurance exercise. To maintain adequate muscle glycogen, athletes should consume 6 to 10 g of carbohydrate per kilogram of body weight daily. By consuming several servings of grains, starchy vegetables, and fruits daily, an athlete can obtain enough carbohydrate to maintain adequate liver and muscle glycogen stores.

14. Answers will vary but should include grains, starchy vegetables, and fruits. Also, see Table 11.4 for high–carbohydrate, low–fat foods.

15. Compared to nonathletes, athletes may need more than the RDA for protein because they need to have amino acids available to repair muscle tissue damaged during intense physical activity and to build muscle tissue.

16. Dehydration and overhydration detract from optimal physical performance and can cause serious health problems.

17. Answers will vary but should include signs and symptoms listed in Table 11.7.

18. According to the IMMDA, sports drinks are necessary when work–outs or events are 10 kilometers or more. Although electrolytes are lost in sweat, the quantities lost in shorter periods can be easily replaced by consuming foods and beverages, such as water or fruit juice, after the event.

19. The practice of taking antioxidant supplements may not be helpful and could be harmful. Free radicals generated during intense exercise may stimulate the body's natural antioxidant defense system. Thus, the oxidative stress produced during exercise might have benefits, and blocking this process by taking antioxidant vitamin supplements may not be desirable.

20. Iron deficiency can negatively affect athletic performance because the body needs iron to produce red blood cells, transport oxygen, and obtain energy.

21. Female athletes who have irregular or no menstrual cycles may lack adequate amounts of the hormone estrogen. Although weight–bearing exercise, such as jogging, improves bone density, estrogen is necessary for maintaining healthy bones. Female athletes who develop menstrual cycle abnormalities should consult a physician to determine the cause.

22. Athletes often use ergogenic aids to improve their physical performance, because they hope to gain the competitive edge over their sports rivals.

23. Answers will vary but should include ephedra–containing supplements, caffeine (high intakes), anabolic steroids, and growth hormone.

24. Coffee, energy drinks, caffeinated soft drinks, chocolate, and tea (see Table 11.9).

25. Caffeine raises the level of fatty acids in blood, and as a result, exercising muscles can use more fat for energy. Caffeine also enhances the ability of skeletal and heart muscles to contract and increases mental alertness.

26. The three key components of an aerobic workout regimen are warm–up, workout, and cool–down.

27. Answers will vary, but the fitness program should include the principles of exercise variety, balance, and moderation. Furthermore, the person should include activities that are enjoyable and easy to incorporate into his or her routine.

Chapter 12

1. Norovirus is responsible for most cases of food-borne illness in the United States.

2. The illness caused by norovirus is usually the result of a food-borne infection.

3. The FDA regulates nearly all domestic and imported food sold in interstate commerce and enforces federal food safety laws. Additionally, the FDA establishes standards for safe food manufacturing practices, such as Hazard Analysis and Critical Control Point programs. FDA officials can take certain enforcement actions, such as requesting that a food manufacturer recall an unsafe item, so that it is removed from store shelves. The FDA also educates the general public about safe food handling practices. The Food Safety and Inspection Service (FSIS) enforces food safety laws for domestic and imported meat and poultry products. Additionally, FSIS staff collect and analyze food samples to check for the presence of microbial and other unwanted and potentially harmful material in foods. FSIS officials can ask meat and poultry processors to recall unsafe products. FSIS also educates people about proper food handling practices. The EPA oversees drinking water quality and assists state officials in their efforts to monitor water quality. Furthermore, EPA staff regulate toxic substances and wastes to prevent their entry into foods and the environment.

4. Local health departments are responsible for inspecting restaurants, grocery stores, dairy farms, and local food processing companies.

5. Three common ways harmful microbes are transmitted to food are by vermin, poor personal hygiene practices, and improper food handling.

6. Cross-contamination occurs when pathogens in one food are transferred to another food, contaminating it.

7. Pasteurization is a special heating process used by many commercial food producers to kill pathogens.

8. To survive and multiply, most microbes need warmth, moisture, and a source of nutrients, and some also require oxygen.

9. In general, high-risk foods are warm, moist, and protein rich, and they have a neutral or slightly acidic pH (see Table 12.1).

10. Signs and symptoms of food-borne illnesses generally involve the digestive tract and include nausea, vomiting, diarrhea, and intestinal cramps.

11. People who suffer from a food-borne illness should consult a physician when an intestinal disorder is accompanied by one or more of the signs that are listed in Table 12.2.

12. Food-borne illness generally causes gastrointestinal tract symptoms, whereas influenza is primarily a respiratory tract infection.

13. Answers will vary but should include bacteria listed in Table 12.3.

14. Answers will vary but should include viruses listed in Table 12.4.

15. Aflatoxins are poisonous substances produced by certain molds.

16. Answers will vary but should include a protozoan and a parasitic worm listed in Table 12.5.

17. Answers will vary but should include points under the "Purchasing Food" section of Chapter 12.

18. Answers will vary but should include points under the "Setting the Stage for Food Preparation" and "Preparing Food" sections of Chapter 12.

19. Answers will vary but should include points under the "Storing and Reheating Food" section of Chapter 12.

20. Ground meats and poultry are often sources of food-borne illness because grinding increases the surface area of the protein-rich food, exposing it to contaminants.

21. Raw fish should be frozen for recommended amounts of time before being eaten.

22. The "danger zone" for rapid pathogen multiplication is between 40°F and 140°F.

23. The Check Your Steps program recommends four simplified actions: clean, separate, cook, and chill.

24. Shelf life is the period of time that a food can be stored before it spoils.

25. Answers will vary but should include methods highlighted in Table 12.8.

26. Boiling home-canned, low-acid foods for 10 minutes can make them safe to eat.

27. Answers may vary but can include meats, fresh fruits and vegetables, spices, dry vegetable mixes, seeds, and shell eggs.

28. Answers will vary but should include points made under the "Preparing for Disasters" section of Chapter 12. Table 12.9 lists foods that can be stored safely for emergency situations.

29. Safe sources of drinking water include bottled water, an undamaged water heater, toilet tanks (not bowls), melted water from ice cubes, and fruit juices. Water from pools, spas, radiators, heating systems, and water beds is unsafe to drink.

30. A food additive is a substance added to food that influences the product's characteristics. Direct food additives may maintain the safety of foods, prevent undesirable changes, or improve taste or color of foods. Indirect additives, such as compounds from a food's wrapper or container, can enter food as it is packaged, transported, or stored. Indirect additives have no purpose.

31. Color additives are dyes, pigments, or other substances that provide color to foods, drugs, or cosmetics.

32. Food ingredients that had been in use prior to 1958 were listed as Generally Recognized as Safe (GRAS) when qualified

experts generally agreed that the substance was safe for its intended use. Food manufacturers can include on the GRAS list as ingredients without testing them for safety or getting prior approval from the FDA.

33. According to the Delaney Clause, food manufacturers cannot add a new compound that causes cancer at any level of intake. Thus, if an additive causes cancer, even though very high doses may be necessary to cause the disease, no amount of the additive is considered to be safe, and none is allowed in food. Evidence for cancer risk could come from either laboratory animal or human studies. The FDA allows very few exceptions to this clause.

34. An unintentional food additive is a substance that accidentally enters food during processing. Common biological and physical food contaminants are insect parts, rodent feces or urine, dust and dirt, and bits of metal or glass from machinery used to process food.

35. A pesticide is any substance that people use to control or kill unwanted insects, weeds, rodents, fungi, or other organisms. Types of pesticides include insecticides, rodenticides, herbicides, and fungicides.

36. Integrated pest management (IPM) involves using a variety of methods for controlling pests while limiting damage to the environment. IPM methods include growing pest-resistant crops, using predatory wasps to control crop-destroying insects, trapping adult insect pests before they can reproduce, and using biologically based pesticides.

37. The EPA regulates the use of pesticides.

38. A pesticide tolerance is the maximum amount of pesticide residue that can be in or on each treated food crop. A pesticide tolerance includes a margin of safety, so the maximum pesticide residue that is allowed to be in or on a food is much lower than amounts that can cause negative health effects.

39. Once a pesticide is applied to cropland, it may remain in the soil, be taken up by plant roots, decompose to other compounds, or enter groundwater and waterways. Winds may carry pesticides in air and dust to distant locations, where the toxic material can land on food crops.

40. Answers will vary but should include using hand sanitizers, drinking only commercially bottled water, boiling water before drinking it, eating foods that are fully cooked and served hot, and not eating locally provided fresh fruits and vegetables that have been washed in unsanitary water.

41. Answers will vary but should include the foods shown in the safe-to-eat category in Figure 12.13.

Chapter 13

1. John is an older adult.

2. For women, lactation is the life stage that involves milk production for breastfeeding.

3. Eight weeks after conception, the developing human being is referred to as a fetus.

4. The role of the placenta is to transfer nutrients and oxygen from the mother's bloodstream to the embryo/fetus. Additionally, the placenta transfers wastes from the embryo/fetus to the mother's bloodstream, so her body can eliminate them.

5. Birth weight is a major factor that determines whether a baby is healthy and survives his or her first year of life.

6. Gestational hypertension can be dangerous because it increases the risk of maternal death and premature delivery.

7. Answers will vary but should include enlarged breasts, "morning sickness," tiredness, swollen feet, constipation, and heartburn.

8. Women whose prepregnancy weights were within the healthy range can expect to gain 25 to 35 pounds. Underweight women should gain 28 to 40 pounds; overweight women should gain 15 to 25 pounds during pregnancy. Obese women should gain 11 to 20 pounds during pregnancy. The recommendations are higher for women who are pregnant with more than one fetus.

9. Pregnant women who are folate deficient have a high risk of giving birth to infants with neural tube defects, such as spina bifida. Pregnant women who are iron deficient can develop iron deficiency anemia, a condition that increases the risk of giving birth prematurely and having low-birth-weight (LBW) infants.

10. Women who drink alcohol during pregnancy are at risk of having a child with a fetal alcohol spectrum disorder. Compared to pregnant women who do not smoke cigarettes, expectant mothers who smoke have higher risk of giving birth too early and having LBW babies. Furthermore, expectant mothers who smoke cigarettes may increase the risk of having babies with birth defects or that die of sudden infant death syndrome.

11. In response to an infant sucking on its mother's nipple, the brain releases oxytocin, a hormone that signals breast tissue to "let down" milk. The let-down reflex enables milk to travel in several tubes to the nipple area. When let-down occurs, the infant removes the milk by continued sucking.

12. Lactation increases a new mother's energy needs by about 300 to 400 kcal more than her prepregnancy energy needs.

13. Colostrum is the first secretion of the breasts that occurs after delivery. Colostrum is a very important first food for babies, because the fluid contains antibodies and immune system cells that can be absorbed by the infant's immature digestive tract. Colostrum also contains substances that encourage the growth of beneficial bacteria in the baby's intestinal tract that reduce the risk of infection.

14. New mothers should exclusively breastfeed their healthy babies for about the first 6 months of life.

15. Answers will vary but should include points in Table 13.5.

16. Answers will vary but should include points in Table 13.5.

17. Compared to whole cow's milk, human milk provides about the same amount of energy, less protein and calcium, and more carbohydrate and fat.

18. Signs indicating a baby is ready physically to eat solid foods include: loss of the extrusion reflex; physiological maturity to digest, metabolize, and excrete a wider range of foods; and ability to sit up with back support and coordinate muscular control over mouth and neck movements.

19. A healthy infant should triple its birthweight during the first year of life.

20. A food jag is a period in which the child refuses to eat a food that was liked in the past or in which the child wants to eat only a particular food.

21. In children, iron deficiency can lead to decreased physical stamina, learning ability, and resistance to infection.

22. Answers will vary but should include brushing teeth with a peasized amount of fluoride–containing toothpaste twice daily; providing routine pediatric dental care; offering fluoridated drinking water; not eating carbohydrate–rich snacks, especially between meals; and offering sugarless chewing gum.

23. Compared to preschoolers, older children often skip breakfast, and they typically consume more foods away from home, larger portions of food, and more fried foods and sweetened beverages. School–age children also tend to consume less milk and fewer fruits and vegetables, except fried potatoes.

24. Answers will vary but should include encouraging children to eat breakfast and other tips from the "Food & Nutrition Tips" feature in the "School–Age Children" section of Chapter 13.

25. Boys usually begin their growth spurt when they are between 12 and 15 years of age. Most girls begin their growth spurt between 10 and 13 years of age.

26. Iron deficiency leads to increased fatigue and decreased ability to concentrate and learn. Inadequate calcium intake during adolescence is associated with decreased bone mass and increased likelihood of bone fractures later in life.

27. Answers should provide the information in Table 13.10. Children and adolescents whose BMI–for–age is greater than or equal to the 85th percentile and less than the 95th percentile are overweight, and youngsters who are at or above the 95th percentile are obese.

28. Answers will vary but should include elevated blood pressure, cholesterol, and glucose levels and the factors listed in Table 13.11.

29. Answers will vary but should include spending too much time on sedentary activities; consuming too many empty calories; and having a family history of obesity, high birth weight, and obese family members.

30. To qualify for bariatric surgery, an adolescent should have extreme obesity, failed to lose weight after 6 months of trying to reduce his or her weight, attained his or her adult height, and developed serious chronic conditions that are associated with obesity.

31. Life expectancy is the length of time a person born in a specific year, such as 1900, can expect to live. Life span refers to the maximum number of years a human can live.

32. Answers will vary but should include points listed in Table 13.13.

33. Compared to younger persons, older adults have greater risk of nutritional deficiencies because of physiological changes associated with the normal aging process. Other factors that can influence an older person's nutritional status include illnesses, medications, low income, and lack of social support.

34. Diets of older adults often provide inadequate amounts of fiber, magnesium, potassium, calcium, zinc, folate, and vitamins A, B–6, C, D, and E.

35. Caregivers can improve nutrient intakes of older persons by adding more spices to foods, making mealtimes social events, and serving energy–dense snacks between meals, such as cheese, milk–shakes, nuts, or oatmeal cookies. If the elderly person has difficulty chewing, serving soft items such as ground meats, cooked vegetables, pureed fruits, and puddings can increase food intake. The "Food & Nutrition Tips" feature in the "Nutrition for Older Adults" section of Chapter 13 presents more suggestions for improving nutrient intakes of elderly persons.

36. Under certain conditions, calorie restriction extends the life expectancies of organisms that include fruit flies and rodents.

37. Answers may vary but should include adopting healthy lifestyles by consuming a nutritionally adequate diet, obtaining regular moderate– to vigorous–intensity physical activity, maintaining a healthy weight, avoiding tobacco products, limiting alcohol consumption, and having regular physical checkups.

Answers to Practice Test Questions

Chapter 1

1. d	2. b	3. d	4. a	5. b
6. c	7. b	8. c	9. b	10. c
11. a	12. d	13. b	14. a	15. b
16. c				

Chapter 2

1. d	2. c	3. a	4. b	5. c
6. d	7. a	8. c	9. b	10. d
11. b	12. a	13. a		

Chapter 3

1. b	2. c	3. c	4. a	5. d
6. a	7. c	8. d	9. b	10. b
11. c	12. b	13. a	14. c	15. d
16. b				

Chapter 4

1. c	2. a	3. b	4. b	5. a
6. c	7. b	8. b	9. d	10. c
11. a	12. c	13. b	14. d	15. a
16. b				

Chapter 5

1. a	2. c	3. b	4. d	5. b
6. c	7. b	8. b	9. c	10. b
11. a	12. c	13. b	14. b	

Chapter 6

1. a	2. b	3. c	4. a	5. b
6. d	7. b	8. c	9. b	10. c
11. c	12. b	13. a	14. d	

Chapter 7

1. c	2. c	3. a	4. a	5. b
6. d	7. c	8. a	9. b	10. a
11. d	12. c	13. a		

Chapter 8

1. d	2. c	3. a	4. d	5. d
6. a	7. b	8. a	9. b	10. c
11. c	12. a	13. b	14. c	15. d
16. a				

Chapter 9

1. c	2. b	3. d	4. d	5. a
6. c	7. d	8. a	9. b	10. c
11. b	12. a			

Chapter 10

1. b	2. d	3. b	4. c	5. b
6. d	7. a	8. b	9. a	10. b
11. d	12. d			

Chapter 11

1. b	2. c	3. a	4. d	5. b
6. a	7. b	8. d	9. a	10. d
11. b	12. c	13. b		

Chapter 12

1. a	2. a	3. c	4. d	5. c
6. b	7. d	8. c	9. c	10. b
11. d	12. b	13. a		

Chapter 13

1. b	2. c	3. b	4. a	5. a
6. c	7. d	8. d	9. a	10. d
11. b				

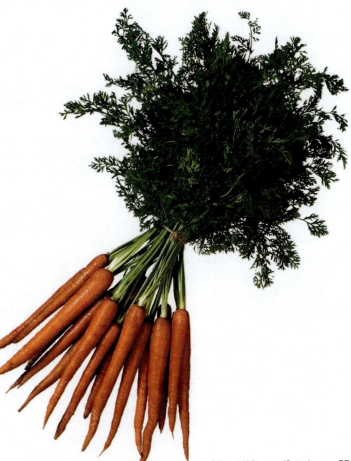

©Brand X Pictures/Getty Images RF

©Wendy Schiff

Chapter 1

1. Harmon BE and others: Associations of key diet–quality indexes with mortality in the Multiethnic Cohort: The Dietary Patterns Methods Project. *American Journal of Clinical Nutrition* 101(3):587, 2015.

2. U.S. Department of Health and Human Services, U.S. Department of Agriculture. 2015–2020 *Dietary Guidelines for Americans*. 2015. www.health.gov/dietaryguidelines/2015/guidelines/executive–summary Accessed: July 5, 2017.

3. Dietary Supplement Health and Education Act of 1994. Public Law 103–417, 103rd Congress. http://ods.od.nih.gov/About/DSHEA_Wording.aspx Accessed: July 7, 2017.

4. National Center for Health Statistics: *Health, United States, 2016*. https://www.cdc.gov/nchs/data/hus/2016/019.pdf Accessed: June 28, 2017.

5. American Cancer Society: *Cancer facts & figures 2017*. 2017. https://www.cancer.org/research/cancer–facts–statistics/all–cancer–facts–figures/cancer–facts–figures–2017.html Accessed: June 28, 2017.

6. American Cancer Society: *American Cancer Society guidelines on nutrition and physical activity for cancer prevention*. Revised: February 2016. https://www.cancer.org/healthy/eat–healthy–get–active/acs–guidelines–nutrition–physical–activity–cancer–prevention/summary.html Accessed: June 28, 2017.

7. U.S. Department of Agriculture, Economic Research Service: *Food availability (per capita) data system*. Last updated: February 2016. https://www.ers.usda.gov/data–products/food–availability–per–capita–data–system/food–availability–per–capita–data–system/#Loss–Adjusted Food Availability Accessed: April 15, 2017.

8. Office of Disease Prevention and Health Promotion, Healthy People.gov: *About Healthy People*. Updated: April 2017. https://www.healthypeople.gov/2020/About–Healthy–People Accessed: April 29, 2017.

9. U.S. Department of Agriculture, Agricultural Research Service: *Solid fats and added sugars in foods*. 2015. https://www.ars.usda.gov/news–events/news/research–news/2015/solid–fats–and–added–sugars–in–foods/ Accessed: June 28, 2017.

10. Huang H–Y and others: The efficacy and safety of multivitamin and mineral supplement use to prevent cancer and chronic disease in adults: A systematic review for a National Institutes of Health State–of–the–Science Conference. *Annals of Internal Medicine* 145(5):372, 2006.

11. Position of the Academy of Nutrition and Dietetics: Functional foods. *Journal of the Academy of Nutrition and Dietetics*. 113(8):1096, 2013.

12. World Health Organization: *Obesity and overweight*. 2016. http://www.who.int/mediacentre/factsheets/fs311/en/ Accessed: June 28, 2017.

13. World Food Program: *Zero Hunger*. http://www1.wfp.org/zero–hunger Accessed: June 28, 2017.

14. World Health Organization: *Progress on sanitation and drinking water: 2015 update and MDG assessment*. 2015. http://www.who.int/water_sanitation_health/publications/jmp–2015–update/en/ Accessed: June 28, 2017.

15. World Food Program: *Nutrition*. http://www1.wfp.org/nutrition Accessed: June 28, 2017.

16. World Health Organization, Micronutrient Deficiencies: *Vitamin A deficiency*. ND. http://www.who.int/nutrition/topics/vad/en/ Accessed: July 11, 2017.

17. World Food Program: *World hunger series: Hunger and markets*. 2009. http://documents.wfp.org/stellent/groups/public/documents/communications/wfp200279.pdf Accessed: June 28, 2017.

18. World Health Organization: *Global nutrition targets 2025: Low birth weight policy brief*. 2014. http://www.who.int/nutrition/publications/globaltargets2025_policybrief_lbw/en/ Accessed: June 28, 2017.

19. World Health Organization: *Infant and young child feeding*. Updated September 2016. http://www.who.int/mediacentre/factsheets/fs342/en/ Accessed: June 28, 2017.

20. U.S. Census Bureau: *Quick facts United States*. ND. http://www.census.gov/quickfacts/table/IPE120214/00 Accessed: June 28, 2017.

21. U.S. Department of Health and Human Services: *Poverty guidelines 2017*. January 2017. https://aspe.hhs.gov/poverty–guidelines Accessed: June 28, 2017.

22. Economic Research Report No. (ERR–194): *Household food security in the United States*. 43 pp. September 2015. https://www.ers.usda.gov/publications/pub–details/?pubid=79760 Accessed: June 28, 2017.

23. United Nations Children's Fund: *Supply annual report 2015*. ND. https://www.unicef.org/publications/index_92018.html Accessed: June 28, 2017.

24. Food and Drug Administration, Food: *Consumer info about food from genetically engineered plants*. Last updated: 2015. https://www.fda.gov/Food/IngredientsPackagingLabeling/GEPlants/ucm461805.htm Accessed: April 16, 2017.

25. Food and Drug Administration, Animal & Veterinary, Genetically Engineered Animals: *AquaAdvantage Salmon*. Last updated: April 12, 2017. https://www.fda.gov/AnimalVeterinary/DevelopmentApprovalProcess/GeneticEngineering/GeneticallyEngineeredAnimals/ucm280853.htm Accessed: April 15, 2017.

26. National Academy of Sciences: *Genetically engineered crops: Experiences and prospects*. 2016. The National Academies Press. https://www.nap.edu/catalog/23395/genetically–engineered–crops–experiences–and–prospects Accessed: April 16, 2017.

27. Foley JA: Can we feed the world and sustain the planet? *Scientific American* 305(5):60, 2011.

Chapter 2

1. Kraut A: *Dr. Joseph Goldberger & the war on pellagra*. Office of NIH History. http://history.nih.gov/exhibits/Goldberger/index.html Accessed: June 5, 2017.

2. Simoni RD and others: Copper as an essential nutrient and nicotinic acid as the anti–black tongue (pellagra) factor: The work of Conrad Arnold Elvehjem. *Journal of Biological Chemistry* 277(34):e22, 2002.

3. Benedetti F and others: How placebos change the patient's brain. *Neuropsychoparmacology* 36(1):339–354, 2011.

4. Centers for Disease Control and Prevention: *2014 National Diabetes Statistics Report*. Last updated: May 2015. https:www.cdc.gov/diabetes/data/statistics/2014StatisticsReport .html Accessed: June 5, 2017.

5. Kearns CE and others: Sugar industry and coronary heart disease research: A historical analysis of internal industry documents. *JAMA Internal Medicine* 2016 Sep 12. doi: 10.1001/jamainternmed .2016.5394.

6. U.S. Federal Trade Commission: Marketers of unproven weight–loss products ordered to pay nearly $2 million. https://www.ftc.gov /news–events/press–releases/2010/01/marketers–unproven–weight –loss–products–ordered–pay–nearly–2 Accessed: July 11, 2017.

7. Dahlstrom E, Bichsel J: *ECAR Study of Undergraduate Students and Information Technology, 2014*. Louisville, CO: ECAR, 2014. https://net.educause.edu/ir/library/pdf/ss14/ERS1406.pdf

8. Coughlin SS and others: Smartphone applications for promoting healthy diet and nutrition: A literature review. *Jacobs Journal of Food and Nutrition* 2(3): 021, 2015.

9. National Institutes of Health, National Center for Complementary and Integrative Health: *Using dietary supplements wisely*. Updated 2014. https://nccih.nih.gov/health/supplements/wiseuse .htm Accessed: May 5, 2017.

10. U.S. Food and Drug Administration: *What is a dietary supplement?* Last Updated 2015. https://www.fda.gov/AboutFDA /Transparency/Basics/ucm195635.htm Accessed: May 5, 2017.

11. National Institutes of Health, National Center for Complementary and Integrative Health: *Use of complementary health approaches in the U.S., National Health Interview Survey (NHIS): Most used natural products*. 2015. https://nccih.nih.gov/research /statistics/NHIS/2012/natural–products Accessed: May 5, 2017.

12. National Institutes of Health, National Center for Complementary and Integrative Health: *Complementary, alternative, or integrative health: What's in a name?* Updated 2016. https://nccih.nih .gov/health/integrative–health Accessed: May 5, 2017.

13. National Institutes of Health, National Center for Complementary and Integrative Health: *Use of complementary health approaches in the U.S., National Health Interview Survey (NHIS): What complementary and integrative approaches do Americans use?* 2015. https://nccih.nih.gov/research/statistics/NHIS/2012/key –findings Accessed: May 5, 2017.

14. Lau CSM, Chamberlain RS: Probiotics are effective at preventing *Clostridium difficile*–associated diarrhea: A systematic review and meta–analysis. *International Journal of General Medicine* 9:27, 2016. doi: 10.2147/IJGM.S98280. eCollection 2016.

15. U.S. Food and Drug Administration: *Dietary supplements*. Last updated: April 2016. http://www.fda.gov/Food/DietarySupplements /default.htm Accessed: May 5, 2017.

16. U.S. Food and Drug Administration: *Dietary supplements: What you need to know*. Last updated May 4, 2017. https://www.fda .gov/Food/ResourcesForYou/Consumers/ucm109760.htm Accessed: May 5, 2017.

17. U.S. Food and Drug Administration: *Dietary supplements*. Last updated: April 2016. https://www.fda.gov/Food/DietarySupplements /default.htm Accessed: May 5, 2017.

18. Daniells S: *Is the $35 billion figure for the dietary supplements industry over–inflated?* http://www.nutraingredients–usa.com /Markets/NBJ–The–US–supplement–industry–is–37–billion –not–12–billion Accessed: May 5, 2017.

19. Liu RH: Potential synergy of phytochemicals in cancer prevention: Mechanism of action. *Journal of Nutrition* 134:3479S, 2004.

20. National Institutes of Health, MedlinePlus: Blueberry. Last reviewed: 2015. https://www.nlm.nih.gov/medlineplus/druginfo /natural/1013.html Accessed: May 5, 2017.

Chapter 3

1. Food Marketing Institute: *Supermarket facts*. ND. https://www .fmi.org/our–research/supermarket–facts Accessed: July 11, 2017.

2. U.S. Department of Agriculture, Economic Research Service: *New products*. April 2016. https://www.ers.usda.gov/topics /food–markets–prices/processing–marketing/new–products.aspx Accessed: May 7, 2017.

3. Institute of Medicine: *Dietary Reference Intakes for vitamin C, vitamin E, selenium, and carotenoids*. Washington, DC: National Academies Press, 2000.

4. Otten JJ and others (eds.): *Dietary Reference Intakes: The essential guide to nutrient requirements*. Institute of Medicine of the National Academies. Washington, DC: National Academies Press, 2006.

5. U.S. Food and Drug Administration: *Draft guidelines: Whole grain label statements*. Updated June 2015. http://www.fda.gov/food /guidanceregulation/guidancedocumentsregulatoryinformation /ucm059088.htm Accessed: May 5, 2017.

6. U.S. Department of Agriculture, ChooseMyPlate: *All about the fruit group*. Updated March 2016. https://www.choosemyplate.gov /fruit Accessed: July 7, 2017.

7. U.S. Department of Agriculture, Choosemyplate.gov: *Tips to help you eat fruits*. Updated January 2016. https://www.choosemyplate .gov/fruits–tips Accessed: May 6, 2017.

8. U.S. Department of Health and Human Services and U.S. Department of Agriculture: *2015–2020 Dietary Guidelines for Americans*. 2015. http://health.gov/dietaryguidelines/2015 /guidelines/ Accessed: July 7, 2017.

9. U.S. Departments of Agriculture and Health and Human Services: *Scientific report of the 2015 Dietary Guidelines advisory committee* 2015. http://health.gov/dietaryguidelines/2015 –scientific–report/PDFs/Scientific–Report–of–the–2015–Dietary –Guidelines–Advisory–Committee.pdf Accessed: July 11, 2017.

10. U.S. Department of Agriculture, ChooseMyPlate.gov: *All about oils*. Updated July 2016. http://www.choosemyplate.gov/oils Accessed: May 7, 2017.

11. U.S. Department of Agriculture, ChooseMyPlate.gov: *Physical activity*. Last updated 2015. http://www.choosemyplate.gov/physical –activity.html Accessed: May 6, 2017.

12. Wilson MM and others: American diet quality: Where it is, where it is heading, and what it could be. *Journal of the Academy of Nutrition and Dietetics* 116(2):302, 2016.

13. U.S. Department of Agriculture, Economic Research Service: *Food availability (per capita) data system: Summary findings*. Last updated: January 2017. https://www.ers.usda.gov/data–products /food–availability–per–capita–data–system/summary–findings /Accessed: May 6, 2017.

14. American Diabetes Association: Exchange system. *Diabetes Forecast* October 2013. http://www.diabetesforecast.org /diabetes–101/exchange–system.html Accessed: May 6, 2017.

15. U.S. Government Publishing Office, Electronic Code of Federal Regulations: *Title 21: Food and drugs, part 101—food labeling*. Current as of June 13, 2016. https://www.ecfr.gov/cgi–bin/retrieveE CFR?gp=1&SID=4bf49f997b04dcacdfbd637db9aa5839&ty=HTML& h=L&mc=true&n=pt21.2.101&r=PART%E2%80%9D Accessed: May 6, 2017.

16. U.S. Food and Drug Administration: *How to understand and use the Nutrition Facts label*. Last updated: February 2017. https://www.fda.gov/Food/IngredientsPackagingLabeling /LabelingNutrition/ucm274593.htm Accessed: July 6, 2017.

17. U.S. Food and Drug Administration: *What is the meaning of 'natural' on a label of food?* April 2017. https://www.fda.gov /aboutfda/transparency/basics/ucm214868.htm Accessed: July 11, 2017.

18. Earles R, Williams P: *Sustainable Agriculture: An Introduction*. 2005. National Center for Appropriate Technology. https://attra.ncat .org/attra–pub/viewhtml.php?id=294 Accessed: May 6, 2017.

19. U.S. Environmental Protection Agency: *Pesticides and food: healthy, sensible food practices*. Last updated March 2017. https://www.epa.gov/safepestcontrol/pesticides–and–food –healthy–sensible–food–practices Accessed: May 7, 2017.

20. U.S. Department of Agriculture, Agricultural Marketing Service: *Agricultural Marketing Service's National Organic Program*. 2015. https://www.ams.usda.gov/sites/default/files/media/About%20 the%20National%20Organic%20Program.pdf Accessed: May 6, 2017.

21. Organic Trade Association, Press Release: *U.S. organic sales post new record of $43.3 billion in 2015*. May 19, 2016. https://www.ota.com/news/press–releases/19031 Accessed: May 6, 2017.

22. Johansson E and others: Contribution of organically grown crops to human health. *International Journal of Environmental Research and Public Health* 11:3870, 2014.

23. Smith–Spangler C and others: Are organic foods safer or healthier than conventional alternatives? A systematic review. *Annals of Internal Medicine*. 157(5):348, 2012.

24. Gavrilova NA, Gavrilov LA: Comments on dietary restriction, Okinawa diet and longevity. *Gerontology* 58:221, 2012.

25. Takase H and others: Dietary sodium consumption predicts future blood pressure and incident hypertension in the Japanese normotensive general population. *Journal of the American Heart Association* 4(8):e001959, 2015.

Chapter 4

1. Saladin KS: *Anatomy & physiology*. 7th ed. Boston: McGraw–Hill Publishing Company, 2015.

2. Kulkarni B, Mattes R: Evidence for presence of nonesterified fatty acids as potential gustatory signaling molecules in humans. *Chemical Senses*. 38(2):119, 2013.

3. Feng P and others: Taste bud homeostasis in health, disease, and aging. *Chemical Senses*. 39: 3, 2014.

4. Vanputte CL and others: *Seeley's Essentials of Anatomy & Physiology*. Boston: McGraw–Hill Publishing Company, 2017.

5. Jayasinghe TN and others: The new era of treatment for obesity and metabolic disorders: Evidence and expectations for Gut Microbiome Transplantation. *Frontiers in Cellular and Infection Microbiology* 6:15, 2016.

6. Marchesi JR and others: The gut microbiota and host health: A new clinical frontier. *Gut* 65(2):330, 2016.

7. The basics of probiotics. *NIH Medline Plus* 10(4): 22, 2016. https://www.nlm.nih.gov/medlineplus/magazine/issues/winter16 /articles/winter16pg22.html Accessed: May 14, 2017.

8. Durchschein F and others: Diet therapy for inflammatory bowel diseases: the established and the new. *World Journal of Gastroenterology* 22(7):2179, 2016.

9. National Institutes of Health, National Institute of Diabetes and Digestive and Kidney Diseases: *Constipation: Definition and facts for constipation*. 2014. https://www.niddk.nih.gov/health –information/health–topics/digestive–diseases/constipation/Pages /definition–facts.aspx Accessed: May 14, 2017.

10. National Institutes of Health, U.S. National Library of Medicine, Medline Plus: *Nausea and vomiting—adults*. 2015. https://www.nlm .nih.gov/medlineplus/ency/article/003117.htm Accessed: July 12, 2017.

11. National Institutes of Health, National Institute of Diabetes and Digestive and Kidney Diseases: *Acid reflux (GER & GERD) in adults*. 2014. https://www.niddk.nih.gov/health–information /digestive–diseases/acid–reflux–ger–gerd–adults Accessed: May 14, 2017.

12. National Institutes of Health, National Institute of Diabetes and Digestive and Kidney Diseases: *Peptic ulcer disease*. 2014. https:// www.niddk.nih.gov/health–information/digestive–diseases /peptic–ulcers–stomach–ulcers Accessed: May 14, 2017.

13. National Institutes of Health, National Institute of Diabetes and Digestive and Kidney Diseases: *Irritable bowel syndrome*. 2015. https://www.nlm.nih.gov/medlineplus/ency/article/000246.htm Accessed: May 14, 2017.

14. Cozma–Petruţ A and others: Diet in irritable bowel syndrome: What to recommend, not what to forbid to patients! *World Journal of Gastroenterology*. 23(21):3771, 2017.

Chapter 5

1. U.S. Department of Agriculture, Economic Research Service: *U.S. sugar supply and use*. Tables 51, 52, and 53. Last updated June 7, 2016. http://www.ers.usda.gov/data–products/sugar–and –sweeteners–yearbook–tables.aspx#25456 Accessed: May 15, 2017.

2. U.S. Food and Drug Administration: *Guidance for industry: Ingredients declared as evaporated cane juice*. May 2016. https://www.fda.gov/food/guidanceregulation/guidancedocuments regulatoryinformation/ucm181491.htm Accessed: May 15, 2017.

3. Centers for Disease Control and Prevention: *Botulism*. Last updated May 2016. https://www.cdc.gov/botulism/index.html Accessed: May 15, 2017.

4. Academy of Nutrition and Dietetics: Position of the Academy of Nutrition and Dietetics: Use of nutritive and nonnutritive sweeteners. *Journal of the Academy of Nutrition and Dietetics* 112 (5):739, 2012.

5. Swithers SE: Artificial sweeteners produce the counterintuitive effect of inducing metabolic derangements. *Trends in Endocrinology & Metabolism* 24(9):431, 2013.

6. U.S. Food and Drug Administration: *High intensity sweeteners.* 2014. https://www.fda.gov/Food/IngredientsPackagingLabeling /FoodAdditivesIngredients/ucm397716.htm Accessed: May 15, 2017.

7. FDA provides guidance on "whole grain" for manufacturers. *FDANews,* P06–23. Updated April 2013. http://www.fda.gov /NewsEvents/Newsroom/PressAnnouncements/2006/ucm108598 .htm Accessed: May 15, 2017.

8. Otten JJ and others (eds.): *Dietary Reference Intakes: The essential guide to nutrient requirements.* Washington, DC: National Academies Press, 2006.

9. U.S. Department of Agriculture, Agricultural Research Service: *What we eat in America, NHANES 2013–2014: Nutrient intakes from food and beverages: Mean amounts consumed by individuals: By gender and age.* 2016. https://www.ars.usda.gov/ARSUserFiles /80400530/pdf/1314/Table_1_NIN_GEN_13.pdf Accessed: May 15, 2017.

10. Patel R, DuPont HL: New approaches for bacteriotherapy: Prebiotics, new–generation probiotics, and synbiotics. *Clinical Infectious Diseases* 60(Suppl 2): S108, 2015. Published online April 28, 2015.

11. U.S. Department of Health and Human Services and U.S. Department of Agriculture: *2015–2020 Dietary Guidelines for Americans.* 2015. http://health.gov/dietaryguidelines/2015/guidelines/ Accessed: May 15, 2017.

12. U.S. Department of Agriculture, Agricultural Research Service: What's in the food you eat *search tool,* 2013–2014. https://www .ars.usda.gov/northeast–area/beltsville–md/beltsville–human –nutrition–research–center/food–surveys–research–group /docs/whats–in–the–foods–you–eat–emsearch–toolem /Accessed: May 15, 2017.

13. Saris WH: Sugars, energy metabolism, and body weight control. *American Journal of Clinical Nutrition* 78(*Suppl*):850S–857S, 2003.

14. U.S. Department of Agriculture, Human Nutrition Information Service: *Nationwide Food Consumption Survey: Food and nutrient intakes by individuals in the United States, 1 day, 1987–88.* Report no. 87–I–1, 1993.

15. Drewnowski A, Rehm CD: Consumption of added sugars among US children and adults by food purchase location and food source. *American Journal of Clinical Nutrition* 100(3):901, 2014.

16. Augustin LSA and others: Glycemic index, glycemic load and glycemic response: An International Scientific Consensus Summit from the International Carbohydrate Quality Consortium (ICQC). *Nutrition, Metabolism & Cardiovascular Diseases* 25:795, 2015.

17. Bray GA, Popkin BM: Dietary sugar and body weight: Have we reached a crisis in the epidemic of obesity and diabetes? *Diabetes Care* 37:950, 2014.

18. Alonso–Alonso M and others: Food reward system: current perspectives and future research needs. *Nutrition Reviews* 73(5):296, 2015.

19. National Institutes of Health, Institute of Diabetes and Digestive and Kidney Diseases: *Nonalcoholic fatty liver disease & NASH.* 2014. https://www.niddk.nih.gov/health–information/liver –disease/nafld–nash Accessed: May 15, 2017.

20. Centers for Disease Control and Prevention: *2014 National diabetes statistics report.* Updated 2015. https://www.cdc.gov/diabetes /data/statistics/2014StatisticsReport.html Accessed: May 15, 2017.

21. Centers for Disease Control and Prevention, National Center for Health Statistics: *Leading causes of death.* Last updated March 2017. https://www.cdc.gov/nchs/fastats/leading–causes –of–death.htm Accessed: May 17, 2017.

22. Pereira PF and others: Does breastfeeding influence the risk of developing diabetes mellitus in children? A review of current evidence. *Jornal de Pediatria* 90(1):7, 2014.

23. American Diabetes Association: *What is gestational diabetes?* Last edited 2016. http://www.diabetes.org/diabetes–basics/gestational /what–is–gestational–diabetes.html?referrer=https://www.google .com/ Accessed: May 15, 2017.

24. American Diabetes Association: *How to treat gestational diabetes.* Last edited 2014. http://www.diabetes.org/diabetes–basics /gestational/how–to–treat–gestational.html Accessed: May 15, 2017.

25. American Diabetes Association: *A1C and eAG.* 2014. http://www .diabetes.org/living–with–diabetes/treatment–and–care/blood –glucose–control/a1c/ Accessed: May 15, 2017.

26. National Institutes of Health, Institute of Diabetes and Digestive and Kidney Diseases: Diabetes prevention program (DPP). ND. https://www.niddk.nih.gov/about–niddk/research–areas/diabetes /diabetes–prevention–program–dpp/Pages/default.aspx Accessed: May 15, 2017.

27. American Diabetes Association: *Improving diet quality reduces risk for type 2 diabetes.* 2014. http://www.diabetes.org/newsroom /press–releases/2014/improving–diet–quality–reduces–risk–for –type–2–diabetes.html Accessed: May 15, 2017.

28. Esposito K and others: A journey into a Mediterranean diet and type 2 diabetes: A systematic review with meta–analyses. *British Medical Journal Open* 2015;5:e008222.

29. Earl J: Dog saves the life of a sleeping boy with type 1 diabetes. *CBS News* March 7, 2016. http://www.cbsnews.com/news/dog –saves–the–life–of–sleeping–boy–with–type–1–diabetes/ Accessed: July 6, 2017.

30. Hardin DS and others: Dogs can be successfully trained to alert to hypoglycemia samples from patients with type 1 diabetes. *Diabetes Therapy* 6 (4): 509, 2015. http://link.springer.com/article/10.1007 %2Fs13300–015–0135–x

31. Neupane S and others: Exhaled breath isoprene rises during hypoglycemia in type 1 diabetes. *Diabetes Care* 39(7):e97, 2016. http://dx.doi.org/10.2337/dc16–0461

32. National Institutes of Health, Institute of Diabetes and Digestive and Kidney Diseases: *Low blood glucose (hypoglycemia).* 2016. https://www.niddk.nih.gov/health–information/diabetes/overview /preventing–problems/low–blood–glucose–hypoglycemia Accessed: May 15, 2017.

33. Baidal DA and others: Correspondence: Bioengineering of an intraabdominal endocrine pancreas. *The New England Journal of Medicine* 376:1887, 2017.

34. National Institutes of Health, National Heart, Lung, and Blood Institute: *How is metabolic syndrome diagnosed?* 2016. https:// www.nhlbi.nih.gov/health/health–topics/topics/ms/diagnosis Accessed: May 18, 2017.

35. National Institutes of Health, U.S. National Library of Medicine, PubMed Health: *Metabolic syndrome.* Updated 2014. https:// www.ncbi.nlm.nih.gov/pubmedhealth/PMH0062969/ Accessed: May 18, 2017.

36. National Institutes of Health, Institute of Diabetes and Digestive and Kidney Diseases: *Lactose intolerance.* 2014. http://www .niddk.nih.gov/health–information/health–topics /digestive–diseases/lactose–intolerance/Pages/facts.aspx Accessed: May 18, 2017.

37. Montalto M and others: Management and treatment of lactose malabsorption. *World Journal of Gastroenterology* 12(2):187, 2006.

38. Centers for Disease Control and Prevention, Attention Deficit/Hyperactivity Disorder: *Facts about ADHD*. Last updated: April 2016. https://www.cdc.gov/ncbddd/adhd/diagnosis.html Accessed: May 18, 2017.

39. Centers for Disease Control and Prevention, Attention Deficit/Hyperactivity Disorder: *Data & Statistics*. Last updated: February 2017. https://www.cdc.gov/ncbddd/adhd/data.html Accessed: May 17, 2017.

40. National Institutes of Health, Institute of Diabetes and Digestive and Kidney Diseases: *Diverticular disease*. 2016. https://www.niddk.nih.gov/health−information/digestive−diseases/diverticulosis−diverticulitis Accessed: May 18, 2017.

41. World Health Organization: *Cancer: fact sheets*. Updated February 2017. http://www.who.int/mediacentre/factsheets/fs297/en/ Accessed: May 18, 2017.

42. Centers for Disease Control and Prevention: *What are the risk factors for colorectal cancer?* Last updated: April 2016. https://www.cdc.gov/cancer/colorectal/basic_info/risk_factors.htm Accessed: May 17, 2017.

43. Maagaard L and others: Follow−up of patients with functional bowel symptoms treated with a low FODMAP diet. *World Journal of Gastroenterology* 22(15):4009, 2016. http://dx.doi.org/10.3748/wjg.v22.i15.4009

44. Barclay AW and others: Glycemic index, glycemic load, and chronic disease risk—a meta−analysis of observational studies. *American Journal of Clinical Nutrition* 87(3):627, 2008.

45. Foster−Powell K and others: International table of glycemic index and glycemic load values. *American Journal of Clinical Nutrition* 76(1):5, 2002.

46. Denova−Gutierrez E and others: Dietary glycemic index, dietary glycemic load, blood lipids, and coronary heart disease. *Journal of Nutrition and Metabolism*. Published online 2010 February 28.

47. Jenkins DJ and others: Effect of low−glycemic index or a high−cereal fiber diet on type 2 diabetes: A randomized trial. *Journal of the American Medical Association* 300(23):2742, 2008.

48. American Diabetes Association: *Glycemic index and diabetes*. 2014. http://www.diabetes.org/food−and−fitness/food/what−can−i−eat/understanding−carbohydrates/glycemic−index−and−diabetes.html Accessed: May 17, 2017.

Chapter 6

1. Position of the Academy of Nutrition and Dietetics: Dietary fatty acids for healthy adults. *Journal of the Academy of Nutrition and Dietetics* 114(1):136, 2014.

2. Otten JJ and others (eds.): *Dietary Reference Intakes: The essential guide to nutrient requirements*. Washington, DC: National Academies Press, 2006.

3. Federal Trade Commission, Press Release: *FTC sends refunds to consumers who purchased Disney− or Marvel Hero−themed children's vitamins*. 2013. https://www.ftc.gov/news−events/press−releases/2013/08/ftc−sends−refunds−consumers−who−purchased−disney−or−marvel−hero Accessed: May 20, 2017.

4. Remig V and others: Trans fat in America: A review of their use, consumption, health implications, and regulation. *Journal of the American Dietetic Association* 110(4):585, 2010.

5. U.S. Food and Drug Administration, FDA News Release: *The FDA takes step to remove artificial trans fat in processed foods*. Updated 2015. https://www.fda.gov/newsevents/newsroom/pressannouncements/ucm451237.htm Accessed: May 20, 2017.

6. Mozaffarian D: Dietary and policy priorities for cardiovascular disease, diabetes, and obesity: A comprehensive review. *Circulation* 33(2):187, 2016.

7. U.S. Department of U.S. Department of Health and Human Services: *2015–2020 Dietary Guidelines for Americans*. 2015. http://health.gov/dietaryguidelines/2015/guidelines/ Accessed: May 20, 2017.

8. Oregon State University, Linus Pauling Institute: *Choline*. Updated 2015. http://lpi.oregonstate.edu/mic/other−nutrients/choline Accessed: May 20, 2017.

9. Bosner MS and others: Percent cholesterol absorption in normal women and men quantified with dual stable isotopic tracers and negative ion mass spectrometry. *Journal of Lipid Research* 40: 302, 1999.

10. U.S. Department of Agriculture, Agricultural Research Service: *What we eat in America, NHANES 2013−2014: Nutrient intakes from food and beverages: Mean amounts consumed by individuals: By gender and age*. 2016. https://www.ars.usda.gov/ARSUserFiles/80400530/pdf/1314/Table_1_NIN_GEN_13.pdf Accessed: May 20, 2017.

11. National Center for Health Statistics: *Health, United States*, 2016. https://www.cdc.gov/nchs/data/hus/2016/019.pdf Accessed: June 28, 2017.

12. Hoogeveen RC and others: Small dense low−density lipoprotein−cholesterol concentrations predict risk for coronary heart disease: The Atherosclerosis Risk in Communities (ARIC) study. *Arteriosclerosis, Thrombosis, and Vascular Biology*, 34:1069, 2014.

13. Zhou M−S and others: Nicotine potentiates proatherogenic effects of oxLDL by stimulating and upregulating macrophage CD36 signaling. *American Journal of Physiology, Heart and Circulatory Physiology* 305(4): H563, 2013.

14. Kohan AB: ApoC−III: A potent modulator of hypertriglyceridemia and cardiovascular disease. *Current Opinion in Endocrinology, Diabetes and Obesity* 22(2): 119, 2015.

15. National Institutes of Health, National Heart, Lung, and Blood Institute: Who is at risk for atherosclerosis? Updated June 22, 2016. http://www.nhlbi.nih.gov/health/health−topics/topics/atherosclerosis/atrisk Accessed: May 20, 2017.

16. National Institutes of Health, National Center for Integrative and Complementary Health: *Hypertension (high blood pressure)*. Page last modified April 2016. https://nccih.nih.gov/health/hypertension Accessed: May 20, 2017.

17. American Heart Association: *Cardiovascular disease & diabetes*. 2015. http://www.heart.org/HEARTORG/Conditions/Diabetes/WhyDiabetesMatters/Cardiovascular−Disease−Diabetes_UCM_313865_Article.jsp/#.V3AyHPkrLIU Accessed: July 12, 2017.

18. Centers for Disease Control and Prevention, Smoking & Tobacco Use: *Health effects of cigarette smoking*. Last updated May 2017. https://www.cdc.gov/tobacco/data_statistics/fact_sheets/health_effects/effects_cig_smoking/index.htm Accessed: July 12, 2017.

19. Centers for Disease Control and Prevention, Smoking & Tobacco Use: *Secondhand smoke (SHS) facts*. Updated February 2017. https://www.cdc.gov/tobacco/data_statistics/fact_sheets/secondhand_smoke/general_facts/index.htm Accessed: July 12, 2017.

20. Rosinger A and others: Trends in total cholesterol, triglycerides, and low−density lipoprotein in US adults, 1999–2014. *JAMA Cardiology*. Published online November 30, 2016.

21. Centers for Disease Control and Prevention, National Center for Health Statistics: *Cholesterol*. Last updated January 2017. https://www.cdc.gov/nchs/fastats/cholesterol.htm Accessed: May 20, 2017.

22. Mayo Clinic: *How important is cholesterol ratio?* April 2015. http://www.mayoclinic.org/cholesterol–ratio/expert–answers/faq–20058006 Accessed: May 20, 2017.

23. Lubrano V, Balzan S: Consolidated and emerging inflammatory markers in coronary artery disease. *World Journal of Experimental Medicine* 5(1):21, 2015.

24. Sun Y and others: Influence of cigarette smoking on burden and characteristics of coronary artery plaques in Chinese men. *Acta Cardiologica Sinica* 31(5): 398, 2015.

25. Fernandez ML, West KL: Mechanisms by which dietary fatty acids modulate plasma lipids. *Journal of Nutrition* 135(9):2075, 2005.

26. National Institutes of Health, National Institute for Complementary and Integrative Health: *Omega–3 supplements: in depth.* 2015. https://nccih.nih.gov/health/omega3/introduction.htm Accessed: May 20, 2017.

27. Shin JY and others: Egg consumption in relation to risk of cardiovascular disease and diabetes: A systematic review and metaanalysis. *American Journal of Clinical Nutrition* 98(1):146, 2013.

28. National Institutes of Health, National Center for Complementary and Integrative Health: *Herbs at a glance: Garlic.* Updated 2016. https://nccih.nih.gov/health/garlic/ataglance.htm Accessed: May 20, 2017.

29. Maji D and others: Safety of statins. *Indian Journal of Endocrinology and Metabolism* 17(4):636, 2013.

30. National Institutes of Health, National Institute on Alcohol Abuse and Alcoholism: *Women and drinking.* 2015. https://pubs.niaaa.nih.gov/publications/brochurewomen/women.htm Accessed: May 20, 2017.

31. Substance Abuse and Mental Health Services Administration, Center for Behavioral Health Statistics and Quality: *Key substance use and mental health indicators in the United States: Results from the* 2015 *National Survey on Drug Use and Health.* 2016. https://www.samhsa.gov/data/sites/default/files/NSDUH–FFR1–2015/NSDUH–FFR1–2015/NSDUH–FFR1–2015.pdf Accessed: May 20, 2017.

32. Centers for Disease Control and Prevention, Alcohol and Public Health: *Fact sheets—binge drinking.* 2016. https://www.cdc.gov/alcohol/faqs.htm#heavy Accessed: May 20, 2017.

33. National Institutes of Health, National Institute on Alcohol Abuse and Alcoholism: *Alcohol use disorder.* ND. https://www.niaaa.nih.gov/alcohol–health/overview–alcohol–consumption/alcohol–use–disorders Accessed: May 20, 2017.

34. Centers for Disease Control and Prevention, Alcohol and Public Health: *Fact sheets—preventing excessive alcohol use.* 2016. https://www.cdc.gov/alcohol/fact–sheets/prevention.htm Accessed: May 20, 2017.

35. American Cancer Society: *Alcohol use and cancer.* Last updated April 2017. https://www.cancer.org/cancer/cancercauses/dietand–physicalactivity/alcohol–use–and–cancer Accessed: May 20, 2017.

36. American Heart Association: *Alcohol & heart health.* 2015. https://www.heart.org/HEARTORG/Conditions/More/MyHeartandStroke News/Alcohol–and–Heart–Disease_UCM_305173_Article.jsp#.V3MzWfkrLlU Accessed: May 20, 2017.

37. Rossi RE and others: Diagnosis and treatment of nutritional deficiencies in alcoholic liver disease: Overview of available evidence and open issues. *Digestive and Liver Disease* 47: 819, 2015.

38. Wilsnack SC and others: Women and the costs of alcohol use. *Alcohol Research* 35(2):219, 2014.

Chapter 7

1. Shier D and others: *Hole's human anatomy & physiology.* 14th ed. Boston: McGraw–Hill Publishing Company, 2017.

2. De Luca A and others: Taurine: The appeal of a safe amino acid for skeletal muscle disorders. *Journal of Translational Medicine* 13:243, 2015.

3. Reeds PJ: Dispensable and indispensable amino acids for humans. *Journal of Nutrition* 130:1835S, 2000.

4. Food and Nutrition Board: *Dietary Reference Intakes for energy, carbohydrate, fiber, fat, fatty acids, cholesterol, protein, and amino acids (macronutrients).* Institute of Medicine of the National Academies, Washington, DC: National Academies Press, 2005.

5. Oelke EA and others: Quinoa. *Alternative Field Crops Manual.* University of Wisconsin–Extension, University of Minnesota: Center for Alternative Plant & Animal Productions, and the Minnesota Extension Service. ND. https://hort.purdue.edu/newcrop/afcm/quinoa.html Accessed: July 12, 2017.

6. Reinwald S and others: Whole versus the piecemeal approach to evaluating soy. *Journal of Nutrition* 140(12):2335S, 2010.

7. Layman DK: Dietary Guidelines should reflect new understandings about adult protein needs. *Nutrition & Metabolism* 6:12, 2009.

8. U.S. Department of Agriculture, Agricultural Research Service: *What we eat in America, NHANES 2013–2014: Nutrient intakes from food and beverages: Mean amounts consumed by individuals: By gender and age.* 2016. https://www.ars.usda.gov/ARSUserFiles/80400530/pdf/1314/Table_1_NIN_GEN_13.pdf Accessed: July 12, 2017.

9. U.S. Department of Agriculture, Center for Nutrition Policy: *Protein contributed from major foods groups.* 2014. https://www.cnpp.usda.gov/reports–publications Accessed: May 28, 2017.

10. U.S. Department of Agriculture: *ChooseMyPlate.gov: All about the protein foods group.* https://www.choosemyplate.gov/protein–foods Accessed: May 28, 2017.

11. Gallup.com: *In U.S., 5% of Americans consider themselves vegetarians.* July 26, 2012. http://www.gallup.com/poll/156215/consider–themselves–vegetarians.aspx Accessed: May 28, 2017.

12. Melina V and others: Position of the Academy of Nutrition and Dietetics: Vegetarian diets. *Journal of the Academy of Nutrition and Dietetics* 116(12):1970, 2016.

13. Rizzo NS and others: Nutrient profiles of vegetarian and nonvegetarian dietary patterns. *Journal of the Academy of Nutrition and Dietetics* 113(12):1610, 2013.

14. Caspero A: *Five myths about building a healthy vegetarian meal.* Reviewed June 2016. http://www.eatright.org/resource/food/nutrition/vegetarian–and–special–diets/building–a–healthy–vegetarian–meal–myths–and–facts Accessed: May 17, 2017.

15. Kocaoglu C and others: Cerebral atrophy in a vitamin B12–deficient infant of a vegetarian mother. *Journal of Health, Population and Nutrition* 32(2):367, 2014.

16. Zuromski KL and others: Increased prevalence of vegetarianism among women with eating pathology. *Eating Behaviors* 19:24, 2015.

17. Rohrmann S and others: Meat consumption and mortality—results from the European prospective investigation into cancer and nutrition. *BMC Medicine* 11:63, 2013. http://www.biomedcentral.com/1741–7015/11/63

18. American Cancer Society: *Colorectal cancer risk factors.* Revised April 2017. https://www.cancer.org/cancer/colonandrectumcancer/detailedguide/colorectal–cancer–risk–factors Accessed: May 28, 2017.

19. Aykan NF: Red meat and colorectal cancer. *Oncology Reviews* 9:288, 2015.

20. American Cancer Society: *Pancreatic cancer risk factors*. Last revised May 2016. https://www.cancer.org/cancer/pancreaticcancer/detailedguide/pancreatic–cancer–risk–factors Accessed: May 28, 2017.

21. American Cancer Society: *What are the risk factors for stomach cancer?* Revised February 2016. http://www.cancer.org/cancer/stomachcancer/detailedguide/stomach–cancer–risk–factors Accessed: May 28, 2017.

22. Cuenca–Sánchez M and others: Controversies surrounding high–protein diet intake: Satiating effect and kidney and bone health. *Advances in Nutrition* 6(3):260, 2015.

23. Delimaris I: Adverse effects associated with protein intake above the recommended dietary allowance for adults. *ISRN Nutrition* 2013. http://dx.doi.org/10.5402/2013/126929

24. National Institutes of Health, National Institute of Diabetes and Digestive and Kidney Diseases: *Eating, diet, & nutrition for kidney stones*. May 2017. https://www.niddk.nih.gov/health–information/health–topics/urologic–disease/diet–for–kidney–stone–prevention/Pages/facts.aspx Accessed: May 28, 2017.

25. Leidy HJ and others: The role of protein in weight loss and maintenance. *American Journal of Clinical Nutrition*. 2015 Apr 29. pii: ajcn084038.

26. World Health Organization: *Double burden of malnutrition*. ND. http://www.who.int/nutrition/double–burden–malnutrition/en/ Accessed: May 28, 2017.

27. National Institutes of Health, National Institute of Allergy and Infectious Diseases, News Releases: *Peanut allergy prevention strategy is nutritionally safe, NIH–funded study shows*. June 10, 2016. https://www.nih.gov/news–events/news–releases/peanut–allergy–prevention–strategy–nutritionally–safe–nih–funded–study–shows Accessed: May 17, 2017.

28. National Institutes of Health, National Institute of Allergy and Infectious Diseases: *Food allergy*. Updated May 2016. https://www.niaid.nih.gov/topics/foodallergy/Pages/default.aspx Accessed: May 28, 2017.

29. American College of Allergy, Asthma, and Immunology: *Food allergy*. ND. http://acaai.org/allergies/types/food–allergies Accessed: May 28, 2017.

30. National Institutes of Health, National Institute of Diabetes and Digestive and Kidney Diseases: *Celiac disease: Definition and facts for celiac disease*. June 16, 2016. https://www.niddk.nih.gov/health–information/health–topics/digestive–diseases/celiac–disease/Pages/overview.aspx Accessed: May 28, 2017.

31. National Institutes of Health, National Library of Medicine, Genetics Home Reference: *Phenylketonuria*. Reviewed 2012. https://ghr.nlm.nih.gov/condition/phenylketonuria# Accessed: May 28, 2017.

32. National Institutes of Health, MedlinePlus: *Phenylketonuria*. Last updated: June 2016. https://www.nlm.nih.gov/medlineplus/ency/article/001166.htm Accessed: May 28, 2017.

33. Prasad C and others: Introducing nutritional genomics teaching in undergraduate dietetic curricula. *Journal of Nutrigenetics and Nutrigenomics* 4(3):165, 2011.

34. Saukko P: State of play in direct–to–consumer genetic testing for lifestyle–related diseases: Market, marketing content, user experiences and regulation. *Proceedings of the Nutrition Society* 72: 53, 2013.

35. U.S. Department of Agriculture, Food Safety and Inspection Service: *Food product dating*. 2016. https://www.fsis.usda.gov/wps/portal/fsis/topics/food–safety–education/get–answers/food–safety–fact–sheets/food–labeling/food–product–dating/food–product–dating Accessed: May 28, 2017.

Chapter 8

1. Bartholomew, M: James Lind's *Treatise of the Scurvy* (1753). *Postgraduate Medicine* 78:695, 2002.

2. Food and Nutrition Board: *Dietary Reference Intakes for vitamin C, vitamin E, selenium, and carotenoids*. Washington, DC: National Academy Press, 2000.

3. Regan L and others: Why US adults use dietary supplements. *JAMA Internal Medicine* 173(5):355, 2013.

4. U.S. Department of Agriculture, Agricultural Research Service: *What we eat in America, NHANES 2013–2014: Nutrient intakes from food and beverages: Mean amounts consumed by individuals: By gender and age*. 2016. https://www.ars.usda.gov/ARSUserFiles/80400530/pdf/1314/Table_1_NIN_GEN_13.pdf Accessed: June 4, 2017.

5. National Institutes of Health, Office of Dietary Supplements: *Vitamin C*. Updated February 2016. https://ods.od.nih.gov/factsheets/VitaminC–HealthProfessional/ Accessed: June 4, 2017.

6. Food and Drug Administration: *Radiation–emitting products: Microwave oven radiation*. Updated 2016. https://www.fda.gov/radiation–emittingproducts/resourcesforyouradiationemittingproducts/ucm252762.htm Accessed: June 4, 2017.

7. National Institutes of Health, Office of Dietary Supplements: *Vitamin A: Fact sheet for health professionals*. Updated 2016. https://ods.od.nih.gov/factsheets/VitaminA–HealthProfessional/ Accessed: June 4, 2017.

8. World Health Organization, Nutrition: *Micronutrient deficiencies*. ND. http://www.who.int/nutrition/topics/vad/en/ Accessed: June 4, 2017.

9. Holick MF: Vitamin D deficiency. *New England Journal of Medicine* 357:266, 2007.

10. National Institutes of Health, Office of Dietary Supplements: *Vitamin D*. Updated: February 2016. https://ods.od.nih.gov/factsheets/VitaminD–HealthProfessional/ Accessed: June 4, 2017.

11. Wacker M, Holick MF: Sunlight and vitamin D: Global perspective for health. *Dermato–Endocrinology* 5(1):51, 2013.

12. Bischoff–Ferrari HA and others: Benefit–risk assessment of vitamin D supplementation. *Osteoporosis International* 21(7): 1121, 2010.

13. National Institutes of Health, Office of Dietary Supplements: *Vitamin E*. Updated May 9, 2016. https://ods.od.nih.gov/factsheets/VitaminE–HealthProfessional/ Accessed: June 4, 2017.

14. National Institutes of Health, Office of Dietary Supplements: *Vitamin K*. Updated 2016. https://ods.od.nih.gov/factsheets/VitaminK–HealthProfessional/ Accessed: June 4, 2017.

15. National Institutes of Health, Office of Dietary Supplements: *Thiamin*. Updated: February 2016. https://ods.od.nih.gov/factsheets/Thiamin–HealthProfessional/ Accessed: June 4, 2017.

16. National Institutes of Health, Office of Dietary Supplements: *Riboflavin*. Updated: February 2016. https://ods.od.nih.gov/factsheets/Riboflavin–HealthProfessional/ Accessed: June 4, 2017.

17. Oregon State University, Linus Pauling Institute, Micronutrient Information Center: *Niacin*. Reviewed: 2013. http://lpi.oregonstate.edu/mic/vitamins/niacin Accessed: June 4, 2017.

18. National Institutes of Health, Medline Plus: *Niacin and niacinamide (vitamin B3)*. 2016. https://www.nlm.nih.gov /medlineplus/druginfo/natural/924.html Accessed: June 4, 2017.

19. National Institutes of Health, Office of Dietary Supplements: *Vitamin B6*. Updated: February 2016. https://ods.od.nih.gov /factsheets/VitaminB6–HealthProfessional/ Accessed: June 4, 2017.

20. Oregon State University, Linus Pauling Institute, Micronutrient Information Center: *Vitamin B–12*. Last updated: June 2015. http://lpi.oregonstate.edu/mic/vitamins/vitamin–B12 Accessed: June 4, 2017.

21. National Institutes of Health, Office of Dietary Supplements: *Folate*. April 2016. https://ods.od.nih.gov/factsheets/Folate –HealthProfessional/ Accessed: June 4, 2017.

22. Centers for Disease Control and Prevention, Folic Acid Homepage: *Data and statistics*. March 2016. http://www.cdc.gov/ncbddd /folicacid/data.html Accessed: June 4, 2017.

23. Dali–Youcef N, Andrès R: An update on cobalamin deficiency in adults. *Quarterly Journal of Medicine* 102(1):17, 2008.

24. National Institutes of Health, Office of Dietary Supplements: *Vitamin B12*. Updated: February 2016. https://ods.od.nih.gov/factsheets /VitaminB12–HealthProfessional/ Accessed: June 4, 2017.

25. Oregon State University, Linus Pauling Institute, Micronutrient Information Center: *Vitamin C*. Updated 2014. http://lpi .oregonstate.edu/mic/vitamins/vitamin–C Accessed: June 4, 2017.

26. Oregon State University, Linus Pauling Institute, Micronutrient Information Center: *Choline*. Updated January 2015. http://lpi .oregonstate.edu/mic/other–nutrients/choline Accessed: June 4, 2017.

27. Ellsworth MA and others: Acute liver failure secondary to niacin toxicity. *Case Reports in Pediatrics* Article ID 692530, 3 pages, 2014.

28. U.S. Preventive Services Task Force: *Final recommendation statement: Vitamin supplementation to prevent cancer and CVD: Counseling, February 2014*. 2014. http://www .uspreventiveservicestaskforce.org/Page/Document /RecommendationStatementFinal/vitamin–supplementation–to –prevent–cancer–and–cvd–counseling Accessed: June 4, 2017.

29. Guallar E and others: Enough is enough: Stop wasting money on vitamin and mineral supplements. *Annals of Internal Medicine* 159(12): 850, 2013.

30. Liu RH: Health benefits of fruits and vegetables are from additive and synergistic combinations of phytochemicals. *American Journal of Clinical Nutrition* 78:517S, 2003.

31. American Cancer Society: *Cancer facts & figures 2017*. http://www. cancer.org/research/cancerfactsstatistics/index Accessed: June 4, 2017.

32. National Institutes of Health, National Cancer Institute: *Risk factors for cancer*. 2015. https://www.cancer.gov/about–cancer /causes–prevention/risk Accessed: June 4, 2017.

33. National Institutes of Health, National Cancer Institute: *Stomach (gastric) cancer prevention (PDQ®)–Health professional version*. March 2017. https://www.cancer.gov/types/stomach/hp /stomach–prevention–pdq Accessed: June 4, 2017.

34. National Institutes of Health, National Cancer Institute: *About cancer: Causes and prevention: Risk factors: Diet*. 2015 https:// www.cancer.gov/about–cancer/causes–prevention/risk/diet Accessed: June 4, 2017.

35. American Cancer Society: *Body weight and cancer risk*. Last revised February 2016. http://www.cancer.org/cancer/cancercauses /dietandphysicalactivity/bodyweightandcancerrisk/body–weight –and–cancer–risk–effects Accessed: June 4, 2017.

36. American Cancer Society, ACS Guidelines on Nutrition and Physical Activity for Cancer Prevention: *Common questions about diet and cancer*. Last revised: February 2016. http://www.cancer. org/healthy/eathealthygetactive/acsguidelinesonnutritionphysica lactivityforcancerprevention/acs–guidelines–on–nutrition–and –physical–activity–for–cancer–prevention–common–questions Accessed: June 4, 2017.

37. American Cancer Society, Bladder Cancer: *Bladder cancer risk factors*. Last revised: May 2016. https://www.cancer.org/ cancer/bladdercancer/detailedguide/bladder–cancer–risk–factors Accessed: June 4, 2017.

Chapter 9

1. Centers for Disease Control and Prevention: Hyperthermia and dehydration–related deaths associated with intentional rapid weight loss in three collegiate wrestlers—North Carolina, Wisconsin, and Michigan, November–December 1997. *Morbidity and Mortality Weekly Report* 47:105, 1998. http://www.cdc.gov/mmwr/preview /mmwrhtml/00051388.htm

2. Negoianu D, Goldfarb S: Just add water. *Journal of the American Society of Nephrology* 19(6):1041, 2008.

3. Food and Nutrition Board, Institute of Medicine: *Dietary Reference Intakes for water, potassium, sodium, chloride, and sulfate*. Washington, DC: National Academy Press, 2004.

4. Saladin KS: *Anatomy & Physiology*. 7th ed. Boston: McGraw–Hill Publishing Company, 2015.

5. Office of Dietary Supplements, National Institutes of Health: *Calcium*. Updated November 2016. https://ods.od.nih.gov /factsheets/Calcium–HealthProfessional/ Accessed: June 14, 2017.

6. Valtrin H: "Drink at least eight glasses of water a day." Really? Is there evidence for "8 × 8"? *American Journal of Physiological Regulation and Integrative Comparative Physiology* 283: R993, 2002.

7. Verster JC, Berthélemy O: Consumer satisfaction and efficacy of the hangover cure After–Effect©. *Advances in Preventive Medicine* 2012. Article ID 617942. http://dx.doi.org/10.1155/2012/617942

8. Casa DJ and others: American College of Sports Medicine roundtable on hydration and physical activity: Consensus statements. *Current Sports Medicine Reports* 4:115, 2005.

9. American College of Sports Medicine: *Selectively and effectively using hydration for fitness*. 2011. https://www.acsm.org/docs /brochures/selecting–and–effectively–using–hydration–for –fitness.pdf Accessed: June 14, 2017.

10. U.S. Department of Health and Human Services: *Bone health and osteoporosis: A report of the Surgeon General*. Rockville, MD: U.S. Department of Health and Human Services, Office of the Surgeon General, 2004. http://www.ncbi.nlm.nih.gov/books /NBK45513/ Accessed: June 14, 2017.

11. Weaver CM and others: Choices for achieving adequate dietary calcium with a vegetarian diet. *American Journal of Clinical Nutrition* 70(suppl):543S, 1999.

12. National Institutes of Health, Medline Plus: *Calcium carbonate with magnesium overdose*. 2015. https://www.nlm.nih .gov/medlineplus/ency/article/002539.htm Accessed: June 14, 2017.

13. U.S. Department of Agriculture, Agricultural Research Service: *What we eat in America, NHANES 2013–2014: Nutrient intakes from food and beverages: Mean amounts consumed by individu– als: By gender and age*. 2016. https://www.ars.usda.gov /ARSUserFiles/80400530/pdf/1314/Table_1_NIN_GEN_13.pdf Accessed: June 14, 2017.

14. National Osteoporosis Foundation: *What is osteoporosis and what causes it?* ND. https://www.nof.org/patients/what–is–osteoporosis/ Accessed: June 14, 2017.

15. National Institute of Arthritis and Musculoskeletal and Skin Diseases: *Osteoporosis overview.* 2015. http://www.niams.nih.gov/Health _Info/Bone/Osteoporosis/overview.asp Accessed: June 14, 2017.

16. National Institutes of Health, NIH Senior Health: *Osteoporosis: frequently asked questions.* 2015. http://nihseniorhealth.gov /osteoporosis/faq/faq18.html Accessed: June 14, 2017.

17. Centers for Disease Control and Prevention: *Most Americans should consume less sodium.* Last updated: June 2016. http:// www.cdc.gov/salt/index.htm Accessed: June 14, 2017.

18. Jackson SL and others: Prevalence of excess sodium intake in the United States—NHANES, 2009–2012. *Morbidity and Mortality Weekly Report* 64(52):1393, 2016.

19. Centers for Disease Control and Prevention: *High blood pressure.* Last updated March 2017. http://www.cdc.gov/bloodpressure/ Accessed: June 14, 2017.

20. National Heart, Lung, and Blood Institute: *Description of the DASH eating plan.* 2015. http://www.nhlbi.nih.gov/health /health–topics/topics/dash Accessed: June 14, 2017.

21. Office of Dietary Supplements, National Institutes of Health: *Magnesium.* Updated: February 2016. http://ods.od.nih.gov/ factsheets/Magnesium–HealthProfessional/ Accessed: June 14, 2017.

22. Food and Nutrition Board: *Dietary Reference Intakes for vitamin A, vitamin K, arsenic, boron, chromium, copper, iodine, iron, manganese, molybdenum, nickel, silicon, vanadium, and zinc.* Washington, DC: National Academy Press, 2000.

23. Ghosh K: Non–haematological effects of iron deficiency—A perspective. *Indian Journal of Medical Sciences* 60:30, 2006.

24. World Health Organization: Miconutrient deficiencies: *Iron deficiency anemia.* ND. http://www.who.int/nutrition/topics/ida/ en/ Accessed: June 14, 2017.

25. Oregon State University, Linus Pauling Institute, Micronutrient Information Center: *Iron.* Updated: April 2016. http://lpi .oregonstate.edu/mic/minerals/iron Accessed: June 14, 2017.

26. American Red Cross: *Blood donors step up; urgent need remains.* 2014. http://www.redcross.org/news/article/Blood–Shortage –Looms–Red–Cross–Issues–Urgent–Call–for–Donors Accessed: June 14, 2017.

27. National Institutes of Health, Office of Dietary Supplements: *Iron.* Updated: February 2016. https://ods.od.nih.gov/factsheets/Iron –HealthProfessional/ Accessed: June 14, 2017.

28. National Institutes of Health, National Institute for Diabetes and Digestive and Kidney Diseases: *Hemochromatosis.* 2014. https:// www.niddk.nih.gov/health–information/health–topics/liver –disease/hemochromatosis/Pages/facts.aspx Accessed: June 14, 2017.

29. Prasad A: Zinc deficiency. *British Medical Journal* 326:409, 2003.

30. Prasad AS and others: Zinc deficiency in sickle cell disease. *Clinical Chemistry* 21:582, 1975.

31. Office of Dietary Supplements, National Institutes of Health: *Dietary supplement fact sheet: Zinc.* Updated: February 2016. https://ods.od.nih.gov/factsheets/Zinc–HealthProfessional/ Accessed: June 14, 2017.

32. Office of Dietary Supplements, National Institutes of Health: *Dietary supplement fact sheet: Iodine.* Updated June 2011. https://ods.od.nih.gov/factsheets/Iodine–HealthProfessional/ Accessed: June 14, 2017.

33. Office of Dietary Supplements, National Institutes of Health: *Dietary supplement fact sheet: Selenium.* Updated: February 2016. https://ods.od.nih.gov/factsheets/Selenium–HealthProfessional/ Accessed: June 14, 2017.

34. Office of Dietary Supplements, National Institutes of Health: *Chromium.* Updated 2013. https://ods.od.nih.gov/factsheets /Chromium–HealthProfessional/ Accessed: June 14, 2017.

35. Oregon State University, Linus Pauling Institute, Micronutrient Information Center: *Manganese.* 2010. http://lpi.oregonstate.edu /mic/minerals/manganese Accessed: June 14, 2017.

36. Oregon State University, Linus Pauling Institute, Micronutrient Information Center: *Molybdenum.* 2013. http://lpi.oregonstate.edu /mic/minerals/molybdenum Accessed: June 15, 2017.

37. Food and Drug Administration: *Questions & answers: Arsenic in rice and rice products.* April 2016. http://www.fda.gov/Food /FoodborneIllnessContaminants/Metals/ucm319948.htm Accessed: June 15, 2017.

38. International Bottled Water Association: Bottled water—the nation's healthiest beverage—sees accelerated growth and consumption. May 24, 2016. http://www.bottledwater.org/bottled –water–%E2%80%93–nation%E2%80%99s–healthiest–beverage –%E2%80%93–sees–accelerated–growth–and–consumption Accessed: June 15, 2017.

39. Environmental Protection Agency: *Water health series: Bottled water basics.* 2005. https://www.epa.gov/sites/production/files /2015–11/documents/2005_09_14_faq_fs_healthseries_bottledwater .pdf Accessed: June 15, 2017.

40. Food and Drug Administration: *FDA regulates the safety of bottled water beverages including flavored water and nutrient– added water beverages.* Updated: April 2016. http://www.fda.gov /Food/ResourcesForYou/Consumers/ucm046894.htm Accessed: June 15, 2017.

41. National Institutes of Health, National Institute of Environmental Health Sciences: *Bisphenol A (BPA).* Last reviewed: March 2017. http://www.niehs.nih.gov/health/topics/agents/sya–bpa/index.cfm Accessed: June 15, 2017.

Chapter 10

1. National Institutes of Health, National Heart Lung and Blood Institute: *Aim for a healthy weight: Why is a healthy weight important?* ND. https://www.nhlbi.nih.gov/health/educational/lose _wt/ Accessed: July 13, 2017.

2. Fryar CD and others: *Prevalence of overweight, obesity, and extreme obesity among adults aged 20 and over: United States, 1960–1962 through 2013–2014.* 2016. https://www.cdc.gov /nchs/data/hestat/obesity_adult_13_14/obesity_adult_13_14.htm Accessed: July 13, 2017.

3. Centers for Disease Control and Prevention: *Adult obesity causes & consequences.* 2016. https://www.cdc.gov/obesity/adult/causes .html Accessed: July 13, 2017.

4. Centers for Disease Control and Prevention: *Childhood obesity facts: Prevalence of childhood obesity in the United States, 2011–2014.* Last updated: April 2017. https:// www.cdc.gov/obesity/data/childhood.html Accessed: July 13, 2017.

5. World Health Organization: *Obesity and overweight.* Updated: June 2016. http://www.who.int/mediacentre/factsheets/fs311/en/ Accessed: July 13, 2017.

6. U.S. Department of Health and Human Services: *Healthy People 2020: Nutrition and weight status.* https://healthypeople.gov/2020/topicsobjectives2020/objectiveslist.aspx?topicId=29 Accessed: July 13, 2017.

7. Warner A, Mittag J: Breaking BAT: Can browning be better than white? *Journal of Endocrinology* 228(1):R19, 2016.

8. Singh P and others: Effects of weight gain and weight loss on regional fat distribution. *American Journal of Clinical Nutrition* 96: 229, 2012.

9. Luebberding S and others: Cellulite: An evidence–based review. *American Journal of Clinical Dermatology* 16(4):243, 2015.

10. Bosch TA and others: Identification of sex–specific thresholds for accumulation of visceral adipose tissue in adults. *Obesity (Silver Spring)* 23(2):375, 2015.

11. Food and Nutrition Board, National Institute of Health: *Dietary Reference Intakes for energy, carbohydrate, fiber, fat, fatty acids, cholesterol, protein, and amino acids (macronutrients).* Washington, DC: National Academies Press, 2005.

12. Williams MH and others: *Nutrition for Health, Fitness & Sport.* 11th ed. New York: McGraw–Hill, 2017.

13. Roberts SB, Dallal GE: Energy requirements and aging. *Public Health Nutrition* 8:1028, 2005.

14. Haugen HA and others: Variability of measured resting metabolic rate. *American Journal of Clinical Nutrition* 78:1141, 2005.

15. Garland T Jr. and others: The biological control of voluntary exercise, spontaneous physical activity and daily energy expenditure in relation to obesity: Human and rodent perspectives. *Journal of Experimental Biology* 214(2):206, 2011.

16. Tremblay MA and others: Systematic review of sedentary behaviour and health indicators in school–aged children and youth. *International Journal of Behavioral Nutrition and Physical Activity* 8:98, 2011.

17. Inoue S and others: Television viewing time is associated with overweight/obesity among older adults, independent of meeting physical activity and health guidelines. *Journal of Epidemiology* 22(1):50, 2012.

18. National Institutes of Health, National Heart, Lung, and Blood Institute: *Reduce screen time.* 2013. https://www.nhlbi.nih.gov/health/educational/wecan/reduce–screen–time/ Accessed: July 13, 2017.

19. Vadeboncoeur C and others: A meta–analysis of weight gain in first year university students: Is freshman 15 a myth? *BMC Obesity* 2: 22, 2015.

20. Fryar CD and others: Anthropometric reference data for children and adults: United States, 2011–2014. *Vital Health Statistics* 3(39):1, 2016.

21. Kitahara CM and others: Association between class III obesity (BMI of 40–59 kg/m²) and mortality: A pooled analysis of 20 prospective studies. *PLoS Medicine* 11(7), 2014.

22. Schvey NA and others: The impact of weight stigma on caloric consumption. *Obesity* 19(10):1957, 2011.

23. Bidulescu A and others: Gender differences in the association of visceral and subcutaneous adiposity with adiponectin in African Americans: The Jackson Heart Study. *BMC Cardiovascular Disorders* 13:9, 2013.

24. Jensen MD and others: 2013 AHA/ACC/TOS Guideline for the management of overweight and obesity in adults: A report of the American College of Cardiology/American Heart Association Task Force on Practice Guidelines and The Obesity Society. *Circulation* November 12, 2013.

25. Münzberg H, Morrison CD: Structure, production and signaling of leptin. *Metabolism* 64(1):13, 2015. Published online September 28, 2014.

26. Softic S and others: Role of dietary fructose and hepatic de novo lipogenesis in fatty liver disease. *Digestive Diseases and Sciences* 61(5):1282, 2016.

27. McNay DEG, Speakman JR: High fat diet causes rebound weight gain. *Molecular Metabolism* 2(2):103, 2013. Published online November 2, 2012.

28. U.S. Department of Agriculture, Agricultural Research Service: *What we eat in America, NHANES 2013–2014: Nutrient intakes from food and beverages: Mean amounts consumed by individuals: By gender and age.* 2016. https://www.ars.usda.gov/ARSUserFiles/80400530/pdf/1314/Table_1_NIN_GEN_13.pdf Accessed: July 13, 2017.

29. U.S. Department of Health and Human Services, Centers for Disease Control and Prevention, National Center for Health Statistics: *Early release of selected estimates based on data from the 2016 National Health Interview Survey: Leisure–time physical activity.* Released: May 2017. https://www.cdc.gov/nchs/nhis/releases/released201705.htm#7 Accessed: June 19, 2017.

30. Morandi A and others: Estimation of newborn risk for child or adolescent obesity: Lessons from longitudinal birth cohorts. *PLoS One* 7(11):e49919, 2012. http://journals.plos.org/plosone/article?id=10.1371/journal.pone.0049919

31. Harrod CS and others: Exposure to prenatal smoking and early–life body composition: The healthy start study. *Obesity (Silver Spring)* 23(1):234, 2015.

32. Hicken MT: Racial and ethnic differences in the association between obesity and depression in women. *Journal of Women's Health* 22(5):445, 2013.

33. Raynor HA, Champagne CM: Position of the Academy of Nutrition and Dietetics: Interventions for the treatment of overweight and obesity in adults. *Journal of the Academy of Nutrition and Dietetics* 116(1):129, 2016.

34. Wilson P: Physical activity and dietary determinants of weight loss success in the US general population. *American Journal of Public Health* 106(2):321, 2016.

35. Hall KD and others: Energy balance and its components: Implications for body weight regulation. *American Journal of Clinical Nutrition* 95(4):989, 2012.

36. Schoeller DA and others: Self–report–based estimates of energy intake offer an inadequate basis for scientific conclusions. *American Journal of Clinical Nutrition* 97(6):1413, 2013.

37. Dyrstad SM and others: Comparison of self–reported versus accelerometer–measured physical activity. *Medicine & Science in Sports & Exercise* 46(1):99, 2014.

38. National Weight Control Registry. ND. http://www.nwcr.ws/ Accessed: July 13, 2017.

39. Neff KJ and others: Bariatric surgery: The challenges with candidate selection, individualizing treatment and clinical outcomes. *BMC Medicine* 11:8, 2013. Published online January 10, 2013.

40. U.S. Food and Drug Administration, FDA News Release: *FDA approves first–of–kind device to treat obesity.* January 14, 2015.

http://www.fda.gov/NewsEvents/Newsroom/PressAnnouncements/ucm430223.htm Accessed: June 17, 2017.

41. U.S. Food and Drug Administration, FDA News Release: *FDA approves AspireAssist obesity device.* June 14, 2016. http://www.fda.gov/newsevents/newsroom/pressannouncements/ucm506625.htm Accessed: June 17, 2017.

42. Nicklas JM and others: Successful weight loss among obese U.S. adults. *American Journal of Preventive Medicine* 42 (5):481, 2012.

43. Johnston BC and others: Comparison of weight loss among named diet programs in overweight and obese adults: A meta−analysis. *Journal of the American Medical Association* 312(9):923, 2014.

44. Bazzano LA and others: Effects of low−carbohydrate and low−fat diets: A randomized trial. *Annals of Internal Medicine* 161(5):309, 2014.

45. Federal Trade Commission, Bureau of Consumer Protection: *Weighing the claims in diet ads.* 2012. http://www.consumer.ftc.gov/articles/0061−weighing−claims−diet−ads Accessed: June 17, 2017.

46. Fryar CD and others: *Prevalence of underweight among adults aged 20 and over: United States, 1960-1962 through 2013-2014.* Last updated: July 18, 2016. http://www.cdc.gov/nchs/data/hestat/underweight_adult_13_14/underweight_adult_13_14.htm Accessed: June 17, 2017.

47. American Psychiatric Association: Feeding and eating disorders. In *Diagnostic and Statistical Manual of Mental Disorders.* 5th ed. 2013.

48. Eating Disorders Victoria: *Eating disorders.* February 2017. https://www.eatingdisorders.org.au/eating−disorders/what−is−an−eating−disorder/risk−factors Accessed: June 18, 2017.

49. National Institutes of Health, National Institute of Mental Health: *Eating disorders.* 2016. https://www.nimh.nih.gov/health/topics/eating−disorders/index.shtml Accessed: June 18, 2017.

50. Ozier AD, Henry BW: Position of the American Dietetic Association: Nutrition intervention in the treatment of eating disorders. *Journal of the American Dietetic Association* 111(8):1236, 2011.

51. Stice E and others: Prevalence, incidence, impairment, and course of the proposed DSM−5 eating disorder diagnoses in an 8−year prospective community study of young women. *Journal of Abnormal Psychology* 122(2):455, 2013.

52. Pinheiro AP and others: The genetics of anorexia nervosa: Current findings and future perspectives. *International Journal of Child and Adolescent Health* 2(2):153, 2009.

53. Mitchison D, Hay PJ: The epidemiology of eating disorders: genetic, environmental, and societal factors. *Clinical Epidemiology* 6:89, 2014.

54. Smink FR and others: Epidemiology of eating disorders: Incidence, prevalence, and mortality rates. *Current Psychiatry Reports* 14:406, 2012.

55. Dimitropoulos G and others: Inpatients with severe anorexia nervosa and their siblings: Non−shared experiences and family functioning. *European Eating Disorders Review* 21:284, 2013.

56. Quiles−Marcos Y and others: Peer and family influence in eating disorders: A meta−analysis. *European Psychiatry* 28:199, 2013.

57. Helfert S, Warschburger P: The face of appearance−related social pressure: Gender, age and body mass variations in peer and parental pressure during adolescence. *Child and Adolescent Psychiatry and Mental Health* 7(16):1, 2013.

58. Centers for Disease Control and Prevention: *About adult BMI.* Updated 2015. http://www.cdc.gov/healthyweight/assessing/bmi/adult_bmi/index.html Accessed: June 17, 2017.

59. Harrington BC and others: Initial evaluation, diagnosis, and treatment of anorexia nervosa and bulimia nervosa. *American Family Physician* 91(1):46, 2015.

60. National Institutes of Health, National Institute of Mental Health: *Eating disorders.* 2016. https://www.nimh.nih.gov/health/topics/eating−disorders/index.shtml Accessed: June 18, 2017

61. Ishigami A and others: Postmortem diagnosis of anorexia nervosa: An endocrinological and immunohistochemical approach. *Journal of Medical Investigation* 63(3−4):305, 2016.

62. Fischer S and others: Night eating syndrome in young adults: Delineation from other eating disorders and clinical significance. *Psychiatry Research* 200:494, 2012.

63. Allison KC and others: An open−label efficacy trial of escitalopram for night eating syndrome. *Eating Behaviors* 14:199, 2013.

64. Gagnon C and others: Comorbid diabetes and eating disorders in adult patients: Assessment and considerations for treatment. *Diabetes Educator* 35:537, 2012.

65. Matheiu J: What is diabulimia? *Journal of the American Dietetic Association* 108(5):769, 2008.

66. Murray SB and others: Muscle dysmorphia and the DSM−V conundrum: Where does it belong? A review paper. *International Journal of Eating Disorders* 43:483, 2010.

67. Tod D and others: Muscle dysmorphia: current insights. *Psychology Research and Behavior Management* 9:179, 2016.

68. Gibbs JC and others: Prevalence of individual and combined components of the female athlete triad. *Medicine and Science in Sports and Exercise* 45(5):985, 2013.

69. Nazem TH, Ackerman KE: The female athlete triad. *Sports Health* 4(4):302, 2012.

70. Thein−Nissenbaum J: Long−term consequences of the female athlete triad. *Maturitas* 75:107, 2013.

71. National Eating Disorder Association: *What Should I Say?* http://www.nationaleatingdisorders.org/what−should−i−say Accessed: June 17, 2017.

Chapter 11

1. U.S. Department of Health and Human Services, Centers for Disease Control and Prevention, National Center for Health Statistics: *Early release of selected estimates based on data from the 2016 National Health Interview Survey: Leisure−time physical activity.* Released: May 2017. https://www.cdc.gov/nchs/nhis/releases/released201705.htm#7 Accessed: June 19, 2017.

2. Centers for Disease Control and Prevention: *Physical activity: How much physical activity do adults need?* Last updated: 2015. https://www.cdc.gov/physicalactivity/basics/adults/index.htm Accessed: June 19, 2017.

3. Centers for Disease Control and Prevention: *Physical activity and health: The benefits of physical activity.* Updated June 2015. https://www.cdc.gov/physicalactivity/everyone/health/index.html Accessed: June 19, 2017.

4. Department of Health and Human Services: *2008 Physical activity guidelines for Americans summary.* 2008. https://health.gov/paguidelines/guidelines/summary.aspx Accessed: June 19, 2017.

5. Centers for Disease Control and Prevention: *Target heart rate and estimated maximum heart rate.* Updated August 2015. https://www.cdc.gov/physicalactivity/everyone/measuring/heartrate.html Accessed: June 19, 2017.

6. Centers for Disease Control and Prevention: *General physical activities defined by level of intensity.* ND. https://www.cdc.gov/nccdphp/dnpa/physical/pdf/PA_Intensity_table_2_1.pdf Accessed: June 19, 2017.

7. Position of the Academy of Nutrition and Dietetics, Dietitians of Canada, and the American College of Sports Medicine: Nutrition and athletic performance. *Journal of the Academy of Nutrition and Dietetics* 116(3):501, 2016.

8. Jeppesen J, Kiens B: Regulation and limitations to fatty acid oxidation during exercise. *Journal of Physiology* 590:1059, 2012.

9. Yeo WK and others: Fat adaptation in well–trained athletes: Effects on cell metabolism. *Applied Physiology, Nutrition, and Metabolism* 36:12, 2011.

10. Economos CD and others: Nutritional practices of elite athletes: Practical recommendations. *Sports Medicine* 16:381, 1993.

11. Otten JJ and others (eds.): *Dietary Reference Intakes: The essential guide to nutrient requirements.* Institute of Medicine of the National Academies. Washington, DC: National Academies Press, 2006.

12. Poole C and others: The role of post–exercise nutrient administration on muscle protein synthesis and glycogen synthesis. *Journal of Sports Science and Medicine* 9:354, 2010.

13. Wismann J, Willoughby D: Gender differences in carbohydrate metabolism and carbohydrate loading. *Journal of the International Society of Sports Nutrition* 3(1):28, 2006.

14. Hulmi JJ and others: Effect of protein/essential amino acids and resistance training on skeletal muscle hypertrophy: A case for whey protein. *Nutrition and Metabolism* 7:51, 2010.

15. National Institutes of Health, National Center for Complementary and Integrative Health: *Asian ginseng.* Updated 2016. https://nccih.nih.gov/health/asianginseng/ataglance.htm Accessed: June 19, 2017.

16. Coyle EF: Fluid and fuel intake during exercise. *Journal of Sports Science* 22:39, 2004.

17. National Library of Medicine: MedLinePlus: *Heat emergencies.* Updated November 2015. https://medlineplus.gov/ency/article/000056.htm Accessed: June 19, 2017.

18. International Marathon Medical Directors Association: *IMMDA's health recommendations for runners & walkers.* 2010. http://immda.org/wp–content/uploads/2015/08/Spring–2010–Health–Recommendations–for–Runners–Walkers.pdf Accessed: June 19, 2017.

19. Powers SK and others: Dietary antioxidants and exercise. *Journal of Sports Sciences* 22:81, 2004.

20. U.S. Food and Drug Administration: *Import alert 66–71.* April 2017. https://www.accessdata.fda.gov/cms_ia/importalert_204.html Accessed: June 19, 2017.

21. National Collegiate Athletic Association: *NCAA 2017–2018 banned drugs.* http://www.ncaa.org/sites/default/files/2017_18_NCAA_Banned_Drugs_20170605.pdf Accessed: June 19, 2017.

22. U.S. Anti–doping Agency: *Prohibited list.* January 2017. https://www.usada.org/substances/prohibited–list/ Accessed: June 19, 2017.

23. U.S. Food and Drug Administration, Food: *Pure powdered caffeine.* Updated 2015. https://www.fda.gov/food/dietarysupplements/productsingredients/ucm460095.htm June 19, 2017.

Chapter 12

1. Centers for Disease Control and Prevention: *The burden of norovirus illness and outbreaks.* 2016. https://www.cdc.gov/norovirus/php/illness–outbreaks.html Accessed: June 26, 2017.

2. Centers for Disease Control and Prevention: *Preventing norovirus infection.* Last updated: July 15, 2016. https://www.cdc.gov/norovirus/preventing–infection.html Accessed: June 26, 2017.

3. Centers for Disease Control and Prevention, Estimates of Foodborne Illness in the United States: *Burden of foodborne illness: An overview.* Updated July 2016. https://www.cdc.gov/foodborneburden/estimates–overview.html Accessed: June 26, 2017.

4. Centers for Disease Control and Prevention: *Food–borne germs and illnesses.* Last updated: December 2015. https://www.cdc.gov/foodsafety/foodborne–germs.html Accessed: June 26, 2017.

5. Food and Drug Administration: *Bad Bug Book: Foodborne Pathogenic Microorganisms and Natural Toxins Handbook.* 2nd ed. 2012. https://www.fda.gov/food/foodborneillnesscontaminants/causesofillnessbadbugbook/default.htm Accesssed: June 26, 2017.

6. National Institutes of Health, National Institute of Diabetes and Digestive and Kidney Diseases: *Foodborne illness.* June 2014. https://www.niddk.nih.gov/health–information/health–topics/digestive–diseases/foodborne–illnesses/Pages/facts.aspx#4 Accessed: June 26, 2017.

7. U.S. Department of Agriculture, Food Safety and Inspection Service: *Molds on Foods: Are they dangerous?* 2013. https://www.fsis.usda.gov/wps/portal/fsis/topics/food–safety–education/get–answers/food–safety–fact–sheets/safe–food–handling/molds–on–food–are–they–dangerous_/ct_index Accessed: June 16, 2017.

8. U.S. Department of Health and Human Services: *Keep foods safe: Cook: Cook to the right temperature.* ND. https://www.foodsafety.gov/keep/basics/cook/index.html Accessed: June 26, 2017.

9. U.S. Department of Agriculture, Food Safety and Inspection Service: *Cooking safely in the microwave oven.* August 2013. https://www.fsis.usda.gov/wps/portal/fsis/topics/food–safety–education/get–answers/food–safety–fact–sheets/appliances–and–thermometers/cooking–safely–in–the–microwave/cooking–safely–in–the–microwave–oven Accessed: June 16, 2017.

10. Miranda RC, Schaffner DW: Longer contact times increase cross–contamination of *Enterobacter aerogenes* from surfaces to food. *Applied and Environmental Microbiology* 82(21):6490, 2016.

11. U.S. Department of Agriculture, Food Safety and Inspection Service: *Basics of handling foods safely: Cold storage chart.* Modified 2015. https://www.fsis.usda.gov/wps/portal/fsis/topics/food–safety–education/get–answers/food–safety–fact–sheets/safe–food–handling/basics–for–handling–food–safely/ct_index/ Accessed: June 26, 2017.

12. U.S. Department of Agriculture, Food Safety and Inspection Service: *Keeping food safe during an emergency.* 2006. https://www.fsis.usda.gov/shared/PDF/Keeping_Food_Safe_During_an_Emergency.pdf Accessed: June 26, 2017.

13. Food and Drug Administration: *Food irradiation: What you need to know.* Last updated June 2016. https://www.fda.gov/Food/ResourcesForYou/Consumers/ucm261680.htm Accessed: June 26, 2017.

14. Casey–Lockyer M and others: Deaths associated with Hurricane Sandy—October–November 2012. *Morbidity and Mortality Weekly Report* 62(20):393, 2013.

15. Federal Emergency Management Agency: *Six months report*: *Superstorm Sandy from pre−disaster to recovery*. 2013. https://www.fema.gov/disaster/4086/updates/6−months−report−superstorm−sandy−pre−disaster−recovery Accessed: June 26, 2017.

16. U.S. Food and Drug Administration: *Food: Overview of food ingredients, additives & colors*. Page last updated 2014. http://www.fda.gov/food/ingredientspackaginglabeling/foodadditivesingredients/ucm094211.htm Accessed: June 23, 2017.

17. U.S. Environmental Protection Agency: *Summary of the Food Quality Protection Act*. Page last updated 2016. https://www.epa.gov/laws−regulations/summary−food−quality−protection−act Accessed: June 23, 2017.

18. U.S. Food and Drug Administration, Food: *Defect levels handbook*. Last revised 2005. https://www.fda.gov/food/guidanceregulation/guidancedocumentsregulatoryinformation/sanitationtransportation/ucm056174.htm Accessed: June 26, 2017.

19. Centers for Disease Control and Prevention: *Fourth national report on human exposure to environmental chemicals*. 2009. http://www.cdc.gov/exposurereport/pdf/FourthReport.pdf Accessed: June 26, 2017.

20. National Institutes of Health, National Cancer Institute: *Agricultural health study*. Last reviewed 2011. https://www.cancer.gov/about−cancer/causes−prevention/risk/ahs−fact−sheet Accessed: June 26, 2017.

21. Connor BA: Chapter 2: The pre−travel consultation: Self−treatable conditions. *CDC health information for international travel* 2018. Last updated June 12, 2017. https://wwwnc.cdc.gov/travel/yellowbook/2018/the−pre−travel−consultation/travelers−diarrhea Accessed: June 26, 2017.

22. Centers for Disease Control and Prevention: *Water disinfection*. 2013. https://wwwnc.cdc.gov/travel/page/water−disinfection Accessed: June 26, 2017.

Chapter 13

1. Otten JJ and others (eds.): Institute of Medicine: *Dietary Reference Intakes: The essential guide to nutrient requirements*. Washington, DC: National Academies Press, 2006.

2. Centers for Disease Control and Prevention: *Unintended pregnancy prevention*. Last update: 2015. https://www.cdc.gov/reproductivehealth/UnintendedPregnancy/index.htm Accessed: July 1, 2017.

3. Thame M and others: Fetal growth is directly related to maternal anthropometry and placental volume. *European Journal of Clinical Nutrition* 58:894, 2004.

4. Centers for Disease Control and Prevention: *Infant mortality*. 2016. https://www.cdc.gov/reproductivehealth/maternalinfanthealth/infantmortality.htm Accessed: July 1, 2017.

5. Martin JA and others: Births: Final data for 2015. *National Vital Statistics Report* 66(1), January 5, 2017. https://www.cdc.gov/nchs/data/nvsr/nvsr66/nvsr66_01.pdf Accessed: July 1, 2017.

6. U.S. Department of Health and Human Services: *The health consequences of smoking—50 years of progress: A report of the Surgeon General*. 2014. https://www.surgeongeneral.gov/library/reports/50−years−of−progress/fact−sheet.html Accessed: July 1, 2017.

7. Kharrazia M and others: California very preterm birth study: Design and characteristics of the population− and biospecimen bank−based nested case control study. *Paediatric and Perinatal Epidemiology* 26(3): 250, 2012.

8. Neville MC, McManaman JL: Milk secretion and composition. In *Neonatal nutrition and metabolism*. 2nd ed. Thureen P, Hay W (eds.) New York, New York: Cambridge University Press, 2006.

9. National Library of Medicine, MedlinePlus: *Morning sickness*. Updated January 2016. https://medlineplus.gov/ency/article/003119.htm Accessed: July 1, 2017.

10. National Library of Medicine, MedlinePlus: *Hyperemesis gravidarum*. 2015. https://medlineplus.gov/ency/article/001499.htm July 1, 2017.

11. Centers for Disease Control and Prevention: *Micronutrient facts*. Last updated: 2015. https://www.cdc.gov/immpact/micronutrients/index.html Accessed: July 1, 2017.

12. Environmental Protection Agency, News releases: *EPA and FDA issue final fish consumption advice*. January 2017. https://www.epa.gov/newsreleases/epa−and−fda−issue−final−fish−consumption−advice−0 Accessed: July 2, 2017.

13. Centers for Disease Control and Prevention, Reproductive health: *Weight gain during pregnancy*. Updated March 2016. https://www.cdc.gov/reproductivehealth/maternalinfanthealth/pregnancy−weight−gain.htm Accessed: July 2, 2017.

14. Mayo Clinic Staff: *Diseases and conditions: Fetal macrosomia*. 2015. http://www.mayoclinic.org/diseases−conditions/fetal−macrosomia/basics/definition/con−20035423 Accessed: July 2, 2017.

15. March of Dimes: *Tracking your weight gain*. ND. http://www.marchofdimes.org/pregnancy/tracking−your−weight−gain.aspx Accessed: July 2, 2017.

16. U.S. Department of Health and Human Services, Office on Women's Health: ePublications: *Prenatal care fact sheet*. Last updated June 12, 2017. https://www.womenshealth.gov/a−z−topics/prenatal−care Accessed: July 2, 2017.

17. DeSisto CL and others: Prevalence estimates of gestational diabetes mellitus in the United States, Pregnancy Risk Assessment Monitoring System (PRAMS), 2007–2010. *Preventing Chronic Disease* 11:130415, 2014. doi: http://dx.doi.org/10.5888/pcd11.130415.

18. National Institutes of Health: *Preeclampsia and eclampsia: Condition information*. https://www.nichd.nih.gov/health/topics/preeclampsia/conditioninfo/Pages/default.aspx Accessed: July 2, 2017.

19. National Heart Lung and Blood Institute: *High blood pressure in pregnancy*. ND. https://www.nhlbi.nih.gov/health/public/heart/hbp/hbp_preg.htm Accessed: July 13, 2017.

20. March of Dimes: Caffeine in pregnancy. 2015. http://www.marchofdimes.org/pregnancy/caffeine−in−pregnancy.aspx Accessed: July 2, 2017.

21. National Institutes of Health: *Sudden infant death syndrome (SIDS): Overview*. https://www.nichd.nih.gov/health/topics/sids/Pages/default.aspx Accessed: July 2, 2017.

22. March of Dimes: *Exercise during pregnancy*. 2012. http://www.marchofdimes.org/pregnancy/exercise−during−pregnancy.aspx Accessed: July 2, 2017.

23. He Y and others: Human colostrum oligosaccharides modulate major immunologic pathways of immature human intestine. *Mucosal Immunology* 7(6):1326. 2014.

24. Lessen R, Kavanagh K: Position of the Academy of Nutrition and Dietetics: Promoting and supporting breastfeeding. *Journal of the Academy of Nutrition and Dietetics* 115(3):444, 2015.

25. Schiff M and others: The impact of cosmetic breast implants on breastfeeding: A systematic review and metaanalysis. *International Breastfeeding Journal* 9:17, 2014.

26. American Academy of Pediatrics: Policy Statement: *Breastfeeding and the use of human milk. Pediatrics* 129 (3):e827, 2012.

27. Centers for Disease Control and Prevention: *Breastfeeding, CDC National Immunization Survey (NIS)*. Last updated: April 2017. https://www.cdc.gov/breastfeeding/data/NIS_data/index.htm Accessed: July 2, 2017.

28. Saarela T and others: Macronutrient and energy contents of human milk fractions during the first six months of lactation. *Acta Paediatricia* 94(9):1176, 2005.

29. Fomon SJ: Infant feeding in the 20th century: Formula and beikost. *Journal of Nutrition* 131:409S, 2001.

30. American Academy of Pediatrics: Expert panel on integrated guidelines for cardiovascular health and risk reduction in children and adolescents: Summary report. *Pediatrics* 128 (S5):S213, 2011.

31. Hayes D: *Reducing the risk of food allergies*. April 2017. http://www.eatright.org/resource/health/allergies-and-intolerances/food-allergies/reducing-the-risk-from-food-allergies Accessed: July 1, 2017.

32. National Institutes of Health, National Institute of Allergies and Infectious Diseases: *Guidelines for clinicians and patients for diagnosis and management of food allergy in the United States. 2017 addendum guidelines for the prevention of peanut allergy in the United States*. January 2017. https://www.niaid.nih.gov/diseases-conditions/guidelines-clinicians-and-patients-food-allergy Accessed: January 7, 2017.

33. American Dental Association: *Chewing gum*. ND. http://www.mouthhealthy.org/en/az-topics/c/chewing-gum Accessed: July 2, 2017.

34. Reedy J, Krebs-Smith S: Dietary sources of energy, solid fats, and added sugars among children and adolescents in the United States. *Journal of the American Dietetic Association* 110(10):1477, 2010.

35. Kranz S: What do we know about dietary fiber intake in children and health? The effects of fiber intake on constipation, obesity, and diabetes in children. *Advances in Nutrition* 3(1):47, 2012.

36. Rampersaud GC and others: Breakfast habits, nutritional status, body weight, and academic performance in children and adolescents. *Journal of the American Dietetic Association* 105:743, 2005.

37. Saladin KS: *Anatomy & Physiology*. 7th ed. Boston: McGraw-Hill Publishing Company, 2015.

38. American Academy of Dermatology: *Growing evidence suggests possible link between diet and acne*. 2013. https://www.aad.org/media/news-releases/growing-evidence-suggests-possible-link-between-diet-and-acne Accessed: July 2, 2017.

39. Centers for Disease Control and Prevention: *Adolescent and Youth Risk Behavior Surveillance System (YRBSS)*. June 2016. https://www.cdc.gov/healthyyouth/yrbs/index.htm Accessed: July 2, 2017.

40. Position of the American Dietetic Association and Dietitians of Canada: Vegetarian diets. *Journal of the American Dietetic Association* 109:748, 2009.

41. Centers for Disease Control and Prevention: *Overweight & Obesity, Childhood Obesity Facts: Prevalence of childhood obesity in the United States, 2011–2014*. Last updated April 2017. https://www.cdc.gov/obesity/data/childhood.html Accessed: June 27, 2017.

42. Lo JC and others: Prevalence of obesity and extreme obesity in children aged 3–5 years. *Pediatric Obesity* 9(3):167, 2014.

43. Centers for Disease Control and Prevention: *Childhood obesity causes & consequences*. Updated December 2016. https://www.cdc.gov/obesity/childhood/causes.html Accessed: June 27, 2017.

44. Dattilo AM and others: Need for early interventions in the prevention of pediatric overweight: A review and upcoming directions. *Journal of Obesity* 2012:123023. Published online May 7, 2012.

45. Xu S, Xue Y: Pediatric obesity: Causes, symptoms, prevention and treatment (Review). *Experimental and Therapeutic Medicine* 11:15, 2016.

46. National Institute of Diabetes and Digestive and Kidney Diseases, Weight Control Information Network: *Bariatric surgery for severe obesity: Bariatric surgery for youth*. 2011. https://www.niddk.nih.gov/health-information/health-topics/weight-control/bariatric-surgery-severe-obesity/Pages/bariatric-surgery-for-severe-obesity.aspx Accessed: July 2, 2017.

47. Centers for Disease Control and Prevention: *Health, United States*, 2016. Table 15. https://www.cdc.gov/nchs/data/hus/hus16.pdf#015 Accessed: July 2, 2017.

48. U.S. Census Bureau: U.S. population aging slower than other countries. *Census Bureau Reports Report* Number: CB16–54. March 28, 2016. https://census.gov/newsroom/press-releases/2016/cb16-54.html Accessed: June 3, 2017.

49. U.S. Census Bureau, Data: *2014 National population projections tables, Table* 6. Last revised May 2017. https://www.census.gov/data/tables/2014/demo/popproj/2014-summary-tables.html Accessed: July 2, 2017.

50. Mokdad AH and others: Actual causes of death in the United States, 2000. *Journal of the American Medical Association* 291:1238, 2004.

51. National Academies of Sciences, Engineering, and Medicine: *Meeting the dietary needs of older adults: Exploring the impact of the physical, social, and cultural environment: Workshop summary*. 2016. Washington, DC: The National Academies Press.

52. Deierlein AL and others: Diet quality of urban older adults aged 60–99: The cardiovascular health of seniors and built environment study. *Journal of the Academy of Nutrition and Dietetics* 114(2):279, 2014.

53. Krebs-Smith SM and others: Americans do not meet federal dietary recommendations. *Journal of Nutrition* 140 (10):1832, 2010.

54. Batsis JA and others: Sarcopenia, sarcopenic obesity, and functional impairments in older adults: National Health and Nutrition Examination Surveys 1999–2004. *Nutrition Research* 35(12):1031, 2015.

55. Centers for Disease Control and Prevention, National Center for Health Statistics: *Dental caries and tooth loss in adults in the United States, 2011–2012*. May 2015. https://www.cdc.gov/nchs/data/databriefs/db197.htm Accessed: July 2, 2017.

56. Savoca MR and others: Severe tooth loss in older adults as a key indicator of compromised diet quality. *Public Health Nutrition* 13(4):466, 2010.

57. Federal Interagency Forum on Aging Related Statistics: *Older Americans 2016: Key indicators of well-being*. 2016. https://agingstats.gov/docs/LatestReport/Older-Americans-2016-Key-Indicators-of-WellBeing.pdf Accessed: July 2, 2017.

58. Centers for Disease Control and Prevention: *Ten leading causes of death and injury: Ten leading causes of death by age group—2015*. Last updated: May 2017. https://www.cdc.gov/injury/wisqars/leadingcauses.html Accessed: June 2, 2017.

59. National Institutes of Health, National Institute on Aging: *Health and aging: Can we prevent aging?* 2012. https://www.nia.nih.gov/sites/default/files/can_we_prevent_aging_0.pdf Accessed: July 2, 2017.

Appendix I

Dietary Reference Intakes (DRIs): Tables

Dietary Reference Intakes (DRIs): Recommended Intakes for Individuals, Vitamins
Food and Nutrition Board, Institute of Medicine, National Academies

Life Stage Group	Vitamin A (µg/d)[a]	Vitamin C (mg/d)	Vitamin D (µg/d)[b,c]	Vitamin E (mg/d)[d]	Vitamin K (µg/d)	Thiamin (mg/d)	Riboflavin (mg/d)	Niacin (mg/d)[e]	Vitamin B-6 (mg/d)	Folate (µg/d)[f]	Vitamin B-12 (µg/d)	Pantothenic Acid (mg/d)	Biotin (µg/d)	Choline (mg/d)[g]
Infants														
0–6 mo	400*	40*	10	4*	2.0*	0.2*	0.3*	2*	0.1*	65*	0.4*	1.7*	5*	125*
7–12 mo	500*	50*	10	5*	2.5*	0.3*	0.4*	4*	0.3*	80*	0.5*	1.8*	6*	150*
Children														
1–3 y	300	15	15	6	30*	0.5	0.5	6	0.5	150	0.9	2*	8*	200*
4–8 y	400	25	15	7	55*	0.6	0.6	8	0.6	200	1.2	3*	12*	250*
Males														
9–13 y	600	45	15	11	60*	0.9	0.9	12	1.0	300	1.8	4*	20*	375*
14–18 y	900	75	15	15	75*	1.2	1.3	16	1.3	400	2.4	5*	25*	550*
19–30 y	900	90	15	15	120*	1.2	1.3	16	1.3	400	2.4	5*	30*	550*
31–50 y	900	90	15	15	120*	1.2	1.3	16	1.3	400	2.4	5*	30*	550*
51–70 y	900	90	15	15	120*	1.2	1.3	16	1.7	400	2.4[h]	5*	30*	550*
>70 y	900	90	20	15	120*	1.2	1.3	16	1.7	400	2.4[h]	5*	30*	550*
Females														
9–13 y	600	45	15	11	60*	0.9	0.9	12	1.0	300	1.8	4*	20*	375*
14–18 y	700	65	15	15	75*	1.0	1.0	14	1.2	400[i]	2.4	5*	25*	400*
19–30 y	700	75	15	15	90*	1.1	1.1	14	1.3	400[i]	2.4	5*	30*	425*
31–50 y	700	75	15	15	90*	1.1	1.1	14	1.3	400[i]	2.4	5*	30*	425*
51–70 y	700	75	15	15	90*	1.1	1.1	14	1.5	400	2.4[h]	5*	30*	425*
>70 y	700	75	20	15	90*	1.1	1.1	14	1.5	400	2.4[h]	5*	30*	425*
Pregnancy														
≤18 y	750	80	15	15	75*	1.4	1.4	18	1.9	600[j]	2.6	6*	30*	450*
19–30 y	770	85	15	15	90*	1.4	1.4	18	1.9	600[j]	2.6	6*	30*	450*
31–50 y	770	85	15	15	90*	1.4	1.4	18	1.9	600[j]	2.6	6*	30*	450*
Lactation														
≤18 y	1200	115	15	19	75*	1.4	1.6	17	2.0	500	2.8	7*	35*	550*
19–30 y	1300	120	15	19	90*	1.4	1.6	17	2.0	500	2.8	7*	35*	550*
31–50 y	1300	120	15	19	90*	1.4	1.6	17	2.0	500	2.8	7*	35*	550*

mg = milligram, µg = microgram

NOTE: This table (taken from the DRI reports; see www.nap.edu) presents Recommended Dietary Allowances (RDAs) in **bold type** and Adequate Intakes (AIs) in ordinary type followed by an asterisk (*). RDAs and AIs may both be used as goals for individual intake. RDAs are set to meet the needs of almost all (97 to 98%) individuals in a group. For healthy breastfed infants, the AI is the mean intake. The AI for other life stage and gender groups is believed to cover needs of all individuals in the group, but lack of data or uncertainty in the data prevents being able to specify with confidence the percentage of individuals covered by this intake.

[a] As retinol activity equivalents (RAEs). 1 RAE = 1 µg retinol, 12 µg β–carotene, 24 µg α–carotene, or 24 µg β–cryptoxanthin. To calculate RAEs from REs of provitamin A carotenoids in foods, divide the REs by 2. For preformed vitamin A in foods or supplements and for provitamin A carotenoids in supplements, 1 RE = 1 RAE.

[b] cholecalciferol. 1 µg cholecalciferol = 40 IU vitamin D.

[c] In the absence of adequate exposure to sunlight.

[d] As α–tocopherol. α–Tocopherol includes RRR–α–tocopherol, the only form of α–tocopherol that occurs naturally in foods, and the 2R–stereoisomeric forms of α–tocopherol (RRR–, RSR–, RRS–, and RSS–α–tocopherol) that occur in fortified foods and supplements. It does not include the 2S–stereoisomeric forms of α–tocopherol (SRR–, SSR–, SRS–, and SSS–α–tocopherol), also found in fortified foods and supplements.

[e] As niacin equivalents (NE). 1 mg of niacin = 60 mg of tryptophan; 0–6 months = preformed niacin (not NE).

[f] As dietary folate equivalents (DFE). 1 DFE = 1 µg food folate = 0.6 µg of folic acid from fortified food or as a supplement consumed with food = 0.5 µg of a supplement taken on an empty stomach.

[g] Although AIs have been set for choline, there are few data to assess whether a dietary supply of choline is needed at all stages of the life cycle, and it may be that the choline requirement can be met by endogenous synthesis at some of these stages.

[h] Because 10 to 30% of older people may malabsorb food–bound B–12, it is advisable for those older than 50 years to meet their RDA mainly by consuming foods fortified with B–12 or a supplement containing B–12.

[i] In view of evidence linking folate intake with neural tube defects in the fetus, it is recommended that all women capable of becoming pregnant consume 400 µg from supplements or fortified foods in addition to intake of food folate from a varied diet.

[j] It is assumed that women will continue consuming 400 µg from supplements or fortified food until their pregnancy is confirmed and they enter prenatal care, which ordinarily occurs after the end of the periconceptional period—the critical time for formation of the neural tube.

Source: Adapted from the *Dietary Reference Intakes series*, National Academies Press, 1997, 1998, 2000, 2001, 2011. The full reports are available from the National Academies Press at www.nap.edu.

Dietary Reference Intakes (DRIs): Recommended Intakes for Individuals, Elements
Food and Nutrition Board, Institute of Medicine, National Academies

Life Stage Group	Calcium (mg/d)	Chromium (µg/d)	Copper (µg/d)	Fluoride (mg/d)	Iodine (µg/d)	Iron (mg/d)	Magnesium (mg/d)	Manganese (mg/d)	Molybdenum (µg/d)	Phosphorus (mg/d)	Selenium (µg/d)	Zinc (mg/d)
Infants												
0–6 mo	200*	0.2*	200*	0.01*	110*	0.27*	30*	0.003*	2*	100*	15*	2*
7–12 mo	260*	5.5*	220*	0.5*	130*	11	75*	0.6*	3*	275*	20*	3
Children												
1–3 y	700	11*	340	0.7*	90	7	80	1.2*	17	460	20	3
4–8 y	1000	15*	440	1*	90	10	130	1.5*	22	500	30	5
Males												
9–13 y	1300	25*	700	2*	120	8	240	1.9*	34	1250	40	8
14–18 y	1300	35*	890	3*	150	11	410	2.2*	43	1250	55	11
19–30 y	1000	35*	900	4*	150	8	400	2.3*	45	700	55	11
31–50 y	1000	35*	900	4*	150	8	420	2.3*	45	700	55	11
51–70 y	1000	30*	900	4*	150	8	420	2.3*	45	700	55	11
>70 y	1200	30*	900	4*	150	8	420	2.3*	45	700	55	11
Females												
9–13 y	1300	21*	700	2*	120	8	240	1.6*	34	1250	40	8
14–18 y	1300	24*	890	3*	150	15	360	1.6*	43	1250	55	9
19–30 y	1000	25*	900	3*	150	18	310	1.8*	45	700	55	8
31–50 y	1000	25*	900	3*	150	18	320	1.8*	45	700	55	8
51–70 y	1200	20*	900	3*	150	8	320	1.8*	45	700	55	8
>70 y	1200	20*	900	3*	150	8	320	1.8*	45	700	55	8
Pregnancy												
≤18 y	1300	29*	1000	3*	220	27	400	2.0*	50	1250	60	12
19–30 y	1000	30*	1000	3*	220	27	350	2.0*	50	700	60	11
31–50 y	1000	30*	1000	3*	220	27	360	2.0*	50	700	60	11
Lactation												
≤18 y	1300	44*	1300	3*	290	10	360	2.6*	50	1250	70	13
19–30 y	1000	45*	1300	3*	290	9	310	2.6*	50	700	70	12
31–50 y	1000	45*	1300	3*	290	9	320	2.6*	50	700	70	12

NOTE: This table presents Recommended Dietary Allowances (RDAs) in **bold type** and Adequate Intakes (AIs) in ordinary type followed by an asterisk (*). RDAs and AIs may both be used as goals for individual intake. RDAs are set to meet the needs of almost all (97 to 98%) individuals in a group. For healthy breastfed infants, the AI is the mean intake. The AI for other life stage and gender groups is believed to cover needs of all individuals in the group, but lack of data or uncertainty in the data prevents being able to specify with confidence the percentage of individuals covered by this intake.

Sources: *Dietary Reference Intakes for Calcium, Phosphorus, Magnesium, Vitamin D, and Fluoride* (1997); *Dietary Reference Intakes for Thiamin, Riboflavin, Niacin, Vitamin B–6, Folate, Vitamin B–12, Pantothenic Acid, Biotin, and Choline* (1998); *Dietary Reference Intakes for Vitamin C, Vitamin E, Selenium, and Carotenoids* (2000); *Dietary Reference Intakes for Vitamin A, Vitamin K, Arsenic, Boron, Chromium, Copper, Iodine, Iron, Manganese, Molybdenum, Nickel, Silicon, Vanadium, and Zinc* (2001); and *Dietary Reference Intakes for Calcium and Vitamin D* (2011). These reports may be accessed via www.nap.edu. Adapted from the Dietary Reference Intake series, National Academies Press, 1997, 1998, 2000, 2001, 2011. The full reports are available from the National Academies Press at www.nap.edu.

Dietary Reference Intakes (DRIs): Recommended Intakes for Individuals, Macronutrients
Food and Nutrition Board, Institute of Medicine, National Academies

Life Stage Group	Carbohydrate (g/d)	Total Fiber (g/d)	Fat (g/d)	Linoleic Acid (g/d)	α–Linolenic Acid (g/d)	Protein[a] (g/d)
Infants						
0–6 mo	60*	ND	31*	4.4*	0.5*	9.1*
7–12 mo	95*	ND	30*	4.6*	0.5*	11.0
Children						
1–3 y	130	19*	ND[b]	7*	0.7*	13
4–8 y	130	25*	ND	10*	0.9*	19
Males						
9–13 y	130	31*	ND	12*	1.2*	34
14–18 y	130	38*	ND	16*	1.6*	52
19–30 y	130	38*	ND	17*	1.6*	56
31–50 y	130	38*	ND	17*	1.6*	56
51–70 y	130	30*	ND	14*	1.6*	56
>70 y	130	30*	ND	14*	1.6*	56
Females						
9–13 y	130	26*	ND	10*	1.0*	34
14–18 y	130	26*	ND	11*	1.1*	46
19–30 y	130	25*	ND	12*	1.1*	46
31–50 y	130	25*	ND	12*	1.1*	46
51–70 y	130	21*	ND	11*	1.1*	46
>70 y	130	21*	ND	11*	1.1*	46
Pregnancy						
14–18 y	175	28*	ND	13*	1.4*	71
19–30 y	175	28*	ND	13*	1.4*	71
31–50 y	175	28*	ND	13*	1.4*	71
Lactation						
14–18 y	210	29*	ND	13*	1.3*	71
19–30 y	210	29*	ND	13*	1.3*	71
31–50 y	210	29*	ND	13*	1.3*	71

NOTE: This table presents Recommended Dietary Allowances (RDAs) in **bold type** and Adequate Intakes (AIs) in ordinary type followed by an asterisk (*). RDAs and AIs may both be used as goals for individual intake. RDAs are set to meet the needs of almost all (97 to 98%) individuals in a group. For healthy breastfed infants, the AI is the mean intake. The AI for other life stage and gender groups is believed to cover needs of all individuals in the group, but lack of data or uncertainty in the data prevents being able to specify with confidence the percentage of individuals covered by this intake.

[a]Based on 0.8g protein/kg body weight for reference body weight.

[b]ND = not determinable at this time.

Sources: *Dietary Reference Intakes for Energy, Carbohydrate, Fiber, Fat, Fatty Acids, Cholesterol, Protein, and Amino Acids* (2002). This report may be accessed via www.nap.edu. Adapted from the Dietary Reference Intake series, National Academies Press, 1997, 1998, 2000, 2001, by the National Academy of Sciences. The full reports are available from the National Academies Press at www.nap.edu.

Dietary Reference Intakes (DRIs): Recommended Intakes for Individuals, Electrolytes and Water
Food and Nutrition Board, Institute of Medicine, National Academies

Life Stage Group	Sodium (mg/d)	Potassium (mg/d)	Chloride (mg/d)	Water (L/d)
Infants				
0–6 mo	120*	400*	180*	0.7*
7–12 mo	370*	700*	570*	0.8*
Children				
1–3 y	1000*	3000*	1500*	1.3*
4–8 y	1200*	3800*	1900*	1.7*
Males				
9–13 y	1500*	4500*	2300*	2.4*
14–18 y	1500*	4700*	2300*	3.3*
19–30 y	1500*	4700*	2300*	3.7*
31–50 y	1500*	4700*	2300*	3.7*
51–70 y	1300*	4700*	2000*	3.7*
> 70 y	1200*	4700*	1800*	3.7*
Females				
9–13 y	1500*	4500*	2300*	2.1*
14–18 y	1500*	4700*	2300*	2.3*
19–30 y	1500*	4700*	2300*	2.7*
31–50 y	1500*	4700*	2300*	2.7*
51–70 y	1300*	4700*	2000*	2.7*
> 70 y	1200*	4700*	1800*	2.7*
Pregnancy				
14–18 y	1500*	4700*	2300*	3.0*
19–50 y	1500*	4700*	2300*	3.0*
Lactation				
14–18 y	1500*	5100*	2300*	3.8*
19–50 y	1500*	5100*	2300*	3.8*

NOTE: The table is adapted from the DRI reports. See www.nap.edu. Adequate Intakes (AIs) are followed by an asterisk (*). These may be used as a goal for individual intake. For healthy breastfed infants, the AI is the average intake. The AI for other life stage and gender groups is believed to cover the needs of all individuals in the group, but lack of data prevent being able to specify with confidence the percentage of individuals covered by this intake; therefore, no Recommended Dietary Allowance (RDA) was set.

Source: *Dietary Reference Intakes for Water, Potassium, Sodium, Chloride, and Sulfate* (2005). This report may be accessed via www.nap.edu.

Acceptable Macronutrient Distribution Ranges

	Range (percent of energy)		
Macronutrient	Children, 1–3 y	Children, 4–18 y	Adults
Fat	30–40	25–35	20–35
omega–6 polyunsaturated fats (linoleic acid)	5–10	5–10	5–10
omega–3 polyunsaturated fats[a] (α–linolenic acid)	0.6–1.2	0.6–1.2	0.6–1.2
Carbohydrate	45–65	45–65	45–65
Protein	5–20	10–30	10–35

[a]Approximately 10% of the total can come from longer–chain n–3 fatty acids.

Source: *Dietary Reference Intakes for Energy, Carbohydrate, Fiber, Fat, Fatty Acids, Cholesterol, Protein, and Amino Acids* (2002). The report may be accessed via www.nap.edu. Adapted from the *Dietary Reference Intakes series*, National Academies Press, 1997, 1998, 2000, 2001, 2011. The full reports are available from the National Academies Press at www.nap.edu.

Dietary Reference Intakes (DRIs): Tolerable Upper Intake Levels (UL[a]), Vitamins
Food and Nutrition Board, Institute of Medicine, National Academies

Life Stage Group	Vitamin A (μg/d)[b]	Vitamin C (mg/d)	Vitamin D (μg/d)	Vitamin E (mg/d)[c,d]	Vitamin K	Thiamin	Riboflavin	Niacin (mg/d)[d]	Vitamin B–6 (mg/d)	Folate (μg/d)[d]	Vitamin B–12	Pantothenic Acid	Biotin	Choline (g/d)	Carotenoids[e]
Infants															
0–6 mo	600	ND	25	ND	ND	ND	ND	ND	ND	ND	ND	ND	ND	ND	ND
7–12 mo	600	ND	38	ND	ND	ND	ND	ND	ND	ND	ND	ND	ND	ND	ND
Children															
1–3 y	600	400	63	200	ND	ND	ND	10	30	300	ND	ND	ND	1.0	ND
4–8 y	900	650	75	300	ND	ND	ND	15	40	400	ND	ND	ND	1.0	ND
Males, Females															
9–13 y	1700	1200	100	600	ND	ND	ND	20	60	600	ND	ND	ND	2.0	ND
14–18 y	2800	1800	100	800	ND	ND	ND	30	80	800	ND	ND	ND	3.0	ND
19–70 y	3000	2000	100	1000	ND	ND	ND	35	100	1000	ND	ND	ND	3.5	ND
>70 y	3000	2000	100	1000	ND	ND	ND	35	100	1000	ND	ND	ND	3.5	ND
Pregnancy															
≤18 y	2800	1800	100	800	ND	ND	ND	30	80	800	ND	ND	ND	3.0	ND
19–50 y	3000	2000	100	1000	ND	ND	ND	35	100	1000	ND	ND	ND	3.5	ND
Lactation															
≤18 y	2800	1800	100	800	ND	ND	ND	30	80	800	ND	ND	ND	3.0	ND
19–50 y	3000	2000	100	1000	ND	ND	ND	35	100	1000	ND	ND	ND	3.5	ND

[a]UL = The maximum level of daily nutrient intake likely to pose no risk of adverse effects. Unless otherwise specified, the UL represents total intake from food, water, and supplements. Due to lack of suitable data, ULs could not be established for vitamin K, thiamin, riboflavin, vitamin B–12, pantothenic acid, biotin, or carotenoids. In the absence of ULs, extra caution may be warranted in consuming levels above recommended intakes.

[b]As preformed vitamin A only.

[c]As α–tocopherol; applies to any form of supplemental α–tocopherol.

[d]The ULs for vitamin E, niacin, and folate apply to synthetic forms obtained from supplements, fortified foods, or a combination of the two.

[e]β–Carotene supplements are advised only due to lack of data of adverse effects in this age group and concern with regard to lack of ability to handle excess amounts. Source of intake should be from food only to prevent high levels of intake.

ND = Not determinable due to lack of data of adverse effects in this age group and concern with regard to lack of ability to handle excess amounts. Source of intake should be from food only to prevent high levels of intake.

Sources: Dietary Reference Intakes for Calcium, Phosphorus, Magnesium, Vitamin D, and Fluoride (1997); Dietary Reference Intakes for Thiamin, Riboflavin, Niacin, Vitamin B–6, Folate, Vitamin B–12, Pantothenic Acid, Biotin, and Choline (1998); Dietary Reference Intakes for Vitamin C, Vitamin E, Selenium, and Carotenoids (2000); and Dietary Reference Intakes for Vitamin A, Vitamin K, Arsenic, Boron, Chromium, Copper, Iodine, Iron, Manganese, Molybdenum, Nickel, Silicon, Vanadium, and Zinc (2001). These reports may be accessed via www.nap.edu. Adapted from the Dietary Reference Intakes series, National Academies Press, 1997, 1998, 2000, 2001, 2011. The full reports are available from the National Academies Press at www.nap.edu.

Dietary Reference Intakes (DRIs): Tolerable Upper Intake Levels (UL[a]), Elements and Electrolytes[b,c]
Food and Nutrition Board, Institute of Medicine, National Academies

Life Stage Group	Arsenic[b]	Boron (mg/d)	Calcium (g/d)	Copper (μg/d)	Fluoride (mg/d)	Iodine (μg/d)	Iron (mg/d)	Magnesium (mg/d)[d]	Manganese (mg/d)	Molybdenum (μg/d)	Nickel (mg/d)	Phosphorus (g/d)	Selenium (μg/d)	Vanadium (mg/d)[e]	Zinc (mg/d)	Sodium (mg/d)	Chloride (mg/d)
Infants																	
0–6 mo	ND[f]	ND	1	ND	0.7	ND	40	ND	ND	ND	ND	ND	45	ND	4	ND	ND
7–12 mo	ND	ND	1.5	ND	0.9	ND	40	ND	ND	ND	ND	ND	60	ND	5	ND	ND
Children																	
1–3 y	ND	3	2.5	1000	1.3	200	40	65	2	300	0.2	3	90	ND	7	1500	2300
4–8 y	ND	6	2.5	3000	2.2	300	40	110	3	600	0.3	3	150	ND	12	1900	2900
Males, Females																	
9–13 y	ND	11	3	5000	10	600	40	350	6	1100	0.6	4	280	ND	23	2200	3400
14–18 y	ND	17	3	8000	10	900	45	350	9	1700	1.0	4	400	ND	34	2300	3600
19–70 y	ND	20	2.5[g]	10000	10	1100	45	350	11	2000	1.0	4	400	1.8	40	2300	3600
>70 y	ND	20	2	10000	10	1100	45	350	11	2000	1.0	3	400	1.8	40	2300	3600
Pregnancy																	
≤18 y	ND	17	3	8000	10	900	45	350	9	1700	1.0	3.5	400	ND	34	2300	3600
19–50 y	ND	20	2.5	10000	10	1100	45	350	11	2000	1.0	3.5	400	ND	40	2300	3600
Lactation																	
≤18 y	ND	17	3	8000	10	900	45	350	9	1700	1.0	4	400	ND	34	2300	3600
19–50 y	ND	20	2.5	10000	10	1100	45	350	11	2000	1.0	4	400	ND	40	2300	3600

[a]UL = The maximum level of daily nutrient intake that is likely to pose no risk of adverse effects. Unless otherwise specified, the UL represents total intake from food, water, and supplements. Due to lack of suitable data, ULs could not be established for arsenic, chromium, and silicon. In the absence of ULs, extra caution may be warranted in consuming levels above recommended intakes.

[b]Although a UL was not determined for arsenic, there is no justification for adding arsenic to food or supplements.

[c]Although silicon has not been shown to cause adverse effects in humans, there is no justification for adding silicon to supplements.

[d]The ULs for magnesium represent intake from a pharmacological agent only and do not include intake from food and water.

[e]Although vanadium in food has not been shown to cause adverse effects in humans, there is no justification for adding vanadium to food and vanadium supplements should be used with caution. The UL is based on adverse effects in laboratory animals and this data could be used to set a UL for adults but not children and adolescents.

[f]ND = Not determinable due to lack of data of adverse effects in this age group and concern with regard to lack of ability to handle excess amounts. Source of intake should be from food only to prevent high levels of intake.

[g]Upper Limit declines to 2 after age 50.

Sources: Dietary Reference Intakes for Calcium and Vitamin D (2011); Dietary Reference Intakes for Calcium, Phosphorus, Magnesium, Vitamin D, and Fluoride (1997); Dietary Reference Intakes for Thiamin, Riboflavin, Niacin, Vitamin B–6, Folate, Vitamin B–12, Pantothenic Acid, Biotin, and Choline (1998); Dietary Reference Intakes for Vitamin C, Vitamin E, Selenium, and Carotenoids (2000); Dietary Reference Intakes for Vitamin A, Vitamin K, Arsenic, Boron, Chromium, Copper, Iodine, Iron, Manganese, Molybdenum, Nickel, Silicon, Vanadium, and Zinc (2001); and Dietary Reference Intakes for Water, Potassium, Sodium, Chloride, and Sulfate (2004). These reports may be accessed via www.nap.edu. Adapted from the Dietary Reference Intakes series, National Academies Press, 1997, 1998, 2000, 2001, 2011. The full reports are available from the National Academies Press at www.nap.edu.

Glossary

A

absorption   process by which substances are taken up from the GI tract and enter the bloodstream or the lymph

Acceptable Macronutrient Distribution Ranges (AMDRs)   macronutrient intake ranges that are nutritionally adequate and may reduce the risk of diet-related chronic diseases

acid-base balance   maintaining the proper pH of body fluids

acid group   acid portion of a compound

acids   substances that donate hydrogen ions

added sugars   sugars added to foods during processing or preparation

adenosine diphosphate (ADP)   high-energy compound; by-product of ATP use

adenosine triphosphate (ATP)   molecule that stores energy

Adequate Intakes (AIs)   dietary recommendations for nutrients that scientists do not have enough information to set RDAs

adipose cells   fat cells; specialized cells that store fat

adolescence   life stage in which a child matures physically into an adult

aerobic   conditions that require free oxygen

aerobic exercise   physical activities that involve sustained, rhythmic contractions of large muscle groups

air displacement   method of estimating body composition by determining body volume

aldosterone   hormone that participates in sodium and water conservation

alpha-linolenic acid   an essential fatty acid

alpha-tocopherol   vitamin E

alternative health care   health care practices that are not widely accepted and used by conventional medical practitioners

alternative sweeteners   substances that sweeten foods while providing few or no kilocalories

amino acids   nitrogen-containing chemical units that comprise proteins

amino or **nitrogen-containing group**   portion of an amino acid that contains nitrogen

anaerobic   conditions that lack free oxygen

anatomy   scientific study of cells and other body structures

anecdotes   reports of personal experiences

anemia   disorder characterized by too few red blood cells and poor oxygen transport in blood

anencephaly   type of neural tube defect in which the brain does not form properly or is missing

anorexia nervosa (AN)   severe psychological disturbance characterized by self-imposed starvation

antibodies   infection-fighting proteins

antidiuretic hormone (ADH)   hormone that participates in water conservation

antioxidant   substance that gives up electrons to radicals to protect cells

appetite   desire to eat appealing food

arterial plaque   lipid-filled deposits that form under the lining of certain arteries

arteries   vessels that carry blood away from the heart

arteriosclerosis   condition that results from atherosclerosis and is characterized by loss of arterial flexibility

ascorbic acid   vitamin C

atherosclerosis   long-term disease process in which plaques build up inside arterial walls

B

bacteria   simple single-celled microorganisms

bariatric medicine   medical specialty that focuses on the treatment of obesity

basal metabolism   minimal number of kilocalories the body uses to support vital activities after fasting and resting for 12 hours

bases   substances that accept hydrogen ions

beriberi   thiamin deficiency disease

beta-carotene   carotenoid that the body can convert to vitamin A

bile   substance that is produced by the liver to prepare fat and fat-soluble vitamins for digestion and absorption

bile salts   components of bile that enhance lipid digestion and absorption

binge eating   consuming a much larger amount of food than is normally eaten in a brief period

binge-eating disorder (BED)   eating disorder featuring recurrent episodes of binge eating that are not followed by purging behaviors

bioavailability   extent to which the digestive tract absorbs a nutrient and how well the body uses it

bioelectrical impedance   technique of estimating body composition in which a device measures the conduction of a weak electrical current through the body

biological activity   describes vitamin's degree of potency or effects in the body

biotechnology   using living things to manufacture new products

blood alcohol concentration (BAC)   percentage of alcohol in the bloodstream

body mass index (BMI)   numerical value of relationship between body weight and risk of certain chronic health problems associated with excess body fat

buffer   substance that can protect the pH of a solution

bulimia nervosa (BN)   severe psychological condition characterized by repeated episodes of binge eating followed by unhealthy behaviors to prevent weight gain

C

caffeine   naturally occurring stimulant drug

calcitonin   hormone secreted by the thyroid gland when blood calcium levels are too high

capillaries   smallest blood vessels

carbohydrate (glycogen) loading   practice of manipulating physical activity and dietary patterns to increase muscle glycogen stores

carbohydrates   class of nutrients that includes glucose, a major source of energy for the body

carcinogen   factor that triggers cancer

cardiovascular disease (CVD)   group of diseases that affect the heart and blood vessels

carotenemia   yellowing of the skin that results from excess beta-carotene in the body

carotenoids   yellow-orange pigments in fruits and vegetables

case-control study   study in which individuals who have a health condition are compared with individuals with similar characteristics who do not have the condition

casein   major protein in cow's milk

cell   smallest living functional unit in an organism

central-body obesity   condition characterized by excessive visceral fat

chemical bond   attraction that holds atoms together

chemical reactions   processes that change the atomic arrangements of molecules

chemistry   study of the composition and characteristics of matter and changes that can occur to it

cholecystokinin (CCK)   hormone that stimulates the gallbladder to release bile and pancreas to secrete digestive enzymes

cholesterol   sterol in animal foods and precursor for steroid hormones, bile, and vitamin D

choline   water-soluble compound in lecithin

chylomicron   particle formed by small intestinal cells that transports lipids in the bloodstream

chyme   mixture of gastric juice and partially digested food

coenzyme   small, organic molecule that interacts with enzymes, enabling the enzymes to function

cofactor metallic ion or small molecule that activates certain chemical reactions

cognitive behavioral therapy (CBT) psychological therapy approaches that address unhealthy emotions and behaviors

cohort study study that measures variables of a group of people over time

collagen fibrous protein that gives strength to connective tissue

color additives dyes, pigments, or other substances that provide color to food

colostrum initial form of breast milk that contains anti-infective properties

complementary combinations mixing certain plant foods to provide all essential amino acids without adding animal protein

complex carbohydrates (polysaccharides) compounds comprised of 10 or more mono-saccharides bonded together

compounds molecules that contain two or more different elements in specific proportions

conception moment when a sperm enters an egg (fertilization)

contaminated food item that is impure or unsafe for human consumption

control group group being studied that does not receive a treatment

conventional medical care health care prac-tices that are widely accepted and used by mainstream medical practitioners

coronary artery disease (CAD) a major form of CVD

correlation relationship between two variables

cretinism condition affecting infants of women who were iodine deficient during pregnancy

cross-contamination unintentional transfer of pathogenic microbes from one food to another

cytochromes group of proteins involved in the release of energy from macronutrients

D

Daily Values (DVs) set of nutrient intake stan-dards developed for labeling purposes

deamination removal of the nitrogen-containing group from an amino acid

deficiency disease state of health that occurs when a nutrient is missing from the diet

dehydration body water depletion

Delaney Clause component of the 1958 Food Additives Amendment that prevents manu-facturers from adding carcinogenic com-pounds to food

denaturation altering a protein's natural shape and function by exposing it to conditions such as heat, acids, and physical agitation

diabetes mellitus (diabetes) group of serious chronic diseases characterized by abnormal glucose, fat, and protein metabolism

diabulimia popular term used to describe people with type I diabetes who skip insulin injections or use less insulin than prescribed to control their body weight

diastolic pressure pressure in an artery that occurs when the ventricles relax between contractions

diet usual pattern of food choices

dietary fiber (fiber) nondigestible plant material; most types are polysaccharides

Dietary Reference Intakes (DRIs) various energy and nutrient intake standards for Americans

dietary supplements nutrient preparations, certain hormones, and herbal products

digestion process by which large food molecules are mechanically and chemically broken down

disaccharide simple sugar comprised of two monosaccharides

disordered eating chaotic and abnormal food-related practices

diuretic substance that increases urine production

diverticula abnormal, small sacs that form in wall of colon

DNA molecule that provides coded instructions for making proteins

double-blind study experimental design in which neither the participants nor the researchers are aware of each participant's group assignment

dual-energy x-ray absorptiometry (DXA) technique of estimating body composition that involves scanning the body with multiple low-energy x-rays

duodenum first segment of the small intestine

E

eating disorders psychological disturbances that lead to certain physiological changes and serious health complications

edema accumulation of fluid in tissues

electrolytes ions of minerals that conduct elec-tricity when they are dissolved in water

electrons small, negatively charged particles that surround the nucleus of an atom

element each type of atom; substance that cannot be separated into simpler substances by ordinary chemical or physical means

embolus thrombus or part of a plaque that breaks free and travels through the bloodstream

embryo human organism from 14 days to 8 weeks after conception

empty calories energy supplied by unhealthy solid fats, added sugars, and/or alcohol

emulsifier substance that helps water-soluble and water-insoluble compounds mix with each other

energy capacity to perform work

energy density energy value of a food in rela-tion to the food's weight

energy equilibrium calorie intake equals calo-rie output

energy intake calories from foods and beverages that contain macronutrients and alcohol

energy output calories cells use to carry out their activities

enrichment replacement of some nutrients that were removed during processing

enterohepatic circulation process that recycles cholesterol in the body

enzyme molecule (usually a protein) that speeds up a particular chemical reaction

epidemiology study of the occurrence, distribution, and causes of health problems in populations

epiglottis flap of tissue that folds down over the windpipe to keep food from entering the respiratory system during swallowing

epithelial cells cells that form protective tissues that line the body

ergogenic aids foods, devices, dietary supple-ments, or drugs used to improve physical performance

esophagus structure of the GI tract that connects the pharynx with the stomach

essential amino acids amino acids the body cannot make or make enough of to meet its needs

essential fatty acids lipids that must be supplied by the diet

essential nutrient nutrient that must be supplied by food

Estimated Average Requirement (EAR) amount of a nutrient that meets the needs of 50% of healthy people in a life stage/sex group

Estimated Energy Requirement (EER) average daily energy intake that meets the needs of a healthy person maintaining his or her weight

estrogen hormone that plays a role in normal bone development and maintenance

evidence based information that is based on results of scientific studies

Exchange System method of classifying foods into lists based on macronutrient composition

exercise physical activities that are usually planned and structured for a purpose

extracellular water water that surrounds cells or is in liquid portion of blood

extrusion reflex involuntary response in which a young infant thrusts its tongue forward when a solid or semisolid object is placed in its mouth

F

fad trendy practice that has widespread appeal for a period, then becomes no longer fashionable

fat-free mass body compartment that is com-prised of body water, mineral-rich tissues, and protein-rich tissues

fat-soluble vitamins vitamins A, D, E, and K

female athlete triad   condition that is characterized by low energy availability, menstrual problems, and reduced bone mineral density in female athletes

fermentation   process used to preserve or produce a variety of foods, including pickles and wine

fetus   human organism from 8 weeks after conception until birth

folic acid   form of folate

food additive   any substance that becomes incorporated into food during production, packaging, transport, or storage

Food Additives Amendment   U.S. legislation that requires evidence that a new food additive is safe before it can be marketed for use

Food and Nutrition Board (FNB)   group of nutrition scientists who develop DRIs

food-borne illness   disorder that is caused by consuming disease-causing agents in food or water

food-borne infection   illness that results when a pathogen in food inflames the intestinal tract or other body tissues

food insecurity   situation in which individuals or families are concerned about running out of food or not having enough money to buy more food

food intoxication   illness that results when poisons produced by certain microbes contaminate food and irritate the intestinal tract

fortification   addition of any nutrient to food to boost its nutritional value

fructose   monosaccharide in fruits, honey, and certain vegetables; "levulose" or "fruit sugar"

fungi   simple organisms that live on dead or decaying organic matter

fungicides   substances used to limit the spread of fungi

G

galactose   monosaccharide that is a component of lactose

gastroesophageal reflux disease (GERD)   condition that can result when acid reflux damages the wall of the lower esophagus and causes ulcers

gastroesophageal sphincter   section of esophagus next to the stomach that controls the opening to the stomach

gastrointestinal (GI) tract   muscular tube that extends from the mouth to the anus

gene   portion of DNA

Generally Recognized as Safe (GRAS)   ingredients considered to be safe

genetic endowment   inherited physical characteristics that can affect physical performance

genetic modification   techniques that alter an organism's DNA

gestational diabetes   form of diabetes that pregnant women can develop

gestational hypertension   type of hypertension that can develop during pregnancy

ghrelin   protein that stimulates eating behavior

glucagon   hormone that helps regulate blood glucose levels

glucose   monosaccharide that is a primary fuel for muscles and other cells; "dextrose" or "blood sugar"

glycogen   storage polysaccharide in animals

glycogenolysis   glycogen breakdown

glycolysis   first stage of glucose oxidation

goitrogens   compounds that inhibit iodide metabolism by the thyroid gland

gut microbiota   various microbes, mostly bacteria, that reside in the GI tract

gut microbiota transplantation   fecal transplants

H

H$^+$ chemical symbol for hydrogen ion

heat cramps   heat-related illness characterized by painful muscle contractions

heat exhaustion   heat-related illness that can occur after intense exercise

heatstroke   most dangerous form of heat-related illness

heme iron   form of iron in hemoglobin and myoglobin

hemoglobin   iron-containing protein in red blood cells that transports oxygen

herbicides   substances used to destroy weeds

hereditary hemochromatosis   most common type of iron overload disease

high-density lipoprotein (HDL)   lipoprotein that transports cholesterol away from tissues and to the liver, where it can be eliminated

high-fructose corn syrup (HFCS)   caloric sweetener that is often added to food

high-intensity sweeteners   group of nonnutritive sweeteners that are extremely sweet tasting compared to the same amount of sugar

high-quality (complete) protein   protein that contains all essential amino acids in amounts that support the deposition of protein in tissues and the growth of a young person

high-sensitivity C-reactive protein (hs-CRP)   protein produced primarily by the liver in response to inflammation

homeostasis   maintenance of an internal chemical and physical environment that is critical for good health and survival

homocysteine   amino acid that may play a role in the development of atherosclerosis

hunger   uncomfortable feeling that drives a person to consume food

hydration   water status

hydrocarbon chain   chain of carbon atoms bonded to each other and to hydrogen atoms

hydrophilic   part of a molecule that attracts water

hydrophobic   part of a molecule that avoids water and attracts lipids

hypercalcemia   condition characterized by higher-than-normal concentration of calcium in blood

hyperglycemia   abnormally high blood glucose level

hypertension   abnormally high blood pressure levels that persist

hyperthermia   very high body temperature

hypoglycemia   condition that occurs when the blood glucose level is abnormally low

I

ileum   last segment of the small intestine

infant formula   synthetic food that simulates human milk

insecticides   substances used to control or kill insects

insoluble fiber   forms of dietary fiber that generally do not dissolve in water

insulin   hormone that helps regulate blood glucose levels

intracellular water   water that is inside cells

intrinsic factor (IF)   substance produced in the stomach that facilitates intestinal absorption of vitamin B-12

ion   atom or group of atoms that has a positive or negative charge

iron deficiency   condition characterized by low body stores of iron

J

jejunum   middle segment of the small intestine

K

keratin   tough protein found in hair, nails, and the outermost layers of skin

ketoacidosis   condition that occurs when the body forms excessive ketone bodies

ketone bodies   chemicals that result from incomplete fat breakdown

kilocalorie or **Calorie**   heat energy needed to raise the temperature of 1 liter of water 1° Celsius; measure of food energy

kwashiorkor   form of undernutrition that results from consuming adequate energy and insufficient high-quality protein

L

lactase   enzyme that splits lactose molecule

lactation   milk production

lacteal   lymph vessel in villus that absorbs most lipids

lactic acid   compound formed from pyruvate during anaerobic metabolism

lactoovovegetarian   vegetarian who consumes milk products and eggs for animal protein

lactose   disaccharide comprised of a glucose and a galactose molecule; "milk sugar"

lactose intolerance   inability to digest lactose properly

lactovegetarian   vegetarian who consumes milk and milk products for animal protein

lecithin   major phospholipid in food

legumes   plants that produce pods with a single row of seeds

leptin   hormone that reduces hunger and inhibits fat storage in the body

life expectancy   length of time an average person born in a specific year can expect to live

life span   maximum number of years an organism can live

lifestyle   usual way of living, including dietary practices and physical activity habits

linoleic acid   an essential fatty acid

lipases   enzymes that break down lipids

lipids   class of nutrients that generally do not dissolve in water

lipolysis   fat breakdown

lipoprotein   water-soluble structure that transports lipids through the bloodstream

lipoprotein lipase   enzyme in capillary walls that breaks down triglycerides

low-birth-weight (LBW)   describes baby generally weighing less than 5½ pounds at birth

low-density lipoprotein (LDL)   lipoprotein that carries cholesterol into tissues

low energy availability   state of negative energy balance

low-quality (incomplete) protein   protein that lacks or has inadequate amounts of one or more of the essential amino acids

lumen   open space within a structure such as the small intestine

lymph   fluid in the lymphatic system

M

macronutrients   nutrients needed in gram amounts daily and that provide energy; carbohydrates, proteins, and fats

major minerals   essential mineral elements required in amounts of 100 mg or more per day

malignant tumor   mass of cancerous cells

malnutrition   state of health that occurs when the body is improperly nourished

maltase   enzyme that splits maltose molecule

maltose   disaccharide comprised of two glucose molecules; "malt sugar"

marasmus   starvation

megadose   amount of a vitamin or mineral that greatly exceeds the recommended amount

metabolic syndrome   condition that increases risk of type 2 diabetes and CVD

metabolic water   water formed by cells as a metabolic by-product

metabolism   total of all chemical processes that take place in living cells

metastasized   spread to other tissues

micelle   lipid-rich particle that is surrounded by bile salts; transports lipids to absorptive cells

micronutrients   vitamins and minerals

minerals   elements that are found in the Earth's crust

mitochondria   cellular structures that release energy from macronutrients

moderation   obtaining adequate amounts of nutrients while balancing calorie intake with calorie expenditure

molecule   matter that forms when two or more atoms interact and are held together by a chemical bond

monoglyceride   single fatty acid attached to a glycerol backbone

monosaccharide   simple sugar that is the basic chemical unit of carbohydrates

monounsaturated fatty acid (MUFA)   fatty acid that has one double bond within the carbon chain

morning sickness   nausea and vomiting associated with pregnancy

mucus   fluid that lubricates and protects certain cells

multivitamin/mineral (MV/M)   describes a dietary supplement that contains vitamins and minerals

muscle dysmorphia   unhealthy preoccupation with the body being too small or not muscular enough

myocardial infarction   heart attack

myoglobin   iron-containing protein in muscle cells that controls oxygen uptake from red blood cells

MyPlate   USDA's interactive Internet dietary and menu planning guide

N

negative energy balance   calorie intake is less than calorie output

negative nitrogen balance   state in which the body loses more nitrogen than it retains

neural tube   embryonic structure that eventually develops into the brain and spinal cord

night eating syndrome (NES)   episodic food binges that are not followed by purging; binges take place after the evening meal or when the person wakens from sleep during the night

nitrogen balance (equilibrium)   balancing nitrogen intake with nitrogen losses

nonessential amino acids   group of amino acids that the body can make

nonalcoholic fatty liver disease (NAFLD)   abnormal accumulation of fat in the liver that is not related to alcohol intake

nonexercise activity thermogenesis (NEAT)   involuntary skeletal muscular activities such as fidgeting

nonheme iron   form of iron that is primarily in vegetables, grains, meats, and supplements

nonnutritive sweeteners   substances that sweeten foods while providing few or no kilocalories

nutrient-dense   describes a food or beverage that contains more key beneficial nutrients in relation to its total calories

nutrients   chemicals necessary for proper body functioning

nutrigenetics   study of how a person's genetic makeup affects the way his or her body responds to food

nutrigenomics   study of how nutrients and other food components can affect one's genetic expression

nutrition   scientific study of nutrients and how the body uses these substances

nutritional genomics   science that investigates the complex interactions among gene functioning, dietary choices, and the environment

nutritive sweeteners   substances that sweeten and contribute energy to foods

O

obesity   condition characterized by excessive and unhealthy amounts of body fat

omega-3 fatty acid   type of polyunsaturated fatty acid

omega end   first carbon of a fatty acid chain that has three hydrogen atoms attached to it

omnivore   organism that can digest and absorb nutrients from plants, animals, fungi, and bacteria

organ   collection of tissues that function in a related fashion

organ system   group of organs that work together for a similar purpose

organelles   structures in cells that have specific functions

organic foods   foods produced without the use of antibiotics, hormones, synthetic fertilizers and pesticides, genetic improvements, or spoilage-killing radiation

osmosis   diffusion of a solvent, such as water, through a selectively permeable membrane

osteoblasts   bone cells that add bone to where the tissue is needed

osteoclasts   bone cells that tear down bone tissue

osteomalacia   adult rickets; condition characterized by poorly mineralized (soft) bones

osteoporosis   chronic disease characterized by loss of bone mass and reduced bone structure

overweight   having extra weight from bone, muscle, body fat, and/or body water

ovovegetarian   vegetarian who eats eggs for animal protein

oxidizing agent   substance that removes electrons from atoms or molecules

oxytocin   hormone that elicits the "let-down" response and causes the uterus to contract

P

pancreatic amylase   enzyme secreted by pancreas that breaks down starch into maltose molecules

pancreatic lipase   digestive enzyme that removes two fatty acids from each triglyceride molecule

parasite   organism that lives in or on another organism, often deriving nourishment from its host

parathyroid hormone (PTH)   hormone secreted by parathyroid glands when blood calcium levels are too low

partial hydrogenation   food manufacturing process that adds hydrogen atoms to some unsaturated fatty acids, forming trans fats

pasteurization   process that kills the pathogens in foods and beverages as well as many microbes responsible for spoilage

pathogens   disease-causing agents

peer review   expert critical analysis of a research article before it is published

pellagra   niacin deficiency disease

pepsin   gastric enzyme that breaks down proteins into smaller polypeptides

peptide bond   chemical attraction that connects two amino acids together

peptides   small chains of amino acids

peristalsis   type of muscular contraction of the gastrointestinal tract

pernicious anemia   condition caused by the lack of intrinsic factor and characterized by vitamin B-12 deficiency, nerve damage, and megaloblastic RBCs

pesticide   substance that people use to kill or control unwanted insects, weeds, or other harmful organisms

pH   measure of the acidity or alkalinity of a solution

phosphocreatine (PCr)   high-energy compound used to reform ATP under anaerobic conditions

phospholipid   type of lipid that is chemically similar to a triglyceride, except it contains phosphorus

physical activity   movement resulting from contraction of skeletal muscles

physical fitness   ability to perform moderate- to vigorous-intensity activities for a reasonable amount of time, without becoming excessively fatigued

physiological dose   amount of a nutrient that is within the range of safe intake and enables the body to function optimally

physiology   scientific study of the functioning of cells and other body structures

phytochemicals   compounds made by plants that are not nutrients

pica   craving nonfood items

placebo   fake treatment, such as a sham pill, injection, or medical procedure

placebo effect   response to a placebo

placenta   organ of pregnancy that connects the uterus to the embryo/fetus via the umbilical cord

polypeptide   protein comprised of two or more amino acids

polyunsaturated fatty acid (PUFA)   fatty acid that has two or more double bonds within the carbon chain

positive energy balance   calorie intake is greater than calorie output

positive nitrogen balance   state in which the body retains more nitrogen than it loses

prebiotics   forms of dietary fiber that are poorly digested by humans but support the growth of beneficial gut microbes

pre-diabetes   condition characterized by fasting blood glucose levels that are 100 to 125 mg/dl

prehypertension   persistent systolic blood pressure readings of 120 mm Hg to 139 mm Hg and diastolic readings of 80 mm Hg to 89 mm Hg

prenatal care   specialized health care for pregnant women

prenatal period   time between conception and birth; pregnancy

probiotics   products that contain healthful microbes; beneficial gut microbes

prolactin   hormone that stimulates milk production after delivery

prooxidant   substance that promotes free radical production

protein-energy malnutrition (PEM)   condition that results from diets that provide inadequate amounts of protein and energy

protein turnover   cellular process of breaking down proteins and recycling their amino acids

proteins   large, complex organic molecules made up of amino acids

protons   positively charged particles in the nucleus of an atom

protozoa   single-celled microorganisms that have complex cell structures

pseudoscience   presentation of information masquerading as factual and obtained by scientific methods

purging   activities that limit calorie intake or increase calorie output

purines   nitrogen-containing chemicals in genetic material

pyruvate   compound that results from anaerobic breakdown of glucose

Q

quackery   promotion of useless medical treatments

R

R group   part of amino acid that identifies the molecule as a particular amino acid

radical   substance with an unpaired electron

Recommended Dietary Allowances (RDAs)   standards for recommending daily intakes of several nutrients

rectum   lower section of the large intestine

registered dietitian (RD) or **registered dietitian nutritionist (RDN)**   college-trained health care professional who has extensive knowledge of foods, nutrition, and dietetics

requirement   smallest amount of a nutrient that maintains a defined level of nutritional health

resting metabolic rate (RMR)   body's rate of energy use a few hours after resting and eating

retinol (preformed vitamin A)   most active form of vitamin A in the body

rhodopsin   vitamin A–containing protein that is needed for vision in dim light

rickets   vitamin D deficiency disorder in children

risk factor   personal characteristic that increases a person's chances of developing a disease

rodenticides   substances used to kill mice and rats

S

salivary amylase   enzyme secreted by salivary glands that begins starch digestion

salt   substance that forms when an acid combines with a base

satiety   sense that enough food or beverages have been consumed to satisfy hunger

saturated fatty acid   fatty acid that has each carbon atom within the chain filled with hydrogen atoms

scurvy   vitamin C–deficiency disease

selectively permeable membrane   barrier that allows the passage of certain substances and prevents the movement of other substances

semivegetarian (or flexitarian)   vegetarian who eats animal products, except red meat

senescence   declining organ functioning and increased vulnerability

set-point theory   scientific notion that body fat content is genetically predetermined

shelf life   period of time that a food can be stored before it spoils

simple carbohydrates   group of carbohydrates that includes sugars

simple diffusion   movement of substances from a region of higher to lower concentration

skinfold thickness measurements   technique of estimating body composition in which calipers are used to measure the width of skinfolds at multiple body sites

solid fats   fats that are fairly hard at room temperature

solubility   describes a substance's ability to dissolve and form a solution

soluble fiber   forms of dietary fiber that dissolve or swell in water

solute   lesser component of a solution that dissolves in solvent

solution   evenly distributed mixture of two or more compounds

solvent   primary component of a solution

spina bifida type of neural tube defect in which the spine does not form properly before birth, and it fails to enclose the spinal cord

starch storage polysaccharide in plants

sterilization process that kills or destroys all microorganisms and viruses

sucrase enzyme that splits sucrose molecule

sucrose disaccharide comprised of a glucose and a fructose molecule; "table sugar"

sustainable agriculture farming methods that do not deplete natural resources or harm the environment while meeting the demand for food

syndrome group of signs and symptoms that occur together and indicate a specific health problem

systolic pressure maximum blood pressure within an artery that occurs when the ventricles contract

T

target heart rate zone heart rate range that reflects intensity of physical exertion

teratogen agent that causes birth defects

testimonial personal endorsement of a product

testosterone hormone needed for normal bone development and maintenance

tetrahydrofolic acid (THFA) folate coenzyme

thermic effect of food (TEF) energy used to digest foods and beverages as well as absorb and further process the macronutrients

thrombus fixed bunch of clots that remains in place

thyroid hormone hormone that regulates the body's metabolic rate

tissues masses of cells that have similar characteristics and functions

Tolerable Upper Intake Level (Upper Level or UL) highest average amount of a nutrient

that is unlikely to be harmful when consumed daily

tolerances maximum amounts of pesticide residues that can be in or on each treated food crop

total body fat essential fat and adipose tissue

total water intake water in beverages and foods

trace minerals essential mineral elements required in amounts that are less than 100 mg per day

trans fatty acid unsaturated fatty acid that has a trans double bond

transamination transfer of the nitrogen-containing group from an unneeded amino acid to a carbon skeleton to form an amino acid

treatment group group being studied that receives a treatment

triglyceride lipid that has three fatty acids attached to a three-carbon compound called glycerol

U

underwater weighing technique of estimating body composition that involves comparing weight on land to weight when completely submerged in a tank of water

underweight describes person with a BMI of less than 18.5

unintentional food additives substances that are accidentally in foods

unsaturated fatty acid fatty acid that is missing hydrogen atoms and has one or more double bonds within the carbon chain

urea waste product of amino acid metabolism

uterus female reproductive organ that protects the developing organism during pregnancy

V

variable personal characteristic or other factor that changes and can influence an outcome

vegan vegetarian who eats only plant foods

vegetarians people who eat plant-based diets

veins vessels that return blood to the heart

very-low-density lipoprotein (VLDL) lipoprotein that carries much of the triglycerides in the bloodstream

villi (singular, villus) tiny, fingerlike projections of the small intestinal lining that participate in digesting and absorbing food

virus microbe consisting of a piece of genetic material coated with protein

vitamin complex organic molecule that regulates certain metabolic processes

W

water intoxication condition that occurs when too much water is consumed in a short time period or the kidneys have difficulty filtering water from blood

water-soluble vitamins thiamin, riboflavin, niacin, vitamin B-6, pantothenic acid, folate, biotin, vitamin B-12, and vitamin C

weaning gradual process of shifting from breastfeeding or bottle-feeding to drinking from a cup and eating solid foods

Wernicke-Korsakoff syndrome degenerative brain disorder resulting from thiamin deficiency that occurs primarily among alcoholics

X

xerophthalmia condition affecting the eyes that results from vitamin A deficiency

Index

Note: Page numbers followed by b indicate boxes; f indicates figures; t indicates tables.